WAVELETS
in Medicine
and Biology

T0136320

Edited by
Akram Aldroubi and Michael Unser

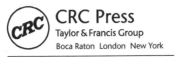

CRC Press
Taylor & Francis Group
Boca Raton London New York

CRC Press is an imprint of the
Taylor & Francis Group, an **informa** business

CRC Press
Taylor & Francis Group
6000 Broken Sound Parkway NW, Suite 300
Boca Raton, FL 33487-2742

© 1996 by Taylor & Francis Group, LLC
CRC Press is an imprint of Taylor & Francis Group, an Informa business

First issued in paperback 2019

No claim to original U.S. Government works

ISBN-13: 978-0-367-44859-2 (pbk)
ISBN-13: 978-0-8493-9483-6 (hbk)

Visit the Taylor & Francis Web site at
http://www.taylorandfrancis.com

and the CRC Press Web site at
http://www.crcpress.com

Library of Congress Card Number 95-46327

Library of Congress Cataloging-in-Publication Data

Wavelets in medicine and biology / edited by Akram Aldroubi, Michael Unser
    p. cm.
Includes bibliographical references and index.
ISBN 0-8493-9483-X (alk. paper)
1. Wavelets (Mathematics). 2. Signal processing. I. Aldroubi, Akram.
II. Unser, Michael A.
R853.M3W38 1996
610′.28—dc20
    95-46327
    CIP

Contents

2 A Practical Guide to the Implementation of the Wavelet Transform

Michael Unser

Part II   Wavelets in Medical Imaging and Tomography

3 An Application of Wavelet Shrinkage to Tomography

Eric D. Kolaczyk

4 Wavelet Denoising of Functional MRI Data

Michael Hilton, Todd Ogden, David Hattery, Guinevere Eden,
and Björn Jawerth

5 Statistical Analysis of Image Differences by Wavelet Decomposition

Urs E. Ruttimann, Michael Unser, Philippe Thévenaz, Chulhee Lee,
Daniel Rio, and Daniel W. Hommer

6 Feature Extraction in Digital Mammography

R. A. DeVore, B. Lucier, and Z. Yang

7 Multiscale Contrast Enhancement and Denoising in Digital Radiographs

Jian Fan and Andrew Laine

8 Using Wavelets to Suppress Noise in Biomedical Images

Maurits Malfait

12 Adapted Wavelet Techniques for Encoding Magnetic Resonance Images

Dennis M. Healy, Jr. and John B. Weaver

Part III Wavelets and Biomedical Signal Processing

13 Sleep Images Using the Wavelet Transform to Process Polysomnographic Signals

*Richard Sartene, Laurent Poupard, Jean-Louis Bernard, and
Jean-Christophe Wallet*

14 Estimating the Fractal Exponent of Point Processes in Biological Systems Using Wavelet- and Fourier-Transform Methods

*Malvin C. Teich, Conor Heneghan, Steven B. Lowen, and
Robert G. Turcott*

15 Point Processes, Long-Range Dependence and Wavelets

Patrice Abry and Patrick Flandrin

16 Continuous Wavelet Transform: ECG Recognition Based on Phase and Modulus Representations and Hidden Markov Models

Lotfi Senhadji, Laurent Thoraval, and Guy Carrault

19 Diagnosis of Coronary Artery Disease Using Wavelet-Based Neural Networks

Metin Akay

Part IV Wavelets and Mathematical Models in Biology

20 A Nonlinear Squeezing of the Continuous Wavelet Transform Based on Auditory Nerve Models

Ingrid Daubechies and Stéphane Maes

21 The Application of Wavelet Transforms to Blood Flow Velocimetry

Lora G. Weiss

22 Wavelet Models of Event-Related Potentials

Jonathan Raz and Bruce Turetsky

23 Macromolecular Structure Computation Based on Energy Function Approximation by Wavelets

Eberhard Schmitt

Preface

This book is the first comprehensive guide to the wavelet transform's applications in medicine and biology. It consists of four main sections:

(1) Wavelet Transform: Theory and Implementation

(2) Wavelets in Medical Imaging and Tomography

(3) Wavelets and Biomedical Signal Processing

(4) Wavelets and Mathematical Models in Biology

The first section presents the theoretical and practical foundations of wavelet methods written for non-experts. It relates the wavelet techniques to more conventional methods and provides the reader with many references. It also fixes the notation for the remainder the book. The next three sections feature contributions from some the most prominent researchers in the field, providing the reader with a comprehensive survey of the use of wavelets in biomedical engineering, and presenting the latest development in this area.

This book is addressed to an audience of scientists, engineers, physicists, and mathematicians who are interested in learning about wavelets and their applications to biomedical problems. Its unified style and standardized notations make it suitable as an undergraduate or graduate textbook on the wavelet transform and its applications.

We would like to thank the authors for their excellent contributions and for the time spent away from the beaches writing about wavelets. We are also grateful to Philippe Thévenaz, Mike Vrhel, and Murray Eden for their constructive criticism and their editorial help. Finally, we would like to thank Wayne Yuhasz, Bob Stern, and Nora Konopka of CRC Press for helping us to produce this book.

Akram Aldroubi
Bethesda, Maryland

Michael Unser
Bethesda, Maryland

Part I

Wavelet Transform: Theory and Implementation

1

The Wavelet Transform: A Surfing Guide

Akram Aldroubi

NIH/BEIP, Building 13/3N17, 13 South DR MSC 5766, Bethesada, MD 20892-5766
`aldroubi@helix.nih.gov`

Dedicated to Richard C. MacCamy on the occasion of his 70th birthday

1.1 Introduction

In any processing system, we first perform measurements to obtain information about a physical quantity. We then analyze this information and eventually take appropriate actions. The physical quantity of interest is often a function of time (e.g., blood pressure $p(t)$), or a function of space (e.g., MRI image of a brain's section $I(x, y)$). The measurements $\{m_k, k = 1, ..., r\}$ that we obtain from a signal $f(t)$ allow us to build some knowledge about $f(t)$. Thus, it is important to choose these measurements carefully so as to acquire as much knowledge as possible while keeping the tasks involved as simple and as cheap as possible. Clearly, the choice of the measurements, their type, and their number depend on the information that we want to extract from our function. For example, the measurements that we will perform to extract the number of heart beats per minute will be different from those that we will perform to detect a diastolic heart murmur signaling a possible heart disease. One way to gain knowledge about a function $f(t)$, is to compare it with a set of test functions $\mathcal{Q} = \{\varphi_q, \ q \in \Lambda\}$ where Λ is some indexing set. This comparison can be carried out by the formula

$$m_q = \int_{-\infty}^{+\infty} f(t)\overline{\varphi_q(t)} \, dt, \qquad (1.1)$$

where $\overline{\varphi_q}$ denotes the complex conjugate of φ_q. The function $f(t)$ may belong to a class $\mathcal{C}$ of finitely many functions. In this case, by choosing sufficiently many test functions, we should be able to distinguish between different functions in $\mathcal{C}$. The class $\mathcal{C}$ can also be infinite. This is, for example, the case when $\mathcal{C}$ consists of all finite energy functions ($\mathcal{C} = L_2$), or when $\mathcal{C}$ consists of the bandlimited functions with bandwidth $W = [-\pi, \pi]$ ($\mathcal{C} = B_{2\pi}$). In both of these examples, the set of test functions $\mathcal{Q}$ must necessarily be infinite in order to distinguish between two functions $f_1(t)$ and $f_2(t)$. This is also the case for all other infinite dimensional function spaces. If we have sufficiently many measurements to distinguish between any two arbitrary functions $f_1(t)$ and $f_2(t)$ in a class $\mathcal{C}$, then we should be able to reconstruct any function $f \in \mathcal{C}$ from the values m_q, $q \in \Lambda$. If the set of test functions in $\mathcal{Q}$ used for our measurements is "very" large, then it can also happen that only a fraction of the measurements m_q, $q \in \Lambda$ are needed to reconstruct any function $f \in \mathcal{C}$. In this case, the values m_q, $q \in \Lambda$ form a redundant set of measurements. This redundancy can be used to our advantage by using the extra elements as control, or to reduce any noise that may have been introduced into our system [3, 4, 13, 30, 31, 41].

If the set of test functions $\mathcal{Q}$ is sufficiently large to distinguish between functions of some fixed class $\mathcal{C}$, then we say that m_q (viewed as a function of the variable q) is a *transform* of $f(t)$. The reason for calling m_q "a transform of $f(t)$" is that all the information in $f(t)$ is captured by the measurements m_q and none is lost. Thus, viewed as a function of the independent variable $q \in \Lambda$, m_q is simply a transformation of $f(t)$. In operator notation we can write $m_q = (T_{\mathcal{Q}} f)(q)$. The inverse transform is the reconstruction of $f(t)$ from m_q, and it can be written as $f(t) = (T_{\mathcal{Q}}^{-1} m_q)(t)$. This last expression can be viewed as a *representation* or *expansion* of $f(t)$.

Clearly, for a given class of signals $\mathcal{C}$, there are many possible transforms and many possible representations. For instance, the Fourier transform and the windowed Fourier transform are two examples of transforms for $\mathcal{C} = L_2$.

The general study of transforms and expansions in various function spaces has a long history in mathematics (see, e.g., [23, 32, 43, 46, 49, 50, 51, 58, 63, 92]). Which space and which transform or expansion to choose is often guided by the problem or application of interest. However, there are several desired features that are shared by many applications:

- Simple algorithms for computing the transform and its inverse.

- Robustness and stability of the algorithms.

The second requirement states that small errors in the data should only produce small errors in the transform.

One way to achieve the first requirement is to choose a set Q of test functions that have a simple structure. For finite energy signals, $C = L_2$, for example, the Fourier transform uses the set of templates $Q = \{\varphi_\omega(t) = e^{i\omega t}, \omega \in R\}$ which consists of all the dilations (or reductions) by a factor ω, of a single periodic function e^{it}:

$$\hat{f}(\omega) = (\mathcal{F}f)(\omega) = \int_{-\infty}^{+\infty} f(t)e^{-i\omega t} dt. \tag{1.2}$$

The reconstruction or inverse Fourier transform is given by

$$f(t) = (2\pi)^{-1} \int_{-\infty}^{+\infty} \hat{f}(\omega)e^{i\omega t} dt. \tag{1.3}$$

For this case, there are no problems of stability or robustness. However, this transform cannot be computed exactly, and a discrete version is used instead, namely, the discrete Fourier transform (DFT).

The Fourier transform is an excellent tool for decomposing a function $f(t)$ in terms of its frequency components. For example, an angular frequency burst of frequency ω_0 in $f(t)$ will show up as a large component at ω_0 in the Fourier transform $\hat{f}(\omega)$. Thus, we can detect or *localize* accurately the frequencies in $f(t)$. This is the frequency localization property of the Fourier transform. However, one drawback is that there is no way to deduce the beginning and the end of the frequency burst by an inspection of $\hat{f}(\omega)$. Moreover, an edge or a singularity in $f(t)$ will not be captured in any simple way by $\hat{f}(\omega)$. In fact, the information on the time (or location) of the events' occurrence in $f(t)$ is spread to all the components of $\hat{f}(\omega)$ (specifically, to the phase), and we say that the Fourier transform is not localized in time (or space). This lack of localization in time makes the Fourier transform unsuitable for designing data processing systems for nonstationary signals or events.

The reason for the lack of time localization in the Fourier transform is that the test functions $e^{i\omega t}$ are periodic, and are not localized in any particular t-region. One way to circumvent this problem is to multiply the function $e^{i\omega t}$ by window functions $\{g(t - b), b \in R\}$ to obtain the new set of templates $Q = \{\varphi_{(\omega,b)}(t) = g(t - b)e^{i\omega t}, (\omega, b) \in R^2\}$. We then obtain what is known as the windowed Fourier transform (WFT) given by

$$(T_g f)(\omega, b) = \int_{-\infty}^{+\infty} f(t)g(t - b)e^{-i\omega t} dt. \tag{1.4}$$

The function $g(t)$ must be chosen to decay rapidly for large values of t (e.g., the rectangular function $g(t) = 1, \forall |t| < 1/2$, and $g(t) = 0, \forall |t| \geq 1/2$). It follows that the frequency component of a function $f(t)$ at frequency $\omega = \omega_0$ and at time $t = b_0$, is captured by the value $(T_g f)(\omega_0, b_0)$. Thus, we are able to obtain the desired t-localization, but at the price of a more complicated transform. In fact, while the Fourier transform is not redundant, the WFT is redundant and maps a function of one variable t into a function of two variables (ω, b). This increases the computational complexity of the algorithms involved in the transform and its inverse. Another drawback of the WFT is that the sizes of the windows $g(t - b)$ are fixed (e.g., the sizes for the rectangular windows mentioned earlier are all equal to 1). As a consequence, the resolution of the WFT will be limited in that it will be difficult to distinguish between successive events that are separated by a distance smaller than the window width. It will also be difficult for the WFT to capture a single large event whose size is larger than the window's size.

One way to decrease the redundancy of the WFT is to sample the variables ω and b on a discrete grid. If we choose $\omega_m = m\omega_0$ and $b_n = nb_0$, we obtain the *generalized Gabor transform*. Thus, the generalized Gabor transform $(\mathbf{G}f)(m, n) = (T_g f)(\omega_m, b_n)$ of a function $f(t)$ uses the set of test function $\mathcal{Q} = \{g^{(m,n)}(t) = g(t - nb_0)e^{im\omega_0 t}, (m, n) \in \mathcal{Z}^2\}$:

$$(\mathbf{G}f)(m, n) = (T_g f)(\omega_m, b_n) = \int_{-\infty}^{+\infty} f(t)g(t - b_n)e^{-i\omega_m t} \, dt. \qquad (1.5)$$

Under appropriate conditions on $g(t)$, the reconstruction is stable and can be carried out using a set of dual Gabor functions $\mathring{g}^{(m,n)}(t) = \mathring{g}(t - b_n)e^{i\omega_m t}$ that are constructed by modulation and translation of a single function $\mathring{g}(t)$ (the original transform of Gabor uses a Gaussian $\mathring{g}(t) = \pi^{-4}e^{-t^2/2}$). The reconstruction formula is given by

$$f(t) = \sum_{(m,n)\in\mathcal{Z}^2} (\mathbf{G}f)(m, n)\mathring{g}^{(m,n)}(t). \qquad (1.6)$$

We can use the inner product notation in L_2 and (1.5) to rewrite the last expansion as

$$f(t) = \sum_{(m,n)\in\mathcal{Z}^2} \left\langle f(t), g^{(m,n)}(t) \right\rangle \mathring{g}^{(m,n)}(t). \qquad (1.7)$$

The above expression can be viewed as an atomic decomposition of a function $f(t)$ in terms of the atoms $g^{(m,n)}(t)$ [2].

As in the case of the WFT, the size of the window $g(t)$ in the Gabor transform limits the size of the structures that can be captured. This happens for example if the signal has "mountain like" structures that are large compared to the sliding window $g(t - nb_0)$. This also happens for signal details that are small compared to the window size. To overcome this limitation, the *dyadic wavelet transform* (DWT) uses the set of atoms

$$\mathcal{Q} = \{\psi_{j,k}(t) = 2^{-j/2}\psi(2^{-j}t - k), (j,k) \in \mathcal{Z}^2\}$$

that are obtained by translation and dilation (or reduction) of a single wavelet function $\psi(t)$ [68, 69]:

$$(W_\psi f)(2^j, 2^j k) = \langle f(t), \psi_{j,k}(t) \rangle = 2^{-j/2} \int_{-\infty}^{+\infty} f(t)\overline{\psi(2^{-j}t - k)}\, dt, \quad (1.8)$$

where $\psi_{j,k}(t) = 2^{-j/2}\psi(2^{-j}t - k)$ (see Figure 1.1). Thus, the DWT uses a set of variable window sizes that are proportional to 2^{-j} and maps a function $f(t)$ into the double sequence $d_j(k) = (W_\psi f)(2^j, 2^j k)$. In effect, like the *Phi*-transform [46], the DWT operates at all dyadic scales to extract information about data structures that live at different scales. Under appropriate conditions on $\psi(t)$ (see Section 1.4.1), this transform can be inverted and we get the stable reconstruction

$$f(t) = \sum_{(j,k)\in\mathcal{Z}^2} d_j(k)\mathring{\psi}_{j,k}(t), \quad (1.9)$$

where $\mathring{\psi}(t)$ is the dual wavelet of $\psi(t)$ (more on this issue in Section 1.4), and where $\mathring{\psi}_{j,k}(t) = 2^{-j/2}\mathring{\psi}(2^{-j}t - k)$. In fact, for the DWT, the set $\{\mathring{\psi}_{j,k}(t), (j,k) \in \mathcal{Z}^2\}$ forms a basis of L_2, and the first orthonormal basis of this form was introduced by Strömberg [82]. Meyer later found another basis of L_2 which belongs to the bandlimited functions [72]; this construction was generalized to higher dimensions in [66]. Daubechies introduced a class of orthonormal wavelet bases with compact support [29]. Since then, many other wavelet bases with various properties have been found [1, 6, 7, 19, 20, 29, 33, 57, 69, 75, 88, 89, 90].

A prototypical example is the Haar wavelet basis. It is formed by all the translations and dilations/contractions of the Haar function ψ^H shown in Figure 1.1. The example of Figure 1.1 shows how a function $f(t)$ can be be expanded in terms of this basis: The L_2-least squares approximation $f_1(t)$ of the piecewise constant function $f_0(t)$ is obtained by averaging two consecutive values of f_0. The error $e_1(t) = f_0(t) - f_1(t)$ is then simply a linear combination of the dilated Haar wavelet $\psi^H(t/2)$ and all of its shifts

$\psi^H \left(\frac{t-2k}{2}\right)$. By approximating f_1 by a coarser function and repeating this process ad infinitum, we obtain the wavelet decomposition of f_0. Since by refining the grid, any finite energy function $f(t) \in L_2$ can be approximated by a piecewise constant function as closely as we wish, we can see that $\psi_{j,k}^H(t)$ is a basis of L_2. In fact, it is an orthogonal basis of L_2 and we have $\overset{\circ}{\psi}^H(t) = \psi^H(t)$.

There are many *wavelet transforms* other than the DWT, and the rest of this chapter will be devoted to the presentation of the various wavelet transforms and their connections to each other. In Section 1.2, we present the notation that, unless otherwise stated, will be used throughout this book. In Section 1.3, we introduce the continuous wavelet transform in one and several variables. In Section 1.4, we review the DWT in more detail and introduce the redundant discrete wavelet transforms. In Section 1.5, we describe the multiresolution approximations (MRA) of L_2 and their related MRA-type wavelets. In particular we examine the orthogonal, biorthogonal and semi-orthogonal wavelet bases (the semi-orthogonal bases are also known as non-orthogonal wavelets). Section 1.6 is devoted to the design of wavelet bases, and we present specific constructions of some useful wavelet bases. In Section 1.7, we give an overview of the applications of the wavelet transform and some generalizations. Finally, Section 1.8 is devoted to the general theory of frames.

1.2   Notations

The set of nonnegative integers is denoted by $\mathcal{N}$. The set of positive and negative integers is denoted by $\mathcal{Z}$. The set of real numbers is denoted by $\mathcal{R}$, and the set of complex numbers is denoted by $\mathcal{C}$. The set $L_2(\mathcal{R})$ denotes the space of measurable, square-integrable functions with the usual norm $||.||_{L_2}$. The space of square-summable sequences (discrete functions) is denoted by l_2.

The symbol "$*$" is used for three slightly different operations that are defined below: the convolution, the mixed convolution, and the discrete convolution. The ambiguity should be easily resolved from the context.

For two functions f and g defined on $\mathcal{R}$, $*$ denotes the usual convolution

$$(f * g)(t) = \int_{-\infty}^{+\infty} f(\xi)g(t - \xi)\,d\xi, \quad t \in \mathcal{R}. \tag{1.10}$$

The mixed convolution between a sequence $\{b(k)\}_{k \in \mathcal{Z}}$ and a function f

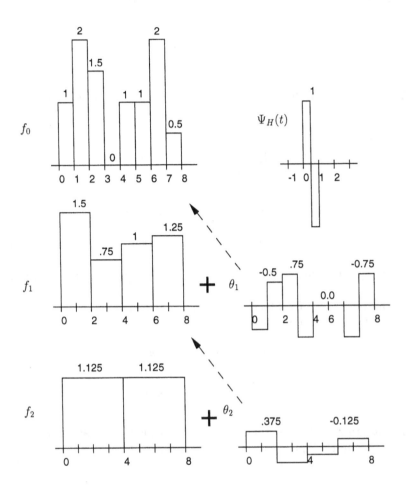

Figure 1.1
A discrete wavelet transform of the function f_0 in terms of the Haar wavelet basis $\psi^H(t)$ (top right). The function f_0 is a piecewise constant function with knot points at the integers (top left). Its approximation is obtained by averaging two consecutive values of f_0 to obtain the coarser piecewise constant function f_1 whose knot points lie on the even integers. Since the approximation f_1 is obtained by averaging neighboring values, the error $e_1 = f_0 - f_1$ for two neighboring values must differ by a sign change only. Therefore, the error e_1 is a linear combination of the Haar function $\psi^H(t/2)$ and its shifts by even integers. We can repeat the process for f_1 to obtain $f_0 = f_2 + e_2 + e_1$. If we repeat the procedure ad infinitum, we obtain the wavelet transform.

defined on $\mathcal{R}$ is the function $b * f$ defined on $\mathcal{R}$ that is given by

$$(b * f)(t) = \sum_{k=-\infty}^{k=+\infty} b(k)f(t-k), \quad t \in \mathcal{R}. \tag{1.11}$$

The discrete convolution between two sequences a and b is the sequence $a * b$ given by

$$(a * b)(l) = \sum_{k=-\infty}^{k=+\infty} a(k)b(l-k), \quad l \in \mathcal{Z}. \tag{1.12}$$

Whenever it exists, the convolution inverse $(b)^{-1}$ of a sequence b is defined to be

$$\left((b)^{-1} * b\right)(k) = \delta_0(k), \tag{1.13}$$

where δ_i is the unit impulse located at i, i.e., $\delta_i(i) = 1$, and $\delta_i(k) = 0$ for $k \neq i$.

The reflection of a function f (resp., a sequence b) is the function $f^\vee$ (resp., the sequence $b^\vee$) given by

$$f^\vee(t) = f(-t), \quad \forall t \in \mathcal{R}, \tag{1.14}$$

$$b^\vee(k) = b(-k), \quad \forall k \in \mathcal{Z}. \tag{1.15}$$

The alternation $\tilde{b}(k)$ of a sequence b (also called modulation) is obtained by changing the signs of the odd components of b:

$$\tilde{b}(k) = (-1)^k b(k), \quad \forall k \in \mathcal{Z}. \tag{1.16}$$

The decimation (or down-sampling) operator by a factor of m, $\downarrow_m [\bullet]$, assigns to a sequence b the sequence $\downarrow_m [b]$ which is given by:

$$\downarrow_m [b](k) = b(mk), \quad \forall k \in \mathcal{Z}. \tag{1.17}$$

The up-sampling operator by a factor m, $\uparrow_m$, assigns to a sequence b a sequence $\uparrow_m [b]$ in which $m-1$ zeroes have been inserted between two successive samples:

$$(\uparrow_m [b])(k) = \begin{cases} b(k'), & k = mk' \\ 0, & \text{otherwise}. \end{cases} \tag{1.18}$$

The Fourier transform of a function $f(t)$ is denoted by $\hat{f}(\omega)$ and is given by

$$\hat{f}(\omega) = \int_{\mathcal{R}} f(t)e^{-i\omega t}\, dt, \quad \omega \in \mathcal{R}, \tag{1.19}$$

where $i = \sqrt{-1}$.

The Z-transform of a sequence $b(k)$ (or its symbol) is denoted by a capital letter $B(z)$ and is given by

$$B(z) = \sum_{k \in \mathcal{Z}} b(k)z^{-k}, \quad z \in \mathcal{C}. \tag{1.20}$$

The Fourier transform of a sequence $b(k)$ is denoted by $\hat{b}(\omega)$. It is given by

$$\hat{b}(\omega) = B(e^{i\omega}) = \sum_{k \in \mathcal{Z}} b(k)e^{-i\omega k}, \quad \omega \in \mathcal{R}. \tag{1.21}$$

Poisson's summation formula is the relation between the Fourier transform $\hat{f}(\omega)$ of a function $f(t)$ and the Fourier transform $\hat{b}(\omega)$ of its samples $b(k) = f(t)|_{t=k}$. It is given by

$$\hat{b}(\omega) = \sum_{k \in \mathcal{Z}} \hat{f}(\omega + 2\pi k). \tag{1.22}$$

1.3 The Continuous Wavelet Transform

1.3.1 The Continuous Wavelet Transform of 1-D Signals

To analyze any finite energy signal, the continuous wavelet transform (CWT) uses the dilation and translation of a single wavelet function $\psi(t)$ called the *mother wavelet*. Specifically, if we choose the set of test functions in (1.1) to be $\mathcal{Q} = \{\psi\left((t-b)/a\right), (a,b) \in (0,\infty) \times \mathcal{R}\}$, then we obtain the continuous wavelet transform $(W_\psi f)(a,b)$ of the signal $f(t) \in L_2(\mathcal{R})$:

$$(W_\psi f)(a,b) = \int_{-\infty}^{+\infty} |a|^{-1/2} f(t)\overline{\psi\left(\frac{t-b}{a}\right)}\, dt, \tag{1.23}$$

where, as before, we have used $\overline{\psi}$ to denote the complex conjugate of ψ, and where $\psi(t) \in L_2(\mathcal{R})$ is an oscillatory function whose Fourier transform must satisfy [31]

$$C_\psi = 2\pi \int_{-\infty}^{+\infty} |\omega|^{-1} \left| \hat{\psi}\left(\omega\right) \right|^2 d\omega < \infty; \qquad (1.24)$$

in effect, if $\psi \in L_1 \cap L_2$, Condition (1.24) specifies that $\psi(t)$ should have zero mean. This last condition allows for the inversion of the wavelet transform. In particular, the signal $f(t) \in L_2(\mathcal{R})$ can be recovered from its transform $(W_\psi f)(a, b)$ by the inverse formula

$$f(t) = C_\psi^{-1} \int_0^\infty \int_{\mathcal{R}} a^{-2} (W_\psi f)(a, b) \psi((t - b)/a) \, da \, db. \qquad (1.25)$$

Using the inner product notation in $L_2(\mathcal{R})$, the continuous wavelet transform can also be written as

$$(W_\psi f)(a, b) = |a|^{-1/2} \langle f(t), \psi_{(a,b)}(t) \rangle, \qquad (1.26)$$

where $\psi_{(a,b)}(t) = \psi((t - b)/a)$, and where $\langle \bullet, \bullet \rangle$ is the inner product in $L_2(\mathcal{R})$. Since the scale factor a is proportional to the inverse of the frequency ω, the value $(W_\psi f)(a_0, b_0)$ exhibits the frequency content of $f(t)$ in a frequency interval centered around $\omega_0 = a_0^{-1}$ at a time interval centered around b_0.

A prototyptical example is generated by the Haar wavelet given by

$$\psi^H(t) = \chi_{[0,1/2]}(t) - \chi_{[1/2,1]}(t)$$

as illustrated in Figure 1.1. This function is clearly in $L_2(\mathcal{R})$, and its Fourier transform $ie^{-i\omega/2}(\omega/4) \operatorname{sinc}^2(\omega/4)$ satisfies Condition (1.24). Moreover, the Haar wavelet has the value zero outside the interval $[0, 1]$. It follows that at scale level a and time b, the integrand $f(t)\overline{\psi^H((t - b)/a)}$ in (1.23) is zero outside the interval $[b, b+a]$. Thus, the functions $\psi^H((t-b)/a)$ are windows supported in $[b, b+a]$, and only the values of $f(t)$ for which $t \in [b, b+a]$ contribute to the wavelet transform $(W_{\psi^H} f)(a, b)$ at scale a and at time b. This is the time localization property of the Haar transform. To see the frequency localization property, we simply note that the Fourier transform $\widehat{\psi^H}(\omega)$ is a bandpass filter concentrated around $[-\pi, -\frac{\pi}{2}] \cup [\frac{\pi}{2}, \pi]$ (see Figure 1.2). As a consequence, the CWT of a signal $f(t)$ consists of a series of bandpass filtering with the bandpass filters concentrated around $\widehat{\psi^H}(a\omega)$ of bandwidth proportional to $BW_a = [-a^{-1}\pi, -a^{-2}\frac{\pi}{2}] \cup [a^{-2}\frac{\pi}{2}, a^{-1}\pi]$. It follows that the value $(W_{\psi^H} f)(a, b)$ measures the frequency content of $f(t)$

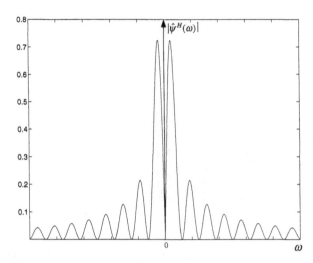

Figure 1.2
The amplitude of the Fourier transform of the Haar wavelet
$(\psi^H)^\wedge(\omega)$. **It can be seen that** $(\psi^H)^\wedge(0) = 0$, **and that** $(\psi^H)^\wedge(\omega)$ **is**
essentially a non-ideal bandpass filter with vanishing side lobes.

in the frequency band of about BW_a within the time interval $[b, b+a]$. Figure 1.3 shows an example of an MRI image and its Haar CWT at scale
$a = 2$. The time-frequency localization is an important feature that we
require for all the wavelet transforms in order to make them useful for analyzing non-stationary signals. For this reason, we will often require our
wavelets $\psi(t)$ to have compact support, or at least to have fast decay as $|t|$
goes to infinity (e.g., $|\psi(t)| = O(1 + |t|^{-2})$). We also require that $\widehat{\psi}(0) = 0$
(actually for L_1 functions, this is a consequence of Condition (1.24)), and
that $\widehat{\psi}(\omega)$ has sufficient decay as $|\omega|$ goes to infinity.

Depending on the application, we may want additional properties. For
example, the discontinuity of the Haar wavelet transform makes it suboptimal for analyzing smooth functions. Therefore, we may want regular
wavelets with a number of derivatives.

1.3.2 Multidimensional Wavelet Transform

There are several ways to define the continuous wavelet transform for
multi-dimensional signals. The simplest way is to use a separable wavelet
obtained by products of one-dimensional wavelets, that is,

$$\psi(\mathbf{x}) = \psi^1(x_1)\psi^2(x_2) \cdots \psi^n(x_n)$$

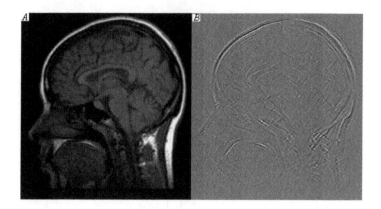

Figure 1.3
MRI image of "Ramses II" (panel A), and a two-dimensional Haar wavelet transform at scale factor $a = 2$ (panel B). This wavelet transform was obtained by two successive 1-D wavelet transforms applied to the rows of the image and then to the columns. Panel B shows the edges of the image of "Ramses II". This is the space-localization property of the wavelet transform. Clearly, there are no low frequency components in panel B. In fact, the Fourier transform of image (B) would contain frequency components that are concentrated near $[-\pi/2, -\pi/4]^2 \cup [\pi/4, \pi/2]^2$. This is the frequency localization property of the wavelet transform.

where $\mathbf{x} = (x_1, \cdots, x_n)$ is a vector in $\mathcal{R}^n$. For this case, the CWT is given by

$$(W_\psi f)(\mathbf{a}, \mathbf{b}) = \int_{\mathcal{R}^n} |a_1 a_2 \cdots a_n|^{-\frac{1}{2}} f(\mathbf{x})$$

$$\overline{\psi^1 \left(\frac{x_1 - b_1}{a_1} \right)} \cdots \overline{\psi^n \left(\frac{x_n - b_n}{a_n} \right)} \, d\mathbf{x}, \qquad (1.27)$$

where $\mathbf{a} = (a_1, \ldots, a_n)$, $\mathbf{b} = (b_1, \ldots, b_n)$, and $d\mathbf{x} = dx_1 \cdots dx_n$. The inverse transform is then given by

$$f(t) = C_\psi^{-1} \int_{\mathcal{R}^n} \int_{\mathcal{R}^n} a_1^{-2} \cdots a_n^{-2} (W_\psi f)(\mathbf{a}, \mathbf{b})$$

$$\psi^1 \left(\frac{x_1 - b_1}{a_1} \right) \cdots \psi^n \left(\frac{x_n - b_n}{a_n} \right) \, d\mathbf{a} \, d\mathbf{b}, \qquad (1.28)$$

where $C_\psi = C_{\psi^1} \cdots C_{\psi^n}$, $d\mathbf{a} = da_1 \cdots da_n$, and $d\mathbf{b} = db_1 \cdots db_n$.

Another way of defining a multidimensional wavelet transform is to choose a spherically symmetric wavelet whose Fourier transform $\hat{\psi}(|\omega|)$, $\omega = (\omega_1, \ldots, \omega_n)$ satisfies Condition (1.24) [31].

Finally, the most general scheme is to introduce rotations and translations in $\mathcal{R}^n$ to obtain all the translations, dilations, and rotations

$$\psi\left(R_\theta\left(\frac{\mathbf{x} - \mathbf{b}}{a}\right)\right)$$

of a wavelet $\psi(\mathbf{x})$, where R_θ is a rotation in $\mathcal{R}^n$, and where $a > 0$ is a scaling factor [31].

1.4   The Discrete Wavelet Transforms

The continuous wavelet transform maps a signal of one independent variable t into a function of two independent variables a, b. Thus, from a computational point of view, this transform is not efficient. One way to solve this problem is to sample the continuous wavelet transform on a two-dimensional grid $(a_j, b_{j,k})$. This will not prevent us from inverting the discretized wavelet transform in general.

1.4.1   The Dyadic Wavelet Transform

If we choose the dyadic scales $a_j = 2^j$, and if we choose $b_{j,k} = k2^j$ to adapt to the scale factors a_j, we obtain the *Phi*-transform of Frazier and Jawerth [46]

$$(W_\psi f)\left(2^j, k2^j\right) = \langle f(t), \psi_{j,k}(t) \rangle. \qquad (1.29)$$

For this choice of grid, and under appropriate conditions on the function $\psi(t)$ [31, 46], the *Phi*-transform of a signal $f(t) \in L_2$ can be inverted by the expansion formula

$$f(t) = \sum_{j,k} \langle f(t), \psi_{j,k}(t) \rangle \, \mathring{\psi}_{j,k}(t),$$

where $\psi_{j,k}(t) = 2^{-j/2}\psi(2^{-j}t - k)$, $\mathring{\psi}(t)$ is the dual wavelet of $\psi(t)$, and $\mathring{\psi}_{j,k}(t) = 2^{-j/2}\mathring{\psi}(2^{-j}t - k)$.

If the sets $\{\psi_{j,k}(t), (j,k) \in \mathcal{Z}^2\}$ and $\{\mathring{\psi}_{j,k}(t), (j,k) \in \mathcal{Z}^2\}$ are unconditional bases of $L_2(\mathcal{R})$, then we say that (1.29) is a DWT [31, 69]. Often

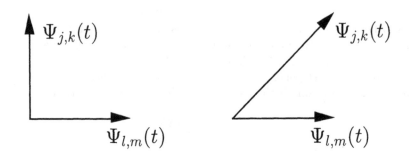

Figure 1.4
**Schematic representation of orthogonal and non-orthogonal
wavelet bases. The space L_2 (represented by the plane) can be
generated by an orthogonal wavelet basis (left), or by the non-
orthogonal wavelet basis (right). Non-orthogonal wavelets generate non-orthogonal bases, e.g., semi-orthogonal wavelets.**

for the DWT, a set of basis functions $\{\psi_{j,k}(t), (j,k) \in \mathcal{Z}^2\}$ is first chosen,
and the goal is then to find the decomposition of a function $f(t)$ as a lin-
ear combination of the given basis functions. The coefficients in this linear
combination are precisely the DWT $W_\psi^\circ f$ with respect to the dual function
$\overset{\circ}{\psi}(t)$:

$$f(t) = \sum_{j,k} \left\langle f(t), \overset{\circ}{\psi}_{j,k}(t) \right\rangle \psi_{j,k}(t). \tag{1.30}$$

For this reason we will sometimes denote the wavelet templates that we
use in the wavelet transform by $\overset{\circ}{\psi}$. However, we should note that this is
only a matter of notation since $\psi(t)$ and $\overset{\circ}{\psi}(t)$ are dual of each other (i.e.,
$\overset{\circ}{\psi}(t)$ is the dual $\psi(t)$ if and only if $\psi(t)$ is the dual of $\overset{\circ}{\psi}(t)$). It should
also be noted that although $\{\psi_{j,k}\}_{(j,k)\in\mathcal{Z}^2}$ is a basis, it is not necessarily
orthogonal. Non-orthogonal bases give greater flexibility and more choice
than orthogonal bases, and they are useful in many applications [1, 6]. This
issue is further discussed in Section 1.5.

REMARK 1   Note that in the literature, non-orthogonal wavelets are
sometimes used to mean redundant. This is not good nomenclature because
non-orthogonal should refer to the angles between vectors and not to the
redundancy of a set of vectors. In fact, most bases are non-orthogonal; see
Figure 1.4.   ∎

1.4.2 The Redundant Discrete Wavelet Transforms

In applications, it is often a subspace $V_0 \subset L_2$ that is considered instead of the whole space L_2. Without loss of generality, this subspace can be chosen to be the span of the wavelet functions $\{\psi_{j,k}(t)\}_{j>0}$ that belong to scales j coarser than the zero scale:

$$V_0 = \left\{ \sum_{j=1}^{\infty} \sum_{k \in \mathcal{Z}} d_j(k) \psi_{j,k}(t) \right\}. \tag{1.31}$$

For example, if the wavelet is an ideal bandpass filter, then V_0 is a space of bandlimited functions. In this case, one important choice of grid is when the scales are still given by $a_j = 2^j$ for $j \geq 0$, but the translation steps are chosen to be $b_k = k$. For a vector $f \in V_0$, the discrete wavelet transform with respect to the dual function $\overset{\circ}{\psi}(t)$ is given by

$$(W_{\overset{\circ}{\psi}} f)(2^{-j}, k) = 2^{-j/2} \left\langle f(t), \overset{\circ}{\psi} \left(2^{-j}(t-k) \right) \right\rangle$$

$$= 2^{-j/2} \int_{\mathcal{R}} f(t) \overline{\overset{\circ}{\psi} \left(\frac{t-k}{2^j} \right)} dt \quad \forall j \geq 1. \tag{1.32}$$

Unlike the DWT, the functions $\{2^{-j/2}\psi(2^{-j}(t-k)), (j,k) \in \mathcal{N}^+ \times \mathcal{Z}\}$ do not constitute a basis of $V_0 \subset L_2(\mathcal{R})$ because they are linearly dependent (here, $\mathcal{N}^+$ is the set of positive integers). However, these functions constitute what is called a *frame* of V_0 (see Section 1.8). This means that any signal $f(t) \in V_0$ can be recovered from its transform by a stable reconstruction algorithm. In particular, if the wavelet ψ is associated with a multiresolution (see Section 1.5), then we have

$$f(t) = \sum_{j=1}^{\infty} \sum_{k \in \mathcal{Z}} 2^{-2j} \left\langle f(t), \overset{\circ}{\psi} \left(2^{-j}(t-k) \right) \right\rangle \psi \left(2^{-j}(t-k) \right). \tag{1.33}$$

Note that, as in the case of wavelet bases, the role of $\psi(t)$ and $\overset{\circ}{\psi}(t)$ can be interchanged, and we have

$$f(t) = \sum_{j=1}^{\infty} \sum_{k \in \mathcal{Z}} 2^{-2j} \left\langle f(t), \psi \left(2^{-j}(t-k) \right) \right\rangle \overset{\circ}{\psi} \left(2^{-j}(t-k) \right).$$

Clearly, from the redundant transform (1.32), we can obtain a DWT (for $j \geq 1$) by down-sampling or ignoring the values that do not lie on the grid points $(2^j, 2^j k)$.

Another important discretization of the (a, b) plane is to choose $a_m = m,\ m > 0$ and $b_n = n$. Similar to the previous case, this discrete wavelet transform is redundant. It is given by

$$(W_{\overset{\circ}{\psi}} f)(m, n) = m^{-1/2} \left\langle f(t), \overset{\circ}{\psi}\left((t - n)/m\right) \right\rangle$$

$$= m^{-1/2} \int_{\mathcal{R}} f(t) \overline{\overset{\circ}{\psi}\left(\frac{t - n}{m}\right)} dt. \tag{1.34}$$

As in the previous case, to obtain the DWT for V_0 (see Definition (1.31)), from the redundant transform (1.34) we need to keep only the values at $m = 2^j, n = k2^j$.

1.5 Multiresolution Approximations and Their Associated Wavelets

1.5.1 Multiresolution Approximations of L_2

There is a class of DWT that can be implemented using extremely efficient algorithms [1, 68, 69]. These types of wavelet transforms are associated with mathematical structures called *multiresolution approximations of L_2* (MRA) [68, 69]. A multiresolution approximation of L_2 is a set of spaces $\{V_j\}_{j \in \mathcal{Z}}$ that are generated by dilating and translating a single function $\varphi(t)$:

$$V_j = \left\{ \sum_{k \in \mathcal{Z}} c_j(k) \varphi_{j,k}(t),\ c_j \in l_2 \right\}, \tag{1.35}$$

where $\varphi_{j,k}(t) = 2^{-j/2} \varphi(2^{-j} t - k)$ are the dilations (or reductions) and translations of the function $\varphi(t)$ called the *scaling function*. Moreover, for fixed j, the set $\{\varphi_{j,k}(t),\ k \in \mathcal{Z}\}$ is required to form an unconditional basis of V_j. If the functions $\{\varphi_{j,k}(t),\ k \in \mathcal{Z}\}$ form an orthogonal basis of V_j, then we call $\varphi(t)$ an *orthogonal scaling function* and we tag the scaling function with the superscript "o": $\varphi^o(t)$. The spaces V_j are also required to satisfy the additional properties:

(i) $\cdots \subset V_1 \subset V_0 \subset V_{-1} \subset \cdots$;

(ii) V_0 is a closed subspace of $L_2(\mathcal{R})$;

(iii) $V_{-\infty} = \text{Clos} \left(\bigcup_{j \in Z} V_j \right) = L_2;$

(iv) $V_{\infty} = \bigcap_{j \in Z} V_j = \{0\}.$

Thus, a multiresolution approximation can be viewed as a ladder of embedded spaces that become coarser and coarser as the index j becomes larger. It follows that if $i > j$, then the orthogonal projections $f_i(t) \in V_i$ of a function $f(t)$ in L_2 is a coarser approximation of f than the projection $f_j \in V_j$.

The construction (1.35) implies that the spaces V_j are similar to each other. For instance, a function $f(t)$ belongs to V_j if and only if $f(t/2)$ belongs to V_{j+1} and vice versa. Thus, the closed subspace property of V_0 (property (ii)) is inherited by all the spaces V_j. This technical property is needed for computing least squares approximations in V_j. The other two technical properties, (iii) and (iv), state that the finest space $V_{-\infty}$ consists of all finite energy functions L_2, and that the coarsest space V_{∞} contains no signal other than the zero function.

Because of properties (i)-(iv), the scaling function $\varphi(t)$ that is used to generate the MRA cannot be chosen arbitrarily. In fact since $V_1 \subset V_0$, and since $2^{-1/2}\varphi(t/2) \in V_1$ and $\varphi(t) \in V_0$, we conclude that the generating function $2^{-1/2}\varphi(t/2)$ must be a linear combination of the basis $\{\varphi(t - k)\}_{k \in Z}$ of V_0:

$$\varphi(t/2) = 2^{1/2} \sum_{k \in Z} h(k)\varphi(t - k). \tag{1.36}$$

This last relation is often called the two-scale relation or the refinement equation, and the sequence $h(k)$ is the generating sequence which is crucial in the implementation of the DWT associated with multiresolutions.

If we take the Fourier transform of (1.36), we obtain the relation

$$\hat{\varphi}(2\omega) = 2^{-1/2}\hat{h}(\omega)\hat{\varphi}(\omega), \tag{1.37}$$

from which, by iteration, we obtain the infinite product

$$\hat{\varphi}(\omega) = 2^{-1/2}\hat{h}\left(\frac{\omega}{2}\right) 2^{-1/2}\hat{h}\left(\frac{\omega}{2^2}\right) 2^{-1/2}\hat{h}\left(\frac{\omega}{2^3}\right) \cdots. \tag{1.38}$$

The above relation suggests a way to construct scaling functions from appropriate sequences. In particular, Mallat showed that if we start from a sequence $h(k)$ with sufficient decay, and if

$$2^{-1/2}\hat{h}(0) = 1, \ \hat{h}(\omega) \neq 0 \quad \forall \omega \in \left[-\frac{\pi}{2}, \frac{\pi}{2}\right]$$

and $\hat{h}(\omega)$ satisfies the quadrature mirror filter condition (QMF)

$$\left|\hat{h}(\omega)\right|^2 + \left|\hat{h}(\omega - \pi)\right|^2 = 2, \qquad (1.39)$$

then the infinite product on the right hand side of Equation (1.38) converges and defines the Fourier transform of an orthogonal scaling function $\varphi^o(t)$ [68, 69]. Other sufficient conditions for obtaining orthogonal scaling functions can be found in [29, 31, 48]. If we remove the QMF condition (1.39), we can still obtain scaling functions by the infinite product (1.38). However, the scaling functions thus obtained are not orthogonal but still form unconditional bases [7].

1.5.2 Orthogonal MRA-Type Wavelets

The orthogonal complement of V_j relative to V_{j-1} is the associated error space W_j:

$$W_j \oplus V_j = V_{j-1}, \qquad (1.40)$$

where $W_j \oplus V_j$ is the set of all vectors obtained by summing a vector from W_j with a vector from V_j. In particular, the difference between the two approximations $f_j(t) \in V_j$ and $f_{j-1}(t) \in V_{j-1}$ of a function $f(t)$ is equal to the orthogonal projection of $f(t)$ on W_j. It can be shown that the associated spaces W_j can also be spanned by an orthonormal basis $\{2^{-j/2}\psi^o(2^{-j}t - k)\}_{k\in\mathbb{Z}}$ generated from a single *orthogonal wavelet* function $\psi^o(t)$, and satisfying Condition (1.24) ($\psi^o(t)$ is not unique; see below) [68, 69]:

$$W_j = \left\{ \sum_{k\in\mathbb{Z}} d_j(k)\psi^o_{j,k}(t), \; d_j \in l_2 \right\}, \qquad (1.41)$$

where $\psi^o_{j,k}(t) = 2^{-j/2}\psi^o(2^{-j}t - k)$. From the properties (i)-(iv) of MRAs, and from (1.40) and (1.41), any function $f(t) \in L_2$ can be expanded as a low resolution approximation $f_J(t) \in V_J$, and error terms in the spaces $\{W_j, \; j = J, J+1, ...\}$:

$$f(t) = f_J(t) + \sum_{j=-\infty}^{J} \sum_{k\in\mathbb{Z}} \langle f(t), \psi^o_{j,k}(t) \rangle \, \psi^o_{j,k}(t). \qquad (1.42)$$

If we let J tend to infinity in the previous equation, and if we use property (iv) of MRAs, we obtain the expansion

$$f(t) = \sum_{(j,k)\in\mathbb{Z}^2} \langle f(t), \psi^o_{j,k}(t) \rangle \, \psi^o_{j,k}(t). \qquad (1.43)$$

It follows that the set $\mathcal{Q} = \{\psi_{j,k}^o(t), (j,k) \in \mathcal{Z}^2\}$ is an orthonormal basis of L_2. Expression (1.43) can be seen to be a particular case of the DWT formula (1.30) in which the dual wavelets $\mathring{\tilde{\psi}}_{j,k}(t)$ are given by $\mathring{\tilde{\psi}}_{j,k}(t) = \psi_{j,k}^o(t)$. Examples of such wavelets are the Battle-Lemarié spline wavelets and the Daubechies wavelets [29, 64].

As will be developed in the next chapter, the DWT of orthogonal MRA-type wavelets can be implemented by the repetitive application of a simple filtering algorithm. In particular, if $c_j(k) = \langle f(t), \varphi_{j,k}(t) \rangle$, and $d_j(k) = (W_{\psi^o} f)(2^j, 2^j k)$, then the algorithm implementing the DWT takes the form

$$c_{j+1}(k) = \sum_{l \in \mathcal{Z}} \mathring{h}(2k - l)c_j(l) = \downarrow_2 \left[\mathring{h} * c_j\right](k) \tag{1.44}$$

$$d_{j+1}(k) = \sum_{l \in \mathcal{Z}} \mathring{g}(2k - l)c_j(l) = \downarrow_2 \left[\mathring{g} * c_j\right](k), \tag{1.45}$$

where $\mathring{h}(k) = h^{\vee}(k)$ is the reflection of the two-scale sequence $h(k)$ underlying the MRA (see Equation (1.36)), and where $\mathring{g}(k) = g^{\vee}(k)$ is the reflection of the wavelet generating sequence $g(k) = \delta_1 * \tilde{h} = (-1)^{k-1}h(k-1)$, which relates the orthogonal wavelet to the orthogonal scaling function:

$$\psi^o(t/2) = 2^{1/2} \sum_{k \in \mathcal{Z}} g(k)\varphi^o(x - k). \tag{1.46}$$

The coefficients $c_j(k)$ at resolution j can be obtained from the coefficients c_{j+1} and d_{j+1} at a coarser resolution by the reconstruction algorithm

$$c_j(k) = \sum_{l \in \mathcal{Z}} h(2l - k)c_{j+1}(l) + \sum_{l \in \mathcal{Z}} g(2l - k)d_{j+1}(l)$$

$$= (\uparrow_2 [c_{j+1}] * h)(k) + (\uparrow_2 [d_{j+1}] * g)(k), \tag{1.47}$$

which is essentially the computational algorithm for inverting the DWT associated with MRAs.

1.5.3 Semi-Orthogonal MRA-Type Wavelet Bases

There are many other bases that generate the wavelet spaces $\{W_j, j \in \mathcal{Z}\}$ defined by (1.40) and characterized by (1.41). In particular, we will say that $\psi(t)$ is a *semi-orthogonal* wavelet (or non-orthogonal wavelet—see Figure 1.4 and Remark 1), if for each $j \in \mathcal{Z}$, the set $\{2^{-j/2}\psi(2^{-j}t-k)\}_{k \in \mathcal{Z}}$ forms a non-orthogonal, unconditional basis of W_j. However, since the spaces W_j remain orthogonal to each other (i.e., $W_j \perp W_l$ for $j \neq l$), we still have the orthogonality of the wavelet functions at different scales:

$$\langle \psi_{j,k}(t), \psi_{l,m}(t) \rangle = 0 \quad \text{for } j \neq l. \tag{1.48}$$

It follows that the approximation error $e = f_{j-1}(t) - f_j(t)$, obtained when we approximate a function $f(t)$ by $f_j(t) \in V_j$ instead of $f_{j-1}(t) \in V_{j-1}$, is still equal to the orthogonal projection of $f(t)$ on W_j, as in the orthogonal wavelet case. The difference is that, instead of the orthogonal expansion (1.43), the expansion of any function $f(t) \in L_2$ in terms of its wavelet coefficients $\langle f(t), \mathring{\psi}_{j,k}(t) \rangle$ is now given by

$$f(t) = \sum_{(j,k) \in \mathbb{Z}^2} \left\langle f(t), \mathring{\psi}_{j,k}(t) \right\rangle \psi_{j,k}(t), \tag{1.49}$$

where $\mathring{\psi}_{j,k}(t)$ is the semi-orthogonal dual wavelet basis. The expression of the semi-orthogonal dual wavelet in terms of $\psi(t)$ is given by

$$\mathring{\psi}(t) = (a_\psi^{-1} * \psi)(t)$$

where $a_\psi(k) = (\psi * \psi^\vee)(k)$ is the sampled autocorrelation of $\psi(t)$ [7, 9]. The computation of the wavelet transform and its inverse can still be performed using a fast filter bank algorithm (cf. Chapter 2) similar to the one described in (1.45) and (1.47) (see [1]). The advantage of the semi-orthogonal wavelets is that we gain flexibility for finding analyzing wavelets suitable to our needs, without losing the fast computational algorithms, or the decoupling between the wavelet spaces at different scales (more on this issue in Section 1.6; see also [1]).

One particularly useful choice of a semi-orthogonal wavelet is the basic wavelet $\psi^b(t)$ which uses for its construction the generating sequence $h(k)$ in (1.36) and the sampled autocorrelation sequence $a(k) = (\varphi * \varphi^\vee)(k)$ of the scaling function $\varphi(t)$:

$$\psi^b(t) = \sum_{k \in \mathbb{Z}} g(k) \varphi(t - k), \tag{1.50}$$

where the wavelet generating sequence $g(k)$ is given by [7]

$$g(k) = (\delta_1 * \tilde{h} * \tilde{a})(k),$$

and where $\tilde{h}(k) = (-1)^k h(k)$ and $\tilde{a} = (-1)^k a(k)$ are the alternations of h and a (see Definition (1.16)). The basic wavelet basis $\{\psi^b_{j,k}(t)\}_{k \in \mathbb{Z}}$ of W_j

generated by the translation of the function $2^{-j/2}\psi^b(2^{-j}t)$ is not orthogonal. However, it has the property of being symmetrical and compactly supported if the associated scaling function has these same properties. In fact, the wavelet $\psi^b(t)$ is the generalization of the B-spline wavelets [19, 88]. It converges to a modulated Gaussian function as the order of smoothness increases [7, Theorem 15].

1.5.4 Bi-Orthogonal MRA-Type Wavelet Bases

Bi-orthogonal MRA-type wavelets are always associated with a pair of MRAs $\{V_j, j \in \mathcal{Z}\}$ and $\{\overset{\circ}{V}_j, j \in \mathcal{Z}\}$, and a pair of complementary spaces $\{W_j, j \in \mathcal{Z}\}$ and $\{\overset{\circ}{W}_j, j \in \mathcal{Z}\}$, instead of a single multiresolution and its associated wavelet spaces in the orthogonal and semi-orthogonal cases. Similar to these two cases, we have that $V_j + W_j = V_{j-1}$ and $\overset{\circ}{V}_j + \overset{\circ}{W}_j = \overset{\circ}{V}_{j-1}$, and there exist two wavelet functions $\psi(t)$ and $\overset{\circ}{\psi}(t)$ that generate the spaces W_j and $\overset{\circ}{W}_j$:

$$W_j = \left\{ \sum_{k \in \mathcal{Z}} d_j(k)\psi_{j,k}(t), \ d_j \in l_2 \right\}, \tag{1.51}$$

$$\overset{\circ}{W}_j = \left\{ \sum_{k \in \mathcal{Z}} d_j(k)\overset{\circ}{\psi}_{j,k}(t), \ d_j \in l_2 \right\}. \tag{1.52}$$

However, unlike the previous cases, we no longer have orthogonality between the wavelet spaces. Instead, we have the bi-orthogonality property

$$W_i \perp \overset{\circ}{W}_j, \quad \forall i \neq j. \tag{1.53}$$

For the bi-orthogonal case, the expansion of a function $f(t) \in L_2$ is given by a formula similar to (1.49), but the approximation error $e = f_{j-1}(t) - f_j(t)$ is no longer the orthogonal projection of $f(t)$ on W_j or $\overset{\circ}{W}_j$. The error is now an oblique projection as described in [20, 31].

1.5.5 Local and Global Characterization of Functions in Terms of Their Wavelet Coefficients

If the mother wavelet $\psi(t)$ is sufficiently regular, then the local behavior of a function $f(t_0)$ at t_0 is completely characterized by its wavelet coefficients $d_j(k) = \langle f(t), \psi_{j,k}(t) \rangle$ near time t_0 [53, 55]. This is essentially the time-localization property of the wavelet transform. For example, if the wavelet coefficients in a neighborhood $[t_0 - \epsilon, t_0 + \epsilon]$ of t_0 are of the order of $\mathcal{O}(2^{-j(\frac{1}{2}+\alpha)})$, then f is Hölder continuous with exponent α at t_0, i.e., at t_0 we have [31]

$$|f(t) - f(t_0)| \leq C |t - t_0|^\alpha. \tag{1.54}$$

The precise conditions that are required to capture the local behavior of $f(t)$ from its wavelet coefficients can be found in [31, 53, 55, 73]. In particular, the regularity of a function can be calculated from the behavior through scales of its wavelet coefficients. This property has been used for signal and image processing [70, 71].

The global behavior of a function can also be captured from the wavelet coefficients. For example, a function $f(t)$ is in the Sobolev space $W^{s,2}$ if and only if

$$\sum_{j,k} |\langle f(t), \psi_{j,k}(t)\rangle|^2 (1 + 2^{-2js}) < \infty.$$

Other characterizations of functional spaces in terms of the wavelet coefficients can be found in, e.g., [31, 36, 68, 73].

1.6   Special Bases of Scaling Functions and Wavelets

As we have discussed in Section 1.5.3, there are many other bases that generate the wavelet spaces W_j defined by (1.40). The same is true for the multiresolution spaces defined in (1.35). In fact, if φ is a scaling function generating V_0, then it is possible to construct another scaling function

$$\varphi^{\approx}(t) = \sum_{k \in \mathcal{Z}} p(k)\varphi(t - k) \tag{1.55}$$

as long as the Fourier transform $\hat{p}(\omega)$ of the real sequence $p(k)$ satisfies (see [7, Proposition 6] and [9, Proposition 1])

$$0 < A \leq \operatorname*{ess\ inf}_{\omega \in [0,\pi]} |\hat{p}(\omega)| \leq \operatorname*{ess\ sup}_{\omega \in [0,\pi]} |\hat{p}(\omega)| \leq B < \infty, \tag{1.56}$$

where A, B are two strictly positive constants, and where ess inf and ess sup are the essential infimum and the essential supremum, respectively. Condition (1.56) is necessary and sufficient. This means that the functions $\varphi^{\approx}_{j,k}(t)$ form an unconditional basis of V_j (not necessarily orthogonal) if and only if (1.56) is satisfied. Moreover, any two functions φ^1 and φ^2 that generate unconditional bases of $\{V_j, j \in \mathcal{Z}\}$ by dyadic translations and dilations are related by the sequence $p(k)$ that satisfies (1.56) [7]:

$$\varphi^1(t) = \sum p(k)\varphi^2(t - k).$$

A sequence $p(k)$ satisfying (1.56) will be called *admissible*, and the admissibility condition (1.56) essentially means that $|\hat{p}(\omega)|$ must be bounded above and below by positive constants A and B.

Similarly, if ψ is an MRA-type wavelet generating W_0, then

$$\psi^{\approx}(t) = \sum_{k \in \mathcal{Z}} q(k)\psi(t - k) \tag{1.57}$$

is a wavelet for W_0 if and only if the sequence $q(k)$ is admissible. Moreover, any two wavelets ψ^1, ψ^2 for W_0 must be related by an admissible sequence $q(k)$ (*i.e.*, $\psi^1 = \sum q(k)\psi^2(t - k)$). Thus, any semi-orthogonal wavelet associated with a fixed multiresolution can be obtained from an orthogonal wavelet by an admissible sequence [7].

Using these facts, it is possible to construct infinitely many scaling and wavelet functions with various desired shapes and properties by choosing the admissible sequences judiciously [1, 7]. In particular, in the next two sections, we will show how to construct interpolating scaling and wavelet functions [6, 7, 86, 89].

1.6.1 Interpolating Scaling Functions

A function φ^I which interpolates between samples on $\mathcal{Z}$ must have a value of zero at all integers except at the origin, where it must be 1:

$$\varphi^I(k) = \delta_0(k) = \begin{cases} 1, & k = 0 \\ 0, & k = \pm 1, \pm 2, \ldots \end{cases} \tag{1.58}$$

In the literature, such a function is sometimes called *fundamental* or *cardinal*. If $\varphi(t)$ is a scaling function satisfying

$$\left| \sum_k \hat{\varphi}(\omega - 2\pi k) \right| \neq 0 \quad \text{for all } \omega \in [0, 2\pi],$$

and $\hat{\varphi}(\omega) \leq \text{Const}(1 + |\omega|)^{-r}$, $r > 1/2$, then we can choose an admissible sequence p_I so that $\varphi^I = p_I * \varphi$ is an interpolating function [7]. The sequence p_I can be specified by its Fourier transform as

$$\hat{p}_I(\omega) = \left(\sum_k \hat{\varphi}(\omega - 2\pi k) \right)^{-1}. \tag{1.59}$$

From Poisson's formula (1.22), the sequence $p_I(k)$ is simply the convolution inverse of the sequence $b(k)$ given by

$$b(k) = \varphi(x)|_{x=k} \, . \tag{1.60}$$

An interpolating scaling function is not necessarily orthogonal. However, by construction, it has the property that any function $f(t) \in V_j$ can be written in terms of its sample values $f(2^k)$ by the interpolation formula

$$f(t) = \sum_{k \in \mathcal{Z}} f(2^k) \varphi_{j,k}^I(t). \tag{1.61}$$

A prototypical example is the function $\mathrm{sinc}(t) = \sin(\pi t)/\pi t$ used in Shannon's sampling theory. In fact, an interpolating scaling function $\varphi^I(t)$ can be viewed as a generalization of the sinc-function, and $\varphi^I(t)$ (under appropriate conditions) converges to $\mathrm{sinc}(t)$ as the order of smoothness goes to infinity [7, Theorem 10]. Interpolating functions that are also orthogonal have been found by Xia and Zhang [94]. Note that, in general, interpolating scaling functions are non-orthogonal.

1.6.2   Interpolating Wavelets

The interpolating wavelet $\psi^I(t)$ must be such that $\psi^I(k + 1/2) = \delta_0(k)$, i.e., $\psi^I(1/2) = 1$, $\psi^I(k + 1/2) = 0$ for all $k \in \mathcal{Z} \setminus \{0\}$ [7]. This definition is a slightly different characterization from the one for $\varphi^I(t)$. Specifically, a function $w \in W_0$ can be expanded in terms of its samples $\{w(k + 1/2), k \in \mathcal{Z}\}$ as

$$w(t) = \sum_{k \in \mathcal{Z}} w(k + 1/2) \psi^I(t - k). \tag{1.62}$$

This definition of the interpolating wavelet $\psi^I(t)$ allows us to obtain interpolating wavelets with axial symmetry (cf., end of this section). To obtain $\psi^I(t)$ from an arbitrary basic wavelet $\psi^b(t)$ (see Definition (1.50)), we choose a sequence q_I as follows:

$$q_I = 2^{-1/2} \left(\downarrow_2 \left[\tilde{h}^{\vee} * \tilde{a} * b, \right] \right)^{-1} \tag{1.63}$$

where $b(k)$ consists of the samples of the scaling function that generates the underlying multiresolution (see Equation (1.60)), and where $\tilde{h}$ and $\tilde{a}$ are the alternations of the two-scale sequence, h, and the autocorrelation function, a, of the underlying scaling function, respectively (see Equations (1.50) and (1.36)). The interpolating wavelet $\psi^I(t)$ is then given by

$$\psi^I(t) = (q_I * \psi^b)(t). \tag{1.64}$$

If the sequence h generating the scaling function $\varphi(t)$ is symmetric (see Equation (1.36)), then $\varphi(t)$ is symmetric. Thus, the corresponding basic wavelet $\psi^b(t)$ given by Expression (1.50), has an axis of symmetry at $t = 1/2$. It follows that, for this case, the wavelet in $\psi^I(t)$ defined by (1.64) and (1.63) has an axis of symmetry at $t = 1/2$ as well.

A prototypical example of interpolating wavelets is the bandpass filter given by the modulated sinc-function $BP(t) = 2\cos(3\pi t/2)\sin(\pi t)/\pi t$. An interpolating wavelet $\psi^I(t)$ can be viewed as a generalization of the ideal bandpass filter $BP(t) = 2\cos(3\pi t/2)\sin(\pi t)/\pi t$, and (under appropriate conditions) $\psi^I(t)$ converges to it as its order of smoothness increases to infinity [7, Theorem 14].

1.7 Applications and Generalizations of the Wavelet Transform

1.7.1 Applications of the Wavelet Transform

The time-frequency localization property of the wavelet transform and the existence of fast algorithms make it a tool of choice for the analysis of nonstationary signals. In particular, the time-frequency localization property gives rise to new algorithms for edge detection and noise reduction in images and signals [36, 37, 38, 61, 69, 76]. The time-frequency localization also gives rise to the characterization and unification of many function spaces [73]. The multiscale and self-similarity properties of the wavelet transform have been used for texture and fractal analysis [11, 35]. They have also been used for speeding up expensive numerical processing tasks, by first finding an approximate solution at low resolution scale and then by refining them at finer scales, a procedure similar to multigrid methods [87]. The ability of the wavelet transform to sort the information into uncorrelated levels of structure at different scales has been used for coding, progressive transmission of images, and statistical inference [10]. The scale sorting property as well as the time-frequency localization property make the wavelet transform an efficient tool for the numerical solution of problems involving pseudo-differential operators [28]. Another important feature of the wavelet transform is that it provides formal links between many different areas in mathematics and engineering, and unifies many seemingly different areas under one simple mathematical framework.

For example, it provides the link between filter bank theory, harmonic analysis, functional analysis, approximation theory, and numerical analysis [36, 54, 68, 58, 69, 73, 56, 85, 81, 93]. The wavelet transform is also related to the sampling theory, the theory of frames, the Gabor transform, and many other representations of analog functions [6, 7, 42, 44, 45].

1.7.2   Generalizations of the Wavelet Transform

There are many other forms and useful generalizations to the wavelet transform. Wavelet bases on finite intervals $I \subset \mathcal{R}$ instead of $\mathcal{R}$ have been constructed to fulfill the need in some applications (e.g., boundary value problems in differential equations) [17, 21, 22, 74]. Wavelet bases for complex domains in higher dimensions can also be found in [34].

MRA-type wavelet bases that have dilation factors other than multiples of 2 can be found in [12, 59]. Wavelet bases with variable dilation and translation factors can be found in [24, 25, 26, 52, 91].

Generalizations of the concept of multiresolutions and associated wavelets to the case of multiple scaling functions and multiple wavelets can be found in [39, 40, 47, 81]. Specifically, the multiresolution and wavelet spaces are generated by the dilations and translations of several scaling functions $\{\phi^1(t), \phi^2(t), \ldots, \phi^r(t)\}$ and several wavelets $\{\psi^1(t), \psi^2(t), \ldots, \psi^r(t)\}$. This gives flexibility on choosing specific wavelets with some desired prescribed properties. For instance, using these types of constructions, it is possible to construct compact, regular, orthonormal wavelet bases that are also symmetrical [39, 40, 81].

The multiresolution and wavelet space theories have also been generalized to spaces other than L_2. For example, they have been generalized to the sphere [27, 79, 80], and to the sequence space l_2 [5, 8, 77].

A more recent advance in the theory of wavelets, *the lifting scheme*, allows the construction of wavelets on curves and surfaces, and their custom-design to suit needs of specific applications [83, 84].

1.8   Frame Representations

Most of the representations that we have discussed so far (and many others) can be viewed as a special instance of frame theory. This theory has been introduced by R. J. Duffin and A. C. Schaeffer in the context of nonharmonic Fourier series [41], and it is the generalization of the concept of bases in Hilbert spaces (complete inner product vector spaces).

In a complete inner product space $\mathcal{H}$ (Hilbert space), a frame is defined to be a set of vectors $Q = \{\varphi_n\}_{n \in \mathbb{Z}}$ such that for any vector $v \in \mathcal{H}$,

$$A \|v\|_{\mathcal{H}}^2 \leq \sum_{n \in \mathbb{Z}} |\langle v, \varphi_n \rangle_{\mathcal{H}}|^2 \leq B \|v\|_{\mathcal{H}}^2, \qquad (1.65)$$

where the *frame bounds* A and B are strictly positive constants. As before, the set Q can be viewed as a set of test vectors with which we can probe an element $v \in \mathcal{H}$ to gain information about it. This is done by the inner products $m_n = \langle v, \varphi_n \rangle_{\mathcal{H}}$. With this interpretation, the lower frame bound in (1.65) says that there must be enough vectors in the set Q, and that these vectors must be sufficiently well-distributed so as to extract some positive information from any vector $v \in \mathcal{H}$ (note that $A > 0$). The upper frame bound says that there is no region in the space $\mathcal{H}$ where there is a cluster of test vectors. If such a cluster existed, there would be a vector v_0 in its vicinity for which all the measurements $m_n = \langle v_0, \varphi_n \rangle_{\mathcal{H}}$ are approximately equal to the same constant $\delta > 0$. This fact would force the infinite sum in (1.65) to blow up, and the upper frame bound to fail. Thus, in a sense, the upper frame bound saves us from repeating the same measurements over and over again, ad infinitum.

It turns out that the Conditions (1.65) are sufficient to have a stable representation of any vector $v \in \mathcal{H}$ in terms of the frame vectors $Q = \{\varphi_n\}_{n \in \mathbb{Z}}$ [41]:

$$v = \sum_{n \in \mathbb{Z}} \left\langle v, \mathring{\varphi}_n \right\rangle_{\mathcal{H}} \varphi_n, \qquad (1.66)$$

where $\{\mathring{\varphi}_n\}_{n \in \mathbb{Z}}$ is a dual frame [41]. Thus, any unconditional basis of $\mathcal{H}$ is also a frame of $\mathcal{H}$, but the converse is not true since a frame can be redundant. In fact, if the frame is not a basis (i.e., it is redundant), then the above expansion is not unique, and there exist other dual frames $\{\mathring{\varphi}_n^{\approx}\}_{n \in \mathbb{Z}}$ (also called pseudo-dual frames) for which a stable representation can be found [67]:

$$v = \sum_{n \in \mathbb{Z}} \left\langle v, \mathring{\varphi}_n^{\approx} \right\rangle_{\mathcal{H}} \varphi_n. \qquad (1.67)$$

Frames can be constructed from other frames or bases by using appropriate operators, and in fact, all frames can be constructed this way [4]. Another construction method uses perturbation of frames to obtain other frames [16]. Redundant frame representations can have advantages over bases. For instance, the redundant wavelet transforms have better time resolution. Moreover, the redundancy of the frames can be used to correct for noise in the reconstruction formula [3, 30]. Multiresolutions and wavelets have been generalized to frame MRAs and frame wavelets [15].

References

[1] P. Abry and A. Aldroubi. Designing multiresolution analysis-type wavelets and their fast algorithms. *J. Fourier Anal. Appl.*, to appear.

[2] A. Aldroubi. Oblique projections in atomic spaces. *Proc. Am. Math. Soc.*, to appear.

[3] A. Aldroubi. Portraits of frames: overcomplete representations with applications to image processing. In [60], pages 322–329.

[4] A. Aldroubi. Portraits of frames. *Proc. Am. Math. Soc.*, 123(6): 1661–1668, 1995.

[5] A. Aldroubi, M. Eden, and M. Unser. Discrete spline filters for multiresolutions and wavelets of ℓ_2. *SIAM J. Math. Anal.*, 25(5): 1412–1432, 1994.

[6] A. Aldroubi and M. Unser. Families of wavelet transforms in connection with Shannon's sampling theory and the Gabor transform. In [18], pages 509–528.

[7] A. Aldroubi and M. Unser. Families of multiresolution and wavelet spaces with optimal properties. *Numer. Funct. Anal. Optimiz.*, 14(5): 417–446, 1993.

[8] A. Aldroubi and M. Unser. Oblique projections in discrete signal subspaces of ℓ_2 and the wavelet transform. In [62], pages 36–45.

[9] A. Aldroubi and M. Unser. Sampling procedure in function spaces and asymptotic equivalence with Shannon's sampling theory. *Numer. Funct. Anal. Optimiz.*, 15(1): 1–21, 1994.

[10] M. Antonini, M. Barlaud, P. Mathieu, and I. Daubechies. Image coding using the wavelet transform. *IEEE Trans. Image Process.*, 1(2): 205–220, 1992.

[11] A. Arneodo, E. Bacry, and J. F. Muzy. The multifractal formalism revisited with wavelets. *Int. J. Bifurcation Chaos*, 42: 245–302, 1994.

[12] P. Auscher. Wavelet bases for $L(\mathcal{R})$ with rational dilation factor. In [78], pages 439–452.

[13] J. J. Benedetto. Irregular sampling and frames. In [18], pages 445–507.

[14] J. J. Benedetto and M.W. Frazier, editors. *Wavelets–Mathematics and Applications.* CRC Press, Boca Raton, FL, 1993.

[15] J. J. Benedetto and S. Li. Multiresolution analysis frames with applications. IEEE-ICASSP-93, 1993. Proc. IEEE-ICASSP-93, Minneapolis, MN, 1993, 304–307.

[16] O. Christensen. A Paley-Wiener theorem on frames. *Proc. Am. Math. Soc.*, 123: 2199–2202, 1994.

[17] C. Chui and E. Quak. Wavelets on a bounded interval. In *Numerical Methods of Approximation Theory*, D. Braess and L.L. Schumaker, editors, Birkhäuser-Verlag, Basel, 1992, pages 1–24.

[18] C. K. Chui, editor. *Wavelets: A Tutorial in Theory and Applications.* Academic Press, San Diego, CA, 1992.

[19] C. K. Chui and J. Z. Wang. A cardinal spline approach to wavelets. *Proc. Am. Math. Soc.*, 113: 785–793, 1991.

[20] A. Cohen, I. Daubechies, and J. C. Fauveau. Biorthogonal bases of compactly supported wavelets. *Comm. Pure Appl. Math.*, 45: 485–560, 1992.

[21] A. Cohen, I. Daubechies, B. Jawerth, and P. Vial. Multiresolution analysis, wavelets and fast algorithms on an interval. *C. R. Acad. Sci. Paris Sér. I Math.*, I(316): 417–421, 1993.

[22] A. Cohen, I. Daubechies, and P. Vial. Multiresolution analysis, wavelets and fast algorithms on an interval. *Appl. Comput. Harmon. Anal.*, 1(1): 54–81, 1993.

[23] R. R. Coifman. A real variable characterization of H^p. *Studia Math.*, 51: 269–274, 1974.

[24] R. R. Coifman and Y. Meyer. Orthonormal wave packet bases. Preprint.

[25] R. R. Coifman, Y. Meyer, S. Quake, and M. V. Wickerhauser. Signal processing and compression with wave packets. In *Proc. Int. Conf. Wavelets, Marseille, 1989*, Y. Meyer, editor, Masson, Paris, 1992.

[26] R. R. Coifman, Y. Meyer, and M. V. Wickerhauser. Size properties of wavelet packets. In [78], pages 453–470.

[27] S. Dahlke, W. Dahmen, E. Schmitt, and I. Weinreich. Multiresolution analysis and wavelets on S^2 and S^3. *Numer. Funct. Anal. Optimiz.*, 16(1&2): 19–41, 1993.

[28] W. Dahmen, S. Prössdorf, and R. Schneider. Wavelet approximation methods for pseudodifferential equations ii: Matrix compression and fast solution. *Adv. Comp. Math.*, 1: 259–335, 1993.

[29] I. Daubechies. Orthonormal bases of compactly supported wavelets. *Comm. Pure Appl. Math.*, 41: 909–996, 1988.

[30] I. Daubechies. The wavelet transform, time-frequency localization and signal analysis. *IEEE Trans. Inform. Theory*, 36: 961–1005, 1990.

[31] I. Daubechies. *Ten Lectures on Wavelets*. Society for Industrial and Applied Mathematics, Philadelphia, 1992.

[32] I. Daubechies, A. Grossmann, and Y. Meyer. Painless nonorthogonal expansions. *J. Math. Phys.*, 27(5): 1271–1283, 1986.

[33] C. de Boor, R. A. DeVore, and A. Ron. On the construction of multivariate pre-wavelets. *Constr. Approx.*, 9(2): 123–166, 1993.

[34] B. Deng, B. Jawerth, G. Peters, and W. Sweldens. Wavelet probing for compression based segmentation. In [60], pages 266–276.

[35] G. Deslauriers and S. Dubuc. Interpolation dyadique. In *Fractals, dimensions non entières et applications*, Masson, Paris, 1987, pages 44–55.

[36] R. A. DeVore, B. Jawerth, and B. J. Lucier. Image compression through wavelet transform coding. *IEEE Trans. Inform. Theory*, 38(2): 719–746, 1992.

[37] R. A. DeVore and B. J. Lucier. Fast wavelet techniques for near-optimal image processing. IEEE Military Communications Conference, New York, NY, 1992, pages 48.3.1–48.3.7.

[38] D. L. Donoho and I. M. Johnstone. Ideal spatial adaptation via wavelet shrinkage. *Biometrika*, to appear.

[39] G. Donovan, D. P. Hardin, and J. S. Geronimo. Fractal functions, splines, intertwining multiresolution analysis, and wavelets. In [60], pages 238–243.

[40] G. C. Donovan, D. P. Hardin, and P. R. Massopust. Fractal functions and wavelet expansions based on several scaling function. *J. Approx. Theory*, 1994.

[41] R. J. Duffin and A. C. Schaeffer. A class of nonharmonic Fourier series. *Trans. Am. Math. Soc.*, 72(2): 341–366, 1952.

[42] H. G. Feichtinger and K. Gröchenig. Non-orthogonal wavelet and Gabor expansions, and group representations. In [78], pages 353–375.

[43] H. G. Feichtinger and K. Gröchenig. Banach spaces related to integrable group representations and their atomic decompositions. *Int. J. Funct. Anal.*, 86: 307–340, 1989.

[44] P. Flandrin. Some aspects of non-stationary signal processing with emphasis on time-frequency and time-scale methods. In *Wavelets, Time-Frequency Methods and Phase Space*, Marseille, 1987.

[45] P. Flandrin. *Temps-fréquence*. Hermes, 1993.

[46] M. Frazier and B. Jawerth. Decomposition of Besov spaces. *Indiana Univ. Math. J.*, 34: 777–799, 1985.

[47] T. N. T. Goodman, S. L. Tang, and W. S. Lee. Wavelet wandering subspaces. *Trans. Am. Math. Soc.*, 338(2): 639–654, 1993.

[48] K. Gröchenig. Orthogonality criteria for compactly supported scaling functions. *Appl. Comput. Harmon. Anal.*, 1: 242–245, 1994.

[49] A. Grossmann and J. Morlet. Decompostion of Hardy functions into square integrable wavelets of constant shape. *SIAM J. Math. Anal.*, 15(4): 723–736, 1984.

[50] A. Grossmann, J. Morlet, and T. Paul. Transforms associated to square integrable group representations. I. General results. *J. Math. Phys.*, 26(10): 2473–2479, 1985.

[51] C. E. Heil and D. F. Walnut. Continuous and discrete wavelet transforms. *SIAM Rev.*, 31(4): 628–666, 1989.

[52] C. Herley and M. Vetterli. Orthogonal time-varying filter banks and wavelet packets. *IEEE Trans. Signal Process.*, 42(10): 2650–2663, 1994.

[53] M. Holschneider and P. Tchamitchian. Regularité locale de la fonction non-différentiable de Riemann. In [65], pages 102–124.

[54] C. Houdré. Wavelets, probability, and statistics: some bridges. In [14], pages 365–398.

[55] S. Jaffard. Exposants de Hölder en des points donnés et coéfficients d'ondelettes. *C. R. Acad. Sci. Paris*, 308(10): 79–81, 1989.

[56] B. Jawerth and W. Sweldens. An overview of wavelet based multiresolution analyses. *SIAM Rev.*, 36(3): 377–412, 1994.

[57] R. Jia and C. A. Micchelli. Using the refinement equation for the construction of pre-wavelets II: Powers of two. In *Curves and Surfaces*, P. J. Laurent, A. le Méhauté, and L. L. Schumaker, editors. Academic Press, New York, 1991, 209–249.

[58] P. T. Jorgensen and S. Pederson. Harmonic analysis of fractal measures induced by representations of a certain C^*-algebra. *Bull. Am. Math. Soc.*, 29: 228–234, 1993.

[59] J. Kovačević and M. Vetterli. Perfect reconstruction filter banks with arbitrary rational sampling rates. *IEEE Trans. Signal Process.*, 41(6): 2047–2066, 1993.

[60] A. F. Laine, editor. *Mathematical Imaging: Wavelet Applications in Signal and Image Processing, Proc. SPIE*, Vol. 2034. SPIE–The International Society for Optical Engineering, Bellingham, WA, 1993.

[61] A. F. Laine, S. Schuler, and J. Fan. Mammographic feature enhancement by multiscale analysis. *IEEE Trans. Medical Imaging*, 13(14), 1994.

[62] A. F. Laine and M. Unser, editors. *Mathematical Imaging: Wavelet Applications in Signal and Image Processing, Proc. SPIE*, Vol. 2303. SPIE–The International Society for Optical Engineering, Bellingham, WA, 1994.

[63] R. Latter. A decomposition of $H^p(\mathcal{R}^n)$ in terms of atoms. *Studia Math.*, 62: 92–101, 1978.

[64] P. G. Lemarié. Ondelettes a localisation exponentielles. *J. Math. Pures Appl.*, 67: 227–236, 1988.

[65] P. G. Lemarié, editor. *Les Ondelettes en 1989*. Number 1438 in Lecture Notes in Math. Springer-Verlag, 1990.

[66] P. G. Lemarié and Y. Meyer. Ondelettes et bases hilbertiennes. *Rev. Math. Iberoam.*, 2, 1986.

[67] S. Li and D. Healy. General frame decompositions, pseudo-duals and its application to Weyl-Heisenberg frames. *Numer. Funct. Anal. Optimiz.*, to appear.

[68] S. Mallat. Multiresolution approximations and wavelet orthonormal bases of $L^2(\mathcal{R})$. *Trans. Am. Math. Soc.*, 315(1): 69–97, 1989.

[69] S. Mallat. A theory for multiresolution signal decomposition: The wavelet representation. *IEEE Trans. Signal Proc.*, II(7): 674–693, 1989.

[70] S. Mallat and W. L. Hwang. Singularity detection and processing with wavelets. *IEEE Trans. Inform. Theory*, 38(2): 617–643, 1992.

[71] S. Mallat and S. Zhong. Characterization of signals from multiscale edges. *IEEE Trans. Patt. Anal. Mach. Intell.*, 14: 710–732, 1992.

[72] Y. Meyer. Principe d'incertitude, bases hilbertiennes et algèbres d'opérateurs. In *Sèmin. Bourbaki*, Vol. 662, 1985.

[73] Y. Meyer. *Ondelettes et opérateurs.* Hermann, Paris, 1990.

[74] Y. Meyer. Ondelettes sur l'intervalle. *Rev. Math. Iberoam.*, 7: 115–133, 1992.

[75] C. A. Micchelli. Using the refinement equation for the construction of pre-wavelet. *Numerical Algorithms*, 1: 75–116, 1991.

[76] T. Olson and J. DeStefano. Wavelet localization of the Radon transform. *IEEE Trans. Signal Process.*, 42(10): 2055–2067, 1994.

[77] O. Rioul. A discrete-time multiresolution theory. *IEEE Trans. Signal Process.*, 41(8): 2591–2606, 1993.

[78] M. B. Ruskai, G. Beylkin, R. R. Coifman, I. Daubechies, S. Mallat, Y. Meyer, and L. Raphael, editors. *Wavelets and their Applications.* Jones and Bartlett, Boston, 1992.

[79] P. Schröder and W. Sweldens. Spherical wavelets: Efficiently representing functions on the sphere. *Computer Graphics, (SIGGRAPH '95 Proceedings)*, to appear.

[80] P. Schröder and W. Sweldens. Spherical wavelets: Texture processing. Tech. Rep. 1995:4, Industrial Mathematics Initiative, Department of Mathematics, University of South Carolina, Columbia, 1995.

[81] V. Strela and G. Strang. Finite element multiwavelets. In [60], pages 202–213.

[82] J. O. Strömberg. A modified Franklin system and higher order spline systems on $\mathcal{R}^n$ as unconditional bases for Hardy spaces. In *Conf. Harmonic Analysis in Honor of Antoni Zygmund*, Beckner, et al., editors, volume II, University of Chicago Press, Chicago, 1981, 475–494.

[83] W. Sweldens. The lifting scheme: A construction of second generation wavelets. Tech. Rep. 1994:6, Industrial Mathematics Initiative, Department of Mathematics, University of South Carolina, Columbia, 1994.

[84] W. Sweldens. The lifting scheme: A custom-design construction of biorthogonal wavelets. Tech. Rep. 1994:7, Industrial Mathematics Initiative, Department of Mathematics, University of South Carolina, Columbia, 1994.

[85] W. Sweldens and R. Piessens. Quadrature formulae and asymptotic error expansions for wavelet x approximations of smooth functions. *SIAM J. Num. Anal.*, 31(4): 1240–1264, 1994.

[86] M. Unser and A. Aldroubi. Polynomial splines and wavelets–a signal processing perspective. In [18], pages 543–601.

[87] M. Unser and A. Aldroubi. Multiresolution image registration procedure using spline pyramids. In [60], pages 160–170.

[88] M. Unser, A. Aldroubi, and M. Eden. On the asymptotic convergence of B-spline wavelets to Gabor functions. *IEEE Trans. Inf. Theory*, 38: 864–872, 1992.

[89] M. Unser, A. Aldroubi, and M. Eden. A family of polynomial spline wavelet transforms. *Signal Process.*, 30:141–162, 1993.

[90] M. Vetterli and C. Herley. Wavelets and filter banks. *IEEE Trans. Signal Process.*, 40: 2207–2231, 1993.

[91] M. V. Wickerhauser. Acoustic signal compression with wavelet packets. In [18], pages 679–700.

[92] J. M. Wilson. On the atomic decomposition for hardy spaces. *Pacific J. Math.*, 116: 201–207, 1985.

[93] H. Woerdeman and A. Aldroubi. Extrapolation in multiresolutions. In [60], pages 120–128.

[94] X. G. Xia and Z. Z. Zhang. On sampling theorem, wavelets, and wavelet transforms. *IEEE Trans. Signal Process.*, 41(12): 3524–3535, 1993.

2

A Practical Guide to the Implementation of the Wavelet Transform

Michael Unser

Biomedical Engineering and Instrumentation Program
Building 13, Room 3N17, National Center for Research Resources,
National Institutes of Health, Bethesda, MD 20892-5766

2.1   Introduction

The wavelet transform (WT) decomposes a signal $f(x)$ by performing inner products with a collection of analysis functions $\{\psi_{(a,b)}\}$, which are scaled and translated version of the wavelet ψ; i.e.,

$$(W_\psi f)(a,b) = \langle f, \psi_{(a,b)} \rangle = \int_{-\infty}^{+\infty} f(x)\overline{\psi_{(a,b)}(x)}\, dx, \qquad (2.1)$$

$$\psi_{(a,b)}(x) = a^{-1/2}\psi\left(\frac{x-b}{a}\right). \qquad (2.2)$$

The amplitude of the WT therefore tends to be maximum at those scales and locations where the signal most resembles the analysis template (matched filter interpretation). The WT also provides a natural tool for time-frequency signal analysis since each template $\psi_{(a,b)}$ is predominantly localized in a certain region of the time-frequency plane with a central frequency that is inversely proportional to a. What distinguishes it from the short-time Fourier transform is the multiresolution nature of the analysis. This property enables the WT to zoom in on singularities and makes it very attractive for the analysis of transient signals [8, 9, 20, 45].

The distinction between the various types of wavelet transforms depends on the way in which the scale and translation parameters in (2.1) are discretized (cf. Chapter 1). At the most redundant end, the definition of the continuous wavelet transform assumes that a and b vary in a continuous fashion. At the other extreme (nonredundant transform), a decomposition into wavelet bases only requires the values of the transform at the dyadic scales: $a = 2^j$, and for translation parameters that are critically sampled: $b = k \cdot 2^j$. In between those two extremes, there are many varieties of overcomplete transforms that use a finer sampling of these parameters; for example, wavelet frames and redundant wavelet analyses.

For a signal of length N characterized by its sample values $\{f(k), k = 0, \ldots, N-1\}$, the direct evaluation of (2.1) for a fixed value of a and b typically requires $O(N)$ operations, if one uses any of the standard numerical integration techniques. Depending on the number of coefficients that need to be computed (N in the nonredundant case, and much more otherwise), such an evaluation can rapidly become prohibitive [21]. Fortunately, there are much more efficient algorithms that achieve an effective $O(1)$ complexity per coefficient.

The purpose of this chapter is to describe the various computational approaches available and to give simple implementation recipes that can be of direct use to the practitioner. The presentation is organized as follows. In Section 2.2, we start by reviewing the basic computational tools. In particular, we show how to compute inner products efficiently using discrete convolutions. We also briefly indicate how to handle boundary conditions. In Section 2.3, we provide a detailed description of Mallat's fast wavelet algorithm that can be applied to the decomposition of a signal into orthogonal, semi-orthogonal or bi-orthogonal wavelet bases. This type of nonredundant wavelet transform provides a representation that is fully reversible. It is often used for performing data reduction, or when the orthogonality of the representation is important. The remainder of the chapter is dedicated to the redundant types of wavelet transforms which are usually preferable for signal analyses, feature extraction, or detection tasks, for they provide a description that is truly shift-invariant. In Section 2.4, we consider a particular type of dyadic wavelet frame representation that has a simple reconstruction algorithm associated with it. In Section 2.5, we concentrate on the analysis aspect of the wavelet transform and describe computational solutions that are not necessarily restricted to scales that are powers of two. In particular, we discuss an efficient implementation of

the complex Morlet or Gabor-type wavelet transform which is well suited
for time-frequency analysis.

2.2 Basic Tools

Inner products with wavelet templates are rarely computed directly. Instead, the wavelet is typically represented as a linear combination of translated versions of a scaling function. Hence, the design of fast wavelet transform algorithms essentially amounts to being able to convolve (or correlate)
a signal with dilated versions of a scaling function efficiently.

In this section, we briefly review the properties of scaling functions which
provide the basic atoms with which signals and wavelets are represented.
We then show how, thanks to this representation, continuous inner products can be evaluated numerically via simple discrete convolutions. Finally,
we discuss the important issue of boundary conditions, which is perhaps the
most delicate and critical point that needs to be dealt with when implementing practical wavelet algorithms.

2.2.1 Scaling Functions and Multiresolution Representations

Multiresolution analysis plays a crucial role in the theory of the wavelet
transform [3, 12, 17]. The basic idea is to obtain a sequence of fine-to-
coarse signal approximations by successive projection on the subspaces V_j,
which are generated from the translates of a scaling function $\varphi(x)$ at the
corresponding resolution (cf. Chapter 1, Section 1.5). What makes this
multiresolution structure work are the properties of the underlying scaling
function $\varphi(x)$. To make this more explicit, we like to use the following
definition:

DEFINITION 1 $\varphi(x) \in L_2$ *is a valid scaling function if and only if it
satisfies the following properties:*

(i)   *Unconditional Riesz basis condition:*

$$0 < A \leq \hat{a}_\varphi(\omega) = \sum_{k \in Z} |\hat{\varphi}(\omega + 2\pi k)|^2 < B < +\infty \qquad (2.3)$$

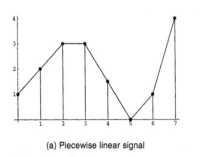
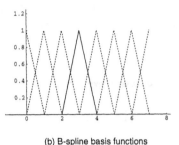

(a) Piecewise linear signal   (b) B-spline basis functions

Figure 2.1
B-spline representation of a piecewise linear signal.

(ii)   Two-scale relation:

$$\varphi(x/2) = \sqrt{2} \sum_{k \in Z} h(k)\varphi(x - k) \tag{2.4}$$

(iii)   Partition of the unity:

$$\forall x \in R, \quad \sum_{k \in Z} \varphi(x - k) = 1. \tag{2.5}$$

Since the spaces $V_j = V_j(\varphi)$ are rescaled versions of each other, we can discuss these properties in terms of the basic space

$$V_0(\varphi) = \left\{ \sum_{k \in Z} c(k)\varphi(x - k), \ c \in l_2 \right\}. \tag{2.6}$$

The first property ensures that $V_0(\varphi)$ is a well-defined subspace of L_2 with $\{\varphi(x - k)\}_{k \in Z}$ as its Riesz basis. Hence, any function $f_0 \in V_0(\varphi)$ has a unique (discrete) representation in terms of its coefficients $c(k)$. The second condition is an indirect statement of the fact that $\varphi(x/2) \in V_0(\varphi)$; it is the key to the multiresolution structure of the decomposition. The last condition is more technical; it essentially guarantees that we can approximate any function $f \in L_2$ as closely as we wish by taking its projection f_j in $V_j(\varphi)$ as $j \to -\infty$ (i.e., as the scale $a = 2^j$ goes to zero) [26, 33]. Note that an equivalent statement of Condition (iii) in the Fourier domain is $\hat{\varphi}(0) = 1$ and $\hat{\varphi}(2\pi k) = 0$, $k \in Z$, $k \neq 0$ [26].

A typical example is the triangular scaling function (or B-spline of degree 1): $\beta^1(x) = 1 - |x|$ for $|x| < 1$, and $\beta^1(x) = 0$ otherwise, which generates the subspace of piecewise linear functions (or splines of degree 1) (cf. Figure 2.1). It is easy to verify that the corresponding h in (2.4) is the 3-tap filter $\frac{1}{\sqrt{2}}(\frac{1}{2}, 1, \frac{1}{2})$ and that the tent function also satisfies Condition (iii).

Definition 1 assumes that φ is known explicitly. There are many instances, however, where φ is only defined indirectly through the specification of the refinement filter h (see also Chapter 1, Section 1.5.1). In this case, the only way to evaluate the scaling function is to apply the basic recursion (2.4) ad infinitum. In the Fourier domain, this leads to the following infinite product representation

$$\hat{\varphi}(\omega) = \prod_{j=1}^{+\infty} \left(\frac{1}{\sqrt{2}} \hat{h}(2^{-j}\omega) \right) \tag{2.7}$$

where $\hat{h}(\omega) = H(z)|_{z=e^{i\omega}}$ is the Fourier transform of h. Obviously, the selection of the filter h can not be completely arbitrary. First, we have to make sure that the infinite product (2.7) converges to a well-defined function. Second, we have to ensure that Conditions (i) and (iii) in our definition are satisfied. The latter one is the simplest to impose because it is equivalent to the following constraint on $\hat{h}(\omega)$:

$$\hat{h}(0) = H(z)|_{z=1} = \sqrt{2} \quad \text{and} \quad \hat{h}(\pi) = H(z)|_{z=-1} = 0. \tag{2.8}$$

Hence, h is essentially a lowpass filter with a gain of $\sqrt{2}$ at the origin.

Interestingly, the zeros of $\hat{h}(\omega)$ at $\omega = \pi$ play a very special role in the theory of the wavelet transform. Their multiplicity L provides the order of the representation and also typically corresponds to the number of vanishing moments of the wavelet. It is an important performance specifier in the sense that it gives the rate of decay of the approximation error as a function of the scale. Specifically, it can been shown that the condition $\hat{h}^{(m)}(\pi) = 0$, $m = 0, \ldots, L - 1$, where $\hat{h}^{(m)}(\omega)$ denotes the mth derivative of $\hat{h}(\omega)$, implies that $\|f - f_j\| = O(2^{jL})$ as $j \to -\infty$ [26, 27, 28, 33]. This Lth order regularity constraint is also necessary (but not sufficient) for constructing scaling functions with $L-1$ continuous derivatives [9]. These are all reasons why most families of scaling functions and wavelets are parameterized by L. Since higher order scaling functions usually result in longer filters, there is always a tradeoff to be made between the approximation power (and smoothness) of the representation and the efficiency of the algorithm.

The z-transform of the refinement filter for the example above (Figure 2.1) is $H(z) = (1 + z^{-1})(1 + z)/(2\sqrt{2})$. It has a zero of multiplicity $L = 2$ at $z = -1$; this is consistent with the well-known property that the approximation error for linear splines decays like $O(T^2)$ where T is the sampling step [24]. This filter is also the shortest one with two zeros at $\omega = \pi$.

2.2.2   Inner Products Via Discrete Convolutions

Even if the wavelet transform is usually expressed mathematically in terms of integrals (or L_2-inner products), it can still be computed exactly through an appropriate sequence of discrete convolutions (digital filters). This is only possible because of the general Hilbert space framework described in Section 2.2.1, which allows one to represent the input signal f and the wavelet (or any other analysis template) in terms of linear combinations of shifted basis functions:

$$f(x) = \sum_{k \in Z} c(k)\varphi_1(x - k) \tag{2.9}$$

$$\psi(x) = \sum_{k \in Z} p(k)\varphi_2(x - k), \tag{2.10}$$

where φ_1 and φ_1 are two scaling functions that are not necessarily identical.

PROPOSITION 1

Given the continuous/discrete representations (2.9) and (2.10), the inner products between f and the various integer shifts of ψ can be determined through the discrete convolution equation

$$\langle f(x), \psi(x - k) \rangle = (a_{12}^{\vee} * \overline{p}^{\vee} * c)(k) \tag{2.11}$$

where $(\cdot)^{\vee}$ denotes the time-reversal operator, and where

$$a_{12}(k) = \langle \varphi_1(x), \varphi_2(x + k) \rangle. \tag{2.12}$$

Note that this process is further simplified if the two scaling functions are bi-orthogonal; i.e., if $a_{12}(0) = 1$, and $a_{12}(k) = 0$ for $k \neq 0$. In this case, the recipe for performing inner products is especially simple: one just needs to correlate the discrete coefficients $c(k)$ and $p(k)$ of the underlying representations.

PROOF   The result is obtained through the following manipulations:

$$\langle f(x), \psi(x - k) \rangle = \int_{-\infty}^{+\infty} \sum_{k_1 \in Z} c(k_1)\varphi_1(x - k_1) \cdot \overline{\sum_{k_2 \in Z} p(k_2)\varphi_2(x - k_2 - k)} \, dx$$

$$= \sum_{k_1 \in Z} c(k_1) \sum_{k_2 \in Z} \overline{p(k_2)} \int_{-\infty}^{+\infty} \varphi_1(x - k_1)\overline{\varphi_2(x - k_2 - k)} \, dx$$

$$= \sum_{k_1 \in Z} c(k_1) \sum_{k_2 \in Z} \overline{p(k_2)}a_{12}(k_1 - k_2 - k)$$

$$= \sum_{k_1 \in Z} c(k_1)q(k_1 - k) = (q^{\vee} * c)(k),$$

where $q^{\vee}(k) = q(-k)$ and $q = a_{12} * \overline{p}$. ∎

2.2.3 Boundary Conditions

The basic wavelet theory assumes that all signals and sequences are defined everywhere. In practice, however, we have to deal with signals that are only specified over a finite interval. Therefore, to apply the basic decomposition formulas over a finite interval, we have to introduce suitable boundary conditions that ensure the transformations are reversible.

Since the basic transformation tool is a discrete convolution (or correlation), we need to use boundary conditions that are not affected by this operation. Specifically, we consider a discrete signal of length N,

$$\{f(k)\}_{k \in I_N} \quad \text{where } I_N = \{0, \cdots, N - 1\},$$

and a digital filter h whose response may or may not be infinite. The convolution between f and h is defined as

$$c(k) = (h * f)(k) = \sum_{l \in Z} h(l)f(k - l). \tag{2.13}$$

In practice, we will only compute $c(k)$ using (2.13) for $k \in I_N$ applying some boundary conditions on $f(k - l)$ whenever $(k - l)$ is not in I_N. The basic requirement for a reversible scheme is to be able to specify a corresponding set of boundary conditions on the ouput $c(k)$ so that the results of this finite computation can be extrapolated to the entire line $k \in Z$. There are three main approaches that can be used (cf. Figure 2.2). Note that a simple zero signal extrapolation for $k \notin I_N$ is not an acceptable solution.

Periodic boundary conditions — The most universal rule, which will work in all cases, is to use a periodic signal extension:

$$f_p(k) = f(k \bmod N). \tag{2.14}$$

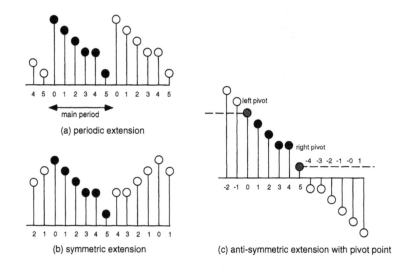

(a) periodic extension

(b) symmetric extension

(c) anti-symmetric extension with pivot point

Figure 2.2
Three primary types of boundary conditions.

In this case, the convolution (2.13) is circular. It can also be computed through the following formula

$$c_p(k) = \sum_{l=0}^{N-1} f(l)h_N(k-l) \qquad (2.15)$$

where h_N is the periodized version of the filter's response

$$h_N(k) = \sum_{n \in Z} h(k+nN). \qquad (2.16)$$

Note that (2.15) involves a finite summation instead of an infinite one as in (2.13). Its direct implementation requires $N_h \times N$ or N^2 operations, depending on whether N_h, the size of the filter h, is finite or not. For larger filter sizes, (2.15) can usually be evaluated more efficiently using a standard N-point FFT convolution algorithm with an $O(N \log N)$ complexity [45].

Symmetric boundary conditions — Although periodic boundary conditions result in a scheme that is mathematically coherent, they have the disadvantage of introducing discontinuities at the boundaries. These typically give rise to large wavelet coefficients near the borders which are not related to the signal itself. If the analysis filter is symmetrical, i.e., if $\forall k \in Z$, $h(k) = h(-k)$, we can avoid these artifacts by using a symmetric

Table 2.1
Various combinations of compatible input/output symmetries.

input: $f(k)$	analysis filter: $h(k)$	output: $c(k) = (h * f)(k)$
Periodic	Arbitrary	Periodic
Symmetric	Symmetric	Symmetric
Anti-symmetric	Anti-symmetric	Symmetric
Symmetric	Anti-symmetric	Anti-symmetric
Anti-symmetric	Symmetric	Anti-symmetric

(or mirror image) signal extension which is defined as follows (cf. Figure 2.2b)

$$f_s(k) = \begin{cases} f(k_s), & \text{if } k_s < N \\ f(2N - 2 - k_s), & \text{otherwise} \end{cases} \tag{2.17}$$

where the auxiliary index k_s is defined as

$$k_s = \begin{cases} k \bmod (2N - 2), & k \geq 0 \\ (2N - 2 - k) \bmod (2N - 2), & k < 0. \end{cases} \tag{2.18}$$

It is important to emphasize that these boundary conditions will only rigorously work for symmetrical analysis templates because the convolution of two symmetrical functions is also symmetrical. Note that the underlying signal model is also periodic with periodicity $N_s = 2N - 2$.

Anti-symmetric boundary conditions—While the previous conditions always result in a smooth signal extension, it may sometimes be more appropriate to use an extrapolation that locally preserves the growth trend of the signal. This is slightly more delicate but can still be achieved by using an anti-symmetric signal extension with a pivot around the boundary signal value $f(k_0)$ (cf. Figure 2.2c). The corresponding definition of anti-symmetry is

$$f(k_0 + k) - f(k_0) = -\left(f(k_0 - k) - f(k_0)\right), \tag{2.19}$$

where one has to consider both $k_0 = 0$ and $k_0 = N - 1$. In this way, we minimize the discontinuity at $k = k_0$ and essentially preserve the values of the odd derivatives on either side of the pivot point. This turns out to be especially useful when dealing with the representation of open curves.

Having such additional anti-symmetric boundary conditions at our disposal, we can also be more general and consider the various combinations in Table 2.1. In this way, it is always possible to obtain implementations of symmetric and anti-symmetric wavelet transforms that are artifact free near the boundaries and yet perfectly reversible.

2.3   Wavelet Bases (Nonredundant Transform)

Even though the construction of wavelet bases is the most constrained mathematically (cf. Chapter 1, Section 1.5), the corresponding transform is the simplest to perform numerically, provided that one takes advantage of the underlying multiresolution structure.

2.3.1   Fast Dyadic Wavelet Transform

The fast wavelet algorithm uses the property that the approximation spaces V_j are nested and that the computations at coarser resolutions can be based entirely on the approximations at the previous finest level [17]. In other words, the scaling and wavelet coefficients at resolution $j+1$ can be computed as

$$c_{j+1}(k) = \langle f, \mathring{\varphi}_{j+1,k} \rangle = \langle f_j, \mathring{\varphi}_{j+1,k} \rangle \tag{2.20}$$

$$d_{j+1}(k) = \langle f, \mathring{\psi}_{j+1,k} \rangle = \langle f_j, \mathring{\psi}_{j+1,k} \rangle, \tag{2.21}$$

where $\mathring{\varphi}$ and $\mathring{\psi}$ are the corresponding analysis functions with the short form convention: $\varphi_{j,k} = 2^{-j/2}\varphi(2^{-j}x - k)$; the function f_j is the projection of f into the finer approximation space V_j and is itself represented as

$$f_j = \sum_{k \in Z} c_j(k)\varphi_{j,k}. \tag{2.22}$$

The algorithm is especially easy to derive if one considers the following representations of the dual scaling function and wavelet

$$2^{-1/2}\mathring{\varphi}(x/2) = \mathring{\varphi}_{1,0} = \sum_{k=-\infty}^{+\infty} \mathring{h}^{\vee}(k)\mathring{\varphi}(x - k) \tag{2.23}$$

$$2^{-1/2}\mathring{\psi}(x/2) = \mathring{\psi}_{1,0} = \sum_{k=-\infty}^{+\infty} \mathring{g}^{\vee}(k)\mathring{\varphi}(x - k). \tag{2.24}$$

To show this, we start with $j = 0$, and rewrite the right-hand side of (2.20) as

$$\langle f_0, \mathring{\varphi}_{1,k} \rangle = \downarrow_2 \left[\left\langle \sum_{l \in Z} c_0(l)\varphi(x - l), \mathring{\varphi}_{1,0}(x - k) \right\rangle \right]$$

where the down-sampling operator $\downarrow_2$ accounts for the fact that we are only computing inner products for integer shifts that are multiples of two. Using (2.23) and the fact that functions φ and $\mathring{\varphi}$ are bi-orthogonal (i.e., $\langle \varphi(x), \mathring{\varphi}(x - k) \rangle = \delta_0(k)$), we can directly apply Proposition 1 to show that

$$\langle f_0, \mathring{\varphi}_{1,k} \rangle = \left(\downarrow_2 [\mathring{h} * c_0] \right)(k). \tag{2.25}$$

We can obviously use the same argument for the corresponding wavelet term. In fact, this reasoning carries over directly for other scales so that we get the wavelet decomposition algorithm

$$c_j(k) = \left(\downarrow_2 [\mathring{h} * c_{j-1}] \right)(k) = \sum_{l \in Z} \mathring{h}(l)c_{j-1}(2k - l) \tag{2.26}$$

$$d_j(k) = \left(\downarrow_2 [\mathring{g} * c_{j-1}] \right)(k) = \sum_{l \in Z} \mathring{g}(l)c_{j-1}(2k - l). \tag{2.27}$$

This analysis process may be interpreted as a succession of filtering and down-sampling by a factor of two (cf. left-hand side of Figure 2.3). It is applied iteratively for $j = 1, \ldots, J$ starting at the finest resolution level.

For reconstructing the coefficients c_j, we use the property that the basis functions at the coarser level are included in the finer approximation space. For the scaling function, this is expressed by the two-scale relation (2.4); for the wavelet, we have the similar relation

$$\psi(x/2) = \sqrt{2} \sum_{k=-\infty}^{+\infty} g(k)\varphi(x - k). \tag{2.28}$$

We then use the fact that the function at the finer level is equal to the sum of its coarser resolution approximation plus the residue

$$f_j = \sum_{k \in Z} c_{j+1}(k)\varphi_{j+1,k} + \sum_{k \in Z} d_{j+1}(k)\psi_{j+1,k}. \tag{2.29}$$

Replacing $\psi_{j+1,k}$ and $\varphi_{j+1,k}$ by their expressions given by (2.4) and (2.28), we find by identification with (2.22) that

$$c_j(k) = (h* \uparrow_2 [c_{j+1}])(k) + (g* \uparrow_2 [d_{j+1}])(k) \tag{2.30}$$

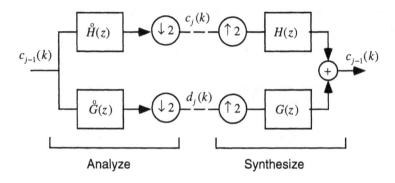

Analyze   Synthesize

Figure 2.3
Perfect reconstruction filter bank for the fast wavelet algorithm.

where the operator $\uparrow_2$ denotes the up-sampling by a factor of two (i.e., insertion of a zero in between signal values). This reconstruction part of algorithm is also applied iteratively, beginning with the coarsest level of the pyramid.

The convolution operators h, g, $\overset{\circ}{h}$, and $\overset{\circ}{g}$ define a perfect reconstruction filter bank which is schematically represented in Figure 2.3. The fact that the decomposition is reversible introduces strong interdependencies among the various filters. A well-known result in multirate filter bank theory [43, 44] is that the z-transforms of the filters must satisfy the constraints

$$\begin{cases} \overset{\circ}{H}(z)H(z) + \overset{\circ}{G}(z)G(z) = 2 \\ \overset{\circ}{H}(z)H(-z) + \overset{\circ}{G}(z)G(-z) = 0, \end{cases} \tag{2.31}$$

which are necessary and sufficient for a perfect reconstruction [45]. In other words, they guarantee the reversibility of the filter bank algorithm.

2.3.2   Implementation Details

In practice, one starts with a signal specified by its sample values $\{f(k), k = 0, \dots, N_0 - 1\}$ at resolution 0 and chooses to perform a wavelet decomposition with a certain depth J, a process that requires N_0 to be a multiple of 2^J. The most frequently used initialization rule is

$$c_0(k) = f(k), \quad k = 0, \dots, N_0 - 1, \tag{2.32}$$

but there are also more sophisticated approaches that find the initial coefficients sequence c_0 such that the continuous signal model perfectly interpolates the initial signal values [39, 40]. Using the decomposition rule specified by (2.26) and (2.27), this sequence is then split into its two half-length subparts

$$\{c_1(k)\}_{k=0,\ldots,N_1-1} \quad \text{and} \quad \{d_1(k)\}_{k=0,\ldots,N_1-1}$$

with $N_1 = N_0/2$. The process is iterated onto the coarser approximation sequence $c_j(k)$ until one reaches the final level J. The wavelet representation of the signal is provided by the detail (or wavelet) sequences $\{d_j(k)\}$, $j = 1, \ldots, J$ (a total of $N_0/2 + \cdots + N_0/2^J = N_0 - N_0/2^J$ coefficients) plus an additional $N_0/2^J$ low-pass coefficient $c_J(k)$ which represents the approximation of the input signal at resolution J. These transformed coefficients provide a one-to-one representation of our initial sequence c_0 (or input signal), which can be recovered exactly by applying the reverse synthesis process described by (2.30) sequentially for $j = J - 1$ down to $j = 0$.

Thus the implementation of the fast wavelet algorithm essentially boils down to the coding of the two complementary subroutines — *Analyze* and *Synthesize* — whose parameters are the filter coefficients $(\mathring{h}, \mathring{g})$, and (h, g), respectively (cf. Figure 2.3). Even if the basis functions and wavelets are symmetrical, the center of the high-pass filter g (resp. $\mathring{g}$) will end up being shifted by one sample to the left (resp. to the right) (cf. Chapter 1, Section 1.5). In practice, it is easier to use centered filters and deal with the offset indirectly by way of an alternating sampling scheme. Typically, the low-pass channel is sampled at the even integers and the high-pass channel at the odd integers.

The only remaining difficulty is to specify boundary conditions that ensure that the transform is reversible. This may seem a trivial issue, but it is by far the major (and often unsuspected) source of problems for those who actually go through the effort of implementing the transform.

Let us consider the low-pass sequence $c_{j-1}(k)$ at resolution $j - 1$ which is of length $N_{j-1} = 2N_j$. If we use the periodic boundary conditions (2.14) and apply the decomposition formulas (2.26)–(2.27), then the resulting subsampled coefficient sequences $c_j(k)$ and $d_j(k)$ are also periodic, with periodicity N_j. It is therefore relatively straightforward to reconstruct the original sequence from the half-length sequences $\{c_j(k), k = 0, \ldots, N_j\}$ and $\{d_j(k), k = 0, \ldots, N_j\}$ using (2.30) and applying the same boundary conditions.

If instead we use the symmetric boundary conditions (2.17) for the decomposition part of the algorithm (downward, or fine-to-coarse direction), the situation in the upward direction becomes more complicated due to previous use of the alternating sampling scheme. The corresponding boundary

Table 2.2
QMF filter coefficients for the orthogonal spline Battle-Lemarié wavelets of degree $n = 1$ and $n = 3$.

k	$n = 1$	$n = 3$
0,	0.578163	0.541736
-1, 1	0.280931	0.30683
-2, 2	-0.0488618	-0.035498
-3, 3	-0.0367309	-0.0778079
-4, 4	0.0120003	0.0226846
-5, 5	0.00706442	0.0297468
-6, 6	-0.00274588	-0.0121455
-7, 7	-0.00155701	-0.0127154
-8, 8	0.000652922	0.00614143
-9, 9	0.000361781	0.00579932
-10, 10	-0.000158601	-0.00307863
-11, 11	-0.0000867523	-0.00274529
-12, 12	$\cdots$	0.00154624
-13, 13		0.00133086
-14, 14		-0.000780468
-15, 15		-0.00065562
-16, 16		0.000395946
-17, 17		0.000326749
-18, 18		-0.000201818
-19, 19		-0.000164264
-20, 20		0.000103307
$\cdots$		$\cdots$

conditions at the coarser scale are

$$c_j(k) = \begin{cases} c_j(k_s), & k_s < N_j \\ c_j(N_s - k_s), & \text{otherwise} \end{cases} \tag{2.33}$$

$$d_j(k) = \begin{cases} d_j(k_s), & k_s < N_j \\ d_j(N_s + 1 - k_s), & \text{otherwise} \end{cases} \tag{2.34}$$

where the auxiliary index is

$$k_s = k \bmod (N_s = 2N_j - 1). \tag{2.35}$$

Note that these sequences are now periodic with periodicity $N_s = 2N_j - 1$. Thus, the simplest solution to get a reversible symmetric wavelet transform is to use the symmetric boundary conditions (2.17) for the direct transform (analysis) and the modified ones (2.33)–(2.34) for the inverse transform

Table 2.3

Filter coefficients for the semi-orthogonal cubic B-spline wavelet transform.

k	$\mathring{h}(k)$	$\mathring{g}(k-1)$	$h(k)$	$g(k+1)$
0,	0.893163	1.47539	0.75	0.601786
−1, 1	0.400681	−0.468423	0.5	−0.458383
−2, 2	−0.282212	−0.742098	0.125	0.196032
−3, 3	−0.232925	0.345771		−0.0415923
−4, 4	0.129084	0.389746		0.0030754
−5, 5	0.126457	−0.196794		−0.0000248016
−6, 6	−0.0664208	−0.207691		
−7, 7	−0.0679036	0.106776		
−8, 8	0.0352261	0.111058		
−9, 9	0.0363736	−0.057331		
−10, 10	−0.0188157	−0.0594334		
−11, 11	−0.0194733	0.0307097		
−12, 12	0.0100667	0.0318118		
−13, 13	0.0104241	−0.0164409		
−14, 14	−0.00538793	−0.017028		
−15, 15	−0.00557984	0.00880084		
−16, 16	0.00288398	0.00911475		
−17, 17	0.00298678	−0.00471096		
−18, 18	−0.00154373	−0.00487894		
−19, 19	−0.00159877	0.00252169		
−20, 20	0.000826327	0.0026116		
−21, 21	0.000855789	−0.00134981		
−22, 22	−0.000442316	−0.00139794		
−23, 23	−0.000458087	0.000722527		
−24, 24	0.000236763	0.000748289		
−25, 25	0.000245205	−0.000386755		
−26, 26	−0.000126735	−0.000400545		
−27, 27	−0.000131254	0.000207022		
	...	...		

(synthesis). Similar modifications can also be made for the anti-symmetric case.

Tables 2.2 and 2.3 provide the filter coefficients for several types of orthogonal and semi-orthogonal spline wavelet transforms that are described in [39]. The cubic B-spline wavelet is particularly interesting because of its near-optimal time-frequency localization properties [35]. Note that the price to pay for symmetry in the (semi-)orthogonal framework is that some of the filters are infinite and may need to be truncated for implementation purposes [30]. The advantage, however, is that these wavelet transforms can all be implemented using symmetric boundary conditions [39]. There are also other examples of symmetric bi-orthogonal wavelet transforms where all filters are FIR (finite impulse response) [6]. The main difference with those reported here is that the coefficients are computed via an oblique projection rather than an orthogonal one [1].

Daubechies wavelets are very popular because they are both orthogonal and compactly supported (i.e., the underlying filters are FIR) [7]. Unfortunately, they are neither symmetric nor anti-symmetric and can only be implemented exactly using periodic boundary conditions, which introduces more artifacts, as we have seen in Section 2.2.3.

2.3.3 Extensions

The basic wavelet decomposition that has been described so far provides a multiresolution representation of a one-dimensional signal. Fortunately, it is also possible to use the same computational tools in higher dimensions. The extension is straightforward if one uses tensor product basis functions [17]. In this case, the wavelet transform is separable and one can simply decompose a higher dimensional signal by successive 1-D splitting along the various dimensions of the data. In p dimension, one iteration of the separable algorithm will decompose a signal into 2^p subparts instead of two as in the 1-D case. The original signal can be reconstructed by applying the corresponding merging process in the exact reverse order. The only practical difficulty is to keep track of the various wavelet components in memory.

We can also use the same basic modules to compute more general wavelet packet decompositions [48]. The essential difference with the conventional wavelet transform is that the iterative splitting process is not restricted to the low-pass components only. In this way, we can use a given set of filters to generate a whole family of wavelet-like bases. Each of these corresponds to a particular tilling of the time-frequency plane which can be described by a binary tree. The most approriate transform is then determined by optimizing an application-dependent criterion (best basis algorithm).

2.4 Dyadic Wavelet Frames

One potential limitation of the nonredundant wavelet transforms discussed so far is that they are not shift-invariant. In other words, a simple translation of the input signal will generally result in a nontrivial modification of the wavelet coefficients. This can be a problem in certain pattern recognition tasks; for example, the detection and characterization of singularities such as edges in images. A simple way around this is to compute the wavelet transform for all shifted versions of the signal, or equivalently, to modify the block diagram in Figure 2.3 by removing the up-sampling and down-down sampling modules. In this way, one obtains a redundant decomposition that is perfectly reversible and is closely related to the redundant discrete wavelet transform discussed in Chapter 1, Section 1.4.2.

Here, we will adopt a slightly different formulation which applies to the wavelet decomposition of any discrete sequence in l_2 (i.e., $V_0 = l_2$). The reason for momentarily switching to a discrete framework is that the constraints on the wavelet filters can be weaker than in the continuous case; in particular, there is no convergence problem since we are only considering a decomposition with a finite number of scales J. The only condition for the specification of the analysis and synthesis filter prototypes — $(\mathring{h}, \mathring{g})$, and (h, g), respectively — is that

$$\mathring{H}(z)H(z) + \mathring{G}(z)G(z) = 1. \tag{2.36}$$

This equation insures that the basic nondecimated analysis/synthesis module acts as the identity operator and that the decomposition in Figure 2.4 is perfectly reversible. Except for the constant on the right, Condition (2.36) is equivalent to the first perfect reconstruction equation in (2.31). Hence, one can always start with a set of perfect reconstruction wavelet filters used in Mallat's algorithm and satisfy (2.36) by adjusting the gain of the synthesis filters (division by a factor of two). Other less constrained solutions may also be considered. In particular, Mallat and co-workers designed FIR filter sets providing a dyadic wavelet analysis in terms of the first or second derivatives of a B-spline [15, 16]; these differential operators are especially suited for the characterization of singularities.

To describe this type of transform, we start from the filter prototypes $H(z)$ and $G(z)$, and generate a sequence of synthesis filters of increasing scale (indexed by j):

$$H_j(z) = H(z^{2^{j-1}})H_{j-1}(z), \quad j = 1, \ldots, J \tag{2.37}$$

$$G_j(z) = G(z^{2^{j-1}})H_{j-1}(z), \quad j = 1, \ldots, J, \tag{2.38}$$

with the initial condition $H_0(z) = 1$. Equivalently, in the signal domain, we have the two-scale relation

$$\begin{cases} h_j(k) = \uparrow_{2^{j-1}} [h] * h_{j-1}(k) \\ g_j(k) = \uparrow_{2^{j-1}} [g] * h_{j-1}(k) \end{cases} \tag{2.39}$$

where the operator $\uparrow_m$ denotes the up-sampling by a factor of m. We also define the same quantities on the analysis side using the filters $\mathring{h}$, $\mathring{g}$.

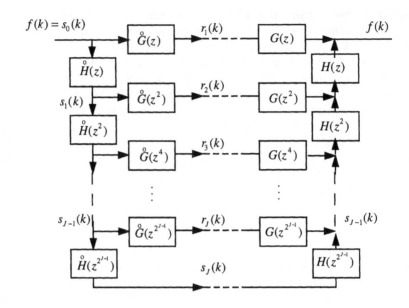

Figure 2.4
Implementation of a dyadic wavelet frame: analysis and synthesis.

The corresponding redundant wavelet decomposition algorithm can now be described as follows

$$r_j(k) := \langle \mathring{g}_j^{\vee}(k-l), f(k) \rangle_{l_2} = \uparrow_{2^{j-1}} [\mathring{g}] * s_{j-1}(k), \quad j = 1, \ldots, J \quad (2.40)$$

$$s_j(k) := \langle \mathring{h}_j^{\vee}(k-l), f(k) \rangle_{l_2} = \uparrow_{2^{j-1}} [\mathring{h}] * s_{j-1}(k), \quad j = 1, \ldots, J, \quad (2.41)$$

where we use the letters s and r to differentiate these redundant coefficients from their subsampled counterparts c and d in (2.26) and (2.27). These equations are applied iteratively from $j = 1$ up to a certain scale J with the initial condition $s_0(k) = f(k)$. This process is equivalent to a filter bank decomposition with J high-pass wavelet channels $(\mathring{G}_1(z), \ldots, \mathring{G}_J(z))$ and one low-pass channel $(\mathring{H}_J(z))$, as illustrated in Figure 2.5. The initial sequence $f(k)$ can then be reconstructed using the complementary resynthesis algorithm, which is shown on the right of Figure 2.4. Using (2.36), it is not difficult to verify that the transfer functions of the equivalent analysis/synthesis filter bank satisfies the identity

$$\sum_{j=1}^{J} \mathring{G}_j(z)G_j(z) + \mathring{H}_J(z)H_J(z) = 1, \quad (2.42)$$

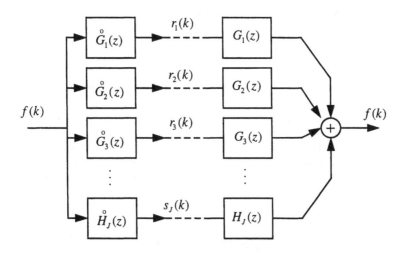

Figure 2.5
Equivalent filter bank representation of the dyadic wavelet frame.

which is a direct expression of the perfect reconstruction property. The reconstruction part of the algorithm can also be described through the expansion formula

$$f(k) = \sum_{j=1}^{J} \sum_{l \in Z} r_j(l) g_j(k - l) + \sum_{l \in Z} s_J(l) h_J(k - l), \qquad (2.43)$$

which states that the input signal has been expressed as a linear combination of the overcomplete family of templates

$$S = \{g_1(k - l), \dots, g_J(k - l), h_J(k - l)\}_{l \in Z}. \qquad (2.44)$$

We can further formalize the properties of this type of wavelet decomposition by using the mathematical notion of frames (cf. Chapter 1, Section 1.8).

PROPOSITION 2

The family of sequences S is a wavelet frame of the Hilbert space l_2.

PROOF   To prove that S constitutes a frame of l_2, we need to show that there exist two strictly positive constants A and B such that (cf. [2])

$$A \cdot \|f\|_{l_2}^2 \leq \sum_{l \in Z} \langle f(k), h_J(k-l) \rangle_{l_2}^2$$

$$+ \sum_{j=1}^{J} \sum_{l \in Z} \langle f(k), g_j(k-l) \rangle_{l_2}^2 \leq B \cdot \|f\|_{l_2}^2 . \qquad (2.45)$$

Since the various inner products can be obtained from the convolution between f and the time-reversed filters $h_J^\vee$, $g_1^\vee$, ..., $g_J^\vee$, we apply Parseval's formula and evaluate the central term in (2.45) by integration in the frequency domain:

$$\sum_{l \in Z} \langle f(k), h_J(k-l) \rangle^2 + \sum_{j=1}^{J} \sum_{l \in Z} \langle f(k), g_j(k-l) \rangle^2 = \frac{1}{2\pi} \int_0^{2\pi} \left| \hat{f}(\omega) \right|^2 K(\omega) \, d\omega$$

where

$$K(\omega) = \left| H_J(e^{i\omega}) \right|^2 + \sum_{j=1}^{J} \left| G_j(e^{i\omega}) \right|^2 \leq B. \qquad (2.46)$$

Our only assumption is that the four prototype filters in (2.36) are stable in the sense that their frequency responses are uniformly bounded. Since the decomposition only involves a finite number of scales, this implies that the constant on the right-hand side of (2.46) is bounded. Hence, we deduce the inequality

$$\inf_{\omega \in [0,2\pi]} [K(\omega)] \cdot \|f\|^2 \leq \frac{1}{2\pi} \int_0^{2\pi} \left| \hat{f}(\omega) \right|^2 K(\omega) d\omega \leq B \cdot \|f\|^2 . \qquad (2.47)$$

The final step is to show that the infimum on the left-hand side of the inequality is strictly positive. For a given $z = e^{i\omega}$, the right-hand sum in (2.42) has the form of an inner product between the synthesis and analysis frequency response vectors. Applying Schwarz inequality, we get

$$1 \leq K(\omega) \cdot \left(\left| \mathring{H}_J(e^{i\omega}) \right|^2 + \sum_{j=1}^{J} \left| \mathring{G}_J(e^{i\omega}) \right|^2 \right). \qquad (2.48)$$

We then use the same stability argument as before to show that the right-hand side factor in (2.48) is bounded: $\mathring{K}(\omega) \leq \mathring{B}$. Combining this result with (2.46), we end up with the inequality

$$0 < \overset{\circ}{B}{}^{-1} \leq K(\omega) \leq B, \tag{2.49}$$

which proves the desired result. ∎

The numerical conditioning of the reconstruction algorithm will depend on the ratio B/A, which should preferably be close to one. Note that we can easily generate a tight frame ($B/A = 1$) if we start with a quadrature mirror $H(z)$ (cf. Equation (1.39) in Chapter 1) and use its modulation $G(z) = H(-z)$ [32]; that is, if we use the digital filter templates associated with an orthogonal wavelet decomposition.

The key features of the dyadic wavelet frame decomposition are its shift-invariance and its reversibility. Mallat and Zhong have used such a decomposition to obtain a signal characterization in terms of the maxima of its wavelet transform [16]. They also showed how to reconstruct a very close approximation of the original from this subset of features. This type of reversible wavelet decomposition can also be the basis for the implementation of noise reduction and image enhancement algorithms. The principle is to insert an additional processing component that selectively modifies the wavelet components prior to reconstruction.

2.5 Nondyadic Wavelet Analyses

For applications where the emphasis is on signal analysis and feature extraction, the issue of the reversibility of the transformation is not so critical. Instead, it is often more important to use a fine sampling of both the translation and scale parameters. Accordingly, we will adopt the following definition of the redundant (or running) wavelet transform (RWT)

$$\forall k \in Z, \quad (W_\psi f)(a, k) := a^{-1/2} \int_{-\infty}^{+\infty} \overline{\psi\left(\frac{x-k}{a}\right)} f(x)\, dx, \tag{2.50}$$

which is now specified for all integer shifts k. Assuming that we can represent the input signal $f(x)$ and the enlarged wavelet $a^{-1/2}\psi(x/a)$ using linear combinations of scaling functions as in Proposition 1, then for a fixed value of a, (2.50) is equivalent to a discrete convolution

$$(W_\psi f)(a, k) = \sum_{l \in Z} w_a(k - l) f_0(l) = (w_a * f_0)(k), \tag{2.51}$$

where $f_0(k)$ are the expansion coefficients of the input signal f; the analysis filter is $w_a(k) = (a_{12}^\vee * \overline{p}_a^\vee)(k)$, where the p_a's are the expansion coefficients of the enlarged wavelet and where a_{12} is the cross-correlation sequence defined in Proposition 1. Note that the standard signal processing approach to the discretization of (2.50) would be to use $\text{sinc}(x)$ as our scaling function —we shall see here that this is usually not the best solution. In any case, for a signal of length N, the computation of (2.51) requires $O(N^2)$ (or, at best, $O(a \cdot N)$) operations per scale for the direct evaluation, or $O(N \log N)$ if one uses a standard FFT-based algorithm [13, 45]. We will now look at more efficient approaches that all achieve the lower $O(N)$ complexity per scale.

2.5.1   Wavelet Representation

Let us consider a wavelet $\psi \in V_0(\varphi)$ represented by the expansion

$$\psi(x) = \sum_{k \in Z} p(k)\varphi(x - k), \qquad (2.52)$$

where p is a given FIR sequence of coefficients. Since we are primarily interested in wavelets that are either symmetric or anti-symmetric, we should select a scaling function that is symmetrical. While there are many possible choices for φ, we tend to prefer the B-splines of degree n. These functions are particularly attractive in the present context because of the following unique features:

(i)   For a given order L, the B-spline of degree $n = L - 1$ corresponds to the shortest possible refinement filter h (binomial kernel of order L) [33].

(ii)   B-splines are smooth and well behaved. They generate the polynomial spline functions which are piecewise polynomials with some additional continuity constraints [22, 23].

(iii)   B-splines have a simple explicit form in both the time and frequency domain [22]; such direct formulas are usually not available for other scaling functions.

(iv)   Splines are flexible enough to approximate any desired wavelet shape. Precise convergence rates and bound constants are also available [42].

(v)   Because of their simple explicit form, B-splines are easy to manipulate. Operations such as differentiation can be performed in a straightforward manner [10].

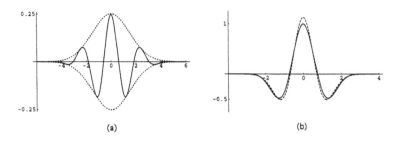

(a)   (b)

Figure 2.6
Two examples of cubic spline wavelets. (a) Semi-orthogonal B-spline wavelet and its Gaussian envelope (dashed line). (b) 2nd derivative of a B-spline of degree $n = 5$ and its Mexican hat approximation (dashed line).

(vi)   Unlike most other multiresolution representations, splines are not restricted to dyadic dilation factors. In particular, it is possible to develop fast algorithms for integer scales [41].

A more detailed treatment of this class of representations is given in Appendix A. If the desired wavelet is not itself a spline, we can still construct its least squares approximation [36], or interpolate the function values in-between the integers. Two examples of cubic spline wavelets ($n = 3$) are shown in Figure 2.6; their corresponding B-spline coefficients can be read from Table 2.4.   The first one is the cubic B-spline wavelet, which is very similar to a cosine-Gabor function and is therefore extremely well localized in time and frequency [35]. The second corresponds to the second derivative of a quintic spline, which provides a very close approximation of a Mexican hat (2nd derivative of a Gaussian).

The next algorithms all rely on the fact that there are efficient digital filtering mechanisms for dilating the underlying basis functions by some specific factors. To make this explicit, we consider the two expansion formulas

$$m^{-1/2}\varphi(x/m) = \sum_{k \in Z} h_m(k)\varphi(x - k) \tag{2.53}$$

$$m^{-1/2}\psi(x/m) = \sum_{k \in Z} p_m(k)\varphi(x - k), \tag{2.54}$$

and use the multiresolution properties of the underlying spaces to characterize the two sequences h_m and p_m which represent the effect of a dilation by a factor of m. First, we will consider the standard case where $m = 2^j$ is a power of two, and then the spline representations where m can be any integer. We will also present an extension of those solutions for the noninteger case (arbitrary scaling factor).

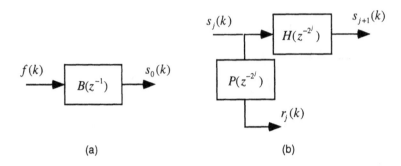

(a)   (b)

Figure 2.7
Schematic representation of the "à-trous" (or zero-padded) RWT
algorithm for dyadic scales. (a) Initialization. (b) Basic process-
ing module.

2.5.2   Fast Redundant Dyadic Wavelet Transform

First, we investigate the simpler dyadic case ($a = 2^j$), where it is possible to use the modified "à trous" (or zero-padded) version of the fast WT
algorithm for the nonsampled case [25, 19]. The procedure is analogous to
the analysis part of the discrete frame decomposition described in Section
2.4, except that the transform is now formulated in the continuous signal
domain. Using the two-scale equation (2.53) for $m = 2$ and the wavelet definition (2.52), it is not difficult to show that the basic expansion coefficients
for the dilated scaling function and wavelets satisfy the recursions

$$h_{2^j}(k) = (\uparrow_{2^{j-1}} [h] * h_{2^{j-1}}) (k) \tag{2.55}$$

$$p_{2^j}(k) = (\uparrow_{2^j} [p] * h_{2^j}) (k), \tag{2.56}$$

where $h = h_2$ is the refinement filter and where p represents the wavelet
coefficients in (2.52). Hence, in order to analyze the discrete signal $f(k)$,
one starts by computing

$$s_0(k) := \langle f(x), \varphi(x - k) \rangle = (a_{12}^{\vee} * f_0) (k) \cong (b^{\vee} * f) (k), \tag{2.57}$$

where a_{12} is the cross-correlation sequence defined in Proposition 1, and
where the left-hand side with $b(k) = \varphi(x)|_{x=k}$ is the Riemman sum ap-
proximation of the inner product. Next, we apply the two-scale equation
iteratively for $j = 1, \ldots, J - 1$ to compute the inner products between the
input signal and the scaling functions at the various dyadic scales

$$s_j(k) := \langle f(x), 2^{-j/2} \varphi ((x - k)/2^{-j}) \rangle = \uparrow_{2^{j-1}} [h^{\vee}] * s_{j-1}(k). \tag{2.58}$$

Table 2.4
Filter parameters for various cubic spline wavelets.

Sequences	z-transform
Initialization filter:	$B(z) = B_1^3(z) = \frac{z+4+z^{-1}}{6}$
Refinement filter:	$H(z) = U_2^3(z) = \frac{z^2+4z+6+4z^{-1}+z^{-2}}{8}$
1st derivative wavelet:	$P_1(z) = 1 - z^{-1}$
2nd derivative wavelet:	$P_2(z) = -z + 2 - z^{-1}$
Cubic B-spline wavelet:	$P_B(z) = \left(\frac{6-4[z+z^{-1}]+[z^2+z^{-2}]}{8}\right) \times$
	$\left(\frac{2416-1191[z+z^{-1}]+120[z^2+z^{-2}]-[z^3+z^{-3}]}{5040}\right)$

This equation involves a convolution with the up-sampled filter: $\uparrow_{2^{j-1}} [h^\vee]$. Note that the complexity of this operation is the same irrespective of j (cf. the function $\mathcal{F}$ in Appendix B). The RWT is then computed by convolving these auxiliary signals with the dilated (zero-padded) version of the wavelet filter p

$$r_j(k) = (W_\psi f)(a = 2^j, k) = (\uparrow_{2^j} [\bar{p}^\vee] * s_j)(k). \qquad (2.59)$$

This algorithm is schematically represented in Figure 2.7. A more detailed step-by-step description is provided in Appendix B. Note that the sequence p may be arbitrary and can be chosen to approximate any desired wavelet shape. The relevant FIR filter parameters (transfer functions) for the cubic spline wavelets in Figure 2.6 are given in Table 2.4.

2.5.3 Fast Redundant Wavelet Transform with Integer Scales

The technique that is described next is more general in the sense that it is valid for all integer scales $a = m$. However, it is limited to B-splines, since these are the only compactly supported scaling functions to satisfy the more general two-scale relation for any integer m (cf. Appendix A). Using the wavelet definition (2.52), it is not difficult to show that the B-spline coefficients in (2.54) of the wavelet dilated by a factor of m are given by

$$p_m(k) = m^{-1/2} \cdot (\uparrow_m [p] * u_m^n)(k), \qquad (2.60)$$

where $u_m^n = m^{1/2} h_m$ represent the B-spline coefficients of a discrete B-spline enlarged by a factor of m (cf. (2.78), in Appendix A). Accordingly,

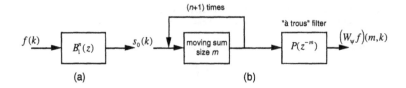

(a)   (b)

Figure 2.8
Schematic representation of the fast RWT algorithm for real spline wavelets and integer scales. (a) Initialization. (b) Individual scale processing.

the RWT can be computed from the following convolution

$$(W_\psi f)(m, k) = m^{-1/2} \cdot (\uparrow_m [\bar{p}^\vee] * u_m^n * s_0)(k) \qquad (2.61)$$

where $s_0(k)$ is the sequence defined by (2.57).

This filtering can be implemented very efficiently since the convolution with u_m^n is equivalent to a cascade of $(n + 1)$ moving sums (cf. Equation (2.78) in Appendix A), each of which can be performed with only two additions per sample. The last step is a convolution with the up-sampled kernel p ("à trous" filter). The whole procedure is summarized in Figure 2.8; for more details, we refer the reader to [41]. This approach has the same complexity per scale as the one in Section 2.5.2 ($O(N)$). What distinguishes it from multiresolution-based approaches is that it is noniterative across scale. Its structure is therefore well suited for a parallel implementation with one processor per scale.

2.5.4 Fast Redundant Wavelet Transform (Arbitrary Scales)

While the possibility of using integer scales is already an improvement over the dyadic case, this form of sampling may still not be appropriate for certain applications. We now consider an extension of the standard dyadic approach for more than one voice per octave [14, 19, 46]. Typically, we want to compute the wavelet transform at the scales $a_{i,j} = a_i \cdot 2^j$ where $a_i = a_0 \cdot 2^{i/M}$ with $i = 0, \ldots, M - 1$. This can be achieved, at least conceptually, by constructing M auxiliary wavelets

$$\left\{ \psi_i(x) \cong a_i^{-1/2} \cdot \psi(x/a_i) \right\}, \quad i = 0, \ldots, M - 1$$

such that these functions are all represented as linear combinations of our scaling function φ

$$\psi_i(x) = \sum_{k \in Z} p_{a_i}(k)\varphi(x - k) \cong a_i^{-1/2} \cdot \psi(x/a_i), \qquad (2.62)$$

where φ is typically a B-spline of degree n. If the sequences $p_{a_i}(k)$ are finite, we can apply a parallel version of the dyadic algorithm described in Section 2.5.2 (or the procedure in Section 2.5.3 with $m = 2^j$) and compute this transform with essentially the same complexity per scale as before $(O(N))$. One major difference, however, is that the computation is nonexact since the wavelet $\psi_i(x)$ is only an approximation of $a_i^{-1/2}\psi(x/a_i)$. We shall see, however, that the error can be made arbitrarily small by adjusting the parameters of the algorithm (i.e., by increasing a_0, or by using higher order splines).

In order to minimize the approximation error, we construct our auxiliary wavelets by performing the least squares approximation of $a_i^{-1/2}\psi(x/a_i)$ in $V_0(\varphi)$. Thus, the optimal expansion coefficients in (2.62) are given by

$$p_{a_i}(k) = \langle a_i^{-1/2}\psi(x/a_i), \mathring{\varphi}(x - k) \rangle, \qquad (2.63)$$

where

$$\mathring{\varphi}(x) = \sum_{k \in Z} (a_\varphi)^{-1}(k)\varphi(x - k) \qquad (2.64)$$

is the dual scaling function (cf. [4]); the sequence $(a_\varphi)^{-1}$ is the convolution inverse of the autocorrelation sequence $a_\varphi(k) = \langle \varphi(x), \varphi(x + k) \rangle$. Since we have assumed that φ is symmetric and compactly supported, the support of its dual will generally be infinite. Consequently, the sequences $p_{a_i}(k)$ are infinite even if the wavelet ψ is compactly supported. To avoid this problem, we use an equivalent wavelet representation in terms of the dual scaling function

$$\psi_i(x) = \sum_{k \in Z} q_{a_i}(k)\mathring{\varphi}(x - k) \qquad (2.65)$$

with

$$q_{a_i}(k) = \langle a_i^{-1/2}\psi(x/a_i), \varphi(x - k) \rangle, \qquad (2.66)$$

where the sequences $q_{a_i}(k)$ are now guaranteed to be finite — assuming that φ and ψ are both compactly supported. Another advantage is that these dual coefficients are much easier to compute numerically, especially when φ is a B-spline of degree n. Using (2.64), we obtain the following decomposition for $p_{a_i}(k)$:

$$p_{a_i}(k) = (a_\varphi)^{-1} * q_{a_i}(k), \qquad (2.67)$$

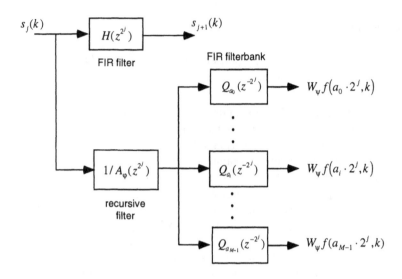

Figure 2.9
Implementation of the redundant wavelet transform with M voices per octave.

where $q_{a_i}(k)$ is FIR and $(a_\varphi)^{-1}$ is infinite. In the B-spline case, we can still get an efficient convolution algorithm because the filter $(a_\varphi)^{-1}$ (or any of its up-sampled versions) can be implemented recursively from a cascade of simple causal and anti-causal exponential filters [38]. Hence, the convolution with $p_{a_i}(k)$ can effectively be computed in $O(N)$ operations. The corresponding block diagram is shown in Figure 2.9. Note that the up-sampled recursive filter $\uparrow_{2^j} [(a_\varphi)^{-1}]$ is only applied once per octave. A more detailed description of this algorithm with specific examples of wavelet design can be found in [47].

One last important issue is the control of the approximation error. Using the basic tools from the Strang-Fix theory of approximation [27, 47], we can show that the L_2 approximation error for a_i sufficiently large (or ψ sufficiently smooth) is such that

$$\left\| \psi_i(x) - a_i^{-1/2} \psi(x/a_i) \right\| = C_\varphi \cdot a_i^{-L} \cdot \left\| \psi^{(L)} \right\| + O(a_i^{-(L+1)}) \qquad (2.68)$$

where L is the order of the scaling function (cf. Section 2.2.1), and $\psi^{(L)}$ denotes the Lth derivative of the wavelet; C_φ is a constant that only depends on φ. In other words, the wavelet approximation error decays like $O(a^{-L})$. For B-splines of degree n, the order is one more than the degree (i.e., $L = n + 1$) and the constant is given by

$$C_\varphi = \sqrt{\frac{|B_{2L}|}{(2L)!}}, \qquad (2.69)$$

where $|B_{2L}|$ is Bernouilli's number of degree $2L$ [42]. Clearly, the error will be maximum at the finer scale a_0. Our design strategy is therefore to select a_0 and L such that this error is below a certain threshold. This determination can be made using the asymptotic relation (2.68). Note that this error analysis is only applicable in the first octave; the error is exactly the same in the higher octaves because all use the same normalized wavelet approximations dilated by a power of two. We have compared several such wavelet approximations using linear and cubic splines [47]. In terms of computational efficiency, cubic splines appear to be more favorable because the wavelet filters for a given error threshold are typically much shorter (smaller a_0). Switching to higher order splines does not seem particularly beneficial because there is a rapid tendency to saturation. In fact, as n increases, the procedure converges to the classical approach dictated by Shannon's sampling theory (bandlimited model) [5, 36]. In this sense, we may look at a_0 as a bandwidth parameter.

2.5.5 Fast Redundant Morlet or Gabor Wavelet Transform

The standard technique for constructing a complex wavelet is to multiply a certain window function $\varphi(x)$ by a complex exponential. The optimum time-frequency localization is achieved when $\varphi(x)$ is a Gaussian (Morlet or Gabor wavelet) [11, 18].

Here, we approximate this Gaussian by a B-spline of order n and define the following complex B-spline wavelet

$$\psi(x) = \beta^n(x)e^{i2\pi x} \quad \overset{\text{Fourier}}{\longleftrightarrow} \quad \hat{\psi}(\omega) = \left(\frac{\sin(\omega/2 - \pi)}{(\omega/2 - \pi)}\right)^{n+1}, \qquad (2.70)$$

which satisfies the usual admissibility condition for the CWT. The localization of this wavelet can be chosen arbitrarily close to the optimum since φ converges to a Gaussian as n goes to infinity. In order to derive our algorithm [31], we now use a discrete (Riemman sum) approximation of the convolution integral (2.50)

$$\left(W_\psi^d f\right)(m, l) = \sum_{k \in Z} f(k)\overline{\psi\left(\frac{k - l}{m}\right)}. \qquad (2.71)$$

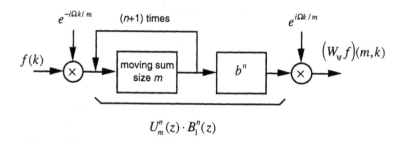

Figure 2.10
Schematic representation of the fast RWT algorithm for Gabor-like complex B-spline wavelets.

Using the wavelet formula (2.70), we can manipulate this expression and rewrite the wavelet transform as

$$\left(W_\psi^d f\right)(m,l) = e^{i\Omega l/m} \sum_{k \in Z} f_m(k) b_m^n(k-l) = e^{i\Omega l/m} \left(b_m^n * f_m\right)(l) \quad (2.72)$$

where the modulated signal $f_m(k)$ is defined as

$$f_m(k) = m^{-1/2} f(k) e^{-i\Omega k/m}, \quad (2.73)$$

and where $b_m^n(k) := \beta^n(k/m) = (u_m^n * b^n)(k)$ is the discrete B-spline enlarged by a factor of m. These two equations suggest the simple computational procedure outlined in Figure 2.10. The input signal is first premultiplied by the complex exponential $e^{-i\Omega k/m}$. This auxiliary signal is then filtered with an enlarged B-spline window function, and finally demodulated. Since the filtering with a B-spline of size m can be performed recursively using the same technique as in Section 2.5.3, we obtain a fast wavelet algorithm with a complexity $O(N)$ independent of m. In practice, the degree of the B-spline window does not need to be very high. For instance, the time-frequency bandwidth product of the complex cubic B-spline wavelet ($n = 3$) is within 0.5% of the limit specified by the uncertainty principle, which should be sufficient for most applications. The corresponding cubic spline WT can be computed with as few as 8 (real) multiplications and 22 additions per output sample.

It is also possible to extend the previous approach for arbitrary scales. For this purpose, we can select a quasi-Gaussian window function φ generated from the n-fold convolution of symmetrical exponentials (instead of a rectangular pulse as in the B-spline case). Each elementary exponential filter can be implemented recursively with as few as 2 adds and 2 multiplies per samples. Here, too, the number of computations is independent of the window size and we have an $O(N)$ algorithm. By increasing the number of elementary filtering modules, the time-frequency localization of the analysis wavelets can be chosen arbitrarily close to the limit specified by the uncertainty principle, a property that follows directly from the central limit theorem. More details on this approach can be found elsewhere [31]. Finally, we should note that the same modulation technique, which has been used for many years in analog spectrum analyzers, can also be applied for computing the windowed Fourier transform [29, 31].

2.6 Conclusion

A very attractive feature of the nonredundant wavelet transform (decomposition into wavelet bases) is the availability of a fast wavelet algorithm with an $O(N)$ complexity. The only delicate issue in the implementation of a generic version of this algorithm is the correct specification of boundary conditions. While the use of a periodic signal extension is always a solution, it is preferable to use the slightly more involved symmetric/antisymmetric boundary conditions whenever they are applicable; that is, when the wavelet is either symmetric or anti-symmetric. In this way, one greatly reduces the boundary artifacts that are typically associated with periodized transforms. While the standard wavelet transform uses a pyramidal decomposition, it is straightforward to obtain more general wavelet packet representations by considering other partitions of the wavelet tree. The basic 1-D decomposition module can also be used directly for implementing separable multidimensional wavelet transforms by successive processing along the various dimensions of the data.

The more redundant versions of the wavelet transform are well suited for signal analysis and feature extraction. Here too, fast algorithms are available with a complexity that is directly proportional to the number of wavelet coefficients produced. The increase in computation is therefore essentially given by the redundancy factor. While computing dyadic redundant wavelet transforms is relatively straightforward, the use of a finer sampling of the scale is slightly more involved and may require a more complicated design. In most cases, the processing is sequential in the sense that the dilation of the filtering templates is achieved by applying the two-scale relation recursively. Two notable exceptions are the procedures described in Sections 2.5.3 and 2.5.5, which are specific to splines. Since there is no iteration across scales, these algorithms are well suited for a parallel implementation with one processor per scale.

Appendix A: Polynomial Spline Representations

A polynomial spline of degree n (n odd) is a function of the continuous variable x that is a polynomial of degree n for each interval $[k, k+1), k \in Z$. The polynomial segments are connected at the integer knots in a way that guarantees the continuity of the function and its derivatives up to order $n-1$ [22]. Any such spline can be represented by a weighted sum of shifted B-splines

$$f(x) = \sum_{k \in Z} c(k)\beta^n(x - k), \qquad (2.74)$$

where the $c(k)$ are the so-called B-spline coefficients [22, 23]. $\beta^n(x)$ is the central B-spline of order n; it is a symmetrical bell-shape function that is obtained from the $(n+1)$-fold convolution of a unit rectangular pulse (i.e., the B-spline of order zero).

Given a discrete signal $f(k) \in l_2$, there is a unique spline of the form (2.74) that provides an exact interpolation; i.e., $f(x)|_{x=k} = f(k)$. This mapping is expressed by the following discrete convolution equation [34, 37]

$$f(k) = (b^n * c)(k) \quad \Longleftrightarrow \quad c(k) = \left((b^n)^{-1} * f\right)(k), \qquad (2.75)$$

where

$$b^n(k) := \beta^n(x)|_{x=k} \quad \overset{z}{\longleftrightarrow} \quad B_1^n(z) \qquad (2.76)$$

is the discrete B-spline kernel of degree n, and where $(b^n)^{-1}$ denotes the inverse filter operator, which exists and is stable for any degree n [5].

A basic spline function enlarged by an integral factor m is still a spline with knots at the integers. This simply follows from the fact that if a dilated function is a polynomial of degree n for each enlarged interval $[k \cdot m, (k+1) \cdot m)$, then it is also polynomial on the smaller integer intervals $[k, (k+1))$. Consequently, there must exist a certain sequence $u_m^n(k)$ such that

$$\beta^n(x/m) = \sum_{k \in Z} u_m^n(k)\beta^n(x - k). \qquad (2.77)$$

It can be shown that the z-transform of $u_m^n(k)$ is given by [41]

$$U_m^n(z) = \frac{z^{k_0}}{m^n}\left(\sum_{k=0}^{m-1} z^{-k}\right)^{n+1}, \qquad (2.78)$$

with $k_0 = (n+1)(m-1)/2$. Thus, this sequence can be generated from the $(n+1)$-fold convolution of a discrete rectangular pulse of length m.

Appendix B: Implementation Example

To illustrate the use of the basic computational techniques, we provide a detailed description of the fast algorithm for the redundant dyadic wavelet transform described in Section 2.5.2.

The input of the algorithm is the discrete signal $f(k)$, $k = 0, \ldots, N-1$. The FIR filter parameters are the initialization kernel $b(k)$, $k = -N_b, \ldots, N_b$; the refinement filter $h(k)$, $k = -N_h, \ldots, N_h$; and the wavelet coefficient sequence $p(k)$, $k = -N_p, \ldots, N_p$. Explicit values can be found in Table 2.4.

First, we define a function that computes $c(k) = \uparrow_m [h^\vee] * f(k)$.

Function $c = \mathcal{F}(f, N, h, N_h, m)$:

For $k \in I_N = \{0, \ldots, N-1\}$, compute

$$c(k) = \sum_{l=-N_h}^{+N_h} h(l)f(k+ml)$$

using boundary conditions (2.14) or (2.18) for $(k+ml) \notin I_N$.

The algorithm can then be described as follows:

(i) $s_0 = \mathcal{F}(f, N, b, N_b, 1)$

(ii) $r_0 = \mathcal{F}(s_0, N, p, N_p, 1)$

(iii) loop: for $j = 1, \ldots, J$
$$s_j = \mathcal{F}(s_{j-1}, N, h, N_h, 2^{j-1})$$
$$r_j = \mathcal{F}(s_j, N, p, N_p, 2^j)$$

Note that the evaluation of the function $\mathcal{F}$ can be accelerated by a factor of two if the filtering templates are symmetric or anti-symmetric.

References

[1] P. Abry and A. Aldroubi. Semi- and bi-orthogonal MRA-type wavelet design and their fast algorithms. *Proc. SPIE, Wavelet Applications in Signal and Image Processing III*, 2569, 452–463, 1995.

[2] A. Aldroubi. Portraits of frames. *Proc. Am. Math. Soc.*, 123(6), 1661–1668, 1995.

[3] A. Aldroubi and M. Unser. Families of multiresolution and wavelet spaces with optimal properties. *Numer. Funct. Anal. Optimiz.*, 14(5-6), 417–446, 1993.

[4] A. Aldroubi and M. Unser. Sampling procedures in function spaces and asymptotic equivalence with Shannon's sampling theory. *Numer. Funct. Anal. Optimiz.*, 15(1-2), 1–21, 1994.

[5] A. Aldroubi, M. Unser, and M. Eden. Cardinal spline filters: stability and convergence to the ideal sinc interpolator. *Signal Process.*, 28(2), 127–138, 1992.

[6] A. Cohen, I. Daubechies, and J. C. Feauveau. Bi-orthogonal bases of compactly supported wavelets. *Commun. Pure Appl. Math.*, 45, 485–560, 1992.

[7] I. Daubechies. Orthogonal bases of compactly supported wavelets. *Commun. Pure Appl. Math.*, 41, 909–996, 1988.

[8] I. Daubechies. The wavelet transform, time-frequency localization and signal analysis. *IEEE Trans. Inform. Theory*, 36(5), 961–1005, 1990.

[9] I. Daubechies. *Ten Lectures on Wavelets*, Society for Industrial and Applied Mathematics, Philadelphia, PA, 1992.

[10] C. de Boor. *A Practical Guide to Splines*, Springer-Verlag, New York, 1978.

[11] D. Gabor. Theory of communication. *J. Inst. Elec. Eng.*, 93(III), 429–457, 1946.

[12] B. Jawerth and W. Sweldens. An overview of wavelet based multiresolution analyses. *SIAM Rev.*, 36(3), 377–412, 1994.

[13] D. L. Jones and R. G. Baraniuk. Efficient approximation of continuous wavelet transforms. *Electron. Lett.*, 27(9), 748–750, 1991.

[14] S. Maes. The Wavelet Transform in Signal Processing, with Application to the Extraction of Speech Modulation Model Features. Ph. D. thesis, Université de Louvain, Belgium, 1994.

[15] S. Mallat and W. L. Hwang. Singularity detection and processing with wavelets. *IEEE Trans. Inform. Theory*, 38(2), 617–643, 1992.

[16] S. Mallat and S. Zhong. Characterization of signals from multiscale edges. *IEEE Trans. Patt. Anal. Mach. Intell.*, 14(7), 710–732, 1992.

[17] S. Mallat. A theory of multiresolution signal decomposition: the wavelet representation. *IEEE Trans. Pattern Anal. Mach. Intell.*, PAMI-11(7), 674–693, 1989.

[18] J. Morlet, G. Arens, I. Fourgeau, and D. Giard. Wave propagation and sampling theory. *Geophysics*, 47, 203–236, 1982.

[19] O. Rioul and P. Duhamel. Fast algorithms for discrete and continuous wavelet transforms. *IEEE Trans. Inform. Theory*, IT-38(2), 569–586, 1992.

[20] O. Rioul and M. Vetterli. Wavelets and signal processing. *IEEE Signal Process. Mag.*, 8(4), 11–38, 1991.

[21] S. J. Schiff, A. Aldroubi, M. Unser, and S. Sato. Fast wavelet transformation of EEG. *Electroencephalogr. Clin. Neurophysiol.*, 91, 442–455, 1994.

[22] I. J. Schoenberg. Contribution to the problem of approximation of equidistant data by analytic functions. *Quart. Appl. Math.*, 4, 45–99, 112–141, 1946.

[23] I. J. Schoenberg. *Cardinal Spline Interpolation*, Society of Industrial and Applied Mathematics, Philadelphia, PA, 1973.

[24] L. L. Schumaker. *Spline Functions: Basic Theory*, Wiley, New York, 1981.

[25] M. J. Shensa. The discrete wavelet transform: wedding the à trous and Mallat algorithms. *IEEE Trans. Signal Process.*, 40(10), 2464–2482, 1992.

[26] G. Strang. Wavelets and dilation equations: a brief introduction. *SIAM Rev.*, 31, 614–627, 1989.

[27] G. Strang and G. Fix. A Fourier analysis of the finite element variational method. In *Constructive Aspect of Functional Analysis*, Edizioni Cremonese, Rome, 1971, 796–830.

[28] W. Sweldens and R. Piessens. Asymptotic error expansions for wavelet approximations of smooth functions II. *Numer. Math.*, 68(3), 377–401, 1994.

[29] M. Unser. Comments on 'A new approach to recursive Fourier transform'. *Proc. IEEE*, 76(10), 1395–1396, 1988.

[30] M. Unser and M. Eden. FIR approximations of inverse filters and perfect reconstruction filter banks. *Signal Process.*, 36(2), 163–174, 1994.

[31] M. Unser. Fast Gabor-like windowed Fourier and continuous wavelet transforms. *IEEE Signal Process. Lett.*, 1(5), 76–79, 1994.

[32] M. Unser. Texture classification and segmentation using wavelet frames. *IEEE Trans. Image Process.*, 1995.

[33] M. Unser. Approximation power of biorthogonal wavelet expansions. *IEEE Trans. Signal Process.*, submitted.

[34] M. Unser, A. Aldroubi, and M. Eden. Fast B-spline transforms for continuous image representation and interpolation. *IEEE Trans. Pattern Anal. Mach. Intell.*, 13(3), 277–285, 1991.

[35] M. Unser, A. Aldroubi, and M. Eden. On the asymptotic convergence of B-spline wavelets to Gabor functions. *IEEE Trans. Inform. Theory*, 38(2), 864–872, 1992.

[36] M. Unser, A. Aldroubi, and M. Eden. Polynomial spline signal approximations: filter design and asymptotic equivalence with Shannon's sampling theorem. *IEEE Trans. Inform. Theory*, 38(1), 95–103, 1992.

[37] M. Unser, A. Aldroubi, and M. Eden. B-spline signal processing. I: Theory. *IEEE Trans. Signal Process.*, 41(2), 821–833, 1993.

[38] M. Unser, A. Aldroubi, and M. Eden. B-spline signal processing. II: Efficient design and applications. *IEEE Trans. Signal Process.*, 41(2), 834–848, 1993.

[39] M. Unser, A. Aldroubi, and M. Eden. A family of polynomial spline wavelet transforms. *Signal Process.*, 30(2), 141–162, 1993.

[40] M. Unser, A. Aldroubi, and M. Eden. The L_2 polynomial spline pyramid. *IEEE Trans. Pattern Anal. Mach. Intell.*, 15(4), 364–379, 1993.

[41] M. Unser, A. Aldroubi, and S. J. Schiff. Fast implementation of the continuous wavelet transform with integer scales. *IEEE Trans. Signal Process.*, 42(12), 3519–3523, 1994.

[42] M. Unser and I. Daubechies. On the approximation power of convolution-based least squares versus interpolation. National Institutes of Health, preprint, 1995.

[43] P. P. Vaidyanathan. Quadrature mirror filter banks, M-band extensions and perfect-reconstruction technique. *IEEE ASSP Mag.*, 4, 4–20, 1987.

[44] M. Vetterli. A theory of multirate filter banks. *IEEE Trans. Acoust. Speech Signal Process.*, ASSP-35(3), 356–372, 1987.

[45] M. Vetterli and J. Kovacevic. *Wavelets and Subband Coding*, Prentice Hall, Englewood Cliffs, NJ, 1995.

[46] M. J. Vrhel, C. Lee, and M. Unser. Fast continuous wavelet transform. in *Proc. Int. Conf. Acoustics, Speech Signal Processing*, 2, 1165–1168, 1995.

[47] M. J. Vrhel, C. Lee, and M. Unser. Fast continuous wavelet transform: a least squares formulation. *Signal Processing*, submitted.

[48] M. V. Wickerhauser. Acoustic signal compression with wavelet packets. In C. K. Chui, Ed., *Wavelets: A Tutorial in Theory and Applications*, Academic Press, New York, 1992, 679–700.

Part II

Wavelets in Medical Imaging and Tomography

3

An Application of Wavelet Shrinkage to Tomography

Eric D. Kolaczyk

Department of Statistics
The University of Chicago
Chicago, IL

3.1 Introduction

3.1.1 Tomography

In this chapter we introduce a wavelet-based method for reconstructing images from certain types of tomographic data. "Tomography" actually refers to a broad class of problems which have in common the fact that their data may be described as noisy observations or approximations of *line integrals*. X-ray computed tomography (CT) and positron emission tomography (PET) are two well-known examples from the field of medical imaging; however, radio and radar astronomy, molecular spectroscopy, and certain stress analysis methods are just a few examples of other areas in which similar data arise. Common to all of these applications are data, often called *projections*, which are indirect, incomplete, and noisy.

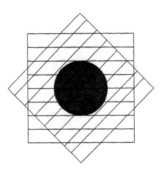

Figure 3.1
Schematic representation of a tomographic sampling pattern.

Here we will consider data of the form

$$D_{a,b} = \int_{L_{\theta_a, u_b}} f(x,y)\, dx\, dy + \sigma z_{a,b}, \qquad (3.1)$$

where

$$L_{\theta, u} = \{(x,y) : x\cos(\theta) + y\sin(\theta) = u\}$$

is a line defined by the polar coordinates (θ, u), f is the object of interest, and the $\{z_{a,b}\}$ represent a Gaussian white noise process with variance 1. The sets $\{\theta_a\}_{a=0}^{N_{ang}-1}$ and $\{u_b\}_{b=1}^{N_{pos}}$ represent discrete samplings of angles in $[0, \pi)$ and positions in $[-1, 1]$, respectively. Figure 3.1 shows a schematic representation of the sampling process for $N_{ang} = 2$ angles, $\theta = 0$ and $\pi/4$, and $N_{pos} = 9$ positions per angle.

3.1.2 Why Wavelets?

The goal in tomography problems is typically to reconstruct the object f from observations $\{D_{a,b}\}$. There are currently a number of fundamental ways in which this task is approached. In medical imaging, commercial machines typically employ Fourier-based methods, such as filtered backprojection (FBP). Maximum likelihood approaches, utilizing the expectation-maximization (EM) algorithm, are fairly common within the research community. Two other approaches are iterative methods and orthogonal series methods.

Our motivation for using wavelets in this problem can be understood by considering Figure 3.2. Figure 3.2(a) shows the Shepp/Logan phantom [15], an idealized version of, say, sections of the brain encountered in X-ray CT and PET studies. Figure 3.2(b) shows a two-dimensional, discrete wavelet transform of the phantom. Note the extreme sparseness of the wavelet representation. This sparseness results from the fact that the phantom is

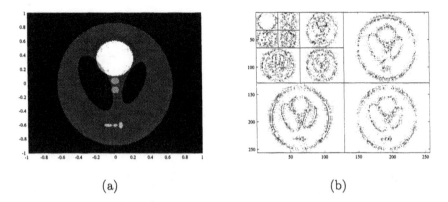

(a)   (b)

Figure 3.2
(a) shows the Shepp/Logan phantom. White corresponds to high intensity, while black corresponds to low. (b) shows the wavelet transform of the phantom. The color scheme has been reversed in (b), to compensate for the large DC component at the coarse level.

characterized primarily by its edges. As a result of their "local" nature in the plane, only wavelets which are located on or near an edge yield large wavelet coefficients. The rest are zero, except for the coarse level coefficients, which pick up the overall gross structure.

The use of wavelets in tomography has been considered by a number of authors recently (see, e.g., [11, 3, 12, 14, 17]). In our approach, we combine a wavelet analogue of the singular value decomposition with a method of denoising called *wavelet shrinkage* to obtain a regularized, 2D-wavelet reconstruction of f.

3.1.3   Wavelet Shrinkage and the Proposed Method

If we were to observe an object f *directly*, with the addition of a Gaussian white noise, say

$$D'_{i,l} = f(x_i, y_l) + \sigma z_{i,l}, \quad i, l = 0, \ldots, N_0 - 1 \tag{3.2}$$

the problem of recovering f would be an ideal candidate for the wavelet shrinkage techniques of Donoho et al. [7] (see [4] [18] for similar approaches). Specifically, by taking the discrete wavelet transform of the data, we obtain a representation which contains the main structure of the image in a relatively few large coefficients, and the noise in the remaining small coefficients. By shrinking the coefficients towards zero in a particular manner, most of the "noise" coefficients are effectively removed, while the "signal" coefficients remain more or less unaffected. Applying the discrete inverse

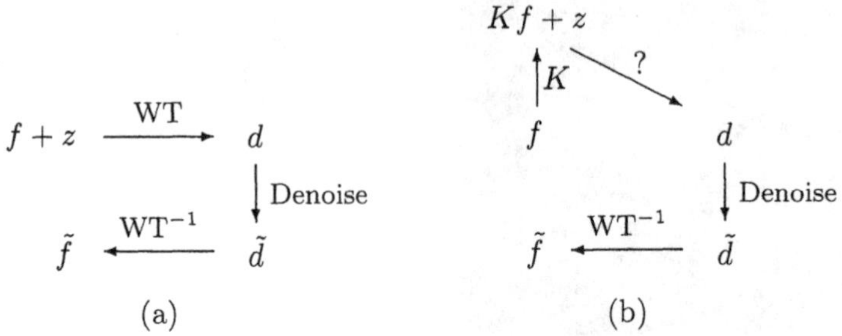

$$Kf + z$$

$$\uparrow K \qquad ?$$

$$f + z \xrightarrow{\quad \text{WT} \quad} d \qquad\qquad f \qquad\qquad d$$

$$\Big\downarrow \text{Denoise} \qquad\qquad\qquad \Big\downarrow \text{Denoise}$$

$$\tilde{f} \xleftarrow{\quad \text{WT}^{-1} \quad} \tilde{d} \qquad\qquad \tilde{f} \xleftarrow{\quad \text{WT}^{-1} \quad} \tilde{d}$$

(a) \qquad\qquad\qquad\qquad (b)

Figure 3.3
Denoising using wavelets. (a) shows the case of direct observations, $D' = f + z$. (b) shows the case of indirect observations,
$D = Kf + z$, where K is some operator having the effect of blurring
or deforming f prior to the addition of noise.

wavelet transform to the resulting matrix of coefficients yields a reconstruction of f.

Unfortunately, in tomography we do not observe the objects directly, but
rather *indirectly*, in the form of line integrals. These line integrals,

$$(\mathcal{R}f)(u, \theta) \equiv \int_{L_{\theta,u}} f(x, y)\, dx\, dy,$$

correspond to the two-dimensional Radon transform, $\mathcal{R}f$, of f. The reconstruction method proposed in this chapter consists of two steps. The
first step involves the inversion of the Radon transform in such a way as to
obtain, not f, but the (noisy) wavelet coefficients of f. In the second step
we apply wavelet shrinkage to the coefficients in order to remove the noise.
However, as a result of the inversion in the first step, the manner in which
we shrink necessarily differs from that of Donoho et al. [7]. Our reconstruction of f is obtained by applying the discrete inverse wavelet transform to
the denoised coefficients.

These two steps will be presented separately in the following two sections,
after which we will examine the results of a small comparison study.

3.2   Inversion

3.2.1   Direct Data Vs. Indirect Data

The indirectness of tomographic data necessitates an additional step in
the typical wavelet-denoising process used with direct data. Figure 3.3(a)
shows a schematic representation of this process, whereby data, $D' = f + z$,

are transformed to a set of wavelet coefficients, d, and denoised to yield a new set of coefficients, $\tilde{d}$. The reconstruction $\tilde{f}$ of f is obtained by applying the discrete inverse wavelet transform to $\tilde{d}$. In this chapter we shall denoise using only wavelet shrinkage methods, but many approaches fit the general framework of Figure 3.3(a).

Figure 3.3(b) shows how the above process is changed when indirect observations are taken. These observations may be expressed formally by writing $D = Kf + z$, where K is an operator which may be thought of as having the effect of blurring or deforming f. In the case of tomography, $K = \mathcal{R}$, the Radon transform. Motivated by the sparseness of the representation in Figure 3.2(b), we would like to work with the coefficients of the unobserved function, f, but the discrete wavelet transform of the actual data obviously does not yield these coefficients. Hence, in order to denoise in the domain of the desired wavelet coefficients, some other operation is necessary, one which has the effect of inverting K.

3.2.2 The Wavelet-Vaguelette Decomposition

The wavelet-vaguelette decomposition (WVD), first introduced by Donoho [5], is a tool specifically designed for the problematic inversion step pictured in Figure 3.3(b). The function f is decomposed with respect to a chosen orthonormal wavelet basis, $\{\psi_{j,k}\}$, and the function Kf is decomposed with respect to a related set of functions, $\{\gamma_{j,k}\}$, such that the respective coefficients are equal, i.e.,

$$[Kf, \gamma_{j,k}] = \langle f, \psi_{j,k} \rangle. \tag{3.3}$$

For certain operators, K, the $\gamma_{j,k}$, when scaled properly, are "almost" wavelets, in the sense that they are smooth, oscillating, local, and nearly orthonormal. Such functions are termed *vaguelettes*. Combining these facts with the additional fact that the sets $\{\psi_{j,k}\}$ and $\{\gamma_{j,k}\}$ are biorthogonal, suggests that the WVD is a wavelet analogue of the singular value decomposition. With respect to the diagram in Figure 3.3(b), when K is an operator for which a vaguelette basis exists, calculating the vaguelette coefficients of Kf will give us the desired wavelet coefficients of f.

Returning to the context of tomography, Donoho [5] showed that if the underlying operator is the Radon transform, a vaguelette basis does indeed exist and is composed of functions of the form

$$\gamma_\lambda(u, \theta) = \frac{1}{(2\pi)^2} \int_{-\infty}^{\infty} |v| \cdot \hat{\psi}_\lambda(v \cos(\theta), v \sin(\theta)) \cdot e^{iuv} \, dv. \tag{3.4}$$

Here $\lambda = (j, (k_x, k_y), \epsilon)$ is used to index the two-dimensional wavelet functions, and hence the vaguelettes as well. The index j refers to the resolution level, (k_x, k_y), to the position, and $\epsilon = 1$, 2, and 3, to the directional sensitivity in the horizontal, vertical, and diagonal directions, respectively.

In order to implement the WVD in the present context of tomography, it is conceivable that one could substitute (3.4) into $[\mathcal{R}f, \gamma_\lambda]$ and calculate these coefficients using numerical integration. However, this approach would be naive and inefficient, considering that in practice 128^2 to 512^2 coefficients will usually need to be calculated. Instead, we introduce a more efficient approach which represents the coefficients as the end product of a sequence of operations.

3.2.3 Efficient Expressions for the Radon Vaguelette Coefficients

We begin by introducing the backprojection operator,

$$\left(\mathcal{B}(\mathcal{R}f)\right)(x, y) = \int_0^\pi (\mathcal{R}f)(u_{(x,y,\theta)}, \theta)\, d\theta = f(x, y) * * \frac{1}{\sqrt{x^2 + y^2}}.$$

Here the symbol "$**$" denotes two-dimensional convolution of functions.

The operation of backprojection is used in tomography to move from the space of the observed projection data to the space of the unobserved object. The specific form of the second equality above suggests that backprojecting the data transforms the reconstruction problem into one of deconvolution. In fact, it is well known that f may be expressed as

$$f(x, y) = \frac{1}{2\pi} \mathcal{F}_2^{-1} \left\{ |\omega| \mathcal{F}_2 \mathcal{B}(\mathcal{R}f) \right\}(x, y), \tag{3.5}$$

where $\mathcal{F}_2$ and $\mathcal{F}_2^{-1}$ denote the operations of taking the two-dimensional Fourier transform and its inverse, respectively, and $|\omega| = (\omega_x^2 + \omega_y^2)^{1/2}$.

The vaguelette coefficients for the Radon transform may be written in a form similar to that of (3.5) if we view the coefficient $[\mathcal{R}f, \gamma_\lambda]$ as a function of its index, $\lambda = (j, (k_x, k_y), \epsilon)$. Specifically, we may write

$$[\mathcal{R}f, \gamma_\lambda] = \frac{1}{2\pi} \mathcal{F}_2^{-1} \left\{ |\omega| h_j^\epsilon(\omega) \mathcal{F}_2 \mathcal{B}(\mathcal{R}f) \right\}(2^j k_x, 2^j k_y), \tag{3.6}$$

where $h_j^\epsilon(\omega) = 2^j \hat{\psi}_{(0,0,\epsilon)}(-2^j \omega)$. See [9] for more details.

3.2.4   Calculation of the Radon Vaguelette Coefficient

The similarity of (3.6) and (3.5), while interesting mathematically, is actually quite helpful from a computational point of view. In practice, researchers replace (3.5) by the approximation

$$\tilde{f}(x,y) \approx \frac{1}{2\pi}\mathcal{F}_2^{-1}\left\{|\omega|h(\omega)\mathcal{F}_2\mathcal{B}(\mathcal{R}f)\right\}(x,y), \tag{3.7}$$

where $h(\cdot)$ is a window function which damps out high frequencies. Equation (3.7) is then applied to real data by discretizing the backprojection operator and replacing $\mathcal{F}_2$ and $\mathcal{F}_2^{-1}$ by the corresponding two-dimensional fast Fourier transforms (FFT). The resulting method has been called the *filtering of backprojected projections* method of reconstruction [2], which we shall denote FBPP. Note that this algorithm differs from the more commonly used filter-backprojection (FBP) algorithm, in which the filtering is done in the Radon domain prior to backprojection.

We now adapt the FBPP algorithm in a straightforward fashion to calculate the necessary vaguelette coefficients from projection data., Let $\mathbf{D}$ be an $N_{ang} \times N_{pos}$ matrix of projection data, obtained according to (3.1). Let $N_0 = 2^{J_0}$ be a power of 2 greater than or equal to N_{pos}, and fix $0 \ll I \le J_0$ to be the depth of the wavelet decomposition. The corresponding $N_0 \times N_0$ matrix of vaguelette coefficients may be obtained using Algorithm 1.

Algorithm 1

1.   Backproject data $\mathbf{D}$ to an $N_0 \times N_0$ matrix.

2.   Take the 2-D FFT.

3.   For each level $j = 1, \ldots, I$,

    (a)   Multiply by the windowed modulus term, $|\cdot|h_{j-J_0}^\epsilon(\cdot)$.

    (b)   Take the 2-D IFFT.

    (c)   Decimate the resulting matrix and store.

Note that although Algorithm 1 resembles a multiresolution analogue of the FBPP algorithm, it is only the filtering step that is done at each of the approximately $3\log_2(N_0)$ resolution levels, while the costly $O(N_{ang}N_{pos}^2)$ backprojection step is done only once. The wavelet window functions in Step 3(a) may be computed either exactly, using the Meyer wavelet basis [1] or spline wavelets [16], or approximately (to any desired accuracy), using Daubechies wavelets [1].

The decimation in Step 3(c) can be understood as follows. The result of Steps 1–3(b) is to take the $N_{ang} \times N_{pos}$ matrix $\mathbf{D}$ and output an $N_0 \times N_0$

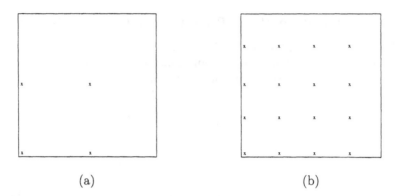

(a)   (b)

Figure 3.4
Matrix sampling scheme for Algorithm 1. (a) shows the case of
$j = J_0 - 1$. **(b) shows the case of** $j = J_0 - 2$.

matrix. However, for each level j and direction ϵ, only $2^{2(J_0-j)}$ coefficients are required. These are obtained by sampling those elements of the output matrix corresponding to positions $(2^{j-J_0}k_x, 2^{j-J_0}k_y)$ on the unit square, for k_x, $k_y = 0, 1, \ldots, 2^{J_0-j} - 1$, as indicated by Equation (3.6).

Figure 3.4 shows this process schematically, interpreting the output matrix as a discretized version of the unit square. At resolution level $j = J_0-1$, we have k_x, $k_y = 0$ and 1, so the four values corresponding to $(0,0)$, $(0,1/2)$, $(1/2,0)$ and $(1/2,1/2)$ are sampled. When $j = J_0 - 2$, k_x, $k_y = 0, 1, 2,$ and 3, so values are sampled at all pairs from the set $\{0, 1/4, 1/2, 3/4\}$.

3.3   Denoising Using Wavelet Shrinkage

Using Algorithm 1, we may calculate a matrix of vaguelette coefficients from projection data. A naive approach to reconstructing f might be to apply the discrete inverse wavelet transform to this matrix immediately. The solution defined by this approach is equivalent to implementing (3.7) with $h(\omega) \equiv 1$ (i.e., FBPP with an unmodified ramp filter) and is typically unstable. Denoising the vaguelette coefficients up to a certain resolution level prior to applying the discrete inverse wavelet transform, as depicted in Figure 3.3(b), will serve to *regularize* the solution. In this section, we briefly outline the method of wavelet shrinkage in its original context of direct data, and then explain how it may be adapted for denoising in tomography.

3.3.1 Wavelet Shrinkage with Direct Data

In the case of direct observations of the object f, as in Equation (3.2), the wavelet transform of the data results in coefficients $\{d_\lambda\}$ of the form

$$d_\lambda = \langle \psi_\lambda, f \rangle + \sigma z_\lambda. \tag{3.8}$$

The $\{z_\lambda\}$ are again a Gaussian white noise process, due to the orthonormality of the underlying wavelets.

We can effectively remove the noise from the data, with little damage to the underlying signal, by applying the nonlinear function

$$\eta_{t_{N_0}}(x) = \begin{cases} x - t_{N_0}, & \text{if } x > t_{N_0} \\ 0, & \text{if } |x| \leq t_{N_0} \\ x + t_{N_0}, & \text{if } x < -t_{N_0} \end{cases}$$

to each of the coefficients, using the threshold value [7]

$$t_{N_0} = \sqrt{2 \log(N_0^2)}\, \sigma. \tag{3.9}$$

The value t_{N_0} is a probabilistic upper bound on the size of the N_0^2 errors

$$|\sigma z_\lambda| = |d_\lambda - \langle f, \psi_\lambda \rangle|.$$

Hence, wavelet shrinkage acts by setting to zero any coefficients smaller than a "maximum error" bound and keeping any coefficients above, after shrinking the latter towards zero by the amount of the bound. It is this shrinking, as opposed to a simple "keep-or-kill" threshold operation, that guarantees a reconstruction of f which is at least as smooth as f itself (with high probability), and is near optimal in a statistical minimax sense. See [7] for details and additional references and [4, 18] for similar threshold-based approaches to denoising with wavelets.

3.3.2 Wavelet Shrinkage with Tomographic Data

The indirect observations of f in Equation (3.1) are transformed via the WVD to vaguelette coefficients of the form

$$v_\lambda \approx [\mathcal{R}f, \gamma_\lambda] + \sigma_{j,\epsilon} z_\lambda = \langle f, \psi_\lambda \rangle + \sigma_{j,\epsilon} z_\lambda. \tag{3.10}$$

To a first approximation, the noise process, $\{z_\lambda\}$, is Gaussian and white within each wavelet channel, due to the near (but not exact) orthogonality of the underlying (rescaled) vaguelettes [5]. The main difference between (3.10) and (3.8) is in the form of the noise level, $\sigma_{j,\epsilon} = 2^{(J_0-j)/2}\sigma c_\epsilon$, which increases as the resolution becomes finer. The value c_ϵ is a constant which depends only on N_{ang}, N_{pos}, and the underlying wavelet.

The increasing noise level is an effect created by the inversion of $\mathcal{R}$ through the WVD. This phenomena is analogous to the increasing nature of the singular values in the singular value decomposition of $\mathcal{R}$, and is similarly related to the need for a window $h(\cdot)$ in the FBPP algorithm. Interpreted another way, the fact that the noise level of the coefficients increases with finer resolution levels indicates that higher frequency components of f will become increasingly difficult to recover, a fact already well-known in the tomographic imaging community.

Nevertheless, as suggested by the form of (3.10), much of the noise may be removed effectively by applying the wavelet shrinkage operator $\eta_t(\cdot)$ to the vaguelette coefficients, but using *level-dependent* thresholds of the form

$$t_{j,\epsilon} = \sqrt{2\log(2^{2(J_0-j)})}\ \sigma_{j,\epsilon}. \tag{3.11}$$

The indexing (j, ϵ) is used to emphasize that a different threshold is used at each level, and each direction within level. Note that the signal-to-noise ratio (SNR) will strongly affect how much, if any, of the signal can be expected to be recovered at the finest resolution (highest frequency) levels. See [9] for more details surrounding the derivation of $t_{j,\epsilon}$.

3.3.3 The Proposed Reconstruction Method

Combining Algorithm 1 and the modifications to the wavelet shrinkage approach described immediately above, we arrive at the following algorithm for reconstructing images from tomographic data of the form found in Equation (3.1). The matrix of vaguelette coefficients will be represented by $\mathbf{V}$, while the submatrix containing coefficients at level j and direction ϵ will be written $\mathbf{V}^{(j,\epsilon)}$.

WVD/WS Reconstruction Algorithm

1. Compute $\mathbf{V}$ from $\mathbf{D}$, using Algorithm 1.

2. For each level $j = 1, \ldots, I$,

    For each direction $\epsilon = 1, 2, 3$

    Compute $\tilde{\mathbf{V}}^{(j,\epsilon)} = \eta_{t_{j,\epsilon}}(\mathbf{V}^{(j,\epsilon)})$

3. Set $\tilde{\mathbf{V}}^{(I,Coarse)} = \mathbf{V}^{(I,Coarse)}$

4. Apply the two-dimensional inverse wavelet transform to $\tilde{\mathbf{V}}$.

Note that no shrinkage is done at the coarsest level of coefficients, as too much signal is lost in doing so. Hence, regularization is accomplished in two steps. First, a coarse resolution level, I, is chosen. The part of the reconstruction based solely on these coarse coefficients is an approximation to f based on certain low-frequency elements of the data, roughly those in the interval $\left[-2^{J_0-I-1}, 2^{J_0-I-1}\right]$. Second, all detail coefficients at levels $j = 1, \ldots, I$ are shrunk. The contributions of the coefficients which remain after shrinkage may be viewed as images of successively finer levels of detail, which are superimposed upon the coarse-level approximation.

3.4   A Short Comparative Study

Data were simulated according to Equation (3.1), taking the Shepp/Logan phantom to be the true underlying object, f. Sampling was done using $N_{ang} = 201$ equispaced angles and $N_{pos} = 129$ positions per angle. The standard deviation of the noise, σ, was set at three different levels, to create three sets of data with SNRs of 20, 30, and 40 decibels (dB).

Our goal was to compare the proposed WVD/WS method with the FBPP method of reconstruction based on Equation (3.7). In Figure 3.5, Figures 5(a–c), in the top row, show 256×256 reconstructions using WVD/WS, while in the bottom row Figures 5(d–f) show the analogous reconstructions using FBPP. The leftmost images are based on data with a 20 dB SNR, the middle, 30 dB, and the rightmost, 40 dB. A decomposition depth of $I = 2$ was chosen, which meant that the top two levels, or 93.75% of the coefficients, were shrunk. Shrinking coefficients at any lower depths tended to oversmooth, as those coefficients contained primary signal. Periodic, Meyer wavelets were used in the reconstructions of Figures 5(a–c), as their simple closed form expression in the frequency domain makes computing the necessary wavelet window functions straightforward [8]. For the FBPP reconstructions in Figures 5(d–f), a Hann window was used, with 0.5 cutoff. Comparison of this window with the coarse level Meyer wavelets at level $I = 2$ (in the frequency domain) suggests that our comparison is being made at similar resolutions.

In examining the two sets of reconstructions, note that the WVD/WS reconstructions display an overall reduction in noise over their FBPP counterparts, especially at the lower SNRs. In fact, the average squared error in the FBPP reconstructions is reduced by approximately 42, 9, and 1%, at 20, 30, and 40 dB, respectively, using the WVD/WS method. With respect to feature detection, consider the reconstructions at 20 dB, where this task

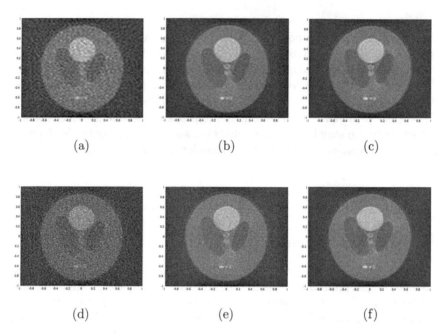

(a)   (b)   (c)

(d)   (e)   (f)

Figure 3.5
(a–c) show WVD/WS reconstructions of the Shepp/Logan phan-
tom from data with SNRs of 20, 30, and 40 dB, respectively.
(d–f) show traditional FBPP reconstructions, using a Hann filter
and 0.5 cutoff.

would be most difficult. There appears to be more evidence of the presence
of each of the eight ellipses in the WVD/WS reconstruction than in that
of the FBPP. At 30 and 40 dB, all features are visible using both methods,
though the texture is less "grainy" using WVD/WS.

As it turns out, the similarity in reconstruction of individual features at
30 and 40 dB is actually somewhat deceiving. Figure 3.6 shows close-up
views of the three small "hot spots" in the lower part of the Shepp/Logan
phantom. Figures 6(a) and (b) correspond to the WVD/WS and FBPP
reconstructions, respectively, at 30 dB, while Figure 6(c) is from the phantom itself. The WVD/WS reconstruction has both removed much of the
noise and preserved the structure and distinctness of the "hot spots." On
the other hand, in the FBPP reconstruction these objects may only be
distinguished poorly against the remaining background noise. Considering
just this reduced region of the phantom, the WVD/WS method achieves an
approximately 28% improvement in average squared error over the FBPP
method. This example suggests that the WVD/WS method of reconstruction may offer marked advantages in recovering small objects at certain
SNRs, due to the ability of wavelets to extract detail at multiple scales.

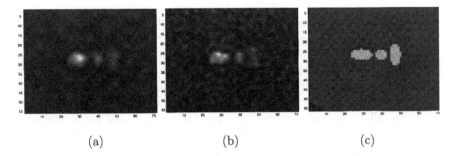

(a)   (b)   (c)

Figure 3.6
**(a) and (b) show a close-up view of the WVD and FBPP recon-
structions, respectively, from data with a 30 dB SNR, in the lower
region of the phantom containing the three small "hot spots". (c)
shows the same region in the phantom itself.**

3.5 Discussion

The reconstructions resulting from the WVD/WS algorithm proposed
herein may actually be viewed as the superposition of two images. The
first image is the result of sampling a rough FBPP reconstruction and "interpolating", via the inverse wavelet transform, to a finer grid. The window
function associated with this rough FBPP is defined in terms of the scale
function or coarse level wavelet. The second image contains the finer details
of the underlying object that were recoverable amid the background noise,
using wavelet shrinkage, and is obtained through the inversion of each level
of detail coefficients. Taking into account the association with FBPP methods, the simple nature of the wavelet shrinkage operation, and the speed
of the inverse wavelet transform algorithms, it seems realistic to suggest
that the WVD/WS method could be implemented efficiently in current or
future tomographic machines.

Our reconstruction algorithm differs from those of other wavelet-based
approaches in two ways. First, most other approaches ([3, 11, 12]) revolve
around a multiresolution analogue of the FBP algorithm, in which at each
level the projections are convolved with a level-dependent filter and then
backprojected to specific locations. In contrast, our approach computes
a single backprojection and then applies different filters for each resolution level, followed by a specific down-sampling operation. We note that it
should be easy to create an analogue of the former approach to compute the
vaguelette coefficients necessary for our WVD/WS algorithm [8]. The second difference between our approach and others is in the use of the simple,
nonlinear thresholding operator, $\eta_{t_{j,\epsilon}}$, within the inversion process, to remove noise at high frequencies. The "shrinkage" aspect of this operator has

lead to its sometimes being called a *soft-threshold* operator, to distinguish it from the *hard-threshold* operator which either returns an input value x or replaces it by zero. Hard-thresholding of wavelet coefficients has been used as a preprocessing tool to denoise projections at each angle, prior to application of the traditional FBP algorithm [14]. Here, however, working within the framework of the wavelet-vaguelette decomposition, our WVD/WS algorithm allows for the inversion and regularization of the projection data without any pre- or postprocessing. Additionally, this framework allows for a careful study of the effects of the inversion on the noise underlying the wavelet coefficients [8, 9].

The improvement of WVD/WS over FBPP observed here is due to the sparseness by which the underlying object may be represented using wavelets, and the efficiency with which wavelet shrinkage exploits this sparseness. It should be noted that the basic thresholds of Donoho et al. [7] presented in this chapter have been expanded upon by these authors and others [6, 10], and that similar expansions may be useful in a suitably modified form in tomography. For example, thresholds could be used which are both level and location dependent or which are adaptive in nature. Furthermore, certain edge-enhancing filters from the engineering literature have been seen to take similar advantage of the wavelet-induced sparseness in other areas of application [13].

As a final note, we mention that Algorithm 1 can be used with complete tomographic geometries other than that depicted in Figure 3.1. However, the characteristics of the noise present in the modalities associated with these geometries may be quite different from that assumed in this chapter. In such cases, careful study is necessary to properly calibrate the thresholds used in shrinking the vaguelette coefficients. See Kolaczyk [8] for some preliminary work in the context of PET data.

References

[1] I. Daubechies. *Ten Lectures on Wavelets.* SIAM, 1992.

[2] S. R. Deans. *The Radon Transform and Some of Its Applications.* John Wiley & Sons, New York, 1983.

[3] A. H. Delaney and Y. Bresler. Multiresolution tomographic reconstruction using wavelets. *IEEE Trans. Image Process.*, 6(6):799–813, 1995.

[4] R. A. DeVore and B. J. Lucier. Fast wavelet techniques for near-optimal image processing. IEEE-ICASSP-93, IEEE Military Communications Conference, New York, 1992, 48.3.1–48.3.7.

[5] D. L. Donoho. Nonlinear solution of linear inverse problems by wavelet-vaguelette decomposition. *Appl. Comput. Harmon. Anal.*, 2:101–126, 1995.

[6] D. L. Donoho and I. M. Johnstone. Adapting to unknown smoothness via wavelet shrinkage. *J. Am. Statist. Assoc.*, 90:1200–1224, 1995.

[7] D. L. Donoho, I. M. Johnstone, G. Kerkyacharian, and D. Picard. Wavelet Shrinkage: Asymptopia? *J. Roy. Statist. Soc. Ser. B*, 57:301–370, 1995.

[8] E. D. Kolaczyk. Wavelet Methods for the Inversion of Certain Homogeneous Linear Operators in the Presence of Noisy Data. Ph.D. thesis, Department of Statistics, Stanford University, Stanford, CA, 1994.

[9] E. D. Kolaczyk. A Wavelet Shrinkage Approach to Tomographic Image Reconstruction. *J. Am. Statist. Assoc.*, 91, 1996.

[10] G. P. Nason. Wavelet regression by cross-validation. Technical report 447, Department of Statistics, Stanford University, Stanford, CA, 1994.

[11] T. Olson and J. DeStefano. Wavelet localization of the Radon transform. *IEEE Trans. Signal. Process.*, 42(8):2055–2067, 1994.

[12] F. Peyrin, M. Zaim, and R. Goutte. Construction of wavelet decompositions for tomographic images. *J. Math. Imag. Vision*, 3(1):105–121, 1993.

[13] W. B. Richardson, Jr. Nonlinear filtering and multiscale texture discrimination for mammograms. *SPIE Vol. 1768, Mathematical Methods in Medical Imaging*, 293–305, 1992.

[14] B. Sahiner and A. E. Yagle. Reconstruction from projections under time-frequency constraints. *IEEE Trans. Med. Imag.*, 14(2):193–204, 1995.

[15] L. A. Shepp and B. F. Logan. The Fourier reconstruction of a head section. *IEEE Trans. Nucl. Sci.*, NS21(3):21–43, 1974.

[16] M. Unser, A. Aldroubi, and M. Eden. A family of polynomial spline wavelet transforms. *Signal Process.*, 30:141–162, 1993.

[17] D. Walnut. Local inversion of the Radon transform in the plane using wavelets. In *Proc. SPIE Conf., Wavelet Applications in Signal and Image Processing*, San Diego, CA, 2034:84–91, 1993.

[18] J. B. Weaver, X. Yansun, D. M. Healy, and L. D. Cromwell. Filtering noise from images with wavelet transforms. *Magn. Reson. Med.*, 21(2):288–295, 1991.

4

Wavelet Denoising of Functional MRI Data

Michael Hilton[1], Todd Ogden[2], David Hattery[3], Guinevere Eden[4], and Björn Jawerth[5]

[1] *Department of Computer Science, University of South Carolina, Columbia, SC*
[2] *Department of Statistics, University of South Carolina, Columbia, SC*
[3] *Washington, DC*
[4] *Functional Brain Imaging, LPP, NIMH, Rockville Pike, MD*
[5] *Department of Mathematics, University of South Carolina, Columbia, SC*

Abstract   Functional MRI is an imaging technique that provides high resolution information about brain blood flow and oxygenation. This information is used to deduce which regions of the brain are activated by various stimuli. Analysis of functional MRI data is complicated by the low signal-to-noise ratios typically encountered. Two different wavelet-based noise removal algorithms are investigated for potential utility in functional MRI analysis.

4.1 Functional MRI and Brain Mapping

In recent years, there has been a tremendous increase in the number of studies that identify the regions of the brain responsible for performing different mental functions. A functional brain mapping study consists of three distinct parts. First, one selects a method of stimulating the brain.

A brain stimulus can be as simple as having the subject touch two fingers together, thereby activating the motor cortex. A tremendous variety of methods exist to evoke a desired functional response, and the stimulus chosen is generally customized for each particular case study. Next, one images, with and without the stimulus, a physiological process that correlates with brain activity. The most common imaging technologies used in brain mapping are positron emission tomography (PET) and magnetic resonance imaging (MRI). Finally, one analyzes the images to determine differences that indicate activated regions.

Brain activity is measured in PET by injecting radioactively tagged molecules that are linked to regional cerebral blood flow or cerebral neural metabolism. PET images capture spatial concentrations of these molecules as they decay. There are a number of limitations to PET imaging. Foremost is the fact that PET images are noisy. Because the changes in regional cerebral blood flow associated with activation of higher order cognitive functions are small, approximately 5% or so [4], they are difficult to distinguish in noisy PET images. To improve the signal-to-noise ratio (SNR) of PET images, results are averaged across a group of individuals. (The hazards associated with the ionizing radiation used in PET imaging prevents repeating experiments multiple times on a single individual.) A second limitation of PET is its low spatial and temporal resolution, which limits the cognitive processes that may be studied and makes it difficult to correlate them with detailed anatomical structures.

Functional MRI (fMRI) is a fairly recent innovation that solves many of the problems associated with PET imaging. MRI systems have spatial and temporal resolutions exceeding that of PET, and MRI does not require invasive procedures or ionizing radiation. In addition, MRI can provide an anatomical image onto which activated regions can be mapped. Unfortunately, fMRI images also suffer from noise problems. The use of wavelet techniques to increase the SNR of fMRI images is the subject of this chapter.

To obtain an MRI image, one applies a strong magnetic field to the material to be imaged. This creates additional energy states in the material that are associated with the magnetic moments of spinning charged particles. These particles will readily absorb energy that is applied at the Larmor (or precession) frequency of the particle, which depends on the charge of the particle and the magnetic field strength. For a proton, the Larmor frequency is 42.58 MHz per Tesla. Thus, radio frequency (RF) pulses are used to excite protons to higher energy states. The energy decay of the particles will occur in quanta related to the Larmor frequency of the net local magnetic field strength. By superimposing a gradient magnetic field over the larger static field, nondirectional radio antennae can determine the spatial source of emissions by determining the frequency. Therefore, the quantity of a particular molecular species in a region of the brain can be determined by the strength and timing of emissions from that region bearing the radio signature of that species.

There are many types of fMRI, each designed to image specific types of physiological activity [21]. The most common fMRI technique used to capture functional images of the brain employs blood oxygenation level-dependent (BOLD) contrast [24]. The link between blood oxygenation levels and functional activation of the brain was revealed by PET studies in the 1980s. During regional brain activation, the blood volume supplied to the region increases. However, the brain does not utilize the additional oxygen, resulting in a higher relative concentration of oxygenated hemoglobin in active regions. Nobel Laureate Linus Pauling established in 1935 that the magnetic susceptibility of hemoglobin changes as a function of oxygen saturation, and this change is used in BOLD-contrast fMRI to measure the ratio of oxygenated to deoxygenated hemoglobin which indicates metabolically active brain regions.

4.2   Image Acquisition

The preferred way to detect blood oxygenation levels is to use MRI RF sequences such as gradient echo or spin echo with echo-planar imaging (EPI) equipment or fast gradient echo imaging (such as fast low angle shot imaging (FLASH)) with traditional MRI equipment [3, 7, 13]. The best SNR for BOLD-related effects is provided by EPI equipment. EPI is a very fast imaging technique that relies on fast magnetic gradient field switching. The BOLD-related signal increases with the square of the magnetic field strength. Pulling the small BOLD signal out of the noise is best accomplished using MRI systems with large magnets, such as 4.0 tesla machines. However, these large machines are very expensive and not readily available. Many of the clinical MRI machines in common use have 1.5 tesla magnetic coils and can be readily modified to perform BOLD imaging. The fMRI data we will examine in this chapter were obtained on such a 1.5 tesla machine. The BOLD-related signal increases are on the order of 1–3% with a 1.5 tesla MRI [13].

MRI images may be captured in a two-dimensional or three-dimensional format. Two-dimensional images are made up of pixels with the image representing a cross-sectional slice of the target. Stacking several of these slices will effectively cover a volume. In three-dimensional images, the image is made up of voxels that represent the material contained in a volume of space. The volumes are collected in layers to cover the region of interest [28]. An EPI system can acquire a 64×64 array of voxels in approximately 40 milliseconds.

Once the images are obtained, there are two distinct steps one must perform to detect regions of activation. The first step is image registration, and the second step is identification of areas of functional activation from the sequential image set. One must register each image in the time series so that it aligns with the other images. Failure to align the images will result in spurious artifacts during the analysis. This is especially true when the area of interest is near a point of high contrast such as the cerebral spinal fluid (CSF) and brain interface. If this is the case, a voxel may be dominated by gray matter in one image and by CSF in the next. The difference between the two voxels may show up in the image analysis as a region of activation. To prevent this, the images must be shifted to compensate for magnetic field inhomogeneities and subject motion during the image sequence. Excessive motion is not always correctable because the plane of the image may tilt in relation to other images. In these cases, one usually discards the data.

4.3   fMRI Time Series Analysis

The analysis software used to detect activation is usually very dependent on the specific study. Most of the fMRI analysis tools are closely related to PET analysis tools. Several studies have been designed to provide data that are directly comparable to previous PET studies [14, 18–20]. These studies set out to demonstrate the value of fMRI on the basis of similarity of results. While the two do have significant commonalities, there are important differences between PET and fMRI. Because PET data contain more noise, PET studies typically require statistical averaging of data across a sampling of patients. By comparison, thresholds for fMRI activation are usually established using less data and can yield valid data for a single patient. As a result, fMRI has more potential to provide diagnostic-quality information for a single patient [20]. With a smaller data set, one must pay close attention to the specific techniques employed. Of particular concern is the relation of regional variances to global data that encompass the entire brain [5, 15].

In the simplest and most common analysis technique, one forms a "baseline" image by averaging approximately ten resting state images together. One then compares the activated images to the baseline by subtracting and looking at the residual. One can also average the activated images together before subtraction, resulting in a fuzzy image with indistinct activation areas. One can show the statistical significance of activated areas by determining the standard deviation of the resting state images and displaying the subtracted residual image in standard deviation units. Although this technique provides interesting results for very simple studies, the activation images are very noisy and suffer from many artifacts. Using this method, Duyn et al. [13] report that under certain conditions, in-flow effects from venous and arterial water and possibly cerebral spinal fluid may dominate the BOLD-related signal increases. Furthermore, Duyn et al. report that it is not possible to identify a priori when those conditions might arise. As a result, this technique is not satisfactory for many studies [3].

One can use Fourier analysis to preserve information that would be lost in statistical averaging and also to eliminate more noise from the image. Simple repetitive physical motions, such as tapping a finger, are well suited to Fourier analysis, as are studies that employ flashing lights or pulsing photic stimulus. This technique can be used for other studies by artificially creating a repetitive environment by alternating resting and activated images. This results in much improved, clearer images than obtained from simple averaging. Fourier techniques, however, do not eliminate noise from multiple, large magnitude, non-related signal changes [3]. In general, Fourier analysis is not suitable for complex stimuli and actions.

More information can be extracted by making a correlation comparison between the stimulus input and the output. In a noisy environment, events that are time-locked to the stimulus rise out of the noncorrelated noise if averaged over many repetitions. Some researchers caution against a simplistic implementation of a correlation analysis [29]. Simple implementations of a correlation comparison can lose information. This is because fMRI images capture neural activity that has been modified by the physiological process of blood oxygen level. The response time delays of this hemodynamic process are well documented (see Section 4.3.1 below). The hemodynamic process is manifested as a low-pass filter between neural activity and the image. One can observe this low-pass effect by having the subject perform a repetitive task such as tapping his fingers while a time-series of fMRI data is collected. One then performs a Fourier analysis on the data which should show a distinct spike at the frequency of finger-tapping. The strength of the signal decreases as the rate of finger-tapping reaches the effective cut-off frequency of the hemodynamic response function. A correlation that fails to account for the time delays of the process can result in a phase cancellation of a significant activation.

4.3.1   The Hemodynamic Response Function

The hemodynamic process that underlies BOLD-contrast imaging does not respond instantaneously to neurological events. There is a 200–400 milliseconds delay following neuronal activity before an increase in oxygen use by the brain cells occurs. Regional blood volume increases 300–400 ms later. About 1 second after neuronal activity starts, the oxygen saturation of the blood rises. The rise is maximal between 4 and 10 s after the process starts. Additionally, the increase in blood oxygen level occurs over a region larger than that of activation. Thus, the hemodynamic process is both dispersing and delayed compared to neural activity [16]. One can capture a single MRI slice in as little as 20 ms and a multislice image in 100 ms to 5 s with EPI equipment. So, although the temporal resolution of fMRI is very good, the information one obtains is limited by the physiological process that filters the neural activity. Furthermore, the effective oversampling of the process results in smooth data that contain autocorrelations. For data collection that is fast compared to the hemodynamic response, the analysis software must locate the significant cross-correlations in the presence of the intrinsic autocorrelations [16].

By oversampling, one can observe features of the hemodynamic response and use them to discriminate the signal from the noise. One can match features from sequential, continuous voxels in the time and frequency domain to identify a response that matches a specified hemodynamic rise function [2].

One can also analyze voxel data from unactivated images through time to determine an intrinsic activity level, forming the basis of a noise characterization. One can then set an activation threshold that provides a fixed false positive rate such as 0.05. The activation threshold may either vary from voxel to voxel or be fixed globally. Next, one convolves the functional stimulus input with an operator that is based on the spatial dispersion and temporal delay properties of the hemodynamic response. A comparison between the convolved functional stimulus input and the observed data can then be made. One considers areas that exceed the activation threshold to be functionally activated by the stimulus. Additionally, by convolving the input function, artifacts that are time-linked to the stimulus but not filtered by the hemodynamic process are prevented [16]. This sort of artifact could otherwise come from physical motion that is part of (or related to) the stimulus, such as in motion studies or those requiring physical feedback.

4.4   Wavelet Denoising of Signals

Collecting many repetitions of activated and nonactivated images eases extraction of the desired signal from the noise. Functional MRI studies have shown that averaging results over a group of individuals loses information due to variations in human brain function. In one study, Binder et al. [3] noted that in direct comparison to PET results, the fMRI data revealed that there were many details of auditory processing that varied in functional location among individuals. This information was not identifiable from the PET data, but was detectable using fMRI [22]. However, even in a single human, functional details of the brain may be lost by repetitive sequences because the brain modifies its structure based on past events. This feature, known as brain plasticity, has been captured by fMRI in both the visual and motor regions of the brain. In the hierarchical structure of the brain, simple or repeated tasks are learned and assumed by lower brain structures. Functional activation studies have revealed cases where the brain relegated a repeated task to a lower region of the brain in later repetitions. Additionally, imaging sequential events or complex actions that are not repeatable will require different analysis techniques. For these reasons, averaging multiple image sequences is not a desirable way to increase the signal-to-noise ratio of fMRI data.

In the last few years, wavelets have emerged as a powerful tool for extracting signals from noisy data. For the case of Gaussian white noise, the signal extraction problem can be stated as follows: how can one determine the true values of a signal f, given a set $f^{\tilde{}}$ of noisy observations

$$f_i^{\tilde{}} = f_i + \sigma z_i, \quad i = 0, \dots, n - 1, \tag{4.1}$$

where $f_i^{\tilde{}} = f^{\tilde{}}(t_i)$ and $f_i = f(t_i)$ at times $t_i = i/n$, σ is the standard deviation of the noise, and the z_i are i.i.d. random variables distributed according to $\mathcal{N}(0, 1)$. In the wavelet domain, we can rewrite (4.1) as

$$W_\psi f_i^{\tilde{}} = (W_\psi)(f_i + \sigma z_i) = W_\psi f_i + \sigma(W_\psi z_i).$$

If the basis functions of our wavelet are orthonormal, the wavelet transform of Gaussian white noise z_i is a Gaussian white noise w_i of the same amplitude, so

$$W_\psi f_i^{\tilde{}} = W_\psi f_i + \sigma w_i.$$

Solving for f_i yields

$$f_i = (W_\psi^{-1})(W_\psi f_i^{\tilde{}} - \sigma w_i).$$

In general we do not know σw_i, so we estimate it by some value λ, giving

$$f_i \approx (W_\psi^{-1})(W_\psi f_i^{\tilde{}} - \lambda).$$

Our desire, then, is to remove the estimated noise contribution λ from each of the wavelet coefficients in $W_\psi f^{\tilde{}}$. An appropriate way to do this is by applying a nonlinear *soft thresholding* operation [9, 8, 30]

$$\eta_\lambda(x) = \begin{cases} x - \lambda, & x \geq \lambda \\ 0, & |x| < \lambda \\ x + \lambda, & x < -\lambda \end{cases}$$

to each coefficient in the detail signals of $W_\psi \tilde{f}$.

A fundamental issue in signal recovery is the choice of the threshold λ, and a variety of methods have been proposed [1, 9–11, 23, 25, 26]. This chapter will consider both a global approach and a data-driven approach for choosing λ. The first method is the "VisuShrink" universal threshold due to Donoho and Johnstone [10]:

$$\lambda = \sigma\sqrt{2\log(n)} \tag{4.2}$$

where n is the number of data samples. This approach has been well developed in [9, 12]. Typically, the true value of the noise standard deviation σ is not known, so σ in (4.2) is replaced by $\hat{\sigma} = MAD/0.6745$, where MAD is the median absolute value of the finest scale wavelet coefficients [10]. The second method uses a data analytic approach that considers both the magnitudes and spatial relationships of empirical wavelet coefficients when determining λ, the development of which is traced here.

4.4.1 Data Analytic Thresholding

We now describe a thresholding technique which considers both the magnitude and location of wavelet coefficients. A threshold λ_ν is selected separately for each level of coefficients according to the two-dimensional analogue of the procedure described in [25]. The method consists of examining empirical wavelet coefficients level-by-level and recursively removing large coefficients until the remaining coefficients resemble a sequence of white noise according to some given criterion.

One-Dimensional Threshold Selection

It is informative to begin with the one-dimensional procedure of [25] before describing its two-dimensional extension. Let $d_j(1), \ldots, d_j(n)$ represent the noisy (one-dimensional) wavelet coefficients at some level j. Unless there is sufficient statistical evidence that there is signal present among these coefficients, all the coefficients are shrunk to zero.

If the data come from a Gaussian distribution and if the wavelet basis is orthogonal, then the empirical coefficients $d_j(1), \ldots, d_j(n)$ have independent normal distributions, each with variance σ^2 and respective means $\mu_1, \ldots, \mu_n$. Note that $\mu_1, \ldots, \mu_n$ could be computed with knowledge of the true function by taking its wavelet transform.

To obtain a parsimonious representation of the signal, most of the coefficients are initially assumed to be essentially zero. The technique described here consists of a statistical test of hypotheses of $H_0 : \mu_1 = \ldots = \mu_n = 0$, with one or more nonzero μ_is comprising the alternative.

The hypotheses can be tested according to the coefficient magnitudes only (as in, e.g., [26] and [1]), but it is possible to take advantage of the spatial clustering of significant coefficients by examining the cumulative sum (CUSUM) process of the (ordered) squared coefficients. The primary question of interest is whether the set of coefficients behaves as white noise. Define the function $B^{\sim}(\cdot)$ to be

$$B^{\sim}\left(\frac{i}{n}\right) = \frac{1}{\sigma\sqrt{2n}} \sum_{k=1}^{i} \left(d_j(k)^2 - \overline{d_j^2}\right) \tag{4.3}$$

for $i = 1, \ldots, n$ where $\overline{d_j^2}$ denotes the mean of the squared $d_j(i)$s. Define $B^{\sim}(0)$ to be zero and linearly interpolate between points defined in (4.3) to get a continuous process on the interval $[0, 1]$. For n large, under the null hypothesis, $B^{\sim}$ behaves asymptotically like a *Brownian bridge stochastic process*, or *pinned down Brownian motion*, so denoted because $B^{\sim}(0) = B^{\sim}(1) = 0$ [27].

Of course, if some signal is present at the current level, the behavior of the function in (4.3) will depart from that of a typical Brownian bridge. The departure can be measured in several ways (most of which have their origins in statistical goodness-of-fit testing), but the one considered here is the supremum functional

$$K = \max_{1 \leq i \leq n} \left| B^{\sim}\left(\frac{i}{n}\right) \right|$$

corresponding to the usual Kolmogorov-Smirnov test statistic. If K is less than the appropriate critical value (≈ 1.36, if $\alpha = 0.05$), then the function is considered to contain only noise.

In essence, the algorithm begins by forming the sample Brownian bridge process and testing to see if there is signal present. If H_0 is rejected (i.e., it is concluded that there is signal present), the coefficient with the largest absolute value is removed from consideration for the time being, the Brownian bridge is recomputed and the test is performed again. Continuing in this way ultimately leads to a set of coefficients that are not judged to have significant signal present, and the threshold λ_j is set to σ times the largest (in absolute value) coefficient in that set, the amount by which all the coefficients at the current level are shrunk.

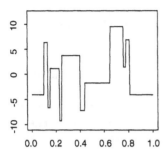 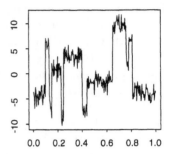

Figure 4.1
Blocky function and blocky function with noise, $n = 256$, SNR = 5dB.

In practical situations, the error variance is unknown, so as in the global thresholding procedure, σ in (4.3) and in the preceding paragraph is replaced by $\hat{\sigma}$.

This approach to denoising in one dimension is illustrated using a simulated example of a function with multiple jumps. The function itself (introduced in [10]) and the function with noise added ($n = 256$, SNR = 5dB) is displayed in Figure 4.1. The de-noising procedure is depicted for level 6 in Figure 4.2: the first plot is the simple cumulative sum of the squared empirical coefficients; the second plot is the Brownian bridge version of the full data set; and the third plot is the Brownian bridge process when the largest 11 coefficients are removed. The results of the VisuShrink and the data analytic ($\alpha = .05$) procedures applied to the simulated dataset are shown in Figure 4.3. An inherent advantage of the data analytic threshold selection technique is that one has some control over the smoothness of the resulting estimator via the level of the tests: a small α would result in a smoother estimate, and a large α would yield a more wiggly result.

Two-Dimensional Threshold Selection

A two-dimensional version of this procedure is introduced in [17], which is briefly outlined here. Let $d_j(k, \ell)$, where $1 \leq k, \ell \leq n$, denote the wavelet coefficients of a particular level of the wavelet transform of a two-dimensional signal. As in the one-dimensional case, we form a cumulative sum process

$$BS^z\left(\frac{k}{n}, \frac{\ell}{n}\right) = \frac{1}{\sigma} \sum_{q=1}^{k} \sum_{r=1}^{\ell} \left(d_j(q, r)^2 - \overline{d_j^2}\right) \tag{4.4}$$

where

$$\overline{d_j^2} = \frac{1}{n^2} \sum_{k=1}^{n} \sum_{\ell=1}^{n} d_j(k, \ell)^2.$$

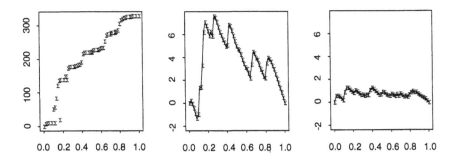

Figure 4.2
Left to right: the CUSUM of the squared coefficients at level 6; the corresponding full Brownian bridge process; and the "cleaned up" Brownian bridge process.

Considered as a function on the unit square $[0, 1] \times [0, 1]$, the process in (4.4) is proportional to a *Brownian sheet*, since $BS^{\sim}(u, 0) = BS^{\sim}(0, v) = BS^{\sim}(1, 1) = 0$. The corresponding test statistic is then

$$K = \max_{1 \leq k, \ell \leq n} \left| BS^{\sim}\left(\frac{k}{n}, \frac{\ell}{n}\right) \right|,$$

which is compared to the appropriate critical value. Simulated critical points for this situation are tabulated in [17].

Again, if the value of σ is unknown, it can be estimated as in the one-dimensional case from the finest-scale wavelet coefficients.

In the one-dimensional case, when it is determined that signal is present, the coefficient with the largest absolute value is removed from consideration and the remaining coefficients are "collapsed" in, with n diminished by one before the Brownian bridge is computed again. In the two-dimensional case, it is not possible to remove a coefficient in such a way, so the largest coefficient is replaced by one (the expected value of the coefficient under the null hypothesis) before the Brownian sheet is recomputed.

The wavelet coefficients at each level are treated separately, so the threshold λ_j depends only on the values of the coefficients at level j. All of the wavelet coefficients at level j are shrunk by the chosen threshold λ_j. If the wavelet decomposition being used yields a set of directionally sensitive detail signals, each detail signal is processed separately.

Figure 4.4 shows the results of applying the two-dimensional wavelet denoising algorithms described here to a 64×64 box function corrupted by $\mathcal{N}(0, 0.2)$ noise. The Haar wavelet was chosen to use in this example because its shape closely matches the box function; other wavelets may be more suitable in other circumstances. Denoising was performed on the

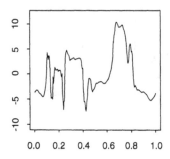 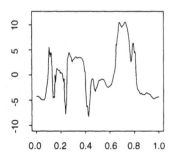

Figure 4.3
Left: VisuShrunk wavelet estimator. Right: Data analytic wavelet estimator with $\alpha = .05$.

three finest levels of the wavelet decomposition, and the standard deviation of the noise was estimated using $\hat{\sigma}$. A low-pass filtering with the kernel

$$\frac{1}{9} \times \begin{bmatrix} 1 & 1 & 1 \\ 1 & 1 & 1 \\ 1 & 1 & 1 \end{bmatrix}$$

is also shown for comparison.

4.5 Experimental Results

This section describes experiments performed on three different fMRI data sets to investigate the effects of wavelet denoising on fMRI analysis. We first describe the data sets used in the experiments, then the analysis technique, and finally, we compare the analysis results of the original and denoised data sets.

4.5.1 Data Set Descriptions

The three fMRI data sets we examined were provided by the Laboratory of Diagnostic Radiology Research, NIH. The data sets were acquired as part of a photic stimulation study which fixated on a small spot for a period of time and then fixated at an 8-Hz reversing red/black checkerboard pattern [14]. The fMRI images were acquired using echo planar imaging on a GE Signa 1.5 tesla system at a rate of approximately one volume per minute. Each volume consists of a number of 64×64 voxel slices, with

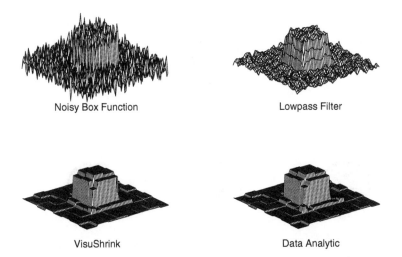

Figure 4.4
Example of 2-D noise removal.

a voxel dimension of 5 mm^3, spanning the occipital and posterior parietal cortex. Because the sampling period is much longer than the hemodynamic response of the brain (1 minute vs. several seconds) we need not worry about the presence of intrinsic autocorrelations.

Each of the three fMRI data sets was obtained from a different subject. Data set 1 consists of 27 volumes of fixation followed by 27 volumes of reversing checkerboard, repeated twice, giving a total of 108 volumes. Each volume in Data set 1 consists of 14 coronal slices; a sample volume is shown in Figure 4.5. Data set 1 is fairly low in noise and has few motion artifacts. Data sets 2 and 3 consist of two cycles of 18 volumes of fixation followed by 18 volumes of reversing checkerboard. Each volume consists of 20 coronal slices. Data sets 2 and 3 are high in noise, with strong motion artifacts. Image registration using Woods' algorithm [31] was performed on the data sets before analysis.

4.5.2 Analysis Technique

The photic stimulation experiment was designed to produce changes in the blood volume of those parts of the brain involved in visual processing. An increase in a region's blood volume is indicated by an increase in the MR signal strength of the region's voxels. To determine if a voxel's mean signal strength has changed in a statistically significant way, we follow the analysis strategy of Eden et al. [14] and use the standard t-test to compare a voxel's values while staring at a fixation point to the voxel's values while staring at the reversing checkerboard.

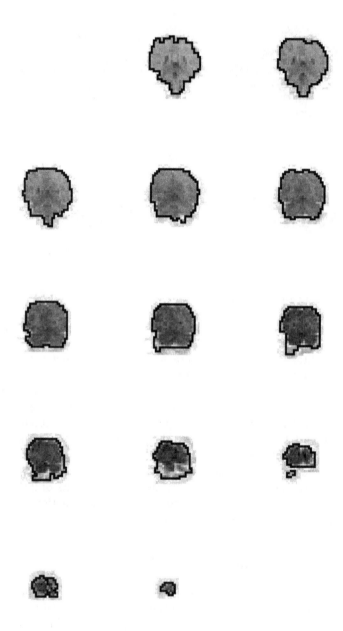

Figure 4.5
A typical volume from data set 1. The dark outlines indicate the
regions included in the statistical analyses.

A complete description of the analysis performed on each data set is as follows:

1. *Mask Generation.* The large amounts of data involved in data set analysis result in a heavy computational burden. To relieve some of this burden, we mask out those voxels that are outside of the brain. A mean volume is formed by averaging, voxel by voxel, the entire volume data set. A masking threshold is set at 20% of the largest voxel value in the mean volume. Every voxel in the mean volume is compared to the masking threshold, and any voxel whose mean value is less than the masking threshold is masked out and will not be considered further in the analysis. After masking, the mean volume is no longer needed and can be discarded.

2. *Create Zero-Mean Volumes.* To remove the effects of any global drifts in signal strength, each volume is independently normalized by subtracting its mean value from each of its voxels.

3. *Statistical Map Generation.* A time series for each voxel is extracted from the data set. Each voxel's time series is split into two groups: those values recorded while staring at the fixation spot, and those values recorded while staring at the reversing checkerboard. A t-test is performed to decide if these two groups have the same mean. The t-statistic for each voxel is recorded into a *statistical map*. The resulting statistical map is thresholded by an appropriate critical value to determine which voxels experience a statistically meaningful change in blood volume during photic stimulation.

Analysis of the statistical map is not as straightforward as it sounds. Because of the large number of t-tests performed, one would normally use a Bonferroni correction to control the number of false positive results. However, many fMRI researchers believe that the Bonferroni-corrected critical value is too large; there is no clear consensus as to what adjustment should be made to the critical value [32]. Another factor complicating the analysis is that brain activity unrelated to the experimental stimulus may result in a significant t-statistic for some voxels. This is especially true for long data sets, such as those examined here. As a result of these complications, somewhat arbitrary rules of thumb are used to threshold the statistical map. The rule of thumb we will follow in this chapter is, after Zeffiro [32], to use one-third of the value of the maximum t-statistic as the critical value *if* this value is larger than the standard critical value for $\alpha = 0.0005$.

The statistical map generated for data set 1 is shown in the left half of Figure 4.6. The maximum t-statistic is 28.8, and the critical value set by the 1/3 maximum rule of thumb is 9.3. A total of 50 voxels exceed this critical value; their locations are shown in the right half of Figure 4.6. The

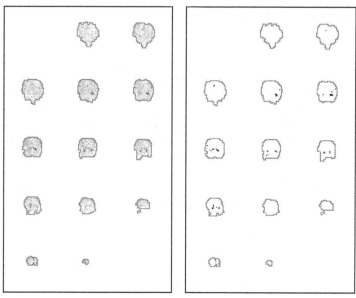

Statistical Map   Tresholded Statistical Map

Figure 4.6
Left: Statistical map for data set 1. Darker voxels correspond to larger *t*-statistics. Right: Thresholded statistical map. The dark voxels indicate regions of the brain activated by the photic stimulus.

maximum *t*-statistic of data sets 2 and 3 is 8.9 and 10.2, respectively.

We note that Ruttimann et al. have also proposed a wavelet-based fMRI analysis procedure, which is described in another chapter of this book. In their technique, the statistical testing is done in the wavelet domain on the empirical wavelet coefficients themselves.

4.5.3   Denoising Results

Each slice of each volume of the fMRI data sets was denoised independently using VisuShrink, the data analytic algorithm of Section 4.4.1, and a simple 3×3 lowpass filter with kernel

$$\frac{1}{9} \times \begin{bmatrix} 1 & 1 & 1 \\ 1 & 1 & 1 \\ 1 & 1 & 1 \end{bmatrix}.$$

Daubechies' six-coefficient orthonormal wavelet [6] was used for denoising the three finest levels of each slice's wavelet decomposition. The denoised

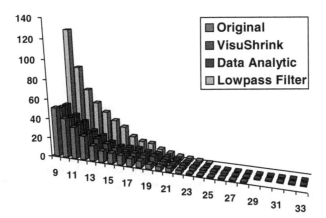

Figure 4.7
Cumulative histogram of data set 1 voxel t-statistics that are above the critical value.

data sets were then analyzed as described above and the resulting statistical maps were compared with the statistical maps of the original data sets.

In order to evaluate our numerical results, we should know what to look for, i.e., what the effect of denoising an fMRI data set *should* be. If we had an ideal data set with a small noise level, the t-statistic for voxels that were not activated by the stimulus would be close to zero, and the t-statistic for those voxels that were activated by the stimulus would be very large. The larger the difference in voxel activation, the larger the t-statistic. Contamination with greater amounts of noise will make it more difficult to distinguish when the mean values are different and thus lower the t-statistics. Denoising a data set, then, should improve the discriminating power of the t-test, increasing the magnitude of the t-statistic for those voxels that have different means.

Data Set 1

Wavelet denoising of data set 1 does indeed produce an increase in t-statistic magnitude for those voxels that were previously determined (by analysis of the noisy data set 1) to be stimulated. The magnitude of the maximum t-statistic was increased 17% by the data analytic algorithm and 14% by the VisuShrink algorithm. At the same time, the number of voxels greater than the original data set's critical value of 9.3 did not change significantly. A cumulative histogram of voxel t-statistics is presented in Figure 4.7. Direct comparison of the statistical maps of the original and denoised data sets indicates a general rise in the magnitude of local maxima.

Low-pass filtering of data set 1 does not perform well. The maximum t-statistic is smaller than that of the noisy original data set, and the number of voxels above the critical value is more than twice that of the original data

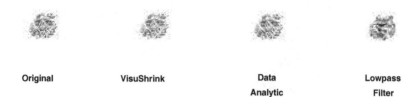

| Original | VisuShrink | Data
Analytic | Lowpass
Filter |

Figure 4.8
Statistical maps of a slice from data set 2 showing quite different results obtained from the wavelet and low-pass filtering noise removal algorithms.

set. Examination of the statistical maps indicates that the local maxima of the low-pass filtered data set are often in different locations than the local maxima of the other data sets.

Data Set 2
Wavelet denoising of data set 2 has very little impact on analysis. The maximum t-statistic value changes by less than one percent, the cumulative histogram of voxel t-statistics is almost identical, and the location and value of local maxima remain approximately the same. Low-pass filtering, on the other hand, raises the maximum t-statistic by 73%, reduces the number of local maxima by a third, and changes their location. Figure 4.8 shows the statistical maps for the slice that experienced the greatest changes in local maxima. A possible explanation for this behavior could lie with the motion artifacts present in this data set.

Data Set 3
Denoising of data set 3, either by the wavelet algorithms or low-pass filtering, results in a general *decrease* in the magnitude of t-statistics: a decrease of 22% for VisuShrink, 13% for the data analytic algorithm, and 14% for low-pass filtering. There is also a drop in the t-statistic cumulative histogram for the denoised data sets (see Figure 4.9) and a reduction in the number of local maxima above the critical value. Again, a possible explanation for this behavior could lie with the motion artifacts present in this data set.

The VisuShrink and data analytic algorithms yield similar results for data sets 1 and 2, but show significant differences for data set 3. For this data set, the maximum t-statistic produced by data analytic denoising is greater than that produced by VisuShrink, but the data analytic algorithm also produces far fewer local maxima than VisuShrink. In fact, the data analytic results for data set 3 resemble those of the low-pass filter much more than those of VisuShrink. This may be due to motion artifacts, since low-pass

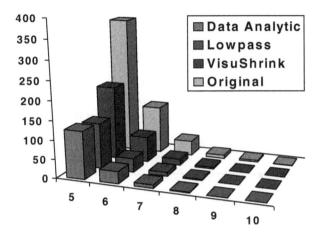

Figure 4.9
Cumulative histogram of data set 3 voxel *t*-statistics that are above the critical value.

filtering and data analytic denoising are both area-sensitive techniques, while VisuShrink is not.

4.6 Conclusions

Based on the analysis results of these three data sets, it is apparent that applying wavelets to the problem of fMRI imaging has the potential to become a useful new analysis tool. Due to the divergent results from these example data sets, it is also evident that there is room for more study to investigate which thresholding strategies are most appropriate overall, and also to identify which methods perform better for special situations (e.g., when there are residual motion artifacts).

The thresholding techniques considered in this study are ones that result in a relatively "smooth" image. Other thresholding techniques could also be considered which have better mean square error properties (but give less smooth results), such as the SURE thresholding method of [11].

The analysis procedure in this paper consisted of two-dimensional denoising of each image slice performed independently of the others before voxels were compared. It would also be interesting to consider smoothing the data set with three-dimensional wavelet bases, and perhaps even four-dimensional bases when appropriate.

4.7   Acknowledgment

The authors would like to thank Tom Zeffiro of the Laboratory of Diagnostic Radiology Research, NIH, and Sensor Systems, Inc., for providing access to fMRI data and sharing his expertise in fMRI data analysis.

References

[1] F. Abramovich and Y. Benjamini. Adaptive thresholding of wavelet coefficients. Preprint, 1994.

[2] P. A. Bandettini, A. Jesmanowicz, E. C. Wong, and J. S. Hyde. Processing strategies for time-course data sets in functional MRI of the human brain. *Magn. Reson. Med.*, 30:161–173, 1993.

[3] J. R. Binder and S. M. Rao. Human brain mapping with functional magnetic resonance imaging. In *Localization and Neuroimaging in Neuropsychology*, A. Kertesz, editor, Academic Press, New York, 185–212, 1994.

[4] H. Chertkow and D. Bub. Functional activation and cognition: The ^{15}o PET subtraction method. In *Localization and Neuroimaging in Neuropsychology*, A. Kertesz, editor, Academic Press, New York, 151–184, 1994.

[5] C. Clark and R. Carson. Analysis of covariance in statistical parametric mapping. *J. Cereb. Blood Flow Metab.*, 13:1038, 1993.

[6] I. Daubechies. Orthonormal bases of compactly supported wavelets. *Commun. Pure Appl. Math.*, 41:909–996, 1988.

[7] R. L. DeLaPaz. Echo-planar imaging. *Radiographics*, 14:1045–1058, 1994.

[8] R. A. DeVore and B. J. Lucier. Fast wavelet techniques for near-optimal processing. In *IEEE Military Commun. Conf.*, pages 48.3.1–48.3.7, 1992.

[9] D. L. Donoho. De-noising by soft-thresholding. *IEEE Trans. Inf. Theory*, 41(3):613–627, 1995.

[10] D. L. Donoho and I. M. Johnstone. Ideal spatial adaptation via wavelet shrinkage. *Biometrika*, 81:425–455, 1994.

[11] D. L. Donoho and I. M. Johnstone. Adapting to unknown smoothness via wavelet shrinkage. *J. Am. Stat. Assoc.*, to appear.

[12] D. L. Donoho, I. M. Johnstone, G. Kerkyacharian, and D. Picard. Wavelet shrinkage: Asymptopia? *J. Roy. Stat. Soc., Ser. B*, 57:301–369, 1995.

[13] J. H. Duyn, V. S. Mattay, R. H. Sexton, G. S. Sobering, F. A. Barrios, G. Liu, J. A. Frank, D. R. Weinbergerm, and C. T. Moonen. 3-dimensional functional imaging of human brain using echo-shifted FLASH MRI. *Magn. Reson. Med.*, 32:150–155, 1994.

[14] G. F. Eden, J. W. vanMeter, J. M. Maisog, P. Jezzard, P. Herscovitch, J. L. Rapoport, and T. A. Zeffiro. A comparison of PET and MRFN techniques using a visual stimulus. *Human Brain Mapping*, S39, 1995.

[15] K. J. Friston. Reply to "Analysis of covariance in statistical parametric mapping". *J. Cereb. Blood Flow Metab..*, 13:1038–1040, 1993.

[16] K. J. Friston, P. Jezzard, and R. Turner. Analysis of functional MRI time-series. *Human Brain Mapping*, 1:153–171, 1994.

[17] M. L. Hilton and R. T. Ogden. Data analytic threshold selection in wavelet image de-noising. Tech. Rep. TR9503, Department of Computer Science, University of South Carolina, Columbia, 1995.

[18] S. G. Kim, J. Ashe, K. Hendrich, J. M. Ellermann, H. Merkle, K. Ugurbil, and A. P. Georgopoulos. Functional magnetic resonance imaging of motor cortex: Hemispheric asymmetry and handedness. *Science*, 261:615–617, 1993.

[19] G. McCarthy, A. M. Blamire, A. Puce, A. C. Nobre, G. Bloch, F. Hyder, P. Goldman-Rakic, and R. G. Shulman. Functional magnetic resonance imaging of human prefrontal cortex activation during a spatial working memory task. *Proc. Natl. Acad. Sci. U.S.A.*, 91:8690–8694, 1994.

[20] G. McCarthy, A. M. Blamire, D. L. Rothman, R. Gruetter, and R. G. Shulman. Echo-planar magnetic resonance imaging studies of frontal cortex activation during word generation in humans. *Proc. Natl. Acad. Sci. U.S.A.*, 90:4952–4956, 1993.

[21] C. T. W. Moonen, P. C. M. van Zijl, J. A. Frank, D. Le Bihan, and E. D. Becker. Functional magnetic resonance imaging in medicine and physiology. *Science*, 250:53–61, 1990.

[22] R. Naeye. The brain at work. *Discover*, 15:30–31, 1994.

[23] G. P. Nason. Wavelet regression by cross-validation. Tech. Rep. 447, Department of Statistics, Stanford University, Stanford, California, 1994.

[24] S. Ogawa, R. S. Menon, D. W. Tank, S.-G. Kim, H. Merkle, J. M. Ellerman, and K. Ugurbil. Functional brain mapping by blood oxygenation level-dependent contrast magnetic resonance imaging. *Biophys. J.*, 64:803–812, 1993.

[25] R. T. Ogden and E. Parzen. Change-point approach to data analytic wavelet thresholding. *Stat. Comput.*, to appear.

[26] R. T. Ogden and E. Parzen. Data dependent wavelet thresholding in nonparametric regression with change-point applications. *Computational Stat. Data Anal.*, to appear.

[27] S. M. Ross. *Stochastic Processes*. Wiley, New York, 1993.

[28] A. W. Song, E. C. Wong, and J. S. Hyde. Echo-volume imaging. *Magn. Reson. Med.*, 32:668–671, 1994.

[29] S. C. Strother, I. Kanno, and D. A. Rottenberg. Principle component analysis, variance partitioning, and "functional connectivity". *J. Cereb. Blood Flow Metab.*, 15:353–360, 1995.

[30] J. B. Weaver, X. Yansun, D. M. Healy, and L. D. Cromwell. Filtering noise from images with wavelet transforms. *Magn. Reson. Med.*, 21(2):288–295, 1991.

[31] R. P. Woods, S. R. Cherry, and J. C. Mazziota. Rapid automated algorithm for aligning and reslicing PET images. *J. Comput. Assist. Tomography*, 16(4):620–633, 1992.

[32] T. Zeffiro. Personal communication.

5

Statistical Analysis of Image Differences by Wavelet Decomposition

Urs E. Ruttimann[1], Michael Unser[2], Philippe Thévenaz[2], Chulhee Lee[2], Daniel Rio[1], and Daniel W. Hommer[1]

[1] *National Institute on Alcohol Abuse and Alcoholism*
[2] *Biomedical Engineering and Instrumentation Program, National Institutes of Health, Bethesda, MD*

5.1 Introduction

Functional neuroimaging is a fast-developing area aimed at studying the dynamic functioning of the brain. Positron emission tomography (PET) [1], single photon emission computed tomography (SPECT) [2], and functional magnetic resonance imaging (fMRI) [3] are some of the modalities currently in use to quantify and localize in space some correlate (e.g., metabolic rate, blood flow) of local neuronal activity. These techniques complement the more familiar static or anatomical imaging modalities used for mapping brain structure, such as X-ray computed tomography (CT), or magnetic resonance imaging (MRI). The value of functional modalities is that they allow for the study of physiological processes in the brain of awake human subjects, either at rest or while they are performing controlled perceptual or cognitive tasks. Of interest is usually the detection of differences in focal neuronal activation patterns, either between different groups of subjects (e.g., normal vs. diseased) or between controlled experimental conditions within the same subject (e.g., rest vs. word generation). The natural variability in the resulting 2-D or 3-D spatial representations of brain activity is large and complex, requiring the use of statistical methods for signal detection. The problem of poor signal-to-noise ratio (SNR) conditions is further complicated in that the location and spatial extent of neuronal activation changes to be detected is in most studies a question of research interest, and thus unknown. Since meaningful neurophysiological interpretation of the data typically requires full use of the spatial resolution provided by the imaging device (in fact, a higher resolution would be preferred, if it only were available), neuroscientists wish to examine the data at the single-voxel level. In addition, in order not to miss any potentially important signal changes at unexpected anatomical locations, the researchers are often led to define a large volume of interest, which then necessitates examination of a very large number of voxels. In engineering terms: both the spatial location and the spatial extent or, equivalently, the frequency bandwidth of the signal to be detected are unknown. It is the needle-in-the-haystack problem where the needle size is unknown, subject to the neuroscientist's desire to find needles as small as possible!

A variety of statistical approaches have been employed to address this problem. Earliest, and still most frequently used methods are all based on subdivisions of the brain into regions of interest (ROIs), defined in terms of neuroanatomical structure [4–6]. Image information is extracted by averaging the functional signal within corresponding ROIs over subject groups of interest. The resulting data are usually analyzed using a battery of univariate statistical tests, investigating a variety of hypotheses that were largely formulated post hoc. While this approach is believed to provide a reasonable solution to the problem of anatomic variability across patients, it is extremely time-consuming and requires the involvement of a skilled operator highly trained in neuroanatomy. It is also problematic because anatomical structure (to define the ROIs) is inferred from a functional image; e.g., it may be difficult to decide whether small spatial extent of a functional signal is due to small structure size, or whether the structure is of normal size, but only partly functional. There occurs also an obvious loss of information because only a subset of the data is analyzed. To offset this loss, investigators are often driven to define more ROIs than they can reliably analyze by multivariate statistical techniques, i.e., the number of chosen ROIs is larger than the number of test subjects or test replications within the same subject [7]. Therefore, in many of these studies a multivariate analysis is abandoned in place of multiple univariate analyses, where, due to insufficient statistical power, the significance levels are usually not adjusted for multiple testing, giving rise to an uncontrolled number of false positive findings. Furthermore, there is typically substantial correlation between data from different ROIs [8], which is incompatible with the assumptions underlying the foregoing statistical approach. At the root of the problem is that ROI analysis is an exploratory data analysis tool that does not require specification of a statistical model. Then, as an afterthought, the same exploratory data are subjected to hypothesis testing, which does require model formulation.

To avoid statistical inconsistencies of that sort, propositional data analysis methods have been developed more recently. They combine observed data with specific mathematical models to attain reliable estimates of model parameters of interest and to yield consistency in hypotheses testing. These methods look at more global solutions to the signal detection problem and refrain from partitioning the images into ROIs. In one approach, Worsley et al. [9] considered the null images (i.e., absence of a signal difference) as realizations of a homogeneous Gaussian random field, which may be thought of as being generated by convolving a white-noise Gaussian random field with a kernel representing the point-spread function of the imaging device. Based on results developed by Adler [10], these workers derived an approximate p-value for the global maximum of such a field to exceed a given threshold. That threshold is much higher than critical values based on the same p-value for the standard normal distribution (z-distribution) because the theory implicitly adjusts for multiple testing. However, the corresponding adjustment may be much smaller than a Bonferroni correction for the total number of voxels in the search volume if, due to a wide point-spread function, adjacent voxels are highly correlated. Heuristically, a supervoxel consistent with the point-spread function, called *resel* for resolution element, was derived from the theory of Gaussian random fields, serving to standardize the spatial correlation in terms of scanner resolution (as opposed to voxel size). It is the number of these resels in the total search volume that is relevant for the p-value adjustment for multiple testing.

While the statistical analysis outlined in this first approach is carried out in the spatial domain, a global propositional analysis performed in the Fourier domain has also been developed [11]. Difficulties arising from spatial correlations are overcome in this approach because the power estimates at the discrete spatial frequencies supplied by the fast Fourier transform are asymptotically uncorrelated. This permits establishment of independent tests of significance in the Fourier domain, using as the null image the spectral density of a zero-mean Gaussian random field with variance estimated from the power spectra of the functional images. Based on the theory for complex multivariate Gaussian distributions [12, 13], rigorous statistical procedures can be formulated that test for significant signal power at a discrete set of spatial frequencies. Fourier coefficients not reaching statistical significance are set to zero and the pruned spectrum is inverse-transformed to display the detected signal differences in the original spatial domain. Within this framework, a Fourier domain model matching the random field constraints employed in the spatial domain approach [9] can also be obtained. This is achieved by specifying the null image as the spectrum of a homogeneous Gaussian random field generated by multiplying a constant (white noise) power density with the squared-magnitude of the Fourier-transformed point-spread function associated with the imaging device.

While the signal decomposition in the Fourier domain permits establishment of independent statistical tests at each discrete spatial frequency, it provides relatively poor localization in the spatial domain because the inverse transform of isolated coefficients of the bandwidth-limited spectrum results in signal components of the form $\sin x/x$, which decay only linearly. Since decorrelated signal components exhibit minimal spectral overlap, the objective is to devise an orthogonal decomposition system providing good localization in both the spatial and Fourier domains. The ideal system with finite support in both domains simultaneously cannot be achieved, as asserted by the theory of analytic functions and the resultant localization trade-off formulations in terms of uncertainty relations [14]. In this view, the spatial domain approach [9] and the Fourier domain approach [10] are at opposite ends of conflicting constraints by employing the smallest possible support in one of the domains, at the loss of localization in the other domain. Since a wavelet decomposition system may retain certain features from both domains (colloquially, the wavelet domain is "in-between the Fourier and the spatial domain"), a trade-off more suitable for the analysis of interest may be negotiated. In particular, narrow spatial support of the decomposition basis (with simultaneously minimal component correlation) is expected to be better adapted to the particular signal detection task than a Fourier analysis because the signal is assumed to be smooth and spatially localized (i.e., nonstationary), while the noise is uniformly distributed across the image (i.e., stationary). Hence, the wavelet transform will concentrate the signal into a small number of local coefficients, yielding favorable local SNR conditions and thus increased statistical signal detection power. This contrasts with the Fourier analysis method, which is optimal for a stationary signal model (matched filter), where the signal coefficients are spatially not localized. The corresponding SNR is therefore global and determined by the signal bandwidth, which in many applications is part of the research inquiry and thus, unknown.

Based on these motivations, we investigated the use of the wavelet transform as a possible method for obtaining simultaneously narrow support in both the spatial and Fourier domains. Then, by imposing regularity and orthogonality conditions on the wavelet transform, we exploited the image component decorrelation so achieved to develop statistical models that enable application of parametric tests of significance on wavelet coefficients directly. Subsequent inverse wavelet transform of significant coefficients only, yielded a noise-reduced reconstruction of the estimated local signals in the original space.

5.2 Wavelet Transform

The wavelet transform performs an orthogonal signal decomposition using the basis functions

$$\psi_{j,k}(t) = 2^{-j/2}\psi(2^{-j}t - k), \tag{5.1}$$

obtained through translation, k, and dilation, j, of a prototype wavelet $\psi(t)$. This permits representation of a bandlimited signal $f(t) \in V_0$ (cf. Section 1.4.2) in terms of these basis functions as

$$f(t) = \sum_{k \in \mathbf{Z}} c_J(k)\varphi_{J,k}(t) + \sum_{j=1}^{J}\sum_{k \in \mathbf{Z}} d_j(k)\psi_{j,k}(t). \tag{5.2}$$

The first term in (5.2) provides a smooth approximation of $f(t)$ at scale J by the so-called scaling function $\varphi_{J,k}(t)$. The second term is the wavelet decomposition per se, and the wavelet coefficients $d_j(k)$ can be interpreted as the residual errors between the successive signal approximations at scales $j-1$ and j, or the signal detail at scale j. Due to orthogonality, the expansion coefficients in (5.2) are obtained by the inner products

$$c_J(k) = \Big\langle f(t), \mathring{\varphi}_{J,k}(t) \Big\rangle, \quad d_j(k) = \Big\langle f(t), \mathring{\psi}_{j,k}(t) \Big\rangle. \tag{5.3}$$

The operations in (5.3) can be interpreted as a filtering operation on the signal $f(t)$ by a pair of two complementary filters h and g. The Fourier transform $\hat{h}(\omega)$ of the low-pass filter $h(n)$ yielding the approximation coefficients $c_J(k)$ must satisfy the quadrature mirror filter (QMF) conditions

$$\left|\hat{h}(\omega)\right|^2 + \left|\hat{h}(\omega + \pi)\right|^2 = 1, \tag{5.4}$$

$$\hat{h}(0) = 1 \quad \Longleftrightarrow \quad \hat{h}(\pi) = 0. \tag{5.5}$$

The filter $g(k)$ producing the wavelet coefficients $d_j(k)$ is the modulated version of $h(k)$, given by

$$g(k) = (-1)^k h(1 - k). \tag{5.6}$$

The constraint (5.5) is necessary to ensure regularity of the digital implementations of $h(k)$ (and $g(k)$); i.e., that in the limit as j indefinitely increases, the sequence $h(k)$ converges to a continuously differentiable function. In general, if there are $p+1$ zeros of $\hat{h}(\omega)$ at $\omega = \pi$, the corresponding wavelet will have vanishing moments up to order p; i.e.,

$$m_q = 0, \quad q = 0, 1, \ldots, p, \text{ where } m_q = \langle t^q, \psi(t) \rangle. \tag{5.7}$$

Constraint (5.5) implies $m_0 = 0$, at least; i.e., from the perspective of signal processing, admissible wavelets must have a zero mean and can be interpreted as impulse functions of specific bandpass filters. From (5.3), these bandpass filters are tuned to the resolution scale j. Hence, the wavelet coefficients in resolution channel j represent the amplitudes of signal components residing in a frequency bandpass that extends up to the bandlimit determined by the Nyquist condition for the sampling rate 2^{-j}. For stationary and ergodic signals, the wavelet coefficients from different channels can be decorrelated to the extent that the bandpass characteristics at different scales can be made nonoverlapping (cf. Section 5.3). Hence, decorrelation is maximized by choosing wavelets whose Fourier transform makes maximum use of the allocated frequency band and suppresses all out-of-band components completely, i.e., best approximates the ideal bandpass filter with support from one-half to the full Nyquist rate. This ideal bandpass decomposition has also been shown to be the wavelet transform that maximizes energy compaction when the spectral density of the signal is nonincreasing [15]. Accordingly, wavelets with good bandpass characteristics are expected to be most efficient for channel decorrelation and signal representation. However, the sharper the bandwidth-limiting characteristics of the wavelets, the larger the spatial support required for their implementation and thus, the larger the loss of spatial localization. The issue of selecting the most suitable wavelet basis is therefore a matter of practical compromise between adequate signal decorrelation and sufficient spatial localization.

In order to investigate the possible trade-offs between decorrelation and spatial localization for images of biomedical interest, we selected the orthogonal spline (or Battle-Lemarié) wavelets as prototypes. This family provides symmetric basis functions, and their regularity can be conveniently controlled by specifying the polynomial order of the spline. In the limit $p \to \infty$, the Battle-Lemarié wavelets (as well as many other wavelet families) approach the ideal bandpass filter, and $\psi(t)$ becomes the modulated sinc function [16, 17]. In this study, the suitability of splines of orders 0 (Haar basis), 1, 3, and 5 was investigated. Explicit filter and wavelet formulas for all spline orders can be found in [18]. The wavelet transform was implemented by the recursive method of Mallat [19] using dyadic scale factors. Extension to two dimensions was achieved by the tensor product representation

$$\Psi_{j,k}^1 = 2^{-j}\varphi(2^{-j}t_1 - k_1)\psi(2^{-j}t_2 - k_2),$$

$$\Psi_{j,k}^2 = 2^{-j}\psi(2^{-j}t_1 - k_1)\varphi(2^{-j}t_2 - k_2), \qquad (5.8)$$

$$\Psi_{j,k}^3 = 2^{-j}\psi(2^{-j}t_1 - k_1)\psi(2^{-j}t_2 - k_2), \quad k = (k_1, k_2) \in \mathbf{Z}^2,$$

defining an orthonormal basis associated with the two-dimensional scaling function

$$\Phi_{j,k} = 2^{-j}\varphi(2^{-j}t_1 - k_1)\varphi(2^{-j}t_2 - k_2), \quad k \in \mathbf{Z}^2. \qquad (5.9)$$

In this decomposition, image detail at resolution j is characterized by three wavelets $\Psi_{j,k}^m$, $m = 1, 2, 3$, called the horizontal, vertical, and diagonal channels, and the low-pass approximation $\Phi_{j,k}$.

A first example of images considered for wavelet analysis is PET images. They represent local cerebral glucose utilization measured with the radioactive tracer ^{18}F-2-fluoro-2-deoxy-D-glucose (FDG), a positron-emitting analogue of glucose. Images for this study were acquired with the Neuro-PET scanner, providing transverse and axial spatial resolution of 7 and 11.5 mm (FWHM), respectively, with an interslice separation of 3.8 mm. Ten patients with alcoholic organic mental disorders and 7 normal volunteers were studied. For each subject, 21 slices with 128×128 pixels of size 2 mm were available. The images were matched to a common standard image at each slice level by global affine transformations involving translation, rotation, anisotropic scaling, and skewing [20, 21], and then averaged for each group separately. Figure 5.1 shows corresponding averages of a cortical slice of the normal (a) and alcoholic (b) subjects. Subtraction of the two group-averages produced the images of clinical interest, depicting the average functional differences between the alcoholic patients and the normal volunteers (c), and the associated standard deviation (d).

Figure 5.2 displays the results of the wavelet decomposition of the difference image in Figure 5.1 (c) using splines of order 0 (a), and order 3 (b). Decomposition into five resolution levels is shown, where the three directional channels at each resolution are represented in the resolution pyramid as introduced by Mallat [19]. A cursory comparison of (a) vs. (b) reveals that edges in the original image are more visible for zero-order splines (Haar wavelets) than for cubic splines. This is best demonstrated in the horizontal and vertical channels at the highest resolution level, where the cubic-spline coefficients display a somewhat more noise-like appearance than the Haar coefficients. Hence, higher-order wavelets may yield more efficient decompositions for images of this kind.

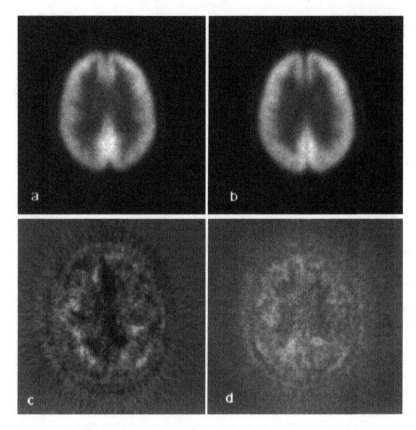

Figure 5.1
Average PET images of (a) alcoholic and (b) normal group; (c)
difference image of group averages (a)–(b); (d) standard deviation
image of the group differences.

The issue of efficiency of the decomposition is addressed more specifically in Figure 5.3. Shown is the fraction of the total power in image Figure 5.1 (c) that can be represented by the vector of the l coefficients with largest amplitudes for Fourier, Haar, and first-order spline decompositions; i.e., using, for simplicity, the one-dimensional notation of (5.2) with the vector $d_j(k)$ ordered by decreasing amplitudes $|d|_{(1)} \geq |d|_{(2)} \geq \ldots$, displayed is $q_l^2/|f(x)|^2$ vs. l, where $q_l^2 = \sum_{i \leq l} |d|_{(i)}^2$. This is a measure of how well the different orthogonal bases are able to compress a given signal into a few large coefficients. In comparison to the Fourier basis, even for a noise-like image as in this example, the wavelet decompositions are more efficient, and first-order splines are more efficient than zero-order splines. The results for third- and fifth-order splines are not shown because they are on this scale indistinguishable from that of the first-order splines. Hence, from the

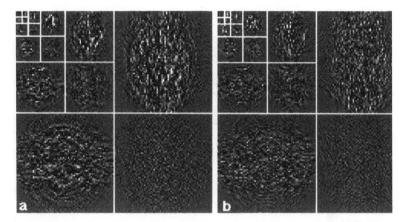

Figure 5.2
2-D wavelet representations of the average PET difference image for five resolution levels using orthogonal polynomial splines of orders (a) zero and (b) three.

cursory aspect of efficient signal representation, the use of wavelets based on at least first-order splines is suggested. A more detailed investigation of the impact of wavelet order on signal decorrelation is addressed in the next section.

5.3 Correlation of Wavelet Coefficients

For notational simplicity, we present the theoretical analysis of the correlation structure for a 1-D signal. For $f(t)$ a signal from a weakly stationary stochastic process with mean value $E[f(t)] = 0$, the autocorrelation between samples at t and s is simply a function of the lag $(s - t)$

$$R(s - t) = \mathbf{E}[f(t)f(s)]. \tag{5.10}$$

Then, from (5.3), the autocorrelation between wavelet coefficients is a random field on $\mathbf{Z}^4$ [22]

$$\mathbf{E}[d_{j_1 k_1} d_{j_2 k_2}] \tag{5.11}$$

$$= 2^{-(j_1+j_2)/2} \iint_{-\infty}^{+\infty} \psi(2^{-j_1}t - k_1)\psi(2^{-j_2}s - k_2)f(t)f(s)\,dt\,ds$$

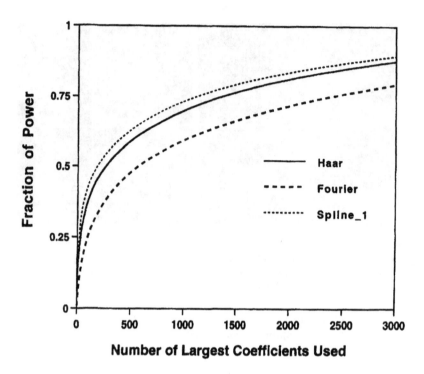

Figure 5.3
Comparison of the signal compression efficiencies for different orthogonal bases.

$$= 2^{-(j_1+j_2)/2} \iint_{-\infty}^{+\infty} \psi(2^{-j_1}t - k_1)\psi(2^{-j_2}s - k_2)R(s - t)\, dt\, ds.$$

With the variable transformations

$$u = 2^{-j_2}s - k_2, \quad \tau = 2^{-j_1}t - 2^{j_2-j_1}u - k_1,$$

and the relation between scales j_1 and j_2 expressed as the ratio $r = 2^{j_2-j_1} \leq 1$, (5.11) can be rewritten as

$$\mathbf{E}\left[d_{j_1k_1}d_{j_2k_2}\right] \tag{5.12}$$

$$= 2^{j_1} \int_{-\infty}^{+\infty} R\left[2^{j_1}(rk_2 - k_1 - \tau)\right] r^{1/2} \int_{-\infty}^{+\infty} \psi(u)\psi(ru + \tau)\, du\, d\tau.$$

Hence, the correlation structure of the coefficients depends on the autocorrelation of the process (first integral) and the wavelet prototype (second integral). Consequently, the analysis wavelet can be chosen to attain some degree of signal decorrelation. Specifically, control is exerted by the correlation between wavelets at different scales

$$k_\psi(r,\tau) = r^{1/2} \int_{-\infty}^{+\infty} \psi(u)\psi(ru+\tau)\, du, \tag{5.13}$$

also called the reproducing kernel of the analysis because it is the wavelet transform of the wavelet itself [23], which is a function of the ratio r of the scales and the relative displacement τ of two wavelets. Since largest correlation (5.12) between wavelet coefficients at different scales $j_1 > j_2$ will occur when the analysis wavelets are positioned at identical spatial locations, the behavior of $k_\psi(r,0)$ for scale changes $r < 1$ is of interest. This behavior can be examined by expanding $\psi(ru)$ into its Taylor series [22]

$$\psi(ru) = \psi(0) + \psi'(0)ru/1! + \psi''(0)(ru)^2/2! + \cdots,$$

yielding for (5.13)

$$k_\psi(r,0) = r^{1/2}\left\{\psi(0)\int_{-\infty}^{+\infty}\psi(u)\,du + \psi'(0)r\int_{-\infty}^{+\infty}u\psi(u)\,du\right.$$

$$\left. +\psi''(0)r^2\int_{-\infty}^{+\infty}u^2\psi(u)/2!\,du + \cdots\right\}$$

$$= r^{1/2}\left\{\psi(0)m_0 + \psi'(0)rm_1 + \psi''(0)r^2 m_2/2! + \cdots\right\},$$

where m_i are the moments as defined in (5.7). Hence, if a wavelet possesses vanishing moments of up to order p, the correlations (5.12) between coefficients of equipositioned ($k_1 = rk_2$, $\tau = 0$) wavelets with different resolutions decay with a power of the scale ratio as

$$\mathbf{E}\left[d_{j_1 k_1} d_{j_2 k_2}\right] \leq Cr^{(p+3/2)}, \quad r = 2^{j_2-j_1} \leq 1. \tag{5.14}$$

A judicious choice of the wavelet basis allows for some control over the decay rate of this correlation. A fast correlation decay becomes particularly important, if the signal autocorrelation R in (5.12) has wide support or, equivalently, the signal power spectrum $S_{ff}(\omega)$ is highly concentrated toward low frequencies, as elaborated below.

The Fourier transform of (5.12) permits a simple interpretation of the coefficient correlation in terms of the cross-spectral density

$$\Gamma_{dd}(\omega,r,j_1) = S_{ff}(2^{-j_1}\omega)r^{1/2}\,\overline{\hat\psi}(\omega)\hat\psi(r\omega), \quad r = 2^{j_2-j_1}. \tag{5.15}$$

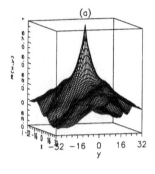
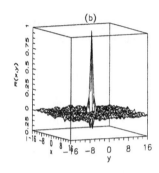

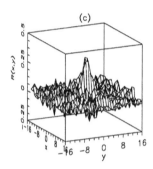
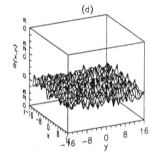

Figure 5.4
Autocorrelation functions of the (a) average PET difference image, and (b) its wavelet representation in the horizontal direction by cubic splines at the highest resolution level. Cross-correlation of the wavelet coefficients between resolution levels 1 and 2 for (c) zero-order and (d) cubic-spline bases.

Hence, cross-power arises only to the extent that the bandpass characteristics $\hat{\psi}(\omega)$ and $\hat{\psi}(r\omega)$ of the wavelet at two different scales overlap. Nonideal bandlimitation causes leakage of the input spectral power at a given frequency through the sidelobes of the nonideal bandpasses of adjacent channels.

In order to assess the regularity of the analysis wavelets required for images of the type shown in Figure 5.1 (c), the investigations shown below were carried out. Specifically, for the Battle-Lemarié wavelets used, it was of particular interest to determine the smallest spline-order, p, that produced sufficient decorrelation between the wavelet coefficients. Figure 5.4 compares the two-dimensional autocorrelation function of the original image (Figure 5.1c) with the correlations found among different sets of wavelet coefficients. Of immediate note are the extended correlations existing in the image domain (Figure 5.4[a]), giving rise to a high signal-power concentration at the low frequency end of the spectrum. The autocorrelation function displays an initial fast decay over a lag of about 8 pixels to values near 0.35. However, for larger lags, particularly in the x-direction, the decay rate is only polynomial. The initial exponential decrease of the autocorrelation results from limitations of the imaging physics of the PET scanner defining the point-spread function, while the slowly decaying part has most likely a biological source; e.g., left/right symmetries of the brain hemispheres introduce "long-range" correlations in the x-direction. In stark contrast, Figure 5.4 (b) shows the autocorrelation of the cubic-spline wavelet coefficients for the horizontal decomposition at the highest resolution level, i.e., the coefficients of $\Psi^1_{j,k}$ (Equation 5.8). The correlation structure is essentially that of white noise, displaying values not significantly different from zero [24] except for the undershoots at lags $(-1,0)$ and $(1,0)$ with values of about -0.185. Figures 5.4 (c) and (d) illustrate the effect of regularity on the suppression of correlation between wavelet coefficients at different scales. Shown are the correlations between resolution levels 1 and 2 for coefficients of the horizontal channels, when splines of order 0 (c) and order 3 (d) are used. The center value shows the correlation between coefficients when the wavelets at the two resolution levels are centered at identical pixel locations in the original image. The lags indicate the relative displacements of the wavelet centers, expressed at the scale of the lower resolution level. As expected from (5.13), the correlation is highest for a zero displacement ($\tau = 0$) between the wavelet centers, reaching a statistically significant value of 0.33 for the Haar wavelets. In contrast, that value is 0.047 for cubic-spline wavelets, which is statistically not different from zero. Hence, the cross-correlation for $p = 3$ is significantly smaller than that for $p = 0$, in agreement with (5.14).

A more detailed investigation of the impact of wavelet order on the correlation across resolution levels is illustrated in Figure 5.5. Bars represent measured correlations derived from the wavelet transform of Figure 5.1(c), and connected symbols depict values computed from (5.14) with, for simplicity, C set to 1. The broken horizontal lines show the size of the correlations required for statistical significance at $p = 0.05$ (two standard errors), where the standard errors were computed by Bartlett's approximation [24]. For $r = 1/2$, averages of the correlations measured for properly centered wavelets ($\tau = 0$) between resolution levels 1–2, 2–3, and 3–4 are shown. Similarly, for $r = 1/4$ the correlations are averages between resolution levels 1–3, and 2–4. The data follow, at least for values significantly above the noise level, the trend indicated by (5.14), with highest correlations occurring between neighboring resolution levels ($r = 1/2$). Splines of order 0 incur statistically significant "leakage" between resolution channels for both $r = 1/2$ and $r = 1/4$. The largest reduction of leakage is achieved by increasing the spline order from 0 to 1, with gradually diminishing im-

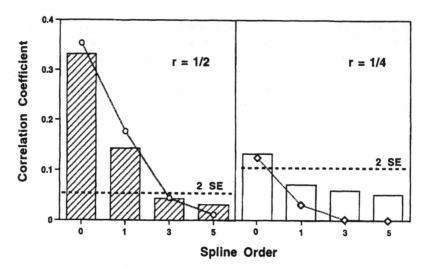

Figure 5.5
Between-channel correlations of orthogonal polynomial-spline
wavelet coefficients for scale ratios 1/2 and 1/4; measured (bars)
and upper bound from Equation (5.14) (connected symbols). 2SE
represents the approximate upper 95th percentile of the null distribution.

provements for higher-order splines. Cross-correlations for cubic splines
were statistically not significantly different from zero. These findings are in
agreement with the results of the compaction efficiency analysis presented
in Figure 5.3. Hence, the relative inefficiency of the Haar compared to the
higher order wavelets can now be interpreted as due to leakage of spectral
power located in low resolution channels into higher resolution channels.
This causes a small decrease in magnitude of the few large wavelet coefficients at low resolution, but increases the magnitude of relatively more
coefficients in the higher resolution channels and thus decreases the compaction efficiency. In conclusion, based on the results of this correlational
analysis cubic-spline wavelets are the optimal choice for the PET images investigated here, i.e., the smallest spline order for which correlation between
all resolution channels was sufficiently suppressed.

5.4   Statistical Tests

The results below are derived for the case where two images per subject,
each acquired under different experimental conditions, are to be compared.

Similar derivations can be made for the comparison of images from different subject groups. Let $x_{il}(t)$, $t = (t_1, t_2) \in \mathbf{Z}^2$, be the (2-D) image of the ith subject acquired under experimental condition l, then of interest are differences between images obtained under two specific conditions l', l'', yielding for each subject the difference images $f_i(t) = x_{il'}(t) - x_{il''}(t)$. These images are assumed to be characterized by the population model

$$f_i(t) = \mu(t) + e_i(t), \quad i = 1, \ldots, N, \quad f_i \in V_0, \qquad (5.16)$$

where $\mu(t)$ represents the underlying (deterministic) spatial pattern to be detected, and $e(t)$ is a Gaussian random field with $E[e(t)] = 0$ and $E[e(t)e(t')] = \sigma^2 \delta(t - t')$, $\forall t \in \mathbf{Z}^2$. To estimate $\mu(t)$, averaging over N subjects is performed, yielding

$$\widehat{\mu}(t) = \frac{1}{N} \sum_{i=1}^{N} f_i(t), \qquad (5.17)$$

$$\widehat{\sigma}^2(t) = \frac{1}{N-1} \sum_{i=1}^{N} \left[f_i(t) - \widehat{\mu}(t) \right]^2, \qquad (5.18)$$

which satisfies

$$E\left[\widehat{\mu}(t)\right] = \mu(t), \quad \text{and} \quad \text{Var}\left[\widehat{\mu}(t)\right] = \sigma^2/N. \qquad (5.19)$$

By pooling $\widehat{\sigma}^2(t)$ over all intracranial (IC) pixels, n_{pix}, a good approximation of σ^2 with a large number of degrees of freedom is obtained [9]. Hence, this parameter is assumed to be given by

$$\overline{\overline{\sigma}}^2 = \frac{1}{n_{pix}} \sum_{t \in IC} \widehat{\sigma}^2(t) \approx \sigma^2, \quad n_{pix} = \#\mathbf{IC}. \qquad (5.20)$$

Since all $f_i \in V_0$, it follows that $\widehat{\mu}(t) \in V_0$, and the orthonormal basis functions defined in Equations (5.8) and (5.9) can be used to decompose the average difference image as

$$\widehat{\mu}(t) = \sum_{k \in \mathbf{Z}} \widehat{c}_{J,k} \, \Phi_{J,k} + \sum_{j=1}^{J} \sum_{m=1}^{3} \sum_{k \in \mathbf{Z}} \widehat{d}_{j,k}^{m} \, \Psi_{j,k}^{m}, \qquad (5.21)$$

where the coefficients $\widehat{c}_{J,k}$ represent the approximation image at resolution level J, and $\widehat{d}_{j,k}^m$ are the wavelet coefficients at resolution level j, encoding horizontally, vertically, and diagonally oriented image detail ($m = 1$, 2, 3, respectively). Following (5.3), the approximation and wavelet coefficients are the projections (inner products) of $\widehat{\mu}(t)$ onto the corresponding orthogonal resolution spaces

$$\widehat{c}_{J,k} = \left\langle \widehat{\mu}(t), \overset{\circ}{\Phi}_{J,k} \right\rangle, \quad k \in \mathbf{Z}^2, \tag{5.22}$$

$$\widehat{d}_{j,k}^m = \left\langle \widehat{\mu}(t), \overset{\circ}{\Psi}_{J,k}^m \right\rangle, \quad k \in \mathbf{Z}^2, \; j = 1, \ldots, J, \; m = 1, 2, 3. \tag{5.23}$$

The null hypothesis H_0 postulates $\widehat{\mu}(t) = 0$; i.e., there is no difference between images acquired under two different experimental conditions. Substituting (5.19) into (5.22) and (5.23), and using the following orthogonality relations implied by (5.8) and (5.9)

$$\langle \varphi(t - h), \varphi(t - l) \rangle = \delta_{hl},$$

$$\langle \psi(t - h), \psi(t - l) \rangle = \delta_{hl}, \tag{5.24}$$

$$\langle \varphi(t - h), \psi(t - l) \rangle = 0, \qquad h, l \in \mathbf{Z},$$

it follows that

$$E\left[\widehat{c}_{J,k}\right] = 0, \quad E\left[\widehat{d}_{j,k}^m\right] = 0, \tag{5.25}$$

and

$$E\left[\widehat{c}_{J,k}\right]^2 = \sigma_N^2, \quad E\left[\widehat{d}_{j,k}^m\right] = \sigma_N^2, \quad j = 1, \ldots, J, \; m = 1, 2, 3, \tag{5.26}$$

where

$$\sigma_N^2 = \sigma^2/N \tag{5.27}$$

is the squared standard error, and σ^2 is obtained from the approximation $\overline{\overline{\sigma}}^2$ in (5.20). Equations (5.22) and (5.23) are linear scaling transforms of $\widehat{\mu}(t)$, which from (5.19) is a Gaussian variate $N(0, \sigma^2/N)$, and thus the standardized coefficients are Gaussian distributed with unitary variance

$$\widehat{c}_{J,k}/\sigma_N \sim N(0,1), \quad \widehat{d}_{j,k}^m/\sigma_N \sim N(0,1). \tag{5.28}$$

Consequently, the square of each standardized coefficient is chi-square distributed with 1 degree of freedom, and due to orthogonality their sum is chi-square with degrees of freedom equal to the number of summation terms

$$\sum_{k \in IC_J} \left[\widehat{c}_{J,k}/\sigma_N\right]^2 \sim \chi^2_{n_J},$$

(5.29)

$$\sum_{k \in IC_j} \left[\widehat{d}^m_{j,k}/\sigma_N\right]^2 \sim \chi^2_{n^m_j}, \quad j = 1, \ldots, J, \ m = 1, 2, 3,$$

where $n^m_j = \#\boldsymbol{IC}_j$ is the number of intracranial pixels at resolution level j and orientation m.

Hence, the decomposition of the squared average difference into orthogonal sums of squares in (5.29) enables testing the null hypothesis by $(3J+1)$ component chi-square tests. By selection of an appropriate wavelet regularity, these tests are under H_0 asymptotically independent due to (5.14). They permit examination of whether the approximation image coefficients $\widehat{c}_{J,k}$ are all simultaneously zero, and whether in each channel, specified by edge orientation m and resolution level j, the wavelet coefficients $\widehat{d}^m_{j,k}$ are all simultaneously zero. Usually, there is no interest in testing the significance of the lowpass approximation coefficients. By assigning to each of the chi-square tests (5.29) for the wavelet coefficients a significance level $\alpha = p/(3J)$ (Bonferroni correction), the overall significance per image can be maintained at the specified level p. Channels where the test outcomes based on (5.29) fall within the acceptance region of the chi-square distribution on n^m_j degrees of freedom are inferred to contain noise only, and their coefficients are all set to zero. Channels associated with test results in the rejection region are presumed to carry signal components, and are thus considered for more specific follow-up testing. To that end, their index pairs (j', m') are entered into a two-dimensional table $\boldsymbol{I}_\alpha$ facilitating the subsequent computations; i.e.,

$$(j', m') \in \boldsymbol{I}_\alpha = \arg_{j,m} \left(\mathrm{Var}\, \widehat{d}^m_{j,k}/\sigma^2_N > \chi^2_{n^m_j;\alpha}/n^m_j \right|$$

(5.30)

$$P\left(\chi^2_{n^m_j;\alpha}/n^m_j\right) = 1 - \alpha \Bigg).$$

The standardized wavelet coefficients in these channels are unitary variance normal according to (5.28), and subjecting each of them to z-tests localizes the significant signal components. This procedure yields the reduced coefficient set

$$\left\{ \widehat{c}_{J,k}, \widehat{d'^{m}_{j,k}} \right\},$$

where

$$\widehat{d'^{m}_{j,k}} = \begin{cases} \widehat{d^{m}_{j,k}} & \text{for } \left| \widehat{d^{m}_{j,k}} \right| > \theta \\ 0 & \text{otherwise} \end{cases}, \quad (j,m) \in \boldsymbol{I}_{\alpha} \tag{5.31}$$

and $\theta = \sigma_N z_{\alpha'}$ is the threshold for a standardized normal variate with the significance level α' adjusted for the total number of follow-up tests performed in the search volume, i.e., the total number of coefficients contained in the channels considered for follow-up testing

$$\alpha' = p \left/ \sum_{j,m \,\in\, \boldsymbol{I}_{\alpha}} \sum n^{m}_{j} \right. \tag{5.32}$$

Finally, application of the inverse wavelet transform to this reduced set of coefficients yields a reconstruction of the estimated difference image that is solely based on significant image components.

From the viewpoint of signal processing, the two-stage approach to signal detection described above has the following interpretation: First, the question is asked whether there are any image differences of a certain spatial extent ("blob size") present in the image (chi-square tests). If the answer is affirmative for some blob size, then the spatial locations of blobs with that size are determined (z-tests). This achieves economy in testing by considerably reducing the search volume compared to the original signal space. Orthogonality of the wavelets with respect to resolution enables an orthogonal partitioning of the signal space in terms of oriented blob sizes, and orthogonality with respect to discrete wavelet locations permits spatial localization of the signal within the resolution channels. This procedure effectively limits the search for signal components to the subspace where significant signal power is located.

5.5   Experimental Results

5.5.1   Functional Magnetic Resonance Images

Application of the wavelet transform and subsequent statistical procedures to a set of fMRI slices is demonstrated below. The images were obtained on a standard clinical 1.5 tesla scanner (SIGNA, General Electric) with standard quadrature head coil. Both structural and functional images were acquired from the same region of the brain to permit subsequent overlay of the two modalities. For the structural images, inversion recovery sequences were used (TI/TR 800/3000 msec), producing a data matrix of 15 slices with 256×128 pixels that represented slices of 3 mm thickness+1 mm gap with an FOV of 240 mm, oriented 45° relative to the AC-PC line. For the functional scans, an Echo-Shifted FLASH sequence was used (TE/TR 29.1/20 ms, flip angle 11°, FOV 64 mm, data matrix 16 slices of 64×64 pixels) [25]. Uniformity limitations of the RF field excitation restricted the image analysis to the 10 innermost slices, covering a 40-mm section with 4 mm thick contiguous slices of in-plane resolution 3.75×3.75 mm. The slice orientation of 45° was selected to minimize artifacts caused by local magnetic field inhomogeneities near the nasal cavity (air/tissue susceptibility difference). The fMRIs were obtained with the subjects either at baseline — breathing room air, or during olfactory stimulation — breathing room air with a pleasant odor added (Coconut or Muguet, International Flavors and Fragrances). The acquisition time for one fMRI volume scan was 20 s. A baseline/stimulation cycle consisted of two consecutive 20-s functional scans, separated by 7 s. Olfactory stimulation was switched on at the end of the first scan, and off at the end of the second scan. Eight stimulation cycles were acquired from each subject, spaced 3 min apart. To minimize motion artifacts, all subsequent fMRI scans were digitally registered to the first scan (3-D rigid-body translation and rotation) by a procedure that minimized the squared gray-level difference over all intracranial voxels, applying the Marquardt-Levenberg optimization procedure to a cubic-spline resolution pyramid representation of the volumes [20, 21].

Hence, in the notation of (5.16) $N = 8$ registered stimulation/baseline difference images were obtained from a subject. Figure 5.6 (a) shows one of the difference images for a center slice of the volume, and Figure 5.6 (b) presents the result after averaging according to (5.17). Using the orthogonal cubic spline basis, the corresponding wavelet coefficients of this average image are displayed in Figure 5.6 (c) for $J = 4$ levels. Results of applying the chi-square tests (5.30) to the variance of the wavelet coefficients in the resulting $4 \times 3 = 12$ channels are summarized in Table 5.1 for wavelets based on spline orders 0, 1, 3, and 5. The significance level was adjusted for the total number of possible tests (120) in the volume of interest comprising 10 slices. Irrespective of the spline order, all channels at resolution level 1 and the diagonal channel at resolution level 2 failed to show signal power above the noise level. The null hypothesis was rejected (overall $p < 0.05$) for all channels at level 3, and the horizontal and diagonal channels at level 4. In these channels, except for the Haar wavelets, which differ in that their first-order derivatives do not exist, the results changed monotonically with the spline order. The number of wavelet coefficients that could be eliminated

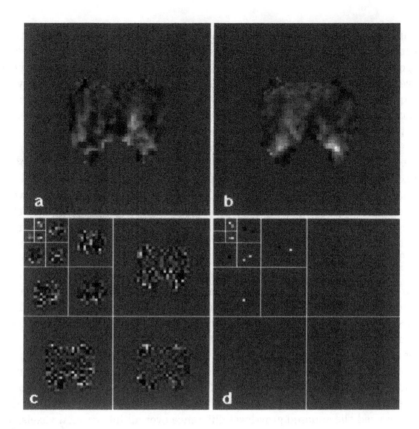

Figure 5.6
(a) **Instance of an fMRI difference image between olfactory stimulus on and off; (b) average difference image for eight stimulation
cycles; (c) wavelet decomposition (four levels) with orthogonal
cubic splines; (d) significant (overall** $p < 0.05$**) wavelet coefficients.**

for this slice (with spline orders > 0) by the chi-square tests is $3 \times 182 + 1 \times 48 + 1 \times 4 = 598$, resulting in about an 81% reduction of the search space. Subjecting the remaining 143 wavelet coefficients to the follow-up z-tests (5.31) produced 12 significant (overall $p < 0.05$) coefficients, or 1.6% of the total of 741. The significant coefficients are displayed in Figure 5.6 (d).

Application of these two-step procedures to the total number of 10 slices encompassing 7001 intracranial voxels resulted in total search space reductions of 88.2, 88.2, 90.0, and 90.1%, for spline wavelets of orders 0, 1, 3, and 5, respectively. The corresponding number of significant ($p < 0.05$) wavelets after applying (5.31) were 95 (1.36%), 77 (1.10%), 76 (1.09%), and 68 (0.97%), respectively. Lower spline orders typically produced a larger number of significant coefficients because of their inferior ability to prevent leakage of the high signal power concentrated at low spectral frequencies

Table 5.1

Ratio of wavelet coefficient variances to the squared standard error in Equation (5.27).

Resolution[a]		Wavelet Spline Order				n_j[b]	χ^2-crit[c]
		0	1	3	5		
	H	.64	.39	.37	.37		
1	V	.56	.38	.34	.34	182	1.39
	D	.33	.18	.17	.17		
	H	2.28	2.87	2.46	2.31		
2	V	2.68	2.58	2.19	1.98	48	1.82
	D	1.48	0.83	1.02	1.12		
	H	16.97	5.49	6.14	6.19		
3	V	9.15	3.54	4.70	4.95	13	2.84
	D	6.45	6.21	5.35	4.71		
	H	10.92	19.86	14.44	12.91		
4	V	13.29	5.01	4.60	4.20	4	5.10
	D	20.89	39.66	30.98	25.75		

[a]H: horizontal, V: vertical, D: diagonal decomposition channel.

[b]Number of intracranial voxels at resolution level j.

[c]Critical value of $\chi^2_{n_j}/n_j$ for $p = 0.05/(12 \times 10) = 0.000417$, Bonferroni adjustment for a volume of 10 slices.

into higher resolution channels, as shown in Section 5.3. This spectral leakage resulted in a few additional coefficients with significant power ιn the higher resolution channels.

Figure 5.7 shows for the same slice the original difference image (a), and the reconstructed difference images (b–d) obtained by applying the inverse wavelet transform to the reduced set of significant coefficients (Equation 5.31). Since most of the deleted coefficients were located in higher resolution channels, a significant amount of noise reduction was achieved, while the main features of the signal were retained. The reconstruction based on Haar wavelets (Figure 5.7 [b]) is perhaps too "blocky" to be of practical use; however, it does provide a valid, cursory abstraction of the main regions of signal change. Both reconstructions employing higher-order wavelets yield reasonable, clear representations of the main focal changes, and there is little visual difference between the results based on first- (c) and third-order (d) wavelets. It is to be reemphasized that these reconstructions were obtained with only about 1% of the total number of coefficients, demonstrating the excellent signal abstraction capability of the wavelets.

In Figure 5.8 regions of functional differences reconstructed from significant cubic-spline wavelets are superimposed over the corresponding set of six contiguous anatomical MRI slices of the same subject (anteroposterior

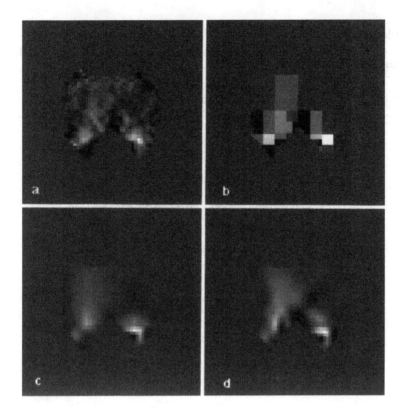

Figure 5.7
(a) **Average difference fMRI; resynthesis of (a) by inverse wavelet transform of only significant (overall $p < 0.05$) coefficients using (b) zero-, (c) first-, and (d) third-order orthogonal spline bases.**

direction from top left to bottom right) [26]. Areas of functional change >1% due to olfactory stimulation are indicated in white for increase and in black for decrease. The maximum signal difference in this subject was a local increase of about 3%. Focal signal increases are demonstrated in regions of the posterior orbitofrontal and pyriform cortices (anterior slices) and of the amygdaloid nuclei, all brain areas that have been found in animal experiments to be associated with the processing of olfactory stimuli. Since the largest fraction of the noise power is distributed into the higher resolution channels due to their wider bandwidths, while the signal proved to be relatively low-pass, application of the statistical test procedures effected a substantial noise suppression. This resulted in resynthesized difference images showing relatively noise-free foci of change, which were not disintegrated into scattered single-pixel regions by the subsequent thresholding step employed to enable the anatomical overlay.

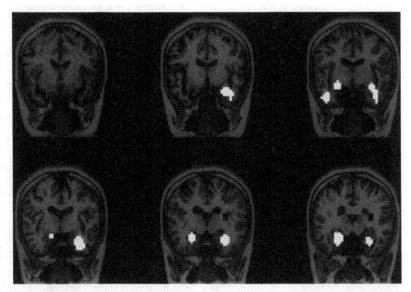

Figure 5.8
Contiguous coronal MRI slices (tilted at an angle of 45° from posterosuperior to anteroinferior), sequence from top left to bottom right proceeds in anteroposterior direction. Superimposed are significant functional signal differences due to olfactory stimulation, thresholded at $>|1\%|$ change (positive, white; negative, black).

5.5.2 Positron Emission Tomography Images

The example of PET image differences between alcoholics and normal subjects shown in Figure 5.1 was also analyzed in a similar way. Application of the chi-square tests (5.30) to $J = 5$ resolution levels (commensurate with the doubled linear dimension of the pixel matrix) yielded results comparable to those shown in Table 5.1. A notable difference was that irrespective of the spline orders, all channels at resolution levels 1 and 2 were eliminated (Bonferroni adjusted $p > 0.05$) by these summary tests, leaving only 9 out of the 15 channels for subsequent analysis. This step achieved a dramatic reduction of the search space from a total of 3988 coefficients to 243, or 6.1%. Furthermore, the elimination of the first two resolution levels, corresponding to a minimum blob size of 8 mm, is consistent with the in-plane resolution of the scanner, specified as FWHM = 7 mm. Follow-up testing by (5.31) yielded 48 (1.20%), 43 (1.08%), 38 (0.95%), and 38 (0.95%) significant (overall $p < 0.05$) coefficients for spline orders 0, 1, 3, and 5, respectively. The reconstructions based on significant coefficients for orders 0, 1, and 3 are compared with the original difference image (i.e., the

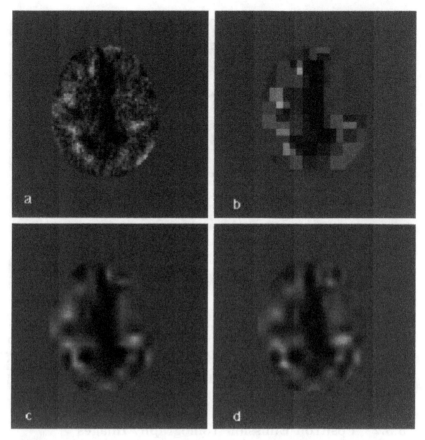

Figure 5.9
Reconstructions of the average PET difference image between alcoholics and normals (a = original difference image) by inverse wavelet transform of only significant (overall $p < 0.05$) coefficients using (b) zero-, (c) first-, and (d) third-order orthogonal spline bases.

use of all coefficients) in Figure 5.9. Again, the resynthesized images are substantially less noisy than the original. The main functional differences are displayed in the medial superior frontal cortex, the cingulate gyri, and the precuneate region, where alcoholics show a relatively depressed glucose utilization rate (dark regions). The zero-order resynthesis (b) exhibits the characteristic "blocky" appearance, while some linear streaking artifacts in high intensity areas are discernible in the first-order spline representation (c). Some small improvement of image quality was obtained with cubic splines (d), while there was very little visual difference between the reconstructions based on third- and fifth-order (not shown) splines.

5.6 Discussion

Wavelet analysis is a flexible tool that is well-suited for the detection of weak signals in noisy images, as they typically arise in the biomedical field. Compared to Fourier analysis, the wavelet bases achieve a superior signal compaction, i.e., they are able to express salient image features by a smaller number of coefficients. In theory, compaction efficiency is expected to increase with the order (regularity), p, of the splines used as prototype wavelet, with the maximum achieved by the modulated-sinc wavelet $(p \to \infty)$. Our investigation of functional images indicated that for the low SNR conditions usually encountered, the selection of spline orders higher than 1 will not substantially improve compaction efficiency. However, a more refined analysis revealed that the cross-correlation between wavelet coefficients at different resolution scales can be further decreased by selecting higher-order splines. This cross-correlation was shown to be due to extended spatial autocorrelations in the original images, exhibiting long, slowly decreasing tails. Selection of appropriate wavelet regularity permitted to control the decay rate of the ensuing cross-channel correlation, imposing a condition on the minimum spline-order for the wavelets as given in (5.14). In the Fourier domain, this condition was shown to be equivalent to controlling the spectral overlap between two resolution channels. This overlap can be made arbitrarily small by selecting the spline-order p sufficiently large, yielding wavelets with Fourier transforms approaching the ideal bandpass filter [16, 17]. In practice, the extent of channel decorrelation realizable must be balanced against the decrease of spatial localization incurred by the larger support required for the implementation of higher-order spline wavelets. Measurement on PET images revealed that it was not necessary to go beyond cubic spline wavelets for suppression of the cross-channel correlation to statistically insignificant values. The fMR images investigated in this study had less inherent blurring (i.e., they were close to optimally sampled), and first-order splines appeared to be sufficient in this particular application.

The decomposition of the image spectrum into a set of minimally overlapping frequency bands permits taking advantage of the high SNR at low frequencies. There, the signal power is highly concentrated, while under the model assumption the noise is uniformly distributed over all resolution channels and remains white within the channels due to the orthogonality of the wavelet bases. This higher SNR results in lower signal detection thresholds at low-resolution channels, compared to a uniform threshold that would be required if the spectrum were not subdivided. Consequently, signal detection performance is improved relative to methods that result in a single threshold, such as detection in the original image domain based on a Gaussian random field model [9]. Since the resolution channels are increasingly narrower as $\omega \to 0$, a relative "whitening" of the signal spectrum within the channels is achieved, creating close to optimal signal detection conditions.

The development of statistical test procedures in the wavelet domain made use of the orthogonality of the decomposition with respect to resolution. By imposing sufficient wavelet regularity, close to ideal channel decorrelation could be achieved. This made it possible to reduce the signal search space to a much smaller subspace with significant spectral power by performing a small number of chi-square tests (5.30). Consequently, the spatial localization of signals could be limited to the substantially reduced set of wavelet coefficients residing in channels with significant power only, thus greatly reducing the total number of statistical tests required. The benefit of a smaller number of follow-up z-tests (5.31) is that a smaller p-value adjustment (Bonferroni correction) (5.32) is needed than if all voxels of interests were to be tested. In fact, detection methods based on individual voxel testing usually do not correct for multiple testing [27], presumably because otherwise, for the large number of voxels that typically arise, the statistical power would become too low. However, the penalty for failing to adjust the significance levels for individual tests is, of course, that an unprotected overall false-positive error rate (type II errors) ensues. For the example images investigated here, the search space reductions achieved by two-stage testing in the wavelet domain amounted to approximately 10:1 for fMR images and 20:1 for PET images. With either modality, about 1% of the coefficients were retained at an overall significance level of 0.05, i.e., a false-positive error rate of 1 in 20 volume scans. The impact of the reduced number of statistical tests on the detection threshold for z-tests is illustrated for the volume set of 10 fMRI slices presented in Section 5.5.1 By applying the Bonferroni correction to the total volume of interest comprising 7001 intracranial voxels, the adjusted p-value (for two-sided tests) is 7.14×10^{-6}, resulting in a detection threshold of 4.49 (this is to be compared with the unprotected threshold of 1.96, which is much too low). Application of the chi-square tests reduced the search space to 699 cubic-spline coefficients, yielding a protected p-level of 7.15×10^{-5} with a corresponding threshold of 3.97. This resulted in a reduction of about 20% along the difference between the thresholds for individual voxel testing with and without Bonferroni correction, without compromising the given overall level of statistical significance. The Bonferroni correction is known to be conservative [28] for tests on correlated data, and in this sense the lower threshold for testing wavelet coefficients can be viewed as the result of taking some of the correlations into proper account.

The process of globally eliminating resolution channels with insufficient power by (5.30) is analogous to applying a filter to the difference image, which, due to the nature of the signal, turned out to be essentially a low-pass. However, the important difference with respect to standard low-pass filtering is that the cutoff frequency does not have to be specified beforehand, but is rather derived from the image itself by statistical testing. This constitutes a flexibility inherent in the wavelet decomposition approach with considerable practical impact. It permits application of the method to images acquired on scanners with ill-specified or unknown point-spread functions. This "blind" filtering is particularly important in the case of fMR imaging, which is still in a phase of development, with new image acquisition techniques continually evolving. Similarly, the testing of coefficients in the significant channels by (5.31) can be viewed as a spatially adaptive filtering process, where a specific bandpass filter (the wavelet) is applied at image locations providing significant edge information, while "flat" image regions are smoothed to the extent permitted by the next lower wavelet resolution band. As a result of these implicit filter operations, resynthesis of the difference images based on significant wavelet coefficients only resulted in smooth, relatively noise-free regions of functional change.

In conclusion, the dyadic resolution decomposition of images implemented by the wavelet transform permits exploiting the usually favorable SNR conditions of functional images at low spatial frequencies. By making use of orthogonality and regularity conditions imposed on the wavelet bases, this decomposition enables application of standard parametric tests of significance on wavelet coefficients directly. The method overcomes the problems associated with large intervoxel correlations in the spatial domain and achieves a vast reduction of the number of statistical tests required, resulting in a lowering of the signal detection threshold for a given significance level. Image resynthesis by using only significant wavelet coefficients for the inverse wavelet transform is equivalent to a spatially adaptive filtering procedure. As a result, compact regions of signal change are produced, which, due to the imposed smoothness, are not disintegrated by subsequent thresholding operations typically required for anatomical overlay of the detected functional changes.

References

[1] K. A. Frey, Positron emission tomography, in *Basic Neurochemistry: Molecular, Cellular, and Medical Aspects*, 5th ed., G. J. Siegel, B. W. Agranoff, R. W. Albers, P. B. Molinoff (eds.), Raven Press, New York, 1994, 935–955.

[2] R. L. Van Heertum and R. S. Tikofsky, *Cerebral SPECT Imaging*, 2nd ed., Raven Press, New York, 1995.

[3] J. W. Prichard and B. R. Rosen, Functional study of the brain by NMR, *J. Cereb. Blood Flow Metab.* 14(1994), 365–372.

[4] K. Herholz, G. Pawlik, K. Wienhard, and W. D. Heiss, Computer assisted mapping in quantitative analysis of cerebral positron emission tomograms, *J. Comput. Assist. Tomogr.* 9(1985), 154–161.

[5] M. B. Schapiro, C. L. Grady, A. Kumar, P. Herscovitch, J. V. Haxby, A. M. Moore, B. White, R. B. Friedland, and S. I. Rapoport, Regional cerebral glucose metabolism is normal in young adults with Down's syndrome, *J. Cereb. Blood Flow Metab.* 10(1990), 199–206.

[6] P. J. Andreason, A. J. Zametkin, A. C. Guo, P. Baldwin, and R. M. Cohen, Gender-related differences in regional cerebral glucose metab-olism in normal volunteers, *Psychiatry Res.* 51(1994), 175–183.

[7] I. Ford, J. H. McColl, A. G. McCormack, and S. J. McCrory, Statistical issues in the analysis of neuroimages, *J. Cereb. Blood Flow Metab.* 11, Suppl. 1(1991), A89–A95.

[8] B. Horowitz, S. E. Swedo, C. L. Grady, P. Pietrini, M. B. Schapiro, J. L. Rapoport, and S. I. Rapoport, Cerebral metabolic pattern in obsessive-compulsive disorder: altered intercorrelations between regional rates of glucose utilization, *Psychiatry Res.: Neuroimaging* 40(1991), 221–237.

[9] K. J. Worsley, A. C. Evans, S. Marrett, and P. Neelin, A three-dimensional statistical analysis for CBF activation studies in human brain, *J. Cereb. Blood Flow Metab.* 12(1992), 900–918.

[10] R. J. Adler, *The Geometry of Random Fields*, Wiley, New York, 1981, 111.

[11] D. E. Rio, R. R. Rawlings, U. E. Ruttimann, and R. Momenan, A study of statistical methods applied in the spatial, wavelet and Fourier domain to enhance and analyze group characteristics of images: applications to PET brain images. *Proc. SPIE, Vol. 2299, Mathematical Methods in Medical Imaging III* (1994), 194–203.

[12] N. Giri, On the complex analogues of T2 and R2 tests, *Ann. Math. Stat.* 36 (1965), 664–670.

[13] H. R. Shumway, Discriminant analysis for time series, in *Handbook of Statistics, Vol. 2, Classification, Pattern Recognition and Reduction*

of Dimensionality, P. R. Krishnaiah and L. N. Kanal (eds.), North-Holland, New York, 1982, 1–46.

[14] R. N. Bracewell, *The Fourier Transform and Its Applications*, 2nd ed., McGraw-Hill, New York, 1986, 160–163.

[15] M. Unser, On the optimality of ideal filters for pyramid and wavelet signal approximation, *IEEE Trans. Signal Process.* 41(1993), 3591–3596.

[16] P.-G. Lemarié, Ondelettes à localisation exponentielles, *J. Math. Pures et Appl.* 67(1988), 227–236.

[17] A. Aldroubi and M. Unser, Families of multiresolution and wavelet spaces with optimal properties, *Numer. Funct. Anal. Optimiz.* 14(1993), 417–446.

[18] M. Unser, A. Aldroubi, and M. Eden, A family of polynomial spline wavelet transform, *Signal Process.* 30(1993), 141–162.

[19] S. G. Mallat, A theory for multiresolution signal decomposition: The wavelet representation, *IEEE Trans. Pattern Anal. Mach. Intell.* PAMI-11 (1989), 674–693.

[20] M. Unser, P. Thévenaz, Ch. Lee, and U. E. Ruttimann, Registration and statistical analysis of PET images using the wavelet transform, *IEEE Eng. Med. Biol. Mag.* (1995), 603–611.

[21] P. Thévenaz, U. E. Ruttimann, and M. Unser, Iterative multi-scale registration without landmarks, *IEEE International Conference on Image Processing* (1995), Vol. III, 228–231.

[22] U. E. Ruttimann, M. Unser, D. Rio, and R. R. Rawlings, The use of the wavelet transform to investigate differences in brain PET images between patients, *Proc. SPIE, Vol. 2035, Mathematical Methods in Medical Imaging II* (1993), 192–203.

[23] P. Flandrin, Wavelet analysis and synthesis of fractal Brownian motion, *IEEE Trans. Inf. Theory* 38(1992), 910–917.

[24] M. S. Bartlett, On the theoretical specification of sampling properties of autocorrelated time series, *J. Roy. Stat. Soc. B* 8, Suppl. (1946), 27–41.

[25] J. Duyn, V. S. Mattay, R. Sexton, G. Sobering, F. Barrios, G. Liu, J. Frank, D. R. Weinberger, and C. T. W. Moonen, Three-dimensional functional imaging of human brain using echo-shifted FLASH MRI, *Magn. Reson. Med.* 32 (1994), 150–155.

[26] U. E. Ruttimann, N. F. Ramsey, D. W. Hommer, P. Thévenaz, Ch. Lee, and M. Unser, Analysis of functional magnetic resonance images by wavelet decomposition, *IEEE International Conference on Image Processing* (1995), Vol. I, 633–636.

[27] M. Ingvar, L. Erikson, T. Greitz, S. Stone-Elander, M. Dahlbom, G. Rosenqvist, P. af Trampe, and C. von Euler, Methodological aspects of brain activation studies: cerebral blood flow determined with [^{15}O]butanol and positron emission tomography, *J. Cereb. Blood Flow Metab.* 14(1994), 628–638.

[28] J. L. Fleiss, *The Design and Analysis of Clinical Experiments*, New York, Wiley, 1986, 103–104.

6

Feature Extraction in Digital Mammography[1]

R. A. DeVore[1], B. Lucier[2], and Z. Yang[3]

[1] *Department of Mathematics, University of South Carolina, Columbia, South Carolina*
[2] *Department of Mathematics, Purdue University, W. Lafayette, Indiana*
[3] *Institute for Scientific Computation, Texas A&M University, College Station, Texas*

6.1 Introduction

The devastating impact of breast cancer in the United States is well documented [1]. This points to the need for early cancer detection. The number of mammograms generated daily is large and therefore it is very desirable to develop image processing tools which facilitate the handling of mammograms (storage and transmission) and aid the radiologist in diagnosis.

We have previously reported [9, 12] on wavelet-based techniques for compression of mammographic images. The purpose of the present paper is to put forward new wavelet-based techniques for the automated detection (using only a computer) and semi-automated detection (interactive with an operator) of certain early signs of cancer. Signs of breast cancer are typically categorized by radiologist in three categories: clusters of microcalci-

---

[1]This research was supported by the Office of Naval Research Contracts N00014-91-J1076 and N00014-91-J1152, and the National Science Foundation Grant EHR 9108772.

fications, stellate lesions, and circumscribed lesions. We shall be primarily concerned with the automated detection of clusters of microcalcifications. However, the techniques we put forward may also have application to the detection of lesions. Moreover, the detection of microcalcification clusters has several features in common with other problems of feature classification and automated detection.

6.2 Mammograms as Digitized Images

While mammograms usually are taken on film, we assume that they have been digitized (typically by a digital scanner). A new generation of mammography will directly produce digitized images.

A digitized image is an array of pixel values. For mammograms, this array is generally not square and this causes some technical difficulties in wavelet-based image processing algorithms. Also the size of mammograms is large when compared with many other images. However, for the convenience of discussion in this paper, we shall assume that the digitized mammogram is not only square but of the size $2^m \times 2^m$. Typical values are $m = 9$, 10. (All examples of digitized mammograms considered in this paper are of size 512×512.)

Thus, a digitized mammogram, for the purposes of this paper, will be an array of nonnegative integers

$$p_k, \quad k = (k_1, k_2), \ k_1, k_2 \in \{0, \dots, 2^m - 1\}.$$

The range of the integer values p_j is related to the scanner and the dynamical range of the film. We shall assume that the p_j take values from $\{0, \dots, 4095\}$ (again for convenience and because all sample images considered will have 12-bit dynamical range). The techniques we develop here are independent of the dynamical range.

The following viewpoint of a digitized image is useful in the analysis that follows. We can view the pixel values as obtained from a bivariate function F defined on the unit square $\Omega := [0, 1]^2$ by taking cell averages

$$p_k = \int_{Q_k} F(x, y) \, dx \, dy, \quad 0 \le k_1, k_2 \le 2^m - 1$$

where $Q_k := [2^{-m}k_1, 2^{-m}k_1 + 2^{-m}] \times [2^{-m}k_2, 2^{-m}k_2 + 2^{-m}]$ is the square with sidelength 2^{-m} and lower left vertex $2^{-m}k = 2^{-m}(k_1, k_2)$. Thus, we view the pixel values as samples of the underlying function F.

In wavelet-based image processing, we need a representation of the image as a wavelet sum. Let φ be a univariate function which generates multiresolution as described in §1.5 of Chapter 1. Since images are bivariate, we shall need the corresponding bivariate multiresolution and bivariate wavelet bases. Let

$$\phi(x, y) := \varphi(x)\varphi(y)$$

be the bivariate function which is the tensor product of φ with itself. As in the univariate case, we have the bivariate ladder of space V_j, $j \in \mathbf{Z}$, with V_j defined as the $L_2(\mathbf{R}^2)$-span of the functions[2]

$$\phi_{j,k} := 2^{-j}\phi(2^{-j}x - k_1, 2^{-j}y - k_2), \quad k := (k_1, k_2) \in \mathbf{Z}^2.$$

Recall that when φ has compact support, the function $\phi_{j,k}$ has support localized near the point $2^j k$. From the pixel values (p_k), we create an approximation f to F from the space V_{-m}:

$$F \approx f = \sum_j c(k)\varphi_{-m,k}. \tag{2.1}$$

We assign the coefficients $c(k)$ so that the portion of the sum (2.1) which is nonzero on Ω is a good approximation to F. This is usually accomplished by defining

$$c(k) := p_k, \quad 0 \le k_1, k_2 \le 2^m - 1,$$

and defining $c(k)$ for other values of k by some extension strategy. Typical extensions are either symmetric (cf. Chapter 2) or chosen to preserve constant or linear sequences. We refer the reader to [2, 4, 13] for general discussions of extension strategies.

The representation (2.1) is not suitable for most tasks in image processing. We therefore convert (2.1) to the more preferable wavelet basis. For our purposes it will be sufficient to restrict our attention to the cases where the univariate wavelet basis is orthogonal, semi-orthogonal, or bi-orthogonal, as described in §1.5 of Chapter 1. If ψ is the univariate function whose shifts are a basis for the wavelet space W_0, then the following bivariate functions span the corresponding bivariate wavelet space:

$$\varphi(x)\psi(y) \quad \psi(x)\varphi(y) \quad \psi(x)\psi(y). \tag{2.2}$$

---

[2] We have conformed to the notation of this book in the definition of the spaces V_j and the functions $\phi_{j,k}$. Our other work on wavelets utilizes slightly different notation with j replaced by $-j$ in the definition of these spaces and functions.

We let Ψ denote the set consisting of the three functions in (2.2) and for $\eta \in \Psi$, we define

$$\eta_{j,k} := 2^{-j}\eta(2^{-j}x - k_1, 2^{-j}x - k_2), \quad k = (k_1, k_2) \in \mathbf{Z}^2.$$

These functions span the corresponding bivariate wavelet space W_j which encodes the detail between V_j and the finer space V_{j-1}. Namely, we have

$$V_{j-1} = V_j + W_j. \tag{2.3}$$

In the case of orthogonal or semi-orthogonal wavelets, the sum in (2.3) is orthogonal, while in the bi-orthogonal case it is generally oblique.

We can use the fast wavelet transform (FWT) to convert the representation (2.1) to the wavelet representation. In this way, we obtain

$$f = \sum_{k \in \mathbf{Z}^2} c(k)\varphi_{-m,k} = \sum_{k \in \mathbf{Z}^2} c_0(k)\phi_{0,k} + \sum_{j=-1}^{-m+1} \sum_{\eta \in \Psi} \sum_{k \in \mathbf{Z}^2} d_{j,\eta}(k)\eta_{j,k}. \tag{2.4}$$

In each of these sums, the k can be restricted to those values for which $\eta_{j,k}$ is nonzero on Ω. The wavelet coefficients $d_{j,\eta}(k)$ can be computed from the pixel values in $O(N)$ operations with $N = 2^{2m}$ the original number of pixel values. We call (2.4) the wavelet representation (cf. Chapter 2) of the image.

6.2.1   Characteristics of Mammographic Images

It will be useful to note some characteristics of mammographic images since these will motivate our algorithms for microcalcification detection. A more detailed exposition of the characteristics of mammographic images as related to the detection of microcalcifications can be found in [3].

A typical mammogram is shown in Figure 6.1. The microcalcifications which we wish to identify appear as small bright spots in the mammogram. Their diameters are up to .7 mm, with an average size of .3 mm. Thus, the microcalcifications can be identified with certain dyadic levels j in the wavelet decomposition — namely, those for which 2^j is comparable with the size of the microcalcification. In the examples of mammograms that we consider in this paper, the dyadic levels $j = -7, -8, -9$ typically correspond to frequencies where microcalcifications occur. It is important not only to retain all microcalcifications but also their shape since these are important in diagnosis.

The remaining part of the mammogram corresponds to breast tissue and film noise. The breast tissue provides a very inhomogeneous background.

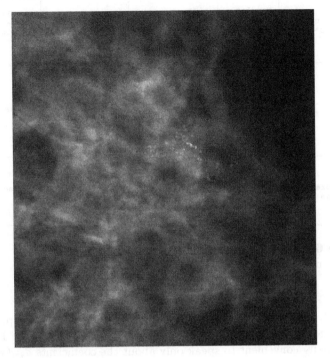

Figure 6.1
A typical mammographic image.

Also, the microcalcifications may be at low contrast to the background and this contrast may vary locally.

6.3 Compression and Noise Removal

While compression and noise removal are important for the storage and transmission of images, in the present paper we are interested in them as a preprocessor for the identification of microcalcification clusters in mammograms. The utilization of compression in this manner has many other related applications such as image registration and object recognition.

We first review briefly the elements of wavelet-based image compression. Figure 6.2 depicts the main steps in wavelet-based compression.

Step I. Computation of wavelet coefficients. We choose a univariate scaling function φ and represent the mammogram as in (2.1). We then use the FWT to change to the wavelet basis representation (2.4). At this stage of the compression algorithm, the file of wavelet coefficients exactly

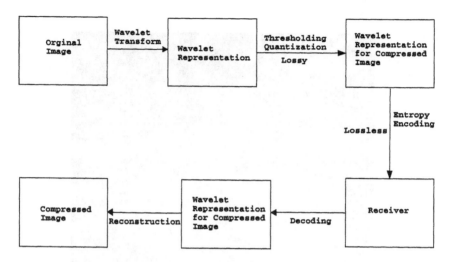

Figure 6.2
A schematic for wavelet-based compression

represents the original image.

Step II. Thresholding/Quantization. We gain lossy compression of the image by reducing the size of the wavelet coefficient file. It will be notationally convenient to speak only about the coefficients $d_{j,\eta}(k)$ of $\eta_{j,k}$. Similar statements apply to the coefficients of $\phi_{0,k}$.

There are two essential (related) methods for compression: thresholding and quantization. Thresholding means that we pick a threshold ϵ_j for each level $j = 0, -1, \ldots, -m+1$ and retain only those coefficients whose absolute value exceeds ϵ_j. Thus, thresholding replaces $d_{j,\eta}(k)$ by $\tau_j(d_{j,\eta}(k))$ where the function τ_j is defined by

$$\tau_j(x) := \begin{cases} x, & |x| \geq \epsilon_j \\ 0, & |x| < \epsilon_j. \end{cases}$$

This is called *hard thresholding*; the function τ_j is not continuous. Soft thresholding would replace τ_j by (for example) the Lipschitz continuous function

$$\tau_j^o(x) := \begin{cases} x, & |x| \geq \epsilon_j \\ 2(|x| - \epsilon_j/2)\,\mathrm{sgn}\,x, & \epsilon_j/2 \leq |x| < \epsilon_j \\ 0, & |x| < \epsilon_j/2. \end{cases}$$

The graph of τ_j^o is given in Figure 6.3. Soft thresholding is numerically stable; a small change in $d_{j,\eta}(k)$ results in a small change in the output $\tau_j^o(d_{j,\eta}(k))$.

Thresholding will replace small wavelet coefficients by zero. This not only has the desired effect of compression but also removes noise. There

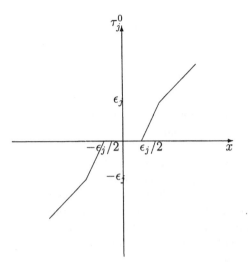

Figure 6.3
The graph of the soft thresholding function τ_j^0.

are several results which show that (soft) thresholding, with a proper choice
of thresholding parameters, gives an optimal (or near optimal) algorithm
for removing Gaussian noise. There are two approaches here. One is statistically based as developed by Donoho and Johnstone (see, e.g., [8]) and
the other is functional analytic as developed by DeVore and Lucier [7].

Quantization is a method for obtaining more compression in the file of
wavelet coefficients. The idea is to economically allocate the number of
bits to represent the coefficient $d_{j,\eta}(k)$. Namely, the coefficients $d_{j,\eta}(k)$ is
replaced by the number $d'_{j,\eta}(k)$ which satisfies

$$|d_{j,\eta}(k) - d'_{j,\eta}(k)| < \epsilon_j$$

and has the fewest number of bits in its binary representation. Note that
$\tau_j(d_{j,\eta}(k) - d'_{j,\eta}(k)) = 0$ which is the motivation for quantization.

The thresholding/quantization parameters ϵ_j can be related to the metric
in which the approximation takes place. We have normalized the wavelets
$\eta_{j,k}$ to have L_2-norm equal to one. Taking $\epsilon_j = \epsilon$ (i.e., thresholding does not
depend on the dyadic level) corresponds to approximation in the L_2 metric.
On the other hand, the choice $\epsilon_j := 2^{(1/2-1/p)2j}\epsilon$ corresponds to approximation in L_p, $0 < p \le \infty$[3]. We refer the reader to [5, 6], where a more
detailed discussion of the connections between thresholding/quantization
and approximation is given.

---

[3]The distance between two functions g, h in L_p is given by $\left(\int |g - h|^p\right)^{1/p}$.

Thresholding in the metric L_1 produces smoother images while thresholding in L_∞ emphasizes edges. We can emphasize edges even more by going to derivative norms. These correspond to increasing ϵ_j at high frequencies and thereby increasing the likelihood that a coefficient at a high frequency is retained.

Step III. Encoding. For the purposes of storage or transmission of the compressed image (and perhaps for further compression), a lossless encoder is applied to the file of wavelet coefficients. While standard arithmetic and runlength encoding can be applied, the best results are obtained with customized encoders (see, e.g., Shapiro [11]) which take into account the spatial correlation of the wavelet coefficients. The encoded wavelet coefficient file is our compressed representation of the image and can be stored or transmitted. Encoding will not play a role in our microcalcification detection, since in this application we are not interested in the storage or transmission of the mammograms.

The last two steps of the image compression schematic are utilized when we want to display the compressed image.

Step IV. Decoding. The encoded file is decoded to obtain the compressed wavelet coefficient file. This is the same file as at the end of Step II.

Step V. Computation of pixel values. We use the inverse fast wavelet transform to compute the pixel values of the compressed image. This step takes again $O(N)$ operations. These are then the pixel values of the compressed image which is our approximation to the original image.

6.4   Some Issues in Compression Algorithms

There are many important considerations in compression algorithms and we mention only a few that relate to the problems of feature extraction and edge detection.

6.4.1   Choice of Wavelet Basis

The performance of compression algorithms depends on the choice of wavelet basis. It is generally agreed upon that the bi-orthogonal wavelets (when combined with a customized encoder [11]) give the best compression with a fixed wavelet basis of the type (2.2). However, this does not necessarily carry over to feature classification, where the criterion for compression is not the visual quality of the compressed image but its effectiveness in the classification. Also, there are variants to the fixed basis given by (2.2) such as hyperbolic wavelet bases and adaptive bases (where the basis is allowed to depend on the image (see [4]).

6.4.2 Choice of Metric

We have noted earlier the effect of the choice of the metric on the thresholding/quantization strategies. In feature classification we have the option of tailoring the compression metric to the feature classification problem.

6.4.3 Level of Compression

We can also adjust the level of compression (compression ratio) to the task at hand. In compression for the purposes of storage or transmission, the visual quality of the image is the driving force behind selecting the compression ratio. However, in certain applications such as image registration, one may want to retain very few features (edges, corners) and therefore utilize high compression. In our application, we use compression primarily to remove noise.

6.5 Algorithms for the Detection of Microcalcification Clusters

We shall now propose a general strategy for constructing algorithms for extracting microcalcification clusters. We wish to distinguish between two types of algorithms. The first are autonomous and do not involve a computer operator. The second are interactive and allow decisions to be made to improve parameter settings which depend on the image. We have applied both approaches to a population of eleven mammograms — nine with microcalcification clusters and two without. The numerical results given in this paper are obtained from an autonomous algorithm. We shall point out where interactive algorithms have provided some improvement over the autonomous algorithm.

Both approaches have the same major steps which we now describe.

Step 1. Compression of the digitized image. An algorithm begins by utilizing compression as a preprocessor to the identification of the microcalcification clusters. The purpose of this step is to remove noise and still retain all microcalcifications. Our earlier results on compression of mammograms show that compression up to 50–1 is viable for this purpose. We have found, however, that a moderate compression (on the order of 10 or 15 to 1) has given the best performance on our limited population of examples.

While the choice of compression metric can be used in interactive algorithms to maximize performance, we have found that compression in the metric of L_2 gives quite satisfactory results. We have implemented compression with various wavelet filters. The six-tap Daubechies filter (corresponding to D_3) and certain bi-orthogonal filters give the best performance of fixed wavelet bases in that they retain all microcalcifications and maintain their shapes as well. We have found the use of hyperbolic wavelets and adaptively chosen wavelet bases to be promising and deserving of further analysis.

The autonomous algorithm used for the numerical examples in this paper are all based on the six-tap Daubechies filter with compression of approximately 13–1 in the L_2 metric.

Step 2. Selecting only high frequency terms. The purpose of this step is to retain only those frequency terms that correspond to the size of the microcalcifications. From the terms retained in the compressed image after step one, we delete all terms corresponding to dyadic levels $0, -1, \ldots,$ -5. Other possible adaptations of this selection are to retain only those terms at levels $j = -6, -7, -8$ corresponding to one or more of the dilated wavelets corresponding to the functions $\varphi(x)\psi(y)$, $\psi(x)\varphi(y)$, or $\psi(x)\psi(y)$ from Ψ. The first two of these choices emphasize edges in the vertical and horizontal directions while the latter emphasizes point singularities. Since microcalcifications are small, the use of $\psi(x)\psi(y)$ might seem preferred. Our numerical experiments show, however, that it is best to retain terms from all three of these wavelet functions.

Step 3. Reconstructing pixel values. This step constructs the image corresponding to the wavelet decomposition after Step 2. While the microcalcifications are very noticeable after this step, the image still has a nontrivial background which will be removed in the next steps.

Step 4. Nonlinear enhancement. The purpose of this step is to remove background and retain only the microcalcifications. Let us denote by $\tilde{p}_j$ the pixel values of the reconstructed image in Step 3. We shall modify these pixel values to obtain the new pixel values p_j^*. The new values p_j^* depend not only on $\tilde{p}_j$ but also on p_j:

$$p_j^* := E(p_j, \tilde{p}_j)$$

where E is some nonlinear enhancement function.

The properties we want for E are the following. If $\tilde{p}_j$ is small then p_j^* should be set to zero. We would also like to enhance $\tilde{p}_j$ in a way that depends on the background brightness of the original pixel values. That is, if $\tilde{p}_j$ is large and the average intensity of the original pixel values p_ν for ν near j is also large, then we would like p_j^* to be an increase of the value of $\tilde{p}_j$. Among all steps in this general algorithm, this step and the next benefit most from interaction.

In our autonomous algorithm, we have utilized the following enhancement function

$$E(p_j, \tilde{p}_j) := \begin{cases} 0, & p_j \le 60 \\ \tilde{p}_j, & 60 < p_j \le 300 \\ \tilde{p}_j + 3\alpha_j, & p_j > 300. \end{cases}$$

The local intensity α_j is defined as

$$\alpha_j := \max_{\nu \in \Lambda_j} \{p_\nu / 256\},$$

where Λ_j is a set of indices near j. In our autonomous algorithm, we take Λ_j to be a 5×5 square array centered at j.

Step 5. Thresholding pixel values. This step thresholds pixel values to retain only the most intense. In the autonomous algorithm this is obtained by retaining only the 300 largest pixel values p_j^*. We denote by $p_j^\#$ the pixel values after this step has been completed. We call the $p_j^\#$ *hot pixel* values. The hot pixels are indications of microcalcifications. However, further processing is necessary to be sure that the entire microcalcification is retained intact and also to eliminate hot pixels that are not part of microcalcification clusters.

Step 6. Removing isolated pixels. This step is intended to remove any isolated hot pixels. A microcalcification should correspond to several hot pixels. In our autonomous algorithm, we remove isolated hot pixels as follows. For each hot pixel $p_j^\#$, we create a 3×3 square of pixels centered at j. If no pixel in this square other than $p_j^\#$ is hot, then we remove $p_j^\#$ from the hot list.

Step 7. Filling out microcalcifications. The purpose of this step is to fill out microcalcifications. It could happen that the thresholding in Step 5 removed pixels which corresponded to microcalcifications and we want to restore these. In our autonomous algorithm, we do this as follows. If $p_j^\#$ is a hot pixel, we form a 3×3 square of pixels centered at j and we consider a ν from this square. If p_ν (the original pixel value corresponding to this location) is greater than $p_j - 5$ and if $p_\nu^\#$ was not one of the hot pixel values, then we change the value of $p_\nu^\#$ from zero to $p_j^\#$ and add it to our list of hot pixels.

Step 8. Test for clusters. Finally, we want to test for clusters. Given a hot pixel value $p_j^\#$, we examine all hot pixels in a 61×61 square of pixels centered at j. If $p_\nu^\#$ is a hot pixel from this square and $|p_\nu^\# - p_j^\#| < 10$, then we say $p_\nu^\#$ is connected to $p_j^\#$ and write $p_\nu^\# \sim p_j^\#$. We say that $p_j^\#$ is related to $p_{j'}^\#$ if there is a sequence $p_{\nu_k}^\#$, $k = 0, \ldots, m$, of hot pixel values with $\nu_0 = j$ and $\nu_m = j'$ and $p_{\nu_k}^{\#} \sim p_{\nu_{k+1}}^{\#}$, $k = 0, \ldots, m-1$. We then choose the smallest rectangle which contains all pixel values $p_{j'}^{\#}$ which are related to $p_j^{\#}$. In this way, we obtain boxes of hot pixel values which correspond to boxing our microcalcification clusters.

6.6   Examples

In Figures 6.4 and 6.5, we give two examples of the autonomous algorithm applied to digitized mammograms which exhibit microcalcification clusters. The upper image in each of these figures is the processed mammogram (after Step 8 has been completed). The lower image is the original mammogram with the clusters boxed.

We have also included an example of the autonomous algorithm applied to a digitized mammogram without microcalcification clusters. Of course, the final image (after Step 8) is completely black (all pixel values $p_j^{\#} = 0$).

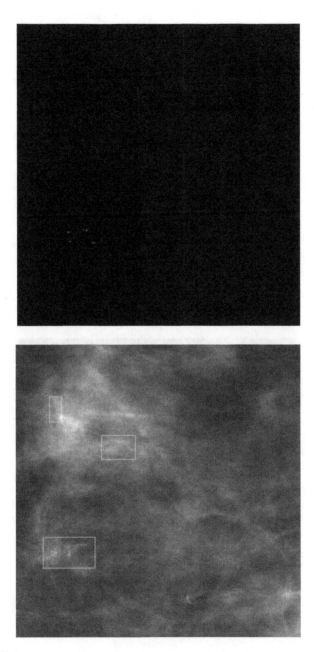

Figure 6.4
The autonomous algorithm applied to a mammogram with microcalcification clusters. Top is the processed image. Bottom is the original image with microcalcification clusters boxed.

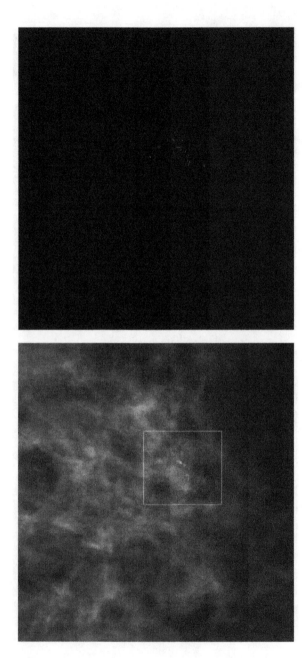

Figure 6.5
The autonomous algorithm applied to a mammogram with microcalcification clusters. Top is the processed image. Bottom is the original image with microcalcification clusters boxed.

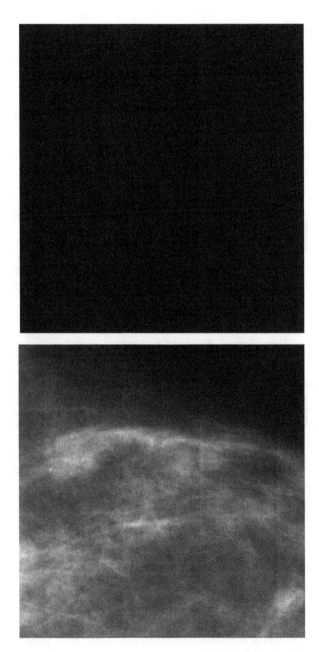

Figure 6.6
The autonomous algorithm applied to a mammogram without microcalcification clusters. Top is the processed image. Bottom is the original image.

References

[1] "Cancer facts & figures", Technical report, American Cancer Society, 1991.

[2] A. Cohen, I. Daubechies, and J. C. Feauveau, Biorthogonal bases of compactly supported wavelet, *Commun. Pure Appl. Math.* **45** (1992), 485–560.

[3] J. Dengler, S. Behrens, and J. F. Desaga, Segmentation of microcalcifications in mammograms, *IEEE Trans. Med. Imaging* **12** (1993), 634–642.

[4] R. DeVore, Adaptive wavelet bases for image compression, *Curves and Surfaces, II*, P. J. Laurent, A. Le Méhauté, and L. L. Schumaker, eds., A. K. Peters, Boston, 1994.

[5] R. DeVore, B. Jawerth, and V. Popov, Compression of wavelet decompositions, *Am. J. Math.* **114** (1992), 737–785.

[6] R. DeVore, B. Jawerth, and B. Lucier, Image compression through transform coding, *IEEE Proc. Inf. Theory* **38** (1992), 719–746.

[7] R. DeVore and B. Lucier, Fast wavelet techniques for near-optimal image processing, *1992 IEEE Military Communications Conference*, IEEE Communications Society, 1992, 1129–1135.

[8] D. L. Donoho and I. M. Johnstone, Ideal spatial adaptation via wavelet shrinkage, *Biometrika* **81** (1994), 425–455.

[9] B. Lucier, M. Kallergi, Wei Qian, R. DeVore, R. Clark, E. Saff, and L. P. Clarke, Wavelet compression and segmentation of mammographic images, *J. Digital Imaging* **7** (1994) 27–38.

[10] Laszlo Taber and Peter B. Dean, Teaching Atlas of Mammography, Georg Thieme Verlag, Stuttgart, 1985.

[11] Jerome Shapiro, An embedded hierarchical image coder using zerotrees of wavelet coefficients, *Data Compression Conference*, J. A. Storer and M. Cohn (eds.), IEEE Computer Society Press, Los Alamitosw, CA, 1993, 214–223.

[12] Z. Yang, M. Kallergi, R. DeVore, B. Lucier, W. Qian, R. A. Clark, and L. P. Clarke, The effect of wavelet bases on compression of digital mammograms, *IEEE Trans. Med. Imaging* (to appear).

[13] Z. Yang, Wavelets and Image Compression, *Ph.D. thesis*, the University of South Carolina, Columbia, 1995.

7

Multiscale Contrast Enhancement and Denoising in Digital Radiographs

Jian Fan[1] and Andrew Laine[2]

[1] *Hewlett-Packard Company, San Diego, California*
[2] *Computer and Information Science and Engineering Department, University of Florida, Gainesville, Florida*

7.1   Introduction

Image enhancement techniques have been widely used in fields such as radiology, where the subjective quality of images is important for human interpretation (diagnosis). Contrast is an important factor in any subjective evaluation of image quality. Many algorithms for accomplishing contrast enhancement have been developed and applied to problems in medical imaging . A comprehensive survey of existing methods can be found in [1]. Among them, histogram modification and edge enhancement techniques have been most commonly used along with traditional methods of image processing.

Histogram modification techniques [2, 3] are attractive due to their simplicity and speed, and have achieved acceptable results for some applications. In general, a transformation function is derived from a desired histogram and the histogram of an input image. In general, the transformation function is almost always nonlinear. For continuous functions, a lossless transformation may be achieved. However, for digital images with some finite number of gray levels, such a transformation results in information loss, due to quantization errors. For example, a subtle edge may be merged with its neighboring pixels and disappear. Attempts to incorporate local context into the transformation process have achieved limited success. For example, simple adaptive histogram equalization [4] supported by fixed contextual regions cannot adapt to features of distinct sizes.

Most edge enhancement algorithms share a common strategy implicitly: detection followed by local "edge sharpening". Unsharp masking is rare in that it has become a popular enhancement algorithm to assist radiologists in diagnosis [5, 6]. "Unsharp masking" sharpens edges by subtracting a portion of a Laplacian filtered component from an original image. Theoretically, this technique was justified as an approximation of a deblurring process in [7]. Loo et al. [8] studied an extension of this technique in the context of radiographs. Another extension based on Laplacian filtering was proposed in [9]. However, these techniques of unsharp masking remain limited by their linear and single scale properties and are less effective for images containing a wide range of salient features typically found in digital mammography. In an attempt to overcome these limitations, a local contrast measure and nonlinear transform functions were introduced in [10], and subsequently refined in [11]. Unfortunately, limitations remained in these nonlinear methods as well: (1) They operated on a single scale; (2) no explicit noise suppression stage was included (in fact noise could be amplified); and (3) ad-hoc nonlinear transform functions were introduced without a rigorous mathematical analysis of their enhancement mechanisms or the possible introduction of artifacts.

Recent advancement of wavelet theory has sparked researchers' interest in the application of image contrast enhancement [12–18]. These early studies showed promise, but were carried out at an experimental level. In this chapter, we give a detailed mathematical analysis of a dyadic wavelet transform and reveal its connection to traditional techniques of unsharp masking. In addition, we propose a simple nonlinear enhancement function and analyze the problem of introducing artifacts, as a result of wavelet processing. Moreover, we describe an explicit denoising stage that preserves edges using wavelet shrinkage [23] and adaptive thresholding.

These techniques are discussed in the following sections of this chapter: Section 7.2 presents a one-dimensional dyadic wavelet transform. Section 7.3 analyzes linear enhancement and its mathematical connection to traditional unsharp masking. Section 7.4 analyzes simple nonlinear enhancement by point-wise functional mapping. Section 7.5 introduces denoising with wavelet shrinkage along with an adaptive approach for finding threshold values. Section 7.6 presents a two-dimensional extension for digital mam-

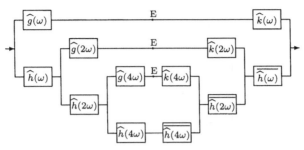

Figure 7.1
Computational structure for a one-dimensional discrete dyadic
wavelet transform (three levels shown).

mography and special procedures developed for denoising and enhancement
that avoid orientation distortions. Section 7.7 presents some sample experimental results and comparisons with existing techniques. Finally, Section
7.8 concludes our discussion and proposes possible future directions of research.

7.2 One-Dimensional Discrete Dyadic Wavelet Transform

7.2.1 General Structure and Channel Characteristics

A fast algorithm [20] for computing a 1-D redundant discrete dyadic
wavelet transform (RDWT) is shown in Figure 7.1. The left side shows its
decomposition structure, and the right, reconstruction. For an N-channel
structure, there are $N-1$ high-pass or bandpass channels and a low-pass
channel. Thus, the decomposition of a signal produces $N-1$ sets of wavelet
coefficients and a coarse signal.

Since there is no down-sampling and up-sampling shown in Figure 7.1,
our redundant discrete dyadic wavelet transform does not correspond to an
orthogonal wavelet basis (see Chapter 1, Section 1.3.2).

For simplicity of analysis, an equivalent multichannel structure is shown
in Figure 7.2. This computational structure also makes obvious the potential for high-speed execution by parallel processing.

We shall refer to filters $\widehat{f}_m(\omega)$ and $\widehat{i}_m(\omega)$ in Figure 7.2 as forward filters
and inverse filters, respectively. Their relationship to filters $\widehat{g}(\omega)$, $\widehat{k}(\omega)$ and

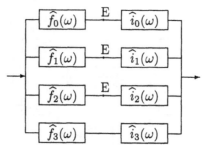

Figure 7.2
An equivalent multichannel structure for a three-level RDWT.

$\widehat{h}(\omega)$ are explicitly given by

$$\widehat{f}_0(\omega) = \widehat{g}(\omega), \quad \widehat{f}_N(\omega) = \prod_{l=0}^{N-1} \widehat{h}(2^l\omega),$$

$$\widehat{f}_m(\omega) = \left[\prod_{l=0}^{m-1} \widehat{h}(2^l\omega)\right]\widehat{g}(2^m\omega), \quad 1 \le m \le N-1.$$

and

$$\widehat{i}_0(\omega) = \widehat{k}(\omega), \quad \widehat{i}_N(\omega) = \prod_{l=0}^{N-1} \overline{\widehat{h}(2^l\omega)},$$

$$\widehat{i}_m(\omega) = \left[\prod_{l=0}^{m-1} \overline{\widehat{h}(2^l\omega)}\right]\widehat{k}(2^m\omega), \quad 1 \le m \le N-1.$$

Since filters $\widehat{h}(\omega)$, $\widehat{g}(\omega)$ and $\widehat{k}(\omega)$ satisfy the condition

$$\left|\widehat{h}(\omega)\right|^2 + \widehat{g}(\omega)\widehat{k}(\omega) = 1, \tag{7.1}$$

filters $\widehat{f}_m(\omega)$ and $\widehat{i}_m(\omega)$ completely cover the frequency domain,

$$\sum_l \widehat{f}_l(\omega)\widehat{i}_l(\omega) = 1.$$

Channel frequency responses $\widehat{c}_m(\omega)$ can be written as

$$\widehat{c}_m(\omega) = \widehat{f}_m(\omega)\widehat{i}_m(\omega) = \begin{cases} 1 - \left|\widehat{h}(\omega)\right|^2, & m = 0, \\ \prod_{l=0}^{m-1}\left|\widehat{h}(2^l\omega)\right|^2\left[1 - \left|\widehat{h}(2^m\omega)\right|^2\right], \\ \qquad\qquad\qquad\qquad 1 \leq m \leq (N-1), \\ \prod_{l=0}^{N-1}\left|\widehat{h}(2^l\omega)\right|^2, & m = N. \end{cases}$$

As an example, we consider an extension of the class of filters proposed by Mallat and Zhang in [20]

$$\widehat{h}(\omega) = e^{ip\frac{\omega}{2}}\left[\cos\left(\frac{\omega}{2}\right)\right]^{2n+p}, \tag{7.2}$$

where $p = 0$, or 1. Let

$$\widehat{\theta}_{m,q}(\omega) = \left[\prod_{l=0}^{m-1}\cos(2^{l-1}\omega)\right]^q,$$

then we can show that

$$\widehat{\theta}_{m,q}(\omega) = \left[\frac{\sin(2^{m-1}\omega)}{2^m\sin(\frac{\omega}{2})}\right]^q, \tag{7.3}$$

and therefore

$$\widehat{c}_m(\omega) = \begin{cases} \widehat{\theta}_{m,4n+2p}(\omega) - \widehat{\theta}_{m+1,4n+2p}(\omega), & 0 \leq m \leq (N-1), \\ \widehat{\theta}_{N,4n+2p}(\omega), & m = N. \end{cases} \tag{7.4}$$

Note that $\widehat{\theta}_{0,n}(\omega) = 1$, and for $0 < m < N$,

$$\widehat{c}_m(\omega) = \widehat{\theta}_{m,4n+2p}(\omega) - \widehat{\theta}_{m+1,4n+2p}(\omega) \tag{7.5}$$

$$= \sin^2\left(\frac{\omega}{2}\right)4^m\widehat{\theta}_{m,4n+2p+2}(\omega)\sum_{l=0}^{2n+p-1}\left[\cos\left(2^{m-1}\omega\right)\right]^{2l},$$

and $\sin^2(\omega/2)$ is the frequency response of the discrete Laplacian operator of impulse response $\{1, -2, 1\}$.

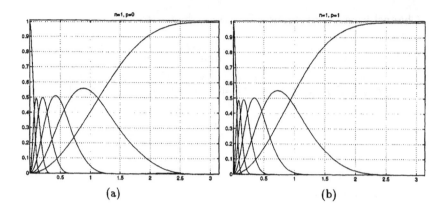

Figure 7.3
Channel frequency responses for $N = 6$, $n = 1$ and (a) $p = 0$ and (b) $p = 1$.

$\widehat{\theta}_{m,q}(\omega)$ with even exponential q is an approximate Gaussian function, while the frequency responses of channels $0 < m < N$ are approximately a Laplacian of Gaussian. Figure 7.3 shows each distinct channel frequency response, and Figure 7.4 compares $\widehat{\theta}_{2,4}(\omega)$ and $\widehat{\theta}_{2,6}(\omega)$ with related Gaussians.

7.2.2   Two Possible Filters

In this framework, the possible choices of filters are constrained by Equation (7.1). For the class of filters defined by Equation (7.2), we can derive

$$\widehat{g}(\omega)\widehat{k}(\omega) = \sin^2\left(\frac{\omega}{2}\right) \sum_{l=0}^{2n+p-1} \left[\cos\left(\frac{\omega}{2}\right)\right]^{2l}.$$

Under the constraint of both $\widehat{g}(\omega)$ and $\widehat{k}(\omega)$ being FIRs, there are two possible choices distinguished by the order of zeros in their frequency responses.

(1) **Laplacian filter.** In this case, $\widehat{g}(\omega) = -4\sin^2(\omega/2)$ or $g(l) = \{1, -2, 1\}$, which defines a discrete Laplacian operator, such that $(g * s)(l) = s(l + 1) - 2s(l) + s(l - 1)$. Accordingly, we can choose both filters $\widehat{h}(\omega)$ and $\widehat{k}(\omega)$ to be symmetric,

$$\widehat{h}(\omega) = \left[\cos\left(\frac{\omega}{2}\right)\right]^{2n}$$

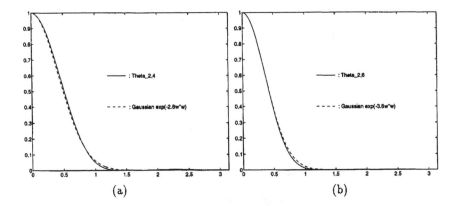

Figure 7.4
(a) $\widehat{\theta}_{2,4}(\omega)$ compared with the Gaussian function $e^{-2.8\omega^2}$. (b) $\widehat{\theta}_{2,6}(\omega)$ compared with the Gaussian function $e^{-3.8\omega^2}$.

and

$$\widehat{k}(\omega) = \frac{1 - \left|\widehat{h}(\omega)\right|^2}{\widehat{g}(\omega)} = -\frac{1}{4}\sum_{l=0}^{2n-1}\left[\cos\left(\frac{\omega}{2}\right)\right]^{2l}.$$

Both forward and inverse filters, $0 \le m \le N - 1$, can be derived by

$$\widehat{f}_m(\omega) = -4\left[\sin(2^{m-1}\omega)\right]^2 \widehat{\theta}_{m,2n}(\omega) \tag{7.6}$$

$$= -4\sin^2\left(\frac{\omega}{2}\right)4^m\widehat{\theta}_{m,2n+2}(\omega) = \widehat{g}(\omega)\widehat{\lambda}_m(\omega)$$

and

$$\widehat{i}_m(\omega) = -\widehat{\theta}_{m,2n}(\omega)\frac{1}{4}\sum_{l=0}^{2n-1}\left[\cos\left(2^{m-1}\omega\right)\right]^{2l} = -\widehat{\gamma}_m(\omega).$$

Note that the forward filters $\widehat{f}_m(\omega)$, $0 < m < N$, can be interpreted as two cascaded operations, a Gaussian averaging of $\widehat{\theta}_{m,2n+2}(\omega)$ and the Laplacian $-4\sin^2(\omega/2)$, while the set of inverse filters $\widehat{i}_m(\omega)$ are low-pass filters. For an input signal $s(l)$, wavelet coefficients at the points "E" (as shown in Figures 7.1 and 7.2) may be written as $w_m(l) = \Delta(s * \lambda_m)(l)$ where Δ is the discrete Laplacian operator, and $\lambda_m(l)$ is approximately a Gaussian filter. This means that each wavelet coefficient $w_m(l)$ is dependent on the local contrast of the original signal at each position l.

(2) **Gradient filter.** In this case, $\widehat{g}(\omega) = 2ie^{-i\omega/2}\sin(\omega/2)$, or $g(0) = 1$, and $g(1) = -1$, such that $(g * s)(l) = s(l) - s(l-1)$. Thus we select the filters

$$\widehat{h}(\omega) = e^{i\frac{\omega}{2}}\left[\cos\left(\frac{\omega}{2}\right)\right]^{2n+1}$$

and

$$\widehat{k}(\omega) = -e^{i\omega}\widehat{g}(\omega)\frac{1}{4}\sum_{l=0}^{2n}\left[\cos\left(\frac{\omega}{2}\right)\right]^{2l}.$$

We then derived the forward filters

$$\widehat{f}_m(\omega) = \widehat{g}(\omega)2^m\widehat{\theta}_{m,2n+2}(\omega) = \widehat{g}(\omega)\widehat{\lambda}_m(\omega)$$

and inverse filters

$$\widehat{i}_m(\omega) = -e^{i\omega}\widehat{g}(\omega)\widehat{\gamma}_m(\omega),$$

where

$$\widehat{\gamma}_m(\omega) = 2^m\widehat{\theta}_{m,2n+2}(\omega)\frac{1}{4}\sum_{l=0}^{2n}\left[\cos\left(2^{m-1}\omega\right)\right]^{2l}$$

is a low-pass filter. In this case, the associated wavelet coefficients may be written as

$$w_m(l) = \nabla(s * \lambda_m)(l)$$

where ∇ is a discrete gradient operator characterized by

$$\nabla s(l) = s(l) - s(l-1).$$

7.3 Linear Enhancement and Unsharp Masking

7.3.1 Review of Unsharp Masking

An early prototype of unsharp masking [7] was

$$s_u(x,y) = s(x,y) - k\Delta s(x,y), \tag{7.7}$$

where $\Delta = \frac{\partial^2}{\partial x^2} + \frac{\partial^2}{\partial y^2}$ is the Laplacian operator. However, this original formula worked only at the level of finest resolution. More versatile formulas were later developed in two distinct ways.

One way to extend this original formula was based on exploiting the averaging concept behind the Laplacian operator. The discrete form of the Laplacian operator may be written as

$$\Delta s(i,j) = [s(i+1,j) - 2s(i,j) + s(i-1,j)]$$

$$+ [s(i,j+1) - 2s(i,j) + s(i,j-1)]$$

$$= -5 \left\{ s(i,j) - \tfrac{1}{5} [s(i+1,j) + s(i-1,j) \right.$$

$$\left. + s(i,j) + s(i,j+1) + s(i,j-1)] \right\}.$$

This formula shows that the discrete Laplacian operator can be implemented by subtracting from the value of a central point its average neighborhood. Thus, an extended formula [8] can be written as

$$s_u(i,j) = s(i,j) + k\left[s(i,j) - (s * h)(i,j)\right], \tag{7.8}$$

where $h(i,j)$ is a discrete averaging filter, and $*$ denotes convolution. In [8], an equal-weighted averaging mask was used:

$$h(x,y) = \begin{cases} 1/N^2, & |x| < N/2, \ |y| < N/2 \\ 0, & \text{otherwise.} \end{cases}$$

Another way to extend the prototype formula [9] came from the idea of a Laplacian-of-Gaussian filter, which expands Equation (7.7) into

$$s_u(x,y) = s(x,y) - k\Delta(s * g)(x,y) = s(x,y) - k(s * \Delta g)(x,y), \tag{7.9}$$

where $g(x,y)$ is a Gaussian function, and $\Delta g(x,y)$ is a Laplacian-of-Gaussian filter.

We mention for future reference, that both extensions shown in Equations (7.8) and (7.9) are limited to a single scale.

7.3.2 Inclusion of Unsharp Masking within RDWT Frame-Work

Next, we shall prove that unsharp masking with a Gaussian low-pass filter is included in a dyadic wavelet framework for enhancement by considering two special cases of linear enhancement.

In the first case, transform coefficients of channels $0 \leq m \leq N - 1$ are enhanced (multiplied) by the same gain $G_0 > 1$, or $G_m = G_0 > 1$, $0 \leq m \leq N - 1$. The system frequency response is thus

$$\widehat{v}(\omega) = \sum_{m=0}^{N-1} G_m \widehat{c}_m(\omega) + \widehat{c}_N(\omega) = G_0 \sum_{m=0}^{N} \widehat{c}_m(\omega) - (G_0 - 1)\widehat{c}_N(\omega)$$

$$= G_0 - (G_0 - 1)\widehat{c}_N(\omega) = 1 + (G_0 - 1)\left[1 - \widehat{c}_N(\omega)\right].$$

This makes the input-output relationship of the system simply

$$s_e(l) = s(l) + (G_0 - 1)\left[s(l) - (s * c_N)(l)\right]. \tag{7.10}$$

Since $\widehat{c}_N(\omega)$ is approximately a Gaussian low-pass filter, Equation (7.10) may be seen as the 1-D counterpart of Equation (7.8).

In the second case, transform coefficients of a single channel p, $0 \leq p < N$ are enhanced by a gain $G_p > 1$, thus

$$\widehat{v}(\omega) = \sum_{m \neq p} \widehat{c}_m(\omega) + G_p \widehat{c}_p(\omega) \tag{7.11}$$

$$= \sum_{m=0}^{N} \widehat{c}_m(\omega) + (G_p - 1)\widehat{c}_p(\omega) = 1 + (G_p - 1)\widehat{c}_p(\omega).$$

Recalling the channel frequency response $\widehat{c}_m(\omega)$ derived previously in 7.5, the input-output relationship of the system (7.11) can be written as

$$s_e(l) = s(l) - (G_p - 1) \cdot \Delta(s * \eta)(l), \tag{7.12}$$

where $\eta(l)$ is the impulse response of an approximate Gaussian filter. Similarly, Equation (7.12) may be seen as the 1-D counterpart of Equation (7.9).

The inclusion of these two forms of unsharp masking demonstrates the flexibility and versatility of a dyadic wavelet framework.

7.4 Nonlinear Enhancement by Functional Mapping

Linear enhancement can be seen as a mapping of wavelet coefficients by a linear function $E_m(x) = G_m x$. Therefore, a direct extension of this is a nonlinear mapping function $E_m(x)$. The main challenges here are how to design a nonlinear function and how to best utilize multichannel information extracted from a dyadic wavelet framework to accomplish contrast enhancement.

7.4.1 Minimum Constraint for an Enhancement Function

A major concern for our enhancement scheme was to introduce no artifacts during processing and reconstruction. For the dyadic wavelet framework adopted, this meant that we could not create new extrema in the channel outputs. This defined a minimum constraint on any enhancement function, that is, such a function must be continuous and monotonically increasing.

7.4.2 Filter Selection

For linear enhancement, selection of filters $\widehat{g}(\omega)$ (and thus $\widehat{k}(\omega)$) made no difference. However, this was not true for the nonlinear case. For this particular nonlinear approach, our analysis showed that a Laplacian filter should be favored.

By selecting a Laplacian filter, we can be assured that positions of extrema will be unchanged and that no new extremum will be created within each channel. This is possible because:

(1) Laplacian filters are zero-phase. No spatial shifting exists in the transform space.

(2) A monotonically increasing function $E(x)$ will not produce new extrema. (At some point x_0, $E[f(x_0)]$ is an extremum if and only if $f(x_0)$ was an extremum.)

(3) The reconstruction filters are simply zero-phase smoothing filters which will not create extrema.

The major difficulty for using a gradient filter is that reconstruction includes another gradient operator. As a result, a monotonically increasing function $E(x)$ alone will no longer guarantee new extrema will not be introduced in each *output channel.* Moreover, it is not difficult to show that any nonlinear mapping will change the positions of original extrema. There-

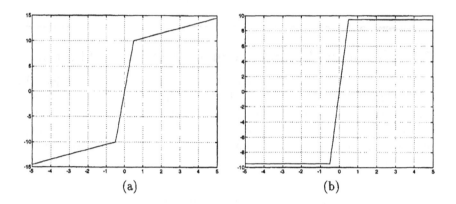

Figure 7.5
(a) $E(x)$ and (b) $\delta(x)$, both with $T = 0.5$ and $K = 20$.

fore, we shall assume the choice of Laplacian filters in the remainder of this section.

7.4.3   A Nonlinear Enhancement Function

Designing a nonlinear enhancement scheme is made difficult due to two reasons: (1) the problem of defining a criteria of optimality for contrast enhancement. (2) complexity of analyzing nonlinear systems. We adopted the following guidelines in designing our nonlinear enhancement functions:

(1)   An area of low contrast should be enhanced more than an area of high contrast. This is equivalent to saying that small values of $w_m[l]$ should have larger gains.

(2)   A sharp edge should not be blurred.

Experimentally, we found the following simple function advantageous:

$$E(x) = \begin{cases} x - (K-1)T \,, & \text{if } x < -T \\ Kx \quad\quad\quad\;, & \text{if } |x| \le T \\ x + (K-1)T \,, & \text{if } x > T \end{cases} = x + \delta(x) \qquad (7.13)$$

where $K > 1$ and

$$\delta(x) = \begin{cases} -(K-1)T, & \text{if } x < -T, \\ (K-1)x, & \text{if } |x| \le T, \\ (K-1)T, & \text{if } x > T. \end{cases}$$

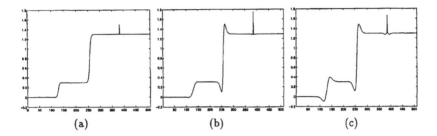

(a)   (b)   (c)

Figure 7.6
1-D contrast enhancement of a synthetic signal (a) by four-level dyadic wavelet analysis with (b) a linear operator with $K_0 = 2.3$, and (c) a nonlinear operator with $t = 0.1$ and $K_0 = 7$.

The enhancement operator δ_m has two free parameters: threshold T_m and gain K_m. In our experimental studies, $K_m = K_0$, $0 \le m \le N-1$, and $T_m = t \times \max\{|w_m[n]|\}$, where $0 < t \le 1$ was user specified. For $t = 1.0$, wavelet coefficients at levels $0 \le m \le N-1$ were multiplied by a gain of K_0, shown previously to be mathematically equivalent to unsharp masking. Thus our nonlinear algorithm includes unsharp masking as a subset. Figure 7.6 shows a numerical example, comparing linear and nonlinear enhancement. Note the lack of enhancement for the leftmost edge, in the case of the linear operator.

Specifically, an enhanced signal $s_e(l)$ can be written as

$$s_e(l) = \sum_{m=0}^{N-1} (E_m [(s * f_m)] * i_m)(l) + (s * f_N * i_N)(l)$$

$$= \sum_{m=0}^{N} (s * f_m * i_m)(l) + \sum_{m=0}^{N-1} (\delta_m [\Delta(s * \lambda_m)] * i_m)(l)$$

or,

$$s_e(l) = s(l) - \sum_{m=0}^{N-1} (\delta_m [\Delta(s * \lambda_m)] * \gamma_m)(l). \qquad (7.14)$$

For completeness, we mention that the formula of Equation (7.14) can be seen as a multiscale and nonlinear extension of the original unsharp masking defined by Equation (7.9). We argue that multiscale unsharp masking as defined by Equation (7.14) makes a marked improvement over traditional techniques in two respects:

(1)   The fast multiscale (or multimask) decomposition efficiently identifies features existing within distinct levels of scale, eliminating the need for search.

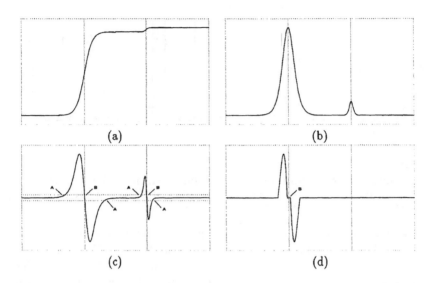

Figure 7.7
(a) Signal with two edges.   (b) First derivative (gradient).
(c) Second derivative (Laplacian). (d) Shrunken second deriva-
tive.

(2)   The nonlinear algorithm enhances small features within each scale
      without blurring the edges of larger features, making possible the
      simultaneous enhancement of features of all sizes.

7.5   A Methodology for Combined Denoising and Enhancement

The nonlinear enhancement methods proposed previously [11] did not
take into account the presence of noise. In general, noise exists in a digitized
image, due to the imaging device (acquisition) and quantization. As a
result of nonlinear processing, noise may be amplified and may diminish
any benefit of enhancement.

Unfortunately, denoising a radiograph (or any medical image) is a very
difficult problem for two reasons. Fundamentally, there is no absolute
boundary to distinguish a feature from noise. Even if there are known
characteristics of a certain type of noise, it may be theoretically impossible
to completely separate the noise from features of interest. Therefore, most
denoising methods may be seen as ways to suppress very high frequency
and incoherent components of an input signal.

A naive method of denoising that is equivalent to low-pass filtering is naturally included in any dyadic wavelet framework. That is, simply discard several channels of highest resolution, and enhance channels confined to lower frequency. The problem associated with this linear denoising approach is that edges are blurred significantly. This flaw makes linear denoising unsuitable within a contrast enhancement scheme targeted for medical imaging. Figure 7.9 (c) shows an example of this approach. In order to achieve edge-preserved denoising, more sophisticated methods based on wavelet analysis were proposed in the literature. Mallat and Hwang [22] connected noise behavior to singularities. Their algorithm relied on a multiscale edge representation. The algorithm traced modulus wavelet maxima to evaluate local Lipschitz exponents and deleted maxima points with negative Lipschitz exponents. Donoho [23] proposed nonlinear wavelet shrinkage. This algorithm reduced wavelet coefficients towards zero, based on a level-dependent threshold.

7.5.1 Incorporating Wavelet Shrinkage into Enhancement

The method of wavelet shrinkage can be incorporated trivially into our nonlinear enhancement framework by simply adding an extra segment to the enhancement function $E(x)$, defined earlier in Equation (7.13).

$$E(x) = \begin{cases} x - (K-1)T_e + KT_n, & \text{if } x \leq -T_e \\ K(x + T_n), & \text{if } -T_e \leq x \leq -T_n \\ 0, & \text{if } |x| \leq T_n \\ K(x - T_n), & \text{if } T_n \leq x \leq T_e \\ x + (K-1)T_e - KT_n, & \text{if } x \geq T_e \end{cases} \qquad (7.15)$$

However, there are two arguments which favor shrinking *gradient coefficients* instead of *Laplacian coefficients*.

First, gradient coefficients exhibit a higher signal-to-noise ratio (SNR). For any shrinkage scheme to be effective, an essential property is that the magnitude of a signal's components be larger than that of existing noise (at least most of the time). It is thus sensible to define the SNR as the maximum magnitude of a signal over the maximum magnitude of noise. For example, consider a soft edge model $f(x) = A/(1 + e^{-2\beta x})$, $A > 0$. Its first and second derivatives are $f'(x) = A\beta/\left[2\cosh^2(\beta x)\right]$ and $f''(x) = -A\beta^2 \sinh(\beta x)/\cosh^3(\beta x)$, with magnitude of local extrema $|f'(x_0)| = A|\beta|/3$ and $|f''(x_0)| = 2A\beta^2/3\sqrt{3}$, respectively. In this simple model, we can assume that noise is characterized by a relatively small A value and large β value. Clearly, gradient coefficients have a higher SNR than that of Laplacian coefficients since β contributes less. Figures 7.7 (b)

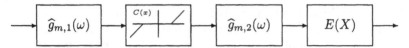

Figure 7.8
Incorporating wavelet shrinkage into an enhancement framework (one level shown).

and (c) show first and second derivatives, respectively, for an input signal (a) with two distinct edges.

In addition, boundary contrast is not affected by shrinking gradient coefficients. As shown in Figure 7.7, coefficients aligned to the boundary of an edge are local extrema in the case of a first derivative (gradient), and zero crossings in the case of a second derivative (Laplacian). For a simple point-wise shrinking operator, there is no way to distinguish the points marked "B" from the points marked "A". As a result, regions around each "A" and "B" point are diminished, while the discontinuity in "B" (Figure 7.7) sacrifices boundary contrast.

In the previous section, we argued that nonlinear enhancement is best performed on Laplacian coefficients. Therefore, in order to incorporate denoising into our enhancement algorithm, we split the Laplacian operator into two cascaded gradient operators. Note that

$$\widehat{g}_m(\omega) = -4 \left[\sin \left(2^{m-1} \omega \right) \right]^2 = \widehat{g}_{m,1}(\omega) \widehat{g}_{m,2}(\omega)$$

where

$$\widehat{g}_{m,1}(\omega) = e^{-i\omega/2} 2i \sin \left(\tfrac{\omega}{2} \right), \widehat{g}_{m,2}(\omega) = e^{i\omega/2} 2i \sin \left(\tfrac{\omega}{2} \right), \quad \text{if } m = 0,$$

$$\widehat{g}_{m,1}(\omega) = \widehat{g}_{m,2}(\omega) = 2i \sin \left(2^{m-1} \omega \right), \quad\quad\quad\quad\quad \text{otherwise.}$$

Denoising by wavelet shrinkage [23] can then be incorporated into this computational structure as illustrated in Figure 7.8, where the shrinking operator can be written as

$$C(x) = sign(x) \cdot \begin{cases} |x| - T_n, & \text{if } |x| > T_n, \\ 0, & \text{otherwise.} \end{cases}$$

Note that the shrinking operator is a piece-wise linear and monotonically nondecreasing function. Thus in practice, the shrinking operator will not introduce artifacts.

7.5.2 Threshold Estimation for Denoising

The threshold T_n is a critical parameter in the shrinking operation. For a white noise model and orthogonal wavelet, Donoho [23] suggested a formula of $T_n = \sqrt{2\log(N)}\,\sigma/\sqrt{N}$, where N is the length of a input signal and σ is the standard deviation of wavelet coefficients. However, the dyadic wavelet we applied is not an orthogonal wavelet. Moreover, in our 2-D applications, a shrinking operation is applied to magnitudes of gradient coefficients instead of wavelet coefficients themselves. Therefore, a method of threshold estimation method proposed in [24] for edge detection may be more suitable.

In our "shrinking" operation, only the magnitudes of the gradient of a Gaussian low-passed signal are modified. As pointed out in [24], for white Gaussian noise, the probability distribution function of the magnitudes of gradient is characterized by the Rayleigh distribution:

$$
Pr_{\|\Delta f\|}(m) = \begin{cases} \frac{m}{\eta^2} e^{-(m/\eta)^2/2}, & m \geq 0, \\ 0, & m < 0. \end{cases}
$$

To estimate η, a histogram (probability) of $\|\Delta f\|$ was computed, and then iterative curve fitting was applied. Under this model, the probability p of noise removal for a particular threshold τ can be calculated by

$$
p = \frac{\int_0^\tau Pr_{\|\Delta f\|}(m)dm}{\int_0^\infty Pr_{\|\Delta f\|}(m)dm},
$$

and thus $\tau = \sqrt{-2\ln(1-p)}\,\eta$. For $p = 0.999$, $\tau = 3.7\eta$.

Figure 7.9 compares the performance of existing approaches. In (b), we observed that enhancement without any denoising results in distracting background noise. In (c), edges were smeared and broadened by low-pass enhancement. Only in (d), with wavelet shrinkage enabled, were we to achieve the remarkable result of denoising and contrast enhancement simultaneously.

To demonstrate the denoising process, Figure 7.10 (a) and (b) shows both nonlinear enhancement of wavelet coefficients without and with denoising, respectively, for the original input signal shown in Figure 7.9 (a). Figure 7.10 (c) shows the associated curve-fitting for threshold estimation.

7.6   Two-Dimensional Extension

For image processing applications, the one-dimensional structures discussed previously were simply extended to two dimensions. In our investigation, we first adopted the method proposed by Mallat [20], shown in Figure 7.11, where filter $\widehat{l}(\omega) = (1 + |\widehat{h}(\omega)|^2)/2$, and $\widehat{h}(\omega)$, $\widehat{k}(\omega)$ and $\widehat{g}(\omega)$ were the same filters constructed for the 1-D case.

However, experimentally we observed that if we simply modified the two oriented wavelet coefficients independently, orientation distortions were introduced. One way to avoid this disastrous artifact is first to apply denoising to the magnitude of gradient coefficients, and then nonlinear enhancement to the sum of the Laplacian coefficients, as shown below in Figure 7.12. For the two oriented gradient coefficients g_x and g_y, the magnitude M and phase P were computed as $M = \sqrt{g_x^2 + g_y^2}$ and $P = \arctan(g_y/g_x)$, respectively. The denoising operation was then applied to M, obtaining M'. The denoised coefficients were then simply restored as $g'_x = M' * \cos(P)$ and $g'_y = M' * \sin(P)$, respectively. For the enhancement operation, notice that the sum of two Laplacian components is *isotropic*. Therefore, we may compute the sum of the two Laplacian components $L = l_x + l_y$ and $F = l_x/L$. A nonlinear enhancement operator was then applied to only L, producing L'. Thus, the restored components were $l'_x = L' * F$ and $l'_y = L' * (1 - F)$.

7.7   Experimental Results and Comparisons

In this section, we present samples of experimental results and compare them with existing state-of-the-art techniques. Figure 7.13 (a) shows a synthetic image with three circular "bumps" and added white noise. The enhancement results shown in (b) and (c) demonstrate amplification of unwanted noise. Moreover, note that histogram equalization processing alters the object's boundary. However, the result shown in (d) accomplished by dyadic wavelet analysis produced a clearer image without orientation distortion.

Figure 7.14 (a) shows an original dense mammogram image with an obvious mass. The boundary of the mass in the enhanced image is more defined and the penetration of spicules into the mass is well delineated.

To study the efficacy of our algorithm, we blended mathematical phantom features into clinically proved cancer-free mammograms. Figures 7.15 (a) and (b) show mathematical phantom features blended into each image M48 and M56 (resulting in Figure 7.16 [a] and Figure 7.17 [a]), respectively.

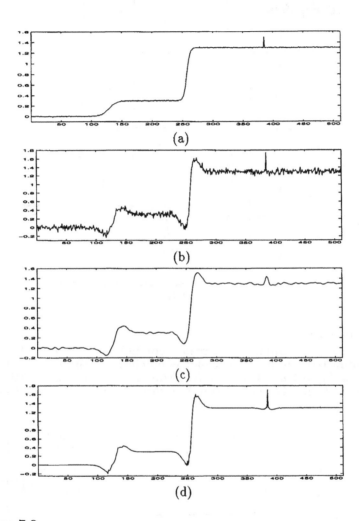

Figure 7.9
(a) Noisy input signal (contaminated by white Gaussian noise).
(b) Nonlinear enhancement without denoising, $G_m = 10$, $N = 4$,
$t = 0.1$. (c) Nonlinear enhancement of levels 2-3, $G_m = 10$, $t = 0.1$;
levels 0–1 zeroed out. (d) Nonlinear enhancement with adaptive
wavelet shrinkage denoising, $G_m = 10$, $N = 4$, $t = 0.1$.

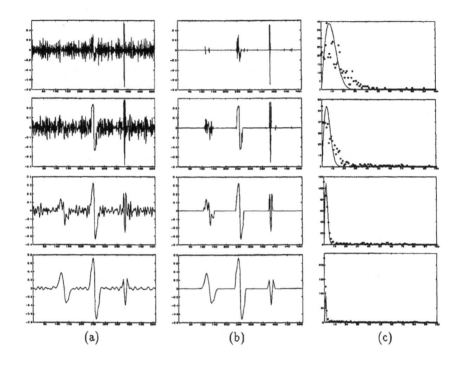

(a)   (b)   (c)

Figure 7.10
Column (a), Enhanced wavelet coefficients without denoising.
Column (b), enhanced wavelet coefficients with adaptive thresholding $T_n = 4.5\eta$. Column (c), the magnitude distribution and
curve-fitting. (Rows 1 through 4 correspond to levels 1 to 4.)

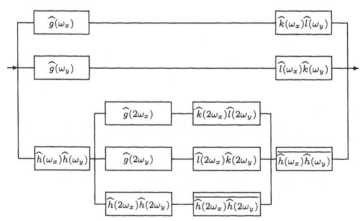

Figure 7.11
Two-dimensional dyadic wavelet transform (two levels shown).

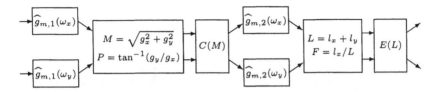

Figure 7.12
Denoising and enhancement for the 2-D case (level one shown).

Figure 7.16 (a) shows a dense mammogram with blended phantom features, and (b) shows an image processed by our nonlinear method. The enhanced image makes more visible the boundary (uncompressed areas) of the breast and its structure. In addition, the phantom features were also well enhanced. Figure 7.17 (a) shows a dense mammogram with blended phantom features, and (b) shows the associated image enhanced.

7.8 Conclusion

We established connections between dyadic wavelet enhancement algorithms and traditional unsharp masking. We proved that two cases of linear enhancement were mathematically equivalent to traditional unsharp masking with Gaussian low-pass filtering. We designed a methodology for accomplishing nonlinear enhancement with a simple nonlinear function to overcome the wide dynamic range usually required for contrast enhancement of digital radiographs. By careful selection of wavelet filters and enhancement functions, we showed that artifacts could be minimized. An additional advantage of our simple enhancement function is that it includes traditional unsharp masking as a subset.

We then showed how an edge-preserved denoising stage (wavelet shrinkage) can be appropriately incorporated into our contrast enhancement framework, and introduced a method for adaptive threshold estimation. Finally, we showed how denoising and enhancement operations should be carried out for two-dimensional images to avoid distortions due to filter orientation.

Our future research plan shall include the systematic study of gain and threshold parameters for nonlinear enhancement. In addition, in the next year we plan to develop localized and complex nonlinear methods to improve the performance of our existing algorithm.

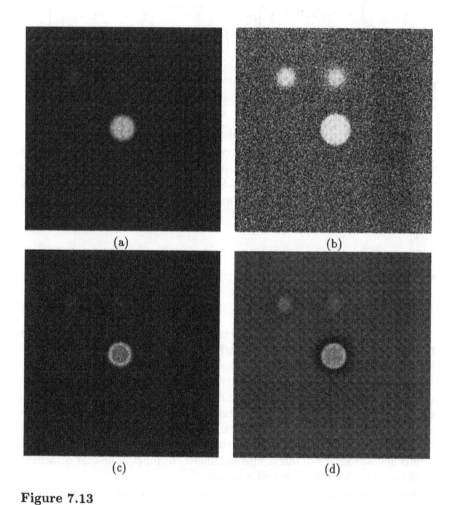

(a)   (b)

(c)   (d)

Figure 7.13
(a) Noisy image (white Gaussian noise contaminated). (b) Histogram equalized. (c) Nonlinear enhancement by Beghdadi and Negrate's algorithm. (d) Nonlinear enhancement with adaptive wavelet shrinkage denoising, $G_m = 20$, $N = 4$, $t = 0.1$.

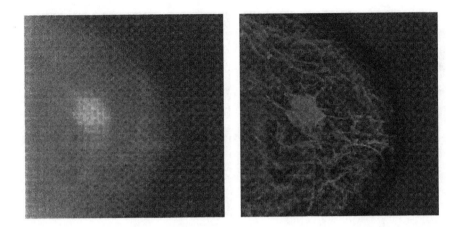

Figure 7.14
(a) Orinial mammogram image M73. (b) Nonlinear enhancement with adaptive wavelet shrinkage denoising, $G_m = 20$, $N = 5$,
$t = 0.1$.

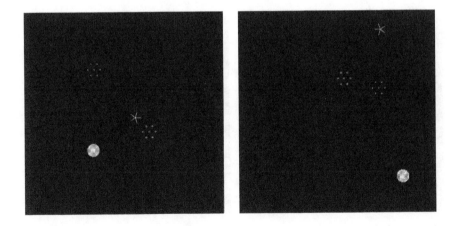

Figure 7.15
(a) Five phantom features blended into M48. (b) Five phantom
features blended into M56.

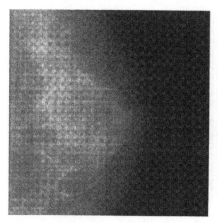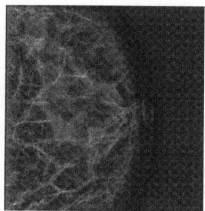

Figure 7.16
(a) Mammogram image M48 with blended phantom features.
(b) Nonlinear enhancement with adaptive wavelet shrinkage denoising, $G_m = 20$, $N = 5$, $t = 0.1$.

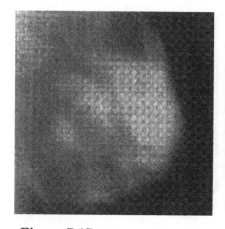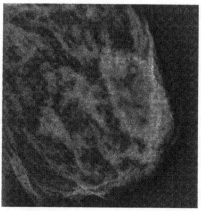

Figure 7.17
(a) Mammogram image M56 with blended phantom features.
(b) Nonlinear enhancement with adaptive wavelet shrinkage denoising, $G_m = 20$, $N = 5$, $t = 0.1$.

7.9 Acknowledgment

This work was sponsored in part by the Whitaker Foundation, and the U.S. Army Medical Research and Development Command, Grant number DAMD17-93-J-3003. The authors wish to thank Doctors Walter Huda, Barbara Steinbach, and Janice Honeyman, of the Department of Radiology, Shands Hospital, University of Florida, Gainesville, for their valuable assistance.

References

[1] D. C. Wang, A. H. Vagnucci, and C. C. Li. Digital image enhancement: a survey. *Comput. Vision, Graphics, Image Process.*, 24:363–381, 1983.

[2] R. Hummel. Histogram modification techniques. *Comput. Graphics Image Process.*, 4:209–224, 1975.

[3] W. Frei. Image enhancement by histogram hyperbolization. *Comput. Graphics Image Process.*, 6:286–294, 1977.

[4] S. M. Pizer, E. P. Amburn, et al. Adaptive histogram equalization and its variations. *Comput. Vision, Graphics, Image Process.*, 39:355–368, 1987.

[5] J. W. Oestmann, R. Greene, et al. High frequency edge enhancement in the detection of fine pulmonary lines: parity between storage phosphor digital images and conventional chest radiograph. *Invest. Radiol.*, 24:643–646, 1989.

[6] M. Prokop, M. Galanski, et al. Storage of phosphor versus screen-film radiography: effect of varying exposure parameters and unsharp mask filtering on the detectability of cortical bone defects. *Radiology*, 177:109–113.

[7] A. Rosenfeld and A. C. Kak. *Digital Picture Processing*, 2nd ed., Academic Press, New York, 1982.

[8] L. D. Loo, K. Doi, and C. E. Metz. Investigation of basic imaging properties in digital radiography. 4. Effect of unsharp masking on the detectability of simple patterns. *Med. Phys.*, 12(2):209–214, 1985.

[9] F. Neycenssac. Contrast enhancement using the Laplacian-of-a-Gaussian filter. *CVGIP: Graphical Models and Image Processing*, 55(6):447–463, 1993.

[10] R. Gordon and R. M. Rangayan. Feature enhancement of film mammograms using fixed and adaptive neighborhood. *Appl. Opt.*, 23:560–564, 1984.

[11] A. Beghdadi and A. L. Negrate. Contrast enhancement technique based on local detection of edges. *Comput. Vision Graphics Image Process.* 46:162–174, 1989.

[12] A. Laine. Multiscale wavelet representations for mammographic feature analysis. In *Image Enhancement Techniques: Computer Science, National Cancer Institute Breast Imaging Workshop: State-of-the-Art and New Technologies*, Bethesda, MD, 1991.

[13] A. Laine and S. Song. Multiscale wavelet representations for mammographic feature analysis. In *Proc. SPIE: Conference on Mathematical Methods in Medical Imaging*, San Diego, CA, 1992.

[14] A. Laine and S. Song. Wavelet processing techniques for digital mammography. In *Proc. SPIE: Conference on Visualization in Biomedical Computing*, Chapel Hill, NC, 1992.

[15] A. Laine, S. Song, and J. Fan. Adaptive Multiscale Processing for Contrast Enhancement. In *Proc. SPIE: Conference on Biomedical Imaging and Biomedical Visualization*, San Jose, CA, 1993.

[16] B. D. Jawerth, M. L. Hilton, and T. L. Huntsberger. Local enhancement of compressed images. *J. Math. Imaging Vision*, 3:39–49, 1993.

[17] A. Laine, S. Schuler, J. Fan, and W. Huda. Mammographic feature enhancement by multiscale analysis. *IEEE Trans. Med. Imaging*, 13(4):725–740, 1994.

[18] J. Lu and D. M. Healy, Jr. Contrast enhancement of medical images using multiscale edge representation. In *Proc. SPIE: Wavelet Applications*, Orlando, FL, 1994.

[19] S. Mallat. A theory for multiresolution signal decomposition: the wavelet representation. *IEEE Trans. Pattern Anal. Mach. Intell.*, 11:674–693, 1989.

[20] S. Mallat and Sifen Zhong. Characterization of signals from multiscale edges. *IEEE Trans. Pattern Anal. Mach. Intell.*, 14:710–732, 1992.

[21] P. Perona and J. Malik. Scale-space and edge detection using aniso-tropic diffusion. *IEEE Trans. Pattern Anal. Mach. Intell.*, 12:629–639, 1990.

[22] S. Mallat and W. L. Hwang. Singularity detection and processing with wavelets. *IEEE Trans. Inform. Theory*, 38(2):617–643, 1992.

[23] D. L. Donoho. Nonlinear wavelet methods for recovery of signals, den-sities, and spectra from indirect and noisy data. *Proc. Symp. Appl. Math.*, 0:173–205, 1993.

[24] H. Voorhees and T. Poggio. Detecting textons and texture boundaries in natural images. *Proc. First Int. Conf. Comput. Vision*, 1987, 250–258.

8

Using Wavelets to Suppress Noise in Biomedical Images

Maurits Malfait

K.U.Leuven, Department of Computer Science
Celestijnenlaan 200 A, B-3001 Heverlee, Belgium
`Maurits.Malfait@cs.kuleuven.ac.be`

Abstract   The influence of various types of noise in biomedical images can not be fully eliminated at the time of image acquisition. This chapter shows how wavelet-based postprocessing methods can be applied to reduce such measurement noise. Noise suppression methods can indeed take full advantage of the localization in both space and frequency that is offered by the wavelet transform. By using this localization, wavelet-based methods can avoid the typical smoothing of fine features that occurs with other methods. The chapter includes an overview of wavelet-based methods that can be used for noise suppression, with the emphasis on methods that are based on a manipulation of the wavelet coefficients. We describe a particular approach that is capable of suppressing most of the noise, while maintaining the relevant fine features in the processed image, which is important for biomedical images. This is illustrated with results for several biomedical images.

191

8.1 Introduction

In spite of the continuing sophistication of medical image acquisition hardware, postprocessing to reduce noise can still be very useful. The noise influences for some different medical imaging techniques can be summarized as follows.

Noise in X-ray computerized tomography (CT) is due to the Poisson statistics of the X-ray photons, to beam hardening, and to photon scatter, in addition to blur by motion and partial volume effects. The raw measurements are transformed into tomographic images via one of the possible reconstruction methods [7]. The particular method evidently influences how the noise on the measurements results in noise in the images. The various phenomena are often studied by reconstruction from simulated projection data, in particular from projections of mathematically described objects called phantoms.

The noise in emission tomography measurements such as positron emission tomography (PET) or single photon emission computerized tomography (SPECT) has a Poisson distribution. Reconstruction from these measurements involves filtering and other convolutions, and for PET, also corrections, followed by a back-projection, which can be iterative. These steps again determine the resulting noise in the images. Simulation is therefore also for PET and SPECT an appropriate way to study noise influences.

Noise in magnetic resonance (MR) images is uncorrelated (*white*). Its distribution depends on the signal-to-noise ratio (SNR) of the image. For SNRs larger than 10 to 15 dB, the distribution is Gaussian. A Rayleigh distribution is an appropriate model [15] for lower SNRs.

Images produced with ultrasound techniques suffer from speckle noise. It is caused by interference of reflected ultrasone pulses at the transducer surface. Noise suppression through image postprocessing seems, at this point, not effective. Current research efforts concern mainly the improvement of ultrasone transducers and models for the reflections in tissue.

Similar noise influences are also involved in the acquisition of biological images. For instance, noise in electron micrographs [1, 16] as well as in gel electropherograms is often modeled as additive Gaussian white noise.

These examples illustrate that it is not straightforward to remove all noise in biomedical images at the time of image acquisition. This chapter will not deal with noise modeling and simulation, but will be restricted to noise suppression as a postprocessing technique for biomedical images. Attention will be paid to the method's ability to maintain fine details in the images during noise removal, since in biology and medicine, even more than in other disciplines, these details can be of critical importance.

8.2 Overview of Wavelet-Based Noise Suppression

Noise suppression methods can use wavelets in various ways. One type of method uses libraries of waveforms, such as described in [17]. The idea is to split the signal into a denoised part that is well represented by a selected waveform and a noisy part that cannot be well represented. Another type of method exploits the redundancy of wavelet frame decompositions to suppress noise. This is further explained in Chapter [18].

This chapter is concerned with another type of method. The idea here is to compute the wavelet decomposition of the noisy signal or image and to manipulate the wavelet coefficients that are obtained. Coefficients that are supposed to be affected by noise are replaced by zero or by another suitable value. Also the other coefficients may be modified. The criteria to distinguish these noisy coefficients are different in each method. Reconstruction from the manipulated coefficients yields the resulting signal or image.

8.2.1 Wavelet Shrinkage

The wavelet shrinkage technique [4, 5] was derived in a statistical framework, using the concept of decisions under uncertainty. The method uses preconditioned, interval-adapted wavelets and applies a soft-threshold nonlinearity to the obtained wavelet coefficients. This means that wavelet coefficients with an absolute value below a certain threshold t are replaced by zero. Coefficients above the threshold are also modified, by shrinking them towards zero with an amount equal to t. In other words, a nonlinear transform maps the wavelet coefficient $d(k)$ to the new coefficient $d(k)^{\text{new}}$, by the formula

$$d(k)^{\text{new}} = \begin{cases} d(k) - t & \text{if } d(k) > t, \\ 0 & \text{if } |d(k)| \leq t, \\ d(k) + t & \text{if } d(k) < -t. \end{cases}$$

When the noise is white, the threshold t

$$t = \sqrt{2 \log(n)}\, \sigma / \sqrt{n}$$

depends only on the global noise variance σ^2 and the number of discrete data points n. It is then kept equal for all levels of the transform. The method can be extended for non-white noise by applying a variance-stabilizing transform to the input data. The threshold then becomes level-dependent, but also in this case it remains fixed within each level.

8.2.2   Correlating Coefficients Between Wavelet Levels

Another recently proposed denoising approach [19] is based on the observation that wavelet coefficients of noise have a much weaker correlation between scales than the coefficients of a noiseless image.

When a two-dimensional signal with an approximately flat power spectrum is decomposed using a square wavelet transform, the power in one level is about one fourth of the power in the level with the next finer scale. One readily sees that most noise power is present at fine-scale levels. Thus, an obvious approach to reduce noise would be to remove most coefficients at these fine scales. However, a noise-free signal may have also have a contribution at these fine, high-frequent levels, particularly where it contains edges or spikes. It is thus necessary to distinguish high-frequency contributions of the signal from those of the noise. Most of the real signal features that contribute to the high-frequency also contribute — at the same location — to lower frequencies. Hence, there will be corresponding wavelet coefficients at different scales. Edges or spikes are clearly features of this type. Consequently, the wavelet contribution of these features is correlated between adjacent levels. However, for noise, this is much less the case. The correlation across scale can thus be used to distinguish the noise high-frequency contribution from that of the signal features. Experiments confirm that noisy coefficients are indeed uncorrelated and meaningful coefficients are correlated, when certain analysing wavelets, such as the *edge-detecting* spline wavelets of Mallat and Zhong, are used.

The algorithm that is proposed in [19], is a modified low-pass filter: the high-frequency contents are mostly suppressed except where highly correlated wavelet coefficients are detected. The algorithm first computes a redundant wavelet transform of the input image (see Section 1.4.1). It then estimates the noise power at each level, which can be done by computing the wavelet transform of a small background part of the given image, where the pixel values are mainly due to noise. Since there is no down-sampling, each scale has the same number of wavelet coefficients. Thus, the coefficients $d_j(k)$ at different scales j always correspond to the same location k as in the subspace V_0. The correlation at level j is then computed as

$$\text{correlation}_j(k) = \left| \prod_{i=j}^{j+\text{corr\_depth}} d_i(k) \right|.$$

At positions k where $\text{correlation}_j(k)$ is small, relative to the coefficient value $d_j(k)$, the coefficient is removed. This is done such that the power of the removed coefficients equals the estimated noise power. Since the coefficient manipulation in this method is specific for each individual coefficient, this method can be called adaptive.

8.2.3 Smoothness Measure from Wavelet Extrema

The method of Mallat and Hwang [13] is also adaptive. The criterion to distinguish noisy from clean coefficients is based on the assumption that the noiseless image is regular and the noise irregular. It particularly exploits the property that a function's regularity is characterized by the behavior of its wavelet coefficients through the levels. In addition, regularity conditions of the image are imposed through a projection procedure during the reconstruction from the modified coefficients.

Practically, the method does not examine the regularity of all wavelet coefficients, but only of their local extrema. In Section 1.4.1 it was explained that the only condition for a numerically stable reconstruction is that the wavelets form a frame. Subsampling in the course of the transform algorithm is the usual way to reduce the redundancy, i.e., the surplus of information available for reconstruction that is generally associated with frames. Mallat and Zhong [14] showed that it is possible to omit the subsampling and reduce the number of wavelet coefficients by retaining only the locally extremal coefficients.

Mallat and Hwang [13] showed that this wavelet extrema approach can also be incorporated in a wavelet denoising algorithm. The distinction between extrema originating from noise and those originating from signal is made by examining the regularity. The characterization property of Section 1.5.5 implies that the Hölder exponent, which is the function's local order of smoothness, can be estimated from the wavelet transform. Based on this information and on additional smoothness measures, Mallat and his co-author derive a criterion to identify wavelet coefficients that correspond to noise: the extrema having the smallest Hölder exponents are supposed to be due to noise and are replaced by zeroes.

Reconstruction from this modified transform can not be done via a fast algorithm but is accomplished through an iterative projection. The procedure yields a function with prescribed wavelet coefficients at a number of locations and with optimal smoothness properties. The iterative projection requires the full computation of a wavelet transform for each iteration step of the reconstruction.

At the price of quite some computation, the method can thus achieve high gains in SNR and a satisfactory visual quality of the obtained images.

8.2.4 Example

This brief overview is concluded with an example that illustrates how this type of methods works. A more extended overview of the above described techniques can be found in [10].

Figure 8.1 shows an MR image of an axial scan of a traumatized human head, the same image with artificially generated Gaussian white noise

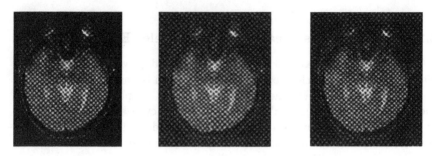

Figure 8.1
Original MR image (238×204 pixels, left), image with noise added (SNR = 12 dB, middle), and result with noise suppression method based on correlation of Section 8.2.2 (SNR = 15.8 dB, right).

added, and the result obtained with our implementation of the method described in [19]. The choices made with the correlation criterion can be conveniently represented in the form of binary labels, which have the value 0 when the corresponding coefficient is replaced by zero, and the value 1 when the corresponding coefficient is kept unmodified. One can thus form binary matrices, containing these labels, that correspond to the different components of the wavelets transform. This is illustrated in Figure 8.2, where the horizontal, diagonal, and vertical component of the finest two levels of the wavelet transform are shown, together with the corresponding binary labels. The depth for this example was corr_depth = 2. The binary matrices can be called *masks*, since one can think of the methods as overlaying a mask on the wavelet coefficients. The masks in Figure 8.2 have a black label when the corresponding wavelet coefficient is kept, and a white label when the coefficient is replaced by zero. Although not all labels are as one would expect, the masks show that most important wavelet coefficients are kept, whereas most noisy coefficients are replaced by zero.

The masks are thus a convenient way to examine a binary noise suppression criterion. The next section will describe an attempt to refine noise suppression criteria by constraining the manner in which the mask is formed.

8.3 Introducing an A Priori Model

8.3.1 Motivation

The techniques described above typically proceed by (1) computing the wavelet decomposition of the image; (2) modifying the obtained wavelet

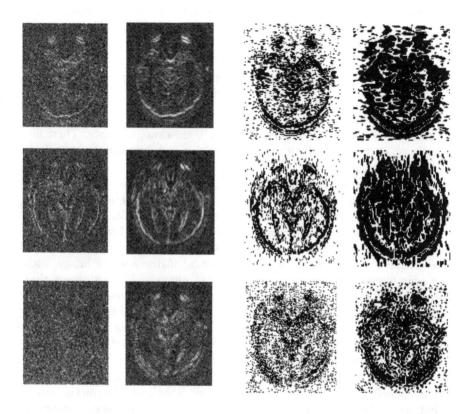

Figure 8.2

The wavelet transform and the corresponding masks obtained with the method of Section 8.2.2 for the noisy image of Figure 8.1. The first column shows the absolute values of the wavelet coefficients at the finest scale; the second those at the next coarser scale. The third and fourth column show the masks corresponding to the first and second column, respectively, whereby black pixels represent binary labels with value 1, and white pixels binary labels with value 0. The first row represents the horizontal components, the second row the vertical components, and the third row the diagonal components.

coefficients according to a specific criterion; (3) reconstructing the cleaned image from the modified coefficients. These techniques rely on a binary decision in the second step: the coefficient is classified as either noisy or clean and is accordingly modified in one of two possible ways. When a particular wavelet coefficient is denoted by $d(k)$, the corresponding binary decision can be represented as a binary label x_k with $x_k \in \{0, 1\}$ and the binary operation as $d(k)^{\text{new}} = x_k \cdot d(k)$, where

$$x_k = \begin{cases} 0, & \text{if } d(k) \text{ is dominated by noise,} \\ 1, & \text{if } d(k) \text{ is sufficiently clean.} \end{cases}$$

These binary labels form masks, as shown in the example above. There are masks on each level and within each level, for each horizontal, vertical, or diagonal component.

The methods described thus far do not consider *geometrical* properties. Meaningful image features usually have some spatial coherence, which also leads to spatial coherence of the wavelet coefficients. Wavelet coefficients indeed compress image information very well: relatively few, but large coefficients carry the essential image information. These coefficients tend to be clustered around the location of important features in the image, such as edge discontinuities, peaks, and corners. One should thus expect that the masks show patterns that correspond to these features. However, the masks shown in the example of Figure 8.2 have some 1 labels that seem inappropriate. On the other hand, some 1 labels are missing at places where one should expect them. This is typical for masks obtained in the presence of noise with methods that do not account for geometrical properties.

One could therefore extend the criteria to remove or retain wavelet coefficients in order to impose spatial continuity or other properties on the masks that are applied. A method using such a model can suppress inappropriate labels and restore missing labels.

8.3.2 Basic Idea and Notation

Just as in [13], the method is based on an approximation to the local Hölder exponent. The wavelet transform used in this method is redundant, which practically means that no down-sampling is applied and that *à trous* filters are used. Details can be found in Sections 1.4.1 and 2.5.2. The algorithm to compute this redundant transform requires more calculations than the usual fast wavelet transform, but has some advantages for noise suppression. The transform has the same number of coefficients in all levels. This makes it easy to compare wavelet coefficients at the same location in two different levels, which is practical in deriving Hölder exponents from the coefficients. It allows input images with sizes that are not powers of two, without any modifications. The redundant wavelet transform is also better for translation-invariance, and the estimates of the local Hölder exponent are more accurate [3, Chapter 9].

However, the local Hölder exponent is only one of two measures that are used in the method. In order to produce better masks, the method incorporates a second criterion. This is used to improve the first measure, by introducing a priori geometrical knowledge, such as the knowledge that meaningful wavelet coefficients for noisy natural images are clustered. The whole approach fits in the framework of Bayesian image processing [2, 6, 18]. The general idea is to consider the unknown output pixels of an image as random variables. Their final values do not only depend on the given (noisy) observations, but also on an a priori model. We apply here a similar idea to the wavelet coefficient masks of an image, rather than directly to the image pixels.

The following notation will be used. Since the method deals with two-dimensional images, a two-dimensional wavelet transform which yields horizontal, vertical, and diagonal components will be used. Coefficients of wavelets that have high frequencies in the x-direction and low frequencies in the y-direction, will be denoted by $d_j(k)^{HL}$. These coefficients represent the vertical components. The notations $d_j(k)^{LH}$ for the horizontal components and $d_j(k)^{HH}$ for the diagonal components are analogous. D denotes a set of wavelet coefficients of one component in a particular level, for instance $D = \{d_j(k)^{HL} \mid j = J\}$. Since the level and component type do not matter for the discussion in this section, the coefficients will have the position k as only index. The set of indices of the coefficients within a level will be denoted by $\mathcal{K}$. Hence, $D = \{d(k) \mid k \in \mathcal{K}\}$. $X = \{x_k \mid k \in \mathcal{K}\}$ represents a mask, i.e., a set of binary labels, such as described above. Each binary label x_k corresponds to a coefficient $d(k)$. The indexing of the labels is the same as the order of the wavelet coefficients. The information of the Hölder criterion, which indicates how noisy the coefficients in D are, is represented as a set $M = \{m_k \mid k \in \mathcal{K}\}$. Each m_k value is based on the local Hölder exponent at the position k in the image and is derived from the wavelet coefficients. Also the criterion values have the same indexing as the coefficients.

8.3.3   Bayesian Method

The method to combine the two measures has its roots in Bayesian statistics. The whole method can therefore be seen as a variant of Bayesian methods for image restoration [6] or of similar methods for other tasks, with the difference that this method deals with wavelet coefficients instead of image pixels. The corresponding models are of course also specific for wavelet coefficients.

Let us now describe how the method deals with one mask for one set of coefficients. The procedure will then be repeated for all masks. For any particular mask X, one can specify how probable it is, taking into account the given image and the chosen criterion. According to *Bayes's rule*, the posterior probability is

$$P(X \mid M) = P(M \mid X) \cdot P(X)/P(M).$$

The probability $P(M)$ can be considered as a constant and therefore

$$P(X \mid M) \propto P(M \mid X) \cdot P(X).$$

The first factor is the *conditional* probability. The second factor is the *a priori* probability.

Both the a priori and the conditional probability are modeled as a Gibbs probability function. This has the advantage that x_k and m_k variables can be directly and conveniently described with a model for interactions between stochastic variables in a field, called a *Markov random field*. The conditional and a priori probabilities are now further described.

8.3.4   The Conditional Probability

To find an expression for the conditional probability $P(M \mid X)$, one needs to translate a classic, binary decision based on the chosen criterion (the Hölder exponent) into a probability. Let us consider a wavelet coefficient $d(k)$ in a set D at position k, and the corresponding binary mask label x_k and local Hölder exponent m_k. When the local Hölder exponent is large, the image is locally regular, and the wavelet coefficients can be kept. When the exponent is small, the function is locally irregular and probably corrupted by noise. The corresponding wavelet coefficients should then be suppressed. In order to practically distinguish "large" and "small" exponents, a threshold t is used. It is calculated from an estimation of the noise energy that is present in the set D, such that the energy of the wavelet coefficients that are replaced by zero is approximately equal to the noise energy.

This can be translated into the conditional probability $P(m_k \mid x_k)$ as follows: if the label $x_k = 1$ (keep coefficient $d(k)$) then Hölder exponents m_k above the threshold t are probable. If the label $x_k = 0$, Hölder exponents m_k below t are probable. Since the prior distributions $P(m_k)$ are assumed to be uniform, the conditional probabilities should meet the condition

$$P(m_k \mid x_k = 0) + P(m_k \mid x_k = 1) = C_1,$$

where C_1 is a constant. A probability function of this type is used for instance in [11].

8.3.5 The A Priori Probability

The conditional probability was only a stochastic equivalent of a previous deterministic method. The a priori probability, however, introduces something new. It expresses that a priori, i.e., when M is not taken into account, the masks are not all equally probable. Any kind of a priori knowledge about masks can in this way be introduced and exploited. As described above, one can a priori expect that 0 and 1 mask labels appear in more or less separated clusters. Via the a priori probability one can assign a higher probability to masks that have this property. The following a priori model is general enough to be valid for a wide class of natural and synthesised images.

The a priori probability $P(X)$ is expressed in terms of small neighborhoods of binary mask variables in the mask X. Such a neighborhood, centred around x_k, is denoted by N_k. The a priori probability is then of the form

$$P(X) = 1/Z \cdot \exp\Big(-\sum_k V_{N_k}(X)\Big),$$

where the $V_{N_k}(X)$ are potential functions that correspond to each of the neighborhoods N_k. Masks in which neighboring state vectors have the same value are now considered as more probable than those with different values. The potential functions $V_{N_k}(X)$ are therefore based on a comparison of the central state with its neighbors, through the definition

$$V_{N_k}(X) = \sum_{x_l \in N_k} V_{k,l}(x_k, x_l) \quad \text{with} \quad V_{k,l}(x_k, x_l) = \begin{cases} -\gamma & \text{if } x_k = x_l, \\ +\gamma & \text{if } x_k \neq x_l. \end{cases}$$

This type of a priori model is very generally applicable and is also used in the direct classification of image pixels [8].

8.3.6 Coefficient Manipulation

Once the a priori and conditional probabilities are specified, it is in principle possible to compute the posterior probability $P(X \mid M)$ for every X. This is not done in practice. What is actually computed is the marginal probability $P(x_k = 1 \mid M)$ for each coefficient $d(k)$ that it is a clean coefficient.

The manipulation of the coefficient is then a multiplication with this probability:

$$d(k)^{\text{new}} = d(k) \cdot P(x_k = 1 \mid M).$$

In addition to the use of two measures, the method thus avoids binary decisions and instead works with probabilities on the wavelet coefficients. This means that it is not binary masks that are applied, but masks with values that continuously vary between 0 and 1. Note that the criterion M is still used, but no longer in a deterministic way as in a classic, binary approach.

The method thus involves a real and fully adaptive shrinkage of wavelet coefficients, with a shrinkage factor that is different for each coefficient. The method is in this sense an extension of nonadaptive wavelet shrinkage methods [5]. The identification and modification of both clean and noisy coefficients are more conservative and less radical than in other methods, such as those mentioned in Section 8.2.

The description in this section had to be rather brief due to space restrictions. Several aspects such as the link between the probability functions and Markov random fields, the calculation of the threshold t, and the computational procedure to derive the marginal probabilities were not explained. Detailed explanations as well as several image processing results and comparisons can be found in [11]. A more concise overview restricted to the statistical aspects of the method is [12].

8.4   Results for Biomedical Images

In this framework, we will not compare in detail the relative performance of the various wavelet-based techniques. For a comparison based on a number of test images, we refer to [9] and [11]. Summarizing the main findings there, we can say that wavelet-based methods outperform the best comparable earlier methods, such as the adaptive Wiener filter. This is demonstrated by quantitative results (SNR gain) and by the qualitative appearance of the images, and it is confirmed by the results of [19]. Among the wavelet-based methods, the probabilistic method of Section 8.3 and the extrema approach of [13] give the best results. The results of the basic soft-thresholding technique [4, 5] are worse. The quantitative results of the probabilistic approach are on a par with, or better than those of the extrema approach, whereas the qualitative performance of the former is better. In addition, the probabilistic method is faster and easier to use. However, when choosing a method, other considerations than the performance can play a role. For instance, soft-thresholding is a relatively simple and easy to implement method, whereas the other methods require more background and greater implementation effort. Evidently, all depends on the requirements of the application. In biomedical imaging it seems com-

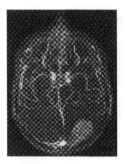 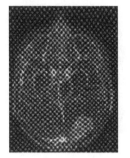 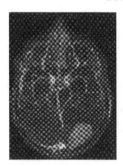

Figure 8.3
Magnetic resonance angiogram of cerebral blood vessels (320×251 pixels, left), image with noise (SNR = 5 dB, middle) and result of new method (SNR = 11.8 dB, right).

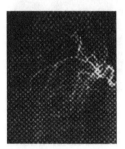 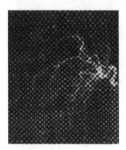 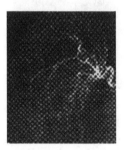

Figure 8.4
Digital subtraction angiogram (351×303 pixels, left), image with noise (SNR = 10 dB, middle) and result of new method (SNR = 16.21 dB, right).

mendable to spend some more effort on the method in return for the best denoising quality.

We now focus on results obtained with the probabilistic method of Section 8.3. The test images are generated by adding Gaussian white noise to medical images obtained under normal conditions. The examples are relevant for all types of biomedical images, but this setting corresponds most closely to the real situation for MR images with a high signal-to-noise ratio, as mentioned in Section 8.1.

Results for four different test images are shown first. Figure 8.3 displays a magnetic resonance angiogram of cerebral blood vessels. It is a maximum intensity projection in the cranial-caudal direction, in which a parietal lesion is clearly visible. The noisy image has a relatively low signal-to-noise ratio of 5 dB. The noise suppression method raises the SNR by almost 7 dB. Almost no visible noise is left in the obtained image, while details such as

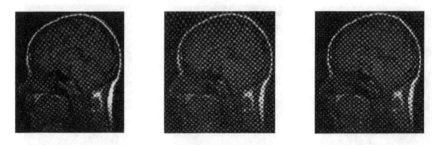

Figure 8.5
MRI image (253 × 238 pixels, left), image with noise (SNR = 10 dB, middle) and result of new method (SNR = 16.49 dB, right).

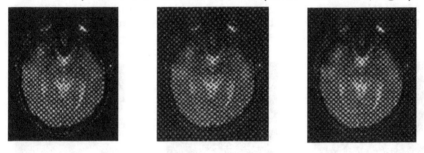

Figure 8.6
Original MR image (238 × 204 pixels, left), image with noise added (SNR = 12 dB, middle) and result of new method (SNR = 17.2 dB, right).

the blood vessels are well maintained. Details that are completely obscured by noise in the noisy image can not be restored. This is the case for some fine blood vessels and the texture of the lesion. The next test image, shown in Figure 8.4, is a digital subtraction angiogram of cerebral blood vessels, taken at the maximal arterial phase in lateral projection. The power of the added noise is smaller than in the previous image. One can see that all visible image details are well retained and that the noise is effectively suppressed. The third test image, shown in Figure 8.5, is one slice of an MRI scan. Some details that are obscured by noise are not well recovered, but the overall quality again seems satisfactory. Figure 8.6 shows the same MR image of a traumatized human head as in Figure 8.1, the noisy version, as well as the result obtained with the new method.

It thus seems that this wavelet-based method is able to maintain important fine details, thanks to the position-frequency localization of wavelets and the use of an additional a priori model.

An overview of quantitative results is shown in Figures 8.7 and 8.8. The figures show the gain in signal to noise ratio (SNR) that is obtained with

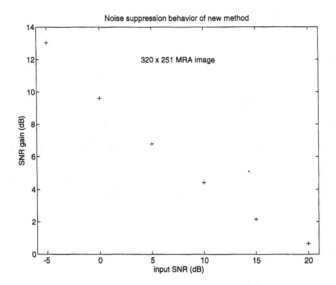

Figure 8.7
Quantitative noise suppression performance for the MRA image
shown in Figure 8.3. The gain in SNR is plotted vs. the SNR of
the noisy image.

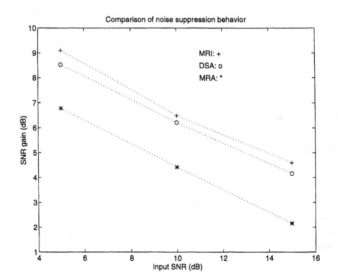

Figure 8.8
Quantitative comparison of noise suppression for a number of
medical images. The gain in SNR is plotted vs. the SNR of the
noisy image.

the method, for a number of input noisy images with different SNRs. The method achieves a higher gain when the input is noisier. This is also typical for other noise suppression methods. Figure 8.7 specifically shows the gains obtained for the MRA image of Figure 8.3. The SNR of the input noisy image is always computed with respect to the given image, without added noise. However, since this is not a phantom image but a real clinical image, it is not completely noise-free. This explains why the method seems incapable of further improvement for an input SNR of 20 dB or higher.

Figure 8.8 compares the gains obtained for the MRA image of Figure 8.3, the DSA image of Figure 8.4 and the MRI image of Figure 8.5. The MRA image seems an inherently more difficult image to denoise, which can be explained partly by its high-frequency, fine detail.

Acknowledgment

This chapter presents research results of the Belgian incentive program Information Technology – Computer Science of the Future (IT/IF/5), initiated by the Belgian State – Prime Minister's Office for Science, Technology and Culture. The scientific responsibility is assumed by its author. MM thanks the members of the medical imaging group at the K.U.Leuven University Hospital Gasthuisberg for providing two of the test images and for additional information. He also thanks the editors for their support.

References

[1] A. Aldroubi, B. L. Trus, M. Unser, F. P. Booy, and A. C. Steven. Magnification mismatches between micrographs: corrective procedures and implications for structural analysis. *Ultramicroscopy*, 46:175–188, 1992.

[2] J. E. Besag. Spatial interaction and the spatial analysis of lattice systems. *J. Royal. Stat. Soc., Ser. B*, 36:192–236, 1974.

[3] I. Daubechies. *Ten Lectures on Wavelets*. CBMS-NSF Regional Conf. Series in Appl. Math., Vol. 61. Society for Industrial and Applied Mathematics, Philadelphia, PA, 1992.

[4] R. A. Devore and B. J. Lucier. Fast wavelet techniques for near-optimal processing. In *Proc. IEEE Military Commun. Conf.*, New York, 1992, 48.3.1–48.3.7.

[5] D. L. Donoho and I. M. Johnstone. Ideal spatial adaptation via wavelet shrinkage. *Biometrika*, 81(3):425, 1994.

[6] S. Geman and D. Geman. Stochastic relaxation, Gibbs distributions, and the Bayesian restoration of images. *IEEE Trans. Patt. Anal. Mach. Intell.*, 6(6):721–741, 1984.

[7] G. T. Herman. Image Reconstruction from Projections. *Computer Science and Applied Mathematics*. Academic Press, New York, 1980.

[8] Z. Kato, M. Berthod, and J. Zerubia. Parallel image classification using multiscale Markov Random Fields. In *Proc. 1993 IEEE Int. Conf. Acoustics, Speech and Signal Processing*, 1993, pages V-137–140, 1993.

[9] M. Malfait. Stochastic Sampling and Wavelets for Bayesian Image Analysis. Ph.D. thesis, Department of Computer Science, K. U. Leuven, Belgium, 1995.

[10] M. Malfait and D. Roose. Wavelet based image denoising I. Preliminaries and existing methods. TW Report 212, Department of Computer Science, K. U. Leuven, Leuven, Belgium, August 1994.

[11] M. Malfait and D. Roose. Wavelet based image denoising II. Wavelet based image denoising using a Markov random field a priori model. TW Report 228, Department of Computer Science, K. U. Leuven, Leuven, Belgium, April 1995.

[12] M. Malfait and D. Roose. Wavelets and Markov Random Fields in a Bayesian framework. In *Wavelets and Statistics*, Lecture Notes in Statistics, A. Antoniadis and G. Oppenheim, editors, 1995, pages 225–238.

[13] S. Mallat and W. L. Hwang. Singularity detection and processing with wavelets. *IEEE Trans. Inform. Theory*, 38(2):617–643, 1992.

[14] S. Mallat and S. Zhong. Characterization of signals from multiscale edges. *IEEE Trans. Patt. Anal. Mach. Intell.*, 14:710–732, 1992.

[15] D. L. Parker and E. M. Haacke. Magnetic resonance angiography: concepts and applications. In *Mosby Year Book*, E. J. Potchen, E. M. Haacke, J. S. Siebert, and A. Gottschalk, editors, chap. 4, St. Louis, 1993.

[16] W. A. Saxton. *Computer Techniques for Image Processing in Electron Microscopy.* Academic Press, New York, 1978.

[17] M. V. Wickerhauser. *Adapted Wavelet Analysis from Theory to Software.* A. K. Peters, Wellesley, MA, 1994.

[18] G. Winkler. *Image analysis, random fields and dynamic Monte Carlo methods.* Applications of Mathematics. Springer, 1995.

[19] Y. Xu, J. B. Weaver, D. M. Healy, and J. Lu. Wavelet transform domain filters: a spatially selective noise filtration technique. *IEEE Trans. Image Process.*, 3(6):747–758, 1994.

9

Wavelet Transform and Tomography: Continuous and Discrete Approaches

F. Peyrin and M. Zaim

CREATIS, URA CNRS # 1216
INSA 502
69621 Villeurbanne Cedex, FRANCE

Abstract   In tomography, an image is reconstructed from its projections from different directions. In this chapter, the relationships between the wavelet decomposition of an image and those of its projections are developed. The problem is first analyzed using a continuous formulation. It may be shown that the images reconstructed from the wavelet transform of the projections provide a 2-D wavelet decomposition of the image. Conversely, an appropriate 1-D filtering may be done on the sinogram prior to reconstruction, in order to recover any 2-D continuous wavelet transform. Then, the application of a multiresolution scheme using a pair of discrete filters is studied. We respectively examine the construction of 2-D filters (resp. 1-D filters) from a pair of 1-D (resp. 2-D) exact reconstruction filters. Both the case of dyadic and quincunx decompositions are considered. For illustration, results on an X-ray CT scan medical image are presented.

9.1 Introduction

A large number of medical images are produced by tomographic reconstruction (X-ray CT, PET, or SPECT ...). Since the wavelet transform (WT) has proved to be an efficient tool in signal and image processing, it may be interesting to study the relationships between tomography and wavelets. The use of wavelets in tomography has been considered by several authors under a number of different aspects, some of which will be examined here.

Tomographic images are produced by the resolution of an inverse problem, and more precisely by the inversion of the so-called Radon transform. In an early theoretical work, Holdshneider considered the Radon transform as a particular wavelet transform, and used this property to propose an inversion formula [1]. A similar study was performed independently by Walnut in a paper where the relationships between the Radon, Gabor and wavelet transforms were presented [2]. In previous works [3, 4], we showed that a 2-D wavelet decomposition of the tomographic image may be constructed from the WT of its projections, and studied the properties of the so-generated 2-D wavelet.

The wavelet transform has also been applied to local tomography, where the goal is to reconstruct accurately only a region of interest (ROI) in a tomographic image. For this purpose, Olson first proposed a procedure based on the use of the wavelet decomposition of the projections, allowing a reduction of radiation exposure [5, 6]. The efficiency of the WT for local tomography was also pointed out in [7]. Multiresolution algorithms have also been proposed in [8], for progressive image reconstruction, and in [9] for reconstruction from noisy data. In both cases, the authors start from a 2-D wavelet decomposition of the tomographic image using separable filters. This results in an approximation image, and three detail images, which may be computed directly from the projections by using "modified ramp filters", including the effect of the wavelet and scale functions. Although a discrete algorithm is proposed, the analysis is essentially performed using a continuous approach.

In general, the use of the wavelet transform for the inversion of ill-posed problems, and denoising has been investigated by Donoho [10]. A particular application of these techniques to the inversion of noisy data in tomography has been developed by Kolaczyk [11]. The use of the WT as a regularization tool for tomographic inversion has also been proposed in particular for applications to emission tomography (ET) in [12, 13].

The review of the recent literature on wavelets and tomography shows that wavelets have a number of potential applications in tomography. The purpose of this paper is to examine precisely the relations between the WTs of the projections and of the tomographic images. Different approaches to WTs will be considered. The 2-D analyzing wavelets are often chosen as separable products of 1-D wavelets or isotropic versions of 1-D wavelets. However, the use of nonseparable wavelets in 2-D is being considered more and more [14–16]. Since a priori there are no privileged directions in tomography, we will focus on nonseparable 2-D wavelets. We will both consider a continuous WT (CWT), and a discrete WT (DWT) derived from a filter bank.

The paper is organized as follows. In Section 9.2, we recall the fundamentals of tomography, i.e., the basis of image reconstruction from projections. In Section 9.3, we derive relationships between the continuous Radon and wavelet transforms. We consider both the case where we start from the 1-D CWT of the projections and the case where we start from the 2-D CWT of an image. For this purpose, we use the general definition of the wavelet transform of image defined as a function of a scale parameter and a rotation angle [17]. In Section 9.4, we consider the use of discrete WT generated from a pair of filters. The relations between the 1-D and 2-D filters are examined precisely for their ability to provide exact reconstruction. Both a dyadic and a quincunx decomposition are considered.

9.2 Basis of Tomography

9.2.1 Problem Position

In tomography an image is reconstructed from measures of its integral over straight lines of a plane, called projections. Since the set of projections constitutes the Radon transform of the image, the reconstruction problem is equivalent to the inversion of the Radon transform. Let us give some precise definitions. Let $f(x, y)$ be a 2-D image, supposed C^∞ with compact support $\mathcal{D}$. A parallel projection $p_\theta(r)$ in direction θ is defined as the integral of $f(x, y)$ on a straight line D of equation $x \cos \theta + y \sin \theta - r = 0$ (Figure 9.1). The projection may be expressed as:

$$p_\theta(r) = \int_{-\infty}^{+\infty} \int_{-\infty}^{+\infty} f(x, y)\, \delta(x \cos \theta + y \sin \theta - r)\, dx\, dy \qquad (9.1)$$

where δ is the Dirac's delta distribution.

The Radon transform $\mathcal{R}$ of the 2-D image maps the image onto the 2-D space of coordinates (r, θ), and is defined by:

$$\mathcal{R}f(r, \theta) = p_\theta(r) \quad \text{for } \theta \in [0, \pi) \text{ and } r \in (-\infty, +\infty). \qquad (9.2)$$

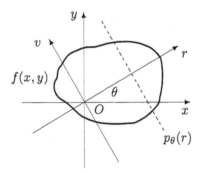

Figure 9.1
Geometry acquisition in tomography

An original inversion formula expressing analytically the image in function of its Radon transform, was proposed by Radon in 1917 [18]. However, due to practical considerations, this latter is rarely used in tomography, and alternative methods have been proposed in this field [19]. Reconstruction methods basically fall into two classes known as transform methods and series expansion methods. In the first case, the solution is obtained by the discretization of an analytic inversion formula, while in the second case a discrete solution is obtained from the resolution of a large dimensionality linear system. When the data are ideal (large number of projections, good sampling, no noise, ...), both approaches give equivalent results, and the choice of a method will rather be dependent on the computing resources. When the data are not ideal, the reconstruction problem may become a severely ill-posed problem, and regularization techniques often have to be included in the reconstruction process. Generally, the second class of methods is more flexible for the introduction of regularization. For the purpose of this paper we simply recall some basic reconstruction methods from the two classes.

9.2.2   Reconstruction Methods: Transform Methods

Transform methods derive from the expression and the resolution of the problem in a transformed space: the Fourier space. The fundamental result is the Fourier slice theorem, which shows that the Radon transform contains all the image information. It states that the 1-D Fourier transform (FT) of a projection in direction θ is a slice of the 2-D Fourier transform of the image on the straight line in direction θ:

$$\mathcal{F}_1 p_\theta(\rho) = \mathcal{F}_2 f(\rho\cos\theta, \rho\sin\theta) \tag{9.3}$$

where $\mathcal{F}_1$ and $\mathcal{F}_2$ are, respectively, the 1-D and 2-D FT operators.

The 2-D FT of the image may thus be obtained from the 1-D FT of the projections. Although this theorem provides itself an inversion formula, it is rarely used in practice because of interpolation problems related to its implementation. However, it permits derivation of the well-known filtered backprojection inversion formula:

$$f(x, y) = \int_0^\pi (p_\theta * k)(x \cos \theta + y \cos \theta) \, d\theta \qquad (9.4)$$

where $*$ denotes 1-D convolution and k is an appropriate 1-D kernel, whose FT satisfies:

$$\mathcal{F}_1 k(\rho) = |\rho|. \qquad (9.5)$$

Inversion formula (9.4) may be rewritten as:

$$f(x, y) = \mathcal{B}(p * k)(x, y) \qquad (9.6)$$

by introducing the adjoint of the Radon transform, the backprojection operator $\mathcal{B}$, applied to the set of projections and defined by:

$$\mathcal{B}p(x, y) = \int_0^\pi p_\theta(x \cos \theta + y \sin \theta) \, d\theta. \qquad (9.7)$$

To allow for regularization, Condition (9.5) may be relaxed and different choices may be selected for the reconstruction kernel k.

9.2.3 Reconstruction Methods: Series Expansion Methods

To make a parallel with Section 9.2.2, it may be said that series expansion methods derive from the expression and the resolution of the problem in a discrete space. If the image is represented by its coordinates f_i in some basis, the problem may be expressed as the resolution of a linear system:

$$R\mathbf{f} = \mathbf{p} \qquad (9.8)$$

where $\mathbf{f}$ is the vector of image coordinates f_i, $\mathbf{p}$ is the vector of data, and R is a 2-D matrix representing an approximation of the Radon transform.

Since matrix R is very large, this system is generally solved by iterative techniques. The ART algorithm (Algebraic Reconstruction Technique), is the most popular series expansion technique in tomography because of its implementation and interpretation simplicity: one new projection ray is processed at each iteration. However, this algorithm may diverge for inconsistent data (noisy projections for instance).

More general solutions are obtained from the solution of the least square system:

$$(R^T R + \lambda W)\mathbf{f} = R^T \mathbf{p} \tag{9.9}$$

where λ is a regularization parameter, W is a ponderation matrix introducing some a priori in the problem, and R^T denotes the transpose of R.

A parallel may be made between transform and series expansion approaches [20]. First, note that R and R^T, respectively, represent the discrete equivalent of the Radon transform and backprojection operator. In the case of ideal regularly sampled data, it may be shown that $R^T R$ is a block Teplitz matrix, which can be diagonalized by the discrete Fourier transform. In this case, the reconstruction may be seen as a 2-D filtering of the backprojection data.

9.3   Continuous Wavelet Decomposition of a Tomographic Image

As was recalled in Section 9.2, the relationships between the Radon and Fourier transforms are well-known and well exploited. In the same way, the purpose of this section is to give the relationships between Radon transform and wavelet transforms. More precisely, we study the relations between the WT of the image and the WT of its projections.

9.3.1   Continuous Wavelet Decomposition of Projections

Each projection p_θ is a 1-D signal which may be decomposed by a 1-D WT. Let us denote $Wp_\theta(a, b)$, the WT of projection p_θ obtained with a 1-D analyzing wavelet $\psi(r)$ satisfying the admissibility condition (cf. Section 9.1.3). For each given scale a, the partial WT with respect to b, $Wp_\theta(a, \cdot)$ is a 1-D signal which may be expressed as the convolution product:

$$Wp_\theta(a, \cdot) = p_\theta * \overline{\psi}_a^\vee \tag{9.10}$$

where

$$\psi_a(r) = \frac{1}{\sqrt{a}} \psi\left(\frac{r}{a}\right),$$

and $^\vee$ denotes the reflection operation $\psi_a^\vee(r) = \psi_a(-r)$.

Let $f_a(x, y)$ be the image reconstructed from the set

$$S_a = \{W_\psi p_\theta(a, \cdot)/\theta \in [0, \pi)\},$$

i.e.,

$$\mathcal{R} f_a(r, \theta) = W_\psi p_\theta(a, r) \quad \text{for } \theta \in [0, \pi) \text{ and } r \in (-\infty, +\infty). \tag{9.11}$$

It may be shown that if we define $W_m f$ as:

$$W_m f(x, y, a) = \sqrt{a}\, f_a(x, y), \tag{9.12}$$

$W_m f$ is a 2-D wavelet transform of the image $f(x, y)$, as a function of scale a, and spatial variables (x, y) [3], with respect to the 2-D wavelet $m(x, y)$. The corresponding 2-D analyzing wavelet $m(x, y)$ is defined by:

$$\mathcal{R} m(r, \theta) = \psi(r) \quad \text{for } \theta \in [0, \pi) \text{ and } r \in (-\infty, +\infty) \tag{9.13}$$

and may be obtained by the filtered backprojection formula:

$$m(x, y) = \mathcal{B}(\psi * k)(x, y). \tag{9.14}$$

Thus, this process allows construction of a 2-D analyzing wavelet from the 1-D analyzing wavelet. If ψ satisfies the 1-D admissibility condition, $m(x, y)$ also satisfies the 2-D admissibility condition. In this case, the so-defined 2-D WT may be inverted and the reconstructed image may be recovered by:

$$f(x, y) = c_m^{-1} \int_0^{+\infty} (W_m f(\cdot, \cdot, a) *_2 m_a)(x, y)\, \frac{da}{a^2} \tag{9.15}$$

where the 2-D convolution $*_2$ is performed with respect to x and y, and m_a is the scaled 2-D wavelet.

The 2-D wavelet so generated is the image having all its projections for θ in $[0, \pi)$ identical and equal to the basic 1-D wavelet $\psi(r)$. In this particular case, the filtered backprojection formula (9.14) may be written:

$$m(x, y) = \int_{-\infty}^{+\infty} \mathcal{F}_1 \psi(\rho)\, |\rho| \left[\int_0^\pi \exp(2i\pi(x\cos\theta + y\cos\theta)\rho)\, d\theta \right] d\rho. \tag{9.16}$$

When $\psi(r)$ is even, $m(x, y)$ is radial, and may be expressed via the Hankel Transform:

$$m(R\cos\alpha, R\sin\alpha) = 2\pi \int_0^{+\infty} \mathcal{F}_1 \psi(\rho)\rho J_0(2\pi R\rho)d\rho, \tag{9.17}$$

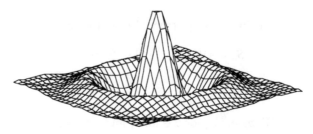

Figure 9.2
2-D wavelet generated from the 1-D Morlet wavelet.

where J_0 is the 0-th order Bessel function. As an example, we show the 2-D wavelet generated from the 1-D Morlet wavelet in Figure 9.2.

From a computational point of view, the filtering on the projections in order to compute their WT, may be included in the filtering process of the filtered backprojection algorithm. The application of this decomposition to an X-ray tomographic image is presented in Figure 9.3. Figure 9.3(a) represents the original image, and the 6-scale wavelet decomposition of the image obtained from the WT of the projections is represented on Figures 9.3(b–g).

We have shown that the set of images reconstructed from the WT of the projections at different scales provides a 2-D WT of the image, associated to a 2-D radial wavelet generated from the 1-D wavelet. In the next section, we examine how this process may be extended to the 2-D wavelet analysis of the image with nonradial wavelets.

9.3.2 Continuous Wavelet Decomposition of the Image

We now directly consider the application of the 2-D continuous wavelet transform (CWT), defined by Murenzi and Antoine [17], to the tomographic image. If $\psi(x, y)$ is a 2-D mother wavelet, the 2-D CWT of an image $f(x, y)$ may be defined as a function of four variables: two translation parameters (x, y), a scale variable a, and a rotation angle β. This representation allows one to introduce a direction parameter in the representation. The 2-D CWT may be expressed as a 2-D convolution by the relation:

$$W_\psi f(x, y, a, \beta) = \left(f *_2 \overline{\psi}^{\vee}_{(a,\beta)} \right)(x, y) \tag{9.18}$$

with

$$\psi_{(a,\beta)}(x, y) = \psi \left(a^{-1} M^{-\beta} \begin{pmatrix} x \\ y \end{pmatrix} \right)$$

where M^β is the rotation matrix of angle β, and $\psi^\vee$ is the reflection operation.

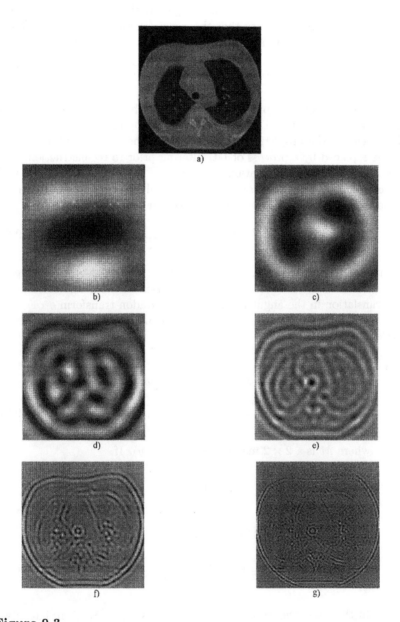

Figure 9.3
(a) original X-ray CT lung image. (b)–(g) 6-scale wavelet decomposition generated from the WT of the projections using 1-D Morlet wavelet.

For a given scale a and rotation angle β, we consider $\mathcal{R}\psi_{(a,\beta)}(r,\theta)$, the Radon transform of the 2-D wavelet $\psi_{(a,\beta)}$. If this later is used to filter each projection, we may show that the reconstruction provides a 2-D WT of the images for scale parameter a and rotation parameter β:

$$W_\psi f(x,y,a,\beta) = \mathcal{B}\left(p_\theta * \mathcal{R}\psi_{(a,\beta)}(\cdot,\theta)\right)(x,y). \qquad (9.19)$$

The difference with the previous case is that each projection has now to be filtered with a different 1-D wavelet, corresponding to the projection of the 2-D wavelet in the projection direction. Thus, the process of 2-D filtering may be replaced by a process of 1-D filtering prior to reconstruction.

Because of the transformation properties of the Radon transform with respect to a change of scale and a rotation, only the projection of the 2-D mother wavelet has to be computed. Indeed, it may be shown that:

$$\mathcal{R}\psi_{(a,\beta)}(r,\theta) = |a|\mathcal{R}\psi(r/a,\theta-\beta). \qquad (9.20)$$

This means that a change of scale in the image corresponds to a change of scale in its Radon transform and that a rotation in the image corresponds to a translation in the angular variable of its Radon transform.

As examples, we examine the 2-D Mexican hat, and the 2-D Morlet wavelet.

- **2-D Mexican hat**
  Let the 2-D Mexican hat be defined by:

$$\psi^{mh}(\mathbf{x}) = (2 - \mathbf{x}^T M \mathbf{x}) \exp\left(-\mathbf{x}^T M \mathbf{x}/2\right) \qquad (9.21)$$

where M is a 2×2 matrix, and $\mathbf{x} = (x,y)$. If

$$M = \begin{pmatrix} 1/\sigma^2 & 0 \\ 0 & 1/\sigma^2 \end{pmatrix},$$

the 2-D Mexican hat becomes radial and is expressed by:

$$\psi^{mh}(\mathbf{x}) = \frac{1}{2\pi\sigma^2}\left(2 - \frac{x^2+y^2}{\sigma^2}\right)\exp\left(-\frac{x^2+y^2}{2\sigma^2}\right). \qquad (9.22)$$

In this case, the resulting 1-D wavelet is also a Mexican hat, given by:

$$\mathcal{R}\psi^{mh}(r,\theta) = \frac{1}{\sqrt{2\pi\sigma^2}}\left(1 - \frac{r^2}{\sigma^2}\right)\exp\left(-\frac{r^2}{2\sigma^2}\right). \qquad (9.23)$$

- **2-D Morlet wavelet**

  The general expression of the 2-D Morlet wavelet [17] is given by:

  $$\psi^{\mathrm{M}}(\mathbf{x}) = \exp\left(2i\pi\,\mathbf{u}_0 \cdot \mathbf{x}\right) \exp\left(-\mathbf{x}^T A \mathbf{x}/2\right), \qquad (9.24)$$

  where A is a 2×2 matrix. It is a 2-D modulated Gaussian, the modulation is given by $\mathbf{u}_0$, and the shape of the Gaussian is given by A. Let us consider the particular case where $A = \begin{pmatrix} 1/\varepsilon & 0 \\ 0 & 1 \end{pmatrix}$ and $\mathbf{u}_0 = (0, v_0)$:

  $$\psi^{\mathrm{M}}(x, y) = \exp(2i\pi\,\mathbf{v}_0 \cdot \mathbf{y}) \exp\left(-(\varepsilon^{-1}x^2 + y^2)\right). \qquad (9.25)$$

  Its 2-D Fourier transform is given by:

  $$\mathcal{F}\psi^{\mathrm{M}}(u, v) = 2\pi\varepsilon \exp\left(-2\pi^2\left(\varepsilon^2 u^2 + (v - v_0)^2\right)\right). \qquad (9.26)$$

  In this case, the corresponding 1-D wavelet is:

  $$\mathcal{R}\psi^{\mathrm{M}}(r, \theta) = \sqrt{2\pi}\,\frac{\varepsilon}{\sqrt{\alpha(\theta)}} \exp\left(\frac{2\pi^2\cos^2\theta\,v_0^2\,\varepsilon^2}{\alpha(\theta)}\right) \qquad (9.27)$$

  $$\exp\left(\frac{-r^2}{2\alpha(\theta)}\right) \exp\left(\frac{2i\pi v_0 \sin\theta\,r}{\alpha(\theta)}\right)$$

  where $\alpha(\theta) = \varepsilon^2\cos^2\theta + \sin^2\theta$, and $r_0 = (v_0\sin\theta)/\alpha(\theta)$.

  It may be seen as a Morlet-type wavelet, the standard deviation of which is $\sigma^2 = \alpha(\theta)$, and the modulation is r_0. Both the standard deviation and the modulation depend on the projection angle. Their evolution in function of the angle is represented in Figure 9.4, for three values of $\varepsilon = 1, 3, 5$.

9.4 Discrete Wavelet Decomposition of the Tomographic Image

We have considered in the first sections, the relationships between the continuous wavelet and Radon transform. We now study their discrete counterparts. In practice, the discrete wavelet transform (DWT) is often

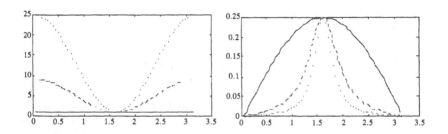

Figure 9.4
**Evolution of (a) the standard deviation and (b) the modulation
as a function of the angle (between 0 and π), for $\varepsilon = 1$ (continuous
line), 3 (dashed line), 5 (point line).**

computed via recursive steps of filtering and subsampling (cf. Chapter 2).
Following the same line as in the continuous case, we can study the case
where we start from the 1-D DWT of the projections, or the case where we
start from the 2-D DWT of the image.

9.4.1   1-D DWT of the Projections

We first consider the application of a 1-D DWT to each projections. For
this purpose, we consider a perfect reconstruction filter bank and a dyadic
scheme. Let h_d and g_d be, respectively, the low-pass and high-pass filters
associated to a 1-D pair of scale and wavelet functions, and h_{r1} and g_{r1} be
the corresponding reconstruction filters.

For one level of decomposition, each N-point discrete projection is, respectively, low- or high-pass filtered, and subsampled. The projections may
be gathered in order to constitute low-frequency and high-frequency sinograms. Let us denote f_H and f_G, the two $(N/2 \times N/2)$ images reconstructed
from the two subsampled sinograms. The two images may be respectively
considered as the detail and the approximation of an $N \times N$ image.

By analogy with the continuous case, the corresponding 2-D filters h_{d2}
and g_{d2} are obtained by tomographic reconstruction from the 1-D filters.
This leads to nonseparable filters. If R now denotes the discrete Radon
transform, the relations between the 1-D and 2-D filters are:

$$Rh_{d2} = h_{d1} \quad \text{and} \quad Rg_{d2} = g_{d1}.$$

The filters may be obtained by any method solving the linear system:

$$h_{d2} = \left(R^T R\right)^{-1} R^T h_{d1} \quad \text{and} \quad g_{d2} = \left(R^T R\right)^{-1} R^T g_{d1}.$$

As an example, we consider the decompositions obtained using 1-D quad-

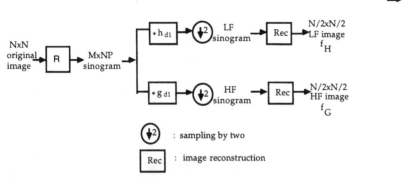

Figure 9.5
Multiresolution scheme from the 1-D DWT of the projections.

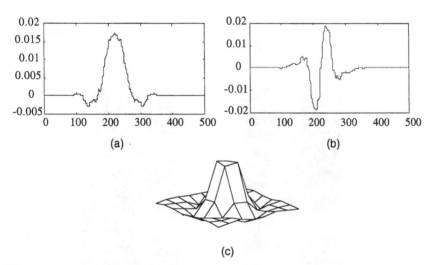

Figure 9.6
Use of the 8-point Johnston QMF filter: (a) scaling function; (b) wavelet function; (c) 2-D low-pass filter generated from the 1-D filter.

rature mirror filter banks (QMF) from Johnston [21]. Figures 9.6 and 9.7, respectively, illustrate the results obtained with Johnston filters of length 8 and 16. The 1-D scale and wavelet functions associated to these filters are presented in Figures 9.6(a–b) (resp., 9.7(a–b)). The corresponding 2-D low-frequency filter wavelets are shown in Figures 9.6(c) and 9.7(c).

The application of this process to a 128×128 lung image is shown in Figure 9.8. The low-pass and high-pass sinograms are presented in Figures 9.8(a) and 9.8(b), the reconstructed low-pass and high-pass images are presented in Figures 9.8(c) and 9.8(d).

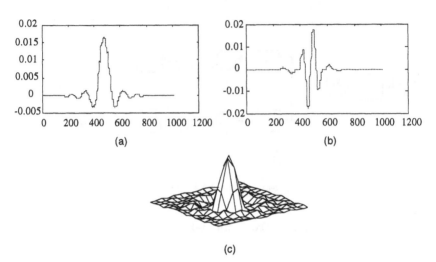

Figure 9.7
Use of the 16-point Johnston QMF filter: (a) scaling function;
(b) wavelet function; (c) 2-D filter generated from the 1-D filter.

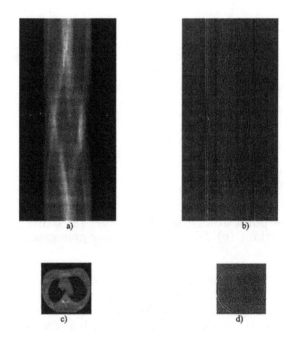

Figure 9.8
Decomposition with the 8-point Johnston filter. (a) LF sinogram;
(b) HF sinogram; (c) reconstructed LF image; and (d) reconstructed HF image.

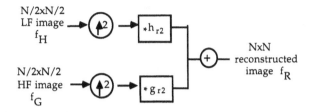

Figure 9.9
Dyadic reconstruction scheme. The oversampling of the images is done by a factor of 2 on x and y.

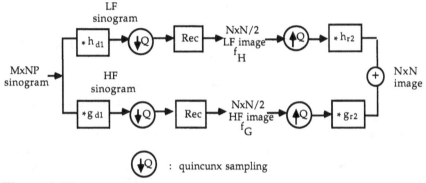

Figure 9.10
Quincunx multiresolution scheme.

To recover the original image, we may study the application of a multiresolution reconstruction scheme (Figure 9.9).

The two images are oversampled, respectively filtered with the filters h_{r2} and g_{r2}, and added. However, the analysis of this process shows that this procedure does not lead to an exact reconstruction. This analysis is developed in Appendix A. It is shown that while the low-frequency part of the image may be correctly reconstructed, the high-frequency part is corrupted by aliasing.

9.4.2   2-D Discrete WT of the Image

Since the dyadic decomposition of the projections does not allow a perfect reconstruction of the tomographic image, we consider the application of a pair of 2-D filters to the image and study the consequences on the projections. As in tomography, there is no reason to give preference to the horizontal or vertical direction, we investigate the use of a 2-D nonseparable decomposition. Indeed, the use of 2-D nonseparable wavelets offers more

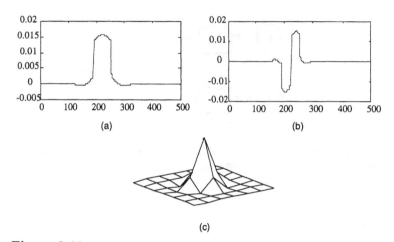

(c)

Figure 9.11
1-D scale function (a) and 1-D wavelet function (b) generated from Feauveau 2-D CQF filter (c).

flexibility for the choice of filters. Feauveau has first presented a multiresolution analysis with a resolution factor $\sqrt{2}$ [14]. He uses nonseparable 2-D wavelets generated by a filter bank associated to a quincunx sub- and oversampling procedures. In this case, the subsampling is obtained by keeping all the lines, and eliminating one point over two on the columns. The quincunx oversampling is obtained by insertion of zero in the same fashion. The 2-D filters used are based on the extension of 2-D CQF (conjugate quadrature filters). Other 2-D filters adapted to this scheme have been generated using the MacCellan Transform. For instance, in [22, 23], 2-D filters have been developed from Daubechies bi-orthogonal filters [24], and in [25], 2-D diamond-shaped filters have been generated from 1-D QMF filters.

The general decomposition and reconstruction schemes are nearly the same as in Section 9.4.1, except that we use a quincunx sampling scheme for the reconstructed images. The 2-D reconstruction filters, h_{r2} and g_{r2}, used are directly those associated to the 2-D analysis. The 1-D filters h_{d1} and g_{d1}, used for the decomposition, are obtained by projection of 2-D decomposition filters h_{d2} and g_{d2}.

Simulations have been performed using different 2-D filters:

- the 2-D CQF given by Feauveau [14]

- the 2-D QMF given by Shah [25]

- the 9/7 bi-orthogonal filters given by Antonini [22]

As an illustration, we show in Figure 9.11 the 1-D scale function (a), the 1-D wavelet function (b) generated from the 2-D filter (c) given by Feauveau

Table 9.1
QME (quadratic mean error) and SNR (signal-to-noise ratio in dB) between the original and reconstructed image for the different filters.

	Biort. 9/7	Feauv.	Shah	John 8
QME	0.12	0.23	0.27	0.31
SNR	66.5	60.9	59.5	58.3

[14]. The corresponding approximation and detail images are presented in Figure 12(a) and (b). The image reconstructed from the approximation and detail images is shown in Figure 12(c), and leads to a satisfying reconstruction. To quantify the reconstruction quality, the quadratic mean error and the SNR between the original and the reconstructed images have been computed. These measures are given for the different filters in Table 9.1.

9.5   Conclusion

In this chapter, we have presented some relations between the wavelet and Radon transforms. The relations established using a continuous formulation have shown that the wavelet and Radon transforms may be equivalently applied prior to or after reconstruction. In this case, the corresponding 1-D or 2-D wavelets are also related by a Radon transform. Then the application of discrete wavelet transforms generated via filter banks has been considered. A decomposition/reconstruction scheme obtained using 1-D and 2-D filters related by a discrete Radon transform has been studied. It has been shown that the dyadic decomposition with a subsampling by a factor of 2 does not lead to a perfect reconstruction. However, the use of quincunx subsampling permits satisfactory results. These relationships may be exploited for the analysis of tomographic images, the reconstruction of region of interest, and denoising.

9.5.1   Acknowledgments

The authors acknowledge the GDR 134 of the Centre National de la Recherche Scientifique for its support.

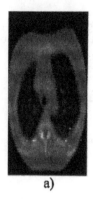

a)

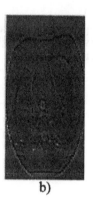

b)

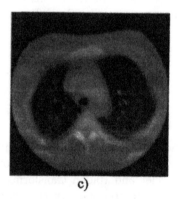

c)

Figure 9.12
Decomposition/reconstruction with the Feauveau filter. (a) reconstructed LF image; (b) reconstructed HF image; (c) reconstructed original image.

9.6   Appendix 1

We show why the dyadic scheme in Section 9.4.1 does not provide an
exact reconstruction of the tomographic image.

The exact reconstruction conditions of a filter bank is generally expressed
in function of the z-transform of the filters. They can be equivalently
expressed in terms of the discrete Fourier transforms of the filters. Let
H_{d1}, G_{d1}, H_{r1}, G_{r1}, be, respectively, the N-points DFT of the low-pass

and high-pass decomposition and reconstruction filters, h_{d1}, g_{d1}, h_{r1}, g_{r1}. The conditions become:

$$H_{d1}(k)H_{r1}(k) + G_{d1}(k)G_{r1}(k) = 2 \tag{A.1}$$

$$H_{d1}(k + N/2)H_{r1}(k) + G_{d1}(k + N/2)G_{r1}(k) = 0 \tag{A.2}$$

for $k = 1, N$, and where the indexes are taken modulo N.

Let us now study the multiresolution scheme considered in Section 9.4.1. For each projection, the low-pass and high-pass subsampled outputs are:

$$P_\theta^H(k) = \frac{1}{2}\left(P_\theta(k)H_{d1}(k) + P_\theta(k + N/2)H_{d1}(k + N/2)\right) \tag{A.3}$$

$$P_\theta^G(k) = \frac{1}{2}\left(P_\theta(k)G_{d1}(k) + P_\theta(k + N/2)G_{d1}(k + N/2)\right) \tag{A.4}$$

for $k = 1, N/2$.

Let f_H and f_G be, respectively, the images reconstructed from the resulting subsampled sinograms. Their 2-D $(N/2 \times N/2)$ DFTs satisfy an approximation of the Fourier slice theorem:

$$F_H(k\cos\theta, k\sin\theta) \approx P_\theta^H(k) \tag{A.5}$$

$$F_G(k\cos\theta, k\sin\theta) \approx P_\theta^G(k) \tag{A.6}$$

for $k = 1, N/2$.

After oversampling, the 2-D DFTs become:

$$F_H'(k,l) = F_H(k\,(\mathrm{mod}\ N/2), l\,(\mathrm{mod}\ N/2)) \tag{A.7}$$

$$F_G'(k,l) = F_G(k\,(\mathrm{mod}\ N/2), l\,(\mathrm{mod}\ N/2)) \tag{A.8}$$

for $k = 1, N$. Let both images be filtered with 2-D reconstruction filters denoted h_{r2}, and g_{r2} and added. The $N \times N$ DFT of the reconstructed image is:

$$F_R(k,l) = F_H'(k,l)H_{r2}(k,l) + F_G'(k,l)G_{r2}(k,l) \tag{A.9}$$

for $k = 1, N$, where H_{r2} and G_{r2} are the DFT of the filters.

If the two 2-D reconstruction filters are reconstructed from the 1-D reconstruction filters, it may be written:

$$H_{r2}(k\cos\theta, k\sin\theta) \approx H_{r1}(k) \tag{A.10}$$

$$G_{r2}(k\cos\theta, k\sin\theta) \approx G_{r1}(k). \tag{A.11}$$

Applying this relation at frequencies $(k\cos\theta, k\sin\theta)$ gives:

$$F_R(k\cos\theta, k\sin\theta) \approx F_H(k\cos\theta, l\sin\theta)H_{r1}(k) \tag{A.12}$$

$$+F_G(k\cos\theta, l\sin\theta)G_{r1}(k).$$

Thus, if k and $l < N/2$, by substituting the expression of P_θ^H and P_θ^G, one obtains:

$$F_R(k\cos\theta, k\sin\theta) \approx P_\theta(k)\left(\frac{1}{2}\big(H_{d1}(k)H_{r1}(k) + G_{d1}(k)G_{r1}(k)\big)\right) \tag{A.13}$$

$$+P_\theta(k+N/2)\left(\frac{1}{2}\big(H_{d1}(k+N/2)H_{r1}(k) + G_{d1}(k+N/2)G_{r1}(k)\big)\right)$$

and since the 1-D filters are supposed to satisfy the exact reconstruction conditions, it results that:

$$F_R(k\cos\theta, k\sin\theta) \approx P_\theta(k). \tag{A.14}$$

However, when k or $l > N/2$, since the indexes $k\cos\theta$ (resp. $k\sin\theta$) mod $N/2$, may be different from $k\,(\text{mod }N/2)\cos\theta$ (resp. $k\,(\text{mod }N/2)\sin\theta$), relation (A.14) may not be proved.

References

[1] M. Holschneider, Inverse Radon transform through inverse wavelet transforms, *Inverse Problems*, 7, 853–861, 1991.

[2] D. Walnut, Applications of Gabor and wavelet expansions to the Radon transform, in *Probabilistic and Stochastic Methods in Analysis with Applications*, J. S. Byrnes et al., Eds., Kluwer Academic Publishers, Boston, 1992, 187–205.

[3] F. Peyrin, M. Zaim, and R. Goutte, Multiscale reconstruction of tomographic images, *IEEE Int. Symp. on Time-Frequency and Time-Scale Analysis*, Victoria, Canada, 1992, 219–222.

[4] F. Peyrin, M. Zaim, and R. Goutte, Construction of wavelet decompositions for tomographic images, *J. Math. Imaging Vision* (special issue on wavelet theory and applications), V.3, 105–121, 1993.

[5] J. DeStefano and T. Olson, Wavelet localization of the Radon transform in even dimension, *Proc. IEEE Int. Symp. on Time-Frequency and Time-Scale Analysis*, 1992, 137–140.

[6] T. Olson, Uncertainty principles, signal recovery, finite Toeplitz forms and approximation theory: connections and applications to limited angle tomography, *Proc. IEEE EMBS*, 1994, 8a–9a.

[7] C. Berenstein and D. Walnut, Local tomography using wavelets, *Proc. IEEE EMBS*, Baltimore, 1994, 6a–7a.

[8] A. Delaney and Y. Bresler, Multiresolution tomographic reconstruction using wavelets, *Proc. ICIP-94, IEEE Int. Conf. on Image Processing*, 2, 830–834, 1994.

[9] B. Sahiner and A. Yagle, Image reconstruction from projections under wavelets constraints, *IEEE Trans. on Signal Process.*, 41, 3579–3584, 1993.

[10] D. Donoho, Wavelet shrinkage and W.V.D: a 10-minute tour, in *Progr. Wavelet Analysis and Applications*, Editiones Frontieres, 1992, 109–128.

[11] E. D. Kolaczyk, Wavelet Methods for the Inversion of Certain Homogeneous Linear Operators in the Presence of Noisy Data, Ph.D. thesis, Stanford University, Stanford, CA, 1994.

[12] P. Charbonnier, L. Blanc-Féraud, and M. Barlaud, An adaptive reconstruction method involving discontinuities, *Proc. IEEE MDSP*, 1993, V.491–V.494.

[13] M. Bhatia, W. C. Karl, and A. S. Willsky, Wavelet based methods for multiscale tomographic reconstruction, *Proc. IEEE EMBS*, Baltimore, 1994, 2a–3a.

[14] J. C. Feauveau, Analyse multirésolution pour les images avec un facteur de résolution $\sqrt{2}$, *Traitement du signal*, v.7, 117–128, 1990.

[15] A. Cohen and I. Daubechies, Non-separable bidimensional wavelet bases, Ten lectures on wavelets, *Rev. Mat. Iberoamericana*, 9, 51–138, 1993.

[16] J. Kovacevic and M. Vetterli, Non-separable multidimensional perfect reconstruction filter banks and wavelet bases for R^n, *IEEE Trans. Inf. Theor.*, 38, 533–555, 1992.

[17] J. P. Antoine, Image analysis with two-dimensional continuous wavelet transform, *Signal Processing*, 31, 241–272, 1993.

[18] J. Radon, Über die Bestimmung von Funktionen durch lhre integralwerte längs gewisser Manningfaltifkeiten. *Ber. Verb. Saechs. Akad. Wiss., Leipzig, Math. Phys. Kl.*, 69, 262–277, 1917.

[19] G. T. Herman, *Image Reconstruction from Projections: the Fundamentals of Computerized Tomography*, Academic Press, New York, 1980, 316 pp.

[20] F. Peyrin, Méthodes de reconstruction d'images 3D à partir de projections coniques de rayons X, Thése de doctorat d'Etat es sciences, INSA/Lyon I, 1990, p. 56.

[21] J. D. Johnston, A filter family designed for use in quadrature mirror filter banks, *Proc. IEEE, Int. Conf. ASSP*, CO, 1980, 291–294.

[22] M. Antonini, Transformée en ondelettes et compression numérique des images, Thèse: Université de Nice-Sophia Antipolis, 1991, 209 p.

[23] J. C. Feauveau, P. Mathieu, M. Barlaud, and M. Antonini, Recursive biorthogonal wavelet transform for image coding, *IEEE ICASSP*, Toronto, 1991, 2649–2652.

[24] I. Daubechies, *Ten lectures on wavelets*, Society for Industrial and Applied Mathematics, Philadelphia, 1992, 357 pp.

[25] I. A. Shah and A. A. C. Kalker, Theory and design of multidimensional QMF sub-band filters from 1D filters using transforms, *Proc. 4th Int. Conf. Image Processing and Applications*, Maastricht, April 1992, 474–477.

10

Wavelets and Local Tomography

Carlos A. Berenstein[1] and David F. Walnut[2]

[1] *Department of Mathematics and Institute for Systems Research, University of Maryland, College Park, MD*
[2] *Department of Mathematical Sciences, George Mason University, Fairfax, VA*

Abstract   In this paper, formulas relating the Radon transform and Radon transform inversion to various wavelet and multiscale transformations, including the continuous wavelet transform, the semi-continuous wavelet transform of Mallat, steerable multiscale filters of Freeman and Adelson, and separable orthogonal and nonorthogonal wavelet bases, are given. The use of wavelets as a valuable tool in the local inversion of the Radon transform in even dimensions is justified, and explicit estimates on the decay of ramp-filtered wavelets is given.

10.1   Introduction

The problem of local tomography can be stated as follows. *Given $a > 0$, compute the values of a function $f(\mathbf{x})$, $\mathbf{x} \in \mathcal{R}^n$, for all $\mathbf{x}$ such that $|\mathbf{x}| \leq a$, from knowledge of the projections of f on lines passing through the ball of radius a about the origin.* In other language, the problem of local tomography is the recovery of the function $f(\mathbf{x})\chi_{\{|\mathbf{x}|\leq a\}}(\mathbf{x})$ from $R_\theta f(s)\chi_{[-a,a]}(s)$, where $\chi_S(t) = 1$ if t is in the set S, and $\chi_S(t) = 0$ otherwise, and $R_\theta f(s)$ is the Radon transform of f (see Equation 10.1). The local tomography problem is also called the *interior problem*, and *region-of-interest* (ROI) *tomography.* The local tomography problem is not uniquely solvable when n is even. This is demonstrated in [22] with the construction of a function $u(\mathbf{x})$, $\mathbf{x} \in \mathcal{R}^2$, with $\text{supp}(u) \subseteq \{\mathbf{x} : |\mathbf{x}| \leq 1\}$ such that for some $0 < a < 1$, $u\chi_{\{|\mathbf{x}|\leq a\}} \not\equiv 0$ but $R_\theta u\chi_{[-a,a]} \equiv 0$. An interpretation of this nonuniqueness in terms of vanishing singular values may be found in [19], where the singular value decomposition of the interior Radon transform is given.

In most practical applications, projections on lines passing through a slightly larger region than the region of interest are known. In this case, the problem may be stated as follows. *Given $0 < a < a'$, compute the values of a function $f(\mathbf{x})$, $\mathbf{x} \in \mathcal{R}^n$, for all $\mathbf{x}$ such that $|\mathbf{x}| \leq a$, from knowledge of the projections of f on lines passing through the ball of radius a' about the origin.* This *semi-local tomography problem* is still not uniquely solvable when n is even, and as before, there exist functions $u(\mathbf{x})$, $\mathbf{x} \in \mathcal{R}^2$ with $R_\theta u\chi_{[-a',a']} \equiv 0$ for all $\theta \in S^1$, but for which $u\chi_{\{|\mathbf{x}|\leq a\}} \not\equiv 0$. However, it has been shown in [22] that such functions do not vary much in $\{\mathbf{x} : |\mathbf{x}| \leq a\}$ if a is small relative to a'.

The purpose of this paper is to show that wavelets and wavelet transforms can be useful tools in the study of the local and semi-local tomography problems. The use of wavelets for such problems was first proposed in [31]. These ideas were modified and successfully implemented in [10], where full recovery of the region of interest was achieved with significant reduction in exposure. The algorithm implemented in [10] was not, strictly speaking, a local tomography algorithm, as measurements far from the region of interest were included at a sparse set of angles to recover the low-resolution components of the image. In [4], the authors use a Radon transform inversion formula based on the continuous wavelet transform (see Section 10.4.1) to obtain explicit error estimates on the recovery within the ball of radius a from integrals on lines through the ball of radius a'. A scheme to reconstruct directly the separable two-dimensional wavelet transform of an image from its projections (see Section 10.4.3) has been implemented in [9]. This algorithm also uses a sparse set of measurements far from the region of interest to recover the low-resolution components of the image. A similar algorithm using only local measurements has been implemented in [26]. Multiresolution reconstruction of tomographic images has also been done in [23], and a general inversion formula in [33].

We also show in this paper that various image analysis techniques that employ wavelet transforms or other multiscale representations, such as those found in [16, 20, 21, 27], intertwine naturally with the Radon transform, and with Radon transform inversion. This allows the possibility of doing image processing, such as compression and edge detection, directly on the tomographic data. The efficiency and localization properties of the wavelet transform allow for efficient implementation.

The paper is organized as follows. In Section 10.2, we provide some background and notation on the Radon transform and on Radon transform inversion. More details may be found in [7] and [22]. In Section 10.3, we motivate the use of wavelets as a tool for local inversion of the Radon transform. We also mention the limitations of the wavelet approach and compare with Λ-tomography ([12–15]). In Section 10.4, we show how Radon transform inversion intertwines with various types of wavelet and multiresolution transforms including the continuous wavelet transform, the semi-continuous wavelet transform of Mallat ([20, 21]), and separable orthonormal and nonorthogonal wavelet bases and frames such as those described in [1, 2, 6, 8, 29, 30]. In Section 10.5, we present estimates showing how the degree of localization depends on the number of vanishing moments and smoothness of the wavelet.

Throughout this paper, $\mathcal{R}^n$ and $\mathcal{C}^n$ denote n-dimensional Euclidean and complex space. A vector $\mathbf{x} \in \mathcal{R}^n$ is written $\mathbf{x} = (x_1, \ldots, x_n)$, with the usual Euclidean inner product denoted by $\mathbf{x} \cdot \mathbf{y} = \sum_{i=1}^n x_i y_i$. $S^{n-1} \subset \mathcal{R}^n$ denotes the $(n-1)$-dimensional sphere, and $\theta \in S^{n-1}$ is written $\theta = (\theta_1, \ldots, \theta_n)$ with $\sum_{i=1}^n \theta_i^2 = 1$. If $n = 2$, we will without comment identify the circle, S^1, in $\mathcal{R}^2$ with the interval $[0, 2\pi)$ in the usual way. All integrals are with respect to Lebesgue measure. $\hat{\mathcal{R}} = \mathcal{R}$, the dual of $\mathcal{R}$, denotes the frequency domain. The Fourier transform of an integrable function $f(\mathbf{x})$ on $\mathcal{R}^n$ is defined by

$$\hat{f}(\xi) = \int_{\mathcal{R}^n} f(\mathbf{x}) \, e^{-2\pi i \mathbf{x} \cdot \xi} \, d\mathbf{x},$$

with the usual generalizations when f is not integrable.

We define the n-dimensional isotropic dilation operator, D_a, $a > 0$, by $D_a f(\mathbf{x}) = a^{-n/2} f(\mathbf{x}/a)$, and we let $f^\vee(\mathbf{x}) = f(-\mathbf{x})$ for $\mathbf{x} \in \mathcal{R}^n$. Hence the continuous wavelet transform of f with $\mathbf{a} = (a, \ldots, a)$, $W_\psi f(\mathbf{a}, \mathbf{b})$, can be written as

$$W_\psi f(\mathbf{a}, \mathbf{b}) = f * D_a \psi^\vee(\mathbf{b}).$$

We will write $W_\psi f(a, \mathbf{b})$ for $W_\psi f(\mathbf{a}, \mathbf{b})$, as we will only consider isotropic dilation in this paper. Note that $(D_a f)^\vee = D_a f^\vee$ and that $\hat{f}^\vee(\xi) = \widehat{f^\vee}(\xi)$. Detailed proofs of all of the results stated in this paper can be found in the Appendix (Section 10.7).

10.2 Background and Notation

The following formulas and notation are standard. More details can be found in [7] and [22].

The *Radon transform*, Rf, of a function $f(\mathbf{x})$, $\mathbf{x} \in \mathcal{R}^n$ is defined by

$$Rf(\theta, s) = R_\theta f(s) = \int_{\theta^\perp} f(s\theta + y)\, dy, \qquad (10.1)$$

where $\theta \in S^{n-1}$, $s \in \mathcal{R}$. $Rf(\theta, s)$ represents the integral of f on the hyperplane in $\mathcal{R}^n$ perpendicular to θ and a directed distance s from the origin. It is easy to see that $Rf(-\theta, s) = Rf(\theta, -s)$.

We define the *backprojection operator* as follows. Given a function $h(\theta, t)$, defined on $S^{n-1} \times \mathcal{R}$, we define the operator $R^\#$ by

$$R^\# h(x) = \int_{S^{n-1}} h(\theta, x \cdot \theta)\, d\theta. \qquad (10.2)$$

We can think of the pair (θ, t) as parametrizing the hyperplane $\{\mathbf{x} : \mathbf{x} \cdot \theta = t\}$, and the function h as being a function defined on $(n-1)$-dimensional hyperplanes in $\mathcal{R}^n$. In this case, $R^\# h(\mathbf{x})$ is the integral of h over all hyperplanes passing through $\mathbf{x}$.

Many of the results in this paper are based on the *filtered backprojection formula*, which is the following. Given $f(\mathbf{x})$, $\mathbf{x} \in \mathcal{R}^n$, and $g(\theta, t) = g_\theta(t)$, $\theta \in S^{n-1}$, $t \in \mathcal{R}$,

$$f * R^\#(g_\theta)(\mathbf{x}) = R^\#(R_\theta f * g_\theta)(\mathbf{x}), \qquad (10.3)$$

where the convolution on the left is with respect to $\mathbf{x} \in \mathcal{R}^n$, and that on the right is with respect to $t \in \mathcal{R}$. Equation (10.3) is the basis for many reconstruction schemes for the Radon transform. If g_θ is determined so that $R^\#(g_\theta)$ approximates a δ-function, then a good approximation of f can be obtained by simple convolution and backprojection. Guédon and Unser have used this approach to compute the least squares projection of $f(\mathbf{x})$ on the space of piecewise polynomial functions with uniformly spaced nodes [17].

The basic inversion formula for the Radon transform comes from the *Fourier slice theorem*, which can be stated as follows. Given $f(\mathbf{x})$, $\mathbf{x} \in \mathcal{R}^n$, and $\theta \in S^{n-1}$ fixed,

$$\widehat{R_\theta f}(\gamma) = \hat{f}(\gamma\theta), \qquad (10.4)$$

for all $\gamma \in \hat{\mathcal{R}}$. Writing the usual Fourier inversion formula in polar coordinates leads to the formula,

$$f(\mathbf{x}) = \int_{S^{n-1}_+} \int_{-\infty}^{\infty} \widehat{R_\theta f}(r)\, e^{2\pi i(x\cdot\theta)r} |r|^{n-1}\, dr\, d\theta, \qquad (10.5)$$

where S_+^{n-1} denotes the upper-half sphere in $\mathcal{R}^n$.

The inversion formula (10.5) can be generalized in the following way. Given $\alpha \in \mathcal{R}$, define the *Riesz potential operator*, I^α by

$$\widehat{I^\alpha f}(\xi) = |\xi|^{-\alpha} \hat{f}(\xi). \tag{10.6}$$

If $\alpha < n$, then

$$f = \frac{1}{2} I^{-\alpha} R^\# (I^{\alpha+1-n} R_\theta f) \tag{10.7}$$

(see [22]).

Note that $I^{-2} = -(2\pi)^{-2} \Delta$, where Δ is the Laplacian operator, and

$$\Delta f = -4\pi^2 I^{-2} f = -2\pi^2 I^{-\alpha-2} R^\# (I^{\alpha+1-n} R_\theta f).$$

We refer to I^{-1} as the *Lambda operator* and write $I^{-1} = \Lambda$. Note that

$$\Lambda f = I^{-1} f = \frac{1}{2} I^{-\alpha-1} R^\# (I^{\alpha+1-n} R_\theta f),$$

so that taking $\alpha = -1$,

$$\Lambda f = \frac{1}{2} R^\# (I^{-n} R_\theta f). \tag{10.8}$$

Similarly, the operator Λ^{-1} satisfies

$$\Lambda^{-1} f = \frac{1}{2} R^\# (I^{2-n} R_\theta f). \tag{10.9}$$

The operators Λ and Λ^{-1} are used in Λ-tomography, an important technique in addressing the problems of local tomography (see Section 10.3.2, and [13], [22]).

10.3 Why Wavelets?

10.3.1 The Nonlocality of the Radon Transform

In order to motivate the usefulness of wavelets in localizing the Radon transform, it is helpful to first explore why the Radon transform is not local in even dimensions. To do this, we consider formula (10.3),

$$f * G(\mathbf{x}) = R^{\#}(R_\theta f * g_\theta)(\mathbf{x}),$$

where $(R^{\#} g_\theta)(\mathbf{x}) = G(\mathbf{x})$. By (10.7) with $\alpha = 0$, G satisfies,

$$G(\mathbf{x}) = R^{\#}\left(\frac{1}{2} I^{1-n} R_\theta G\right)(\mathbf{x}),$$

so that we may take

$$g_\theta = \frac{1}{2} I^{1-n} R_\theta G.$$

By the definition of the Riesz potential operator I^{1-n}, and by (10.4), $g_\theta(t)$ satisfies

$$\widehat{g_\theta}(\gamma) = \frac{1}{2}|\gamma|^{n-1}\hat{G}(\gamma\theta).$$

Now, in order for the Radon transform to be locally invertible from local measurements, it would be sufficient that both g_θ and G be compactly supported. If this were the case, then we could choose $a' > a$ in such a way that $\operatorname{supp}(G) \subseteq \{\mathbf{x}: |\mathbf{x}| \leq a' - a\}$, and $\operatorname{supp}(g_\theta) \subseteq [-a' + a, a' - a]$ for each $\theta \in S^{n-1}$. This would allow us to recover exactly $f * G(\mathbf{x})$ for $|\mathbf{x}| \leq a$ from $R_\theta f(s)$ for $s \in [-a', a']$. Assuming that $\iint_{\mathcal{R}^2} G(\mathbf{x}) \, d\mathbf{x} = 1$, and by dilating G, we can recover f as accurately as desired in $\{\mathbf{x}: |\mathbf{x}| \leq a\}$ since defining $G_\epsilon(\mathbf{x}) = \epsilon^{-n} G(\mathbf{x}/\epsilon)$,

$$f * G_\epsilon \to f, \text{ as } \epsilon \to 0,$$

in some appropriate sense.

However, both g_θ and G cannot be compactly supported for the following reason. Suppose that G were compactly supported. In this case, it is well known that $\hat{G}(\xi)$ can be extended to an entire function in $\mathcal{C}^n$, so that at each angle, θ, $\hat{G}(\gamma\theta)$ is the restriction to $\mathcal{R}$ of an entire function in $\mathcal{C}$. Now, in order that $g_\theta(t)$ have compact support, it is necessary that $|\gamma|^{n-1}\hat{G}(\gamma\theta)$ be the restriction to $\mathcal{R}$ of an entire function. If n is even, and assuming that $\iint_{\mathcal{R}^2} G(\mathbf{x}) \, d\mathbf{x} = \hat{G}(0) = 1$, then this is impossible, since $|\gamma|^{n-1}$ has a discontinuity in its $(n-1)$st derivative at $\gamma = 0$. Therefore, g_θ will not be compactly supported and local inversion is not possible. If n is odd, then $|\gamma|^{n-1} = \gamma^{n-1}$, so that analyticity is preserved. In fact, inversion of the Radon transform is local in odd dimensions.

10.3.2   Wavelets, Vanishing Moments, and Λ-Tomography

Even though compact support of the $g_\theta(t)$ cannot be achieved with a compactly supported $G(\mathbf{x})$, one can ask that $g_\theta(t)$ have rapid decay at

$\pm\infty$. This is accomplished by requiring that $|\gamma|^{n-1}\hat{G}(\gamma\theta)$ be as smooth as possible. Since $|\gamma|^{n-1}\hat{G}(\gamma\theta)$ is infinitely differentiable away from $\gamma = 0$, the only issue is smoothness at $\gamma = 0$, and in order that $|\gamma|^{n-1}\hat{G}(\gamma\theta)$ be smooth at $\gamma = 0$, $\hat{G}(\gamma\theta)$ must vanish to high order at $\gamma = 0$. In fact, if $G(\mathbf{x})$ has compact support and if $\hat{G}(\gamma\theta)$ vanishes to order m at $\gamma = 0$, then $\hat{g_\theta}(\gamma)$ will have $n + m - 1$ continuous derivatives at $\gamma = 0$ (Lemma 1). Assuming good decay on $\hat{G}(\gamma\theta)$ and its derivatives, $g_\theta(t)$ will decay like t^{-n-m+1} at $\pm\infty$ (Theorem 7).

The above suggests that the most one can expect to recover locally in even dimensions is $f * G(\mathbf{x})$, where G has a large number of vanishing moments. By rescaling G and by sampling the convolution appropriately, one obtains a wavelet transform of f. Such tools have been used for some time in compression, edge detection, and other image-processing problems.

The notion of detecting edges locally from local projections is a motivation for the technique of Λ–tomography (see [13], [14], and [15] for details). In this technique, the functions Λf, and $\Lambda^{-1}f$ are recovered locally by (10.8) and (10.9). This can be done since the operators I^{-n} and I^{2-n} preserve compact support as multiplication by $|\gamma|^n = \gamma^n$, and $|\gamma|^{2-n} = \gamma^{2-n}$ preserve analyticity (since n is even). The function $\Lambda f + \alpha\Lambda^{-1}f$ for some appropriately chosen parameter α gives a good edge picture of the original image f. The technique has been extended to estimate density differences at jump discontinuities of f [12] (see also [34]).

The method of Λ-tomography to detect edges has also been extended to the attenuated Radon transform by Kuchment et. al. [18]. The attenuated Radon transform in dimension two is defined as follows. Given $\theta \in [0, 2\pi)$, $s \in \mathcal{R}$,

$$R_\mu f(\theta, s) = \int_{-\infty}^{\infty} f(s\theta + t\theta^\perp)\,\mu(s\theta + t\theta^\perp, \theta)\,dt,$$

where $\mu(\mathbf{x}, \theta) \geq 0$ is assumed to be real analytic on $\mathcal{R}^2 \times S^1$. The key point is that if $R^\#$ is the usual backprojection operator, then $R^\# R_\mu$ is an elliptic Fourier integral operator. This fact has been used very effectively by many people, most notably Boman and Quinto [5], and lies at the heart of the work of Quinto [28], and of Ramm and Zaslavsky [24, 25].

10.4 Wavelet Inversion of the Radon Transform

10.4.1 The Continuous Wavelet Transform

In this subsection, we show how the continuous wavelet transform of a function can be recovered from the wavelet transform of its projections. For convenience, we consider a separable n-dimensional wavelet and isotropic dilation, that is, the same dilation factor in all variables. The radial wavelet case is considered in [4] where error estimates on recovery are given, and the general case for dimension two is considered in [32].

THEOREM 1

Given a separable n-dimensional wavelet $(n > 1)$ of the form

$$\psi(\mathbf{x}) = \psi^1(x_1)\psi^2(x_2)\cdots\psi^n(x_n), \tag{10.10}$$

where the $\psi^i(t)$ satisfy $|\widehat{\psi^i}(\gamma)| \le C_i(1 + |\gamma|)^{-1}$ for all γ, define the family of one-dimensional functions $\{\rho_\theta\}_{\theta \in S^{n-1}}$ by

$$\widehat{\rho_\theta}(\gamma) = \frac{1}{2}|\gamma|^{n-1}\,\widehat{\psi^1}(\gamma\theta_1)\widehat{\psi^2}(\gamma\theta_2)\cdots\widehat{\psi^n}(\gamma\theta_n), \tag{10.11}$$

where $\theta = (\theta_1, \ldots, \theta_n) \in S^{n-1}$. Then for every $f \in L^1 \cap L^2(\mathcal{R}^n)$,

$$(W_\psi f)(a, \mathbf{b}) = a^{(1-n)/2} \int_{S^{n-1}} (W_{\rho_\theta} R_\theta f)(a, \mathbf{b} \cdot \theta)\, d\theta. \tag{10.12}$$

The point of Theorem 1 is the observation that the wavelet transform of a function $f(\mathbf{x})$ with any mother wavelet and at any scale and location can be obtained by backprojecting the wavelet transform of the Radon transform of f using wavelets that vary with each angle, but which are admissible for each angle. The formula (10.12) follows immediately from the filtered backprojection formula (10.3) with an appropriate choice of g_θ and a determination of how dilation commutes with backprojection.

The following result also holds.

THEOREM 2

Given a one-dimensional wavelet $\rho(t)$ satisfying $\rho(t) = \rho(-t)$, $\rho(t) \in \mathcal{R}$, all t, and

$$\int_0^\infty \frac{|\hat{\rho}(r)|^2}{r^{2n-1}}\, dr < \infty, \tag{10.13}$$

define the radial function $\psi(\mathbf{x})$ by

$$\hat{\psi}(\xi) = 2|\xi|^{1-n}\hat{\rho}(|\xi|). \tag{10.14}$$

Then

$$(W_\psi f)(a, \mathbf{b}) = a^{(1-n)/2} \int_{S^{n-1}} (W_\rho R_\theta f)(a, \mathbf{b} \cdot \theta) \, d\theta. \qquad (10.15)$$

Theorem 2 is similar to Theorem 1 except that in Theorem 2 the one-dimensional wavelet ρ is fixed beforehand for all angles θ. This determines the n-dimensional wavelet ψ. In Theorem 1, ψ was fixed beforehand determining $\{\rho_\theta\}_{\theta \in [0,2\pi)}$ for each θ. The interplay between the one- and n-dimensional wavelets in formulas (10.12) and (10.15) is important in understanding how wavelets may be used in local tomography and image processing. In local tomography, we seek ρ with small support and many vanishing moments. In this case (cf. Theorem 7), ψ will have essentially the same radius of support as ρ. Therefore, according to formula (10.15), the wavelet coefficients of f can be recovered locally from local measurements of its Radon transform. For the purposes of image processing, one typically would like to fix the two-dimensional wavelet ψ appropriately to the desired task, then consider the properties of ρ_θ for each θ. An example of this idea is found in Section 10.4.2.

Once the wavelet transform of the function $f(\mathbf{x})$ has been computed, one can now recover the original function $f(\mathbf{x})$ using standard inversion formulas for the continuous wavelet transform.

10.4.2   The Semi-Continuous Wavelet Transform

In this subsection, we consider the planar ($n = 2$) case only. The semi-continuous wavelet transform has been used by Mallat in the compression and edge detection of images via wavelet transform maxima. For more details on Mallat's algorithm, see [21, 20]. The transform can be described briefly as follows. Let $G(\mathbf{x})$ be a radial function on $\mathcal{R}^2$ satisfying $\iint_{\mathcal{R}^2} G(\mathbf{x}) \, d\mathbf{x} = 1$. Define

$$\psi^1(\mathbf{x}) = \frac{\partial}{\partial x_1} G(\mathbf{x}), \quad \psi^2(\mathbf{x}) = \frac{\partial}{\partial x_2} G(\mathbf{x}). \qquad (10.16)$$

Then the *semi-continuous wavelet transform* of a function $f(\mathbf{x})$, is defined by

$$\{(W_{\psi^1} f)(2^j, \mathbf{x}), (W_{\psi^2} f)(2^j, \mathbf{x})\}_{j \in \mathcal{Z}, \mathbf{x} \in \mathcal{R}^2}.$$

THEOREM 3

Given a one-dimensional wavelet $\rho(t)$ satisfying $\rho(t) = \rho(-t)$, $\rho(t) \in \mathcal{R}$, *all t, and with $\lim_{\gamma \to 0} |\gamma|^{-1} \hat{\rho}(\gamma) = 1/2$, define the radial function $G(\mathbf{x})$ by*

$$\hat{G}(\xi) = 2|\xi|^{-1}\hat{\rho}(|\xi|), \tag{10.17}$$

and define $\psi^1(\mathbf{x})$ and $\psi^2(\mathbf{x})$ as in (10.16). Then given $f(\mathbf{x})$,

$$(W_{\psi^1} f)(2^j, \mathbf{x}) = 2^{j/2} \int_0^{2\pi} \cos\theta \, (W_{d\rho/dt} R_\theta f)(2^j, \mathbf{x} \cdot \theta) \, d\theta, \tag{10.18}$$

and

$$(W_{\psi^2} f)(2^j, \mathbf{x}) = 2^{j/2} \int_0^{2\pi} \sin\theta \, (W_{d\rho/dt} R_\theta f)(2^j, \mathbf{x} \cdot \theta) \, d\theta. \tag{10.19}$$

Freeman and Adelson ([16], cf. [27]) have used the notion of *steerable* and *scalable filters* to do image processing, using a wavelet transform in which the analyzing wavelets have an arbitrary orientation in the following sense. Given $G(\mathbf{x})$, $\psi^1(\mathbf{x})$, and $\psi^2(\mathbf{x})$ as before, and given $\beta \in [0, 2\pi)$, define $\psi^\beta(\mathbf{x})$ by

$$\psi^\beta(\mathbf{x}) = \cos\beta \, \psi^1(\mathbf{x}) + \sin\beta \, \psi^2(\mathbf{x}).$$

In other words, $\psi^\beta(\mathbf{x})$ is the directional derivative of $G(\mathbf{x})$ in the direction β. The following theorem holds.

THEOREM 4
Let $\rho(t)$ and $G(\mathbf{x})$ be given as in Theorem 3, and let $\beta \in [0, 2\pi)$. Then

$$(W_{\psi^\beta} f)(2^j, \mathbf{x}) = 2^{j/2} \int_0^{2\pi} \cos(\beta - \theta)(W_{d\rho/dt} R_\theta f)(2^j, \mathbf{x} \cdot \theta) \, d\theta. \tag{10.20}$$

Theorems 3 and 4 say that the semi-continuous wavelet transform of Mallat and a directional wavelet transform described by Freeman and Adleson can be computed directly by means of a weighted backprojection of the wavelet transform of $R_\theta f$ at each θ. The use of a single one-dimensional wavelet independent of θ guarantees that G will be radially symmetric. The weights $\cos\theta$ and $\sin\theta$ in (10.18) and (10.19) are consistent with the notion that $W_{\psi^1} f$ should emphasize vertical edges (corresponding to projections on angles θ near zero and π) and that $W_{\psi^2} f$ should emphasize horizontal edges (corresponding to projections on angles θ near $\pi/2$ and $3\pi/2$). Similarly, the weight $\cos(\beta - \theta)$ in (10.20) is consistent with the notion that the directional wavelet transform $W_{\psi^\beta} f$ should emphasize edges with direction β.

10.4.3   The Discrete Wavelet Transform

In this subsection, we investigate the recovery of a function from its Radon transform by means of the discrete wavelet transform. First, we prove a Radon transform inversion formula based on the separation of the angular and radial components of $R_\theta f(s)$ using a one-dimensional discrete wavelet transform in each direction. This inversion formula first appeared in [31] and was the basis of the local tomography algorithm described in [10]. Next, we show how the separable two-dimensional discrete wavelet transform of a function, f, can be obtained by backprojection of an irregularly sampled one-dimensional wavelet transform of $R_\theta f$, for each θ. A similar formulation is used in [9] as the basis of a local tomography algorithm.

THEOREM 5
Let $\psi(t)$ be a one-dimensional wavelet such that

$$\{\psi_{j,k}\} = \{2^{-j/2}\psi(2^{-j}x - k)\}$$

is a Riesz basis or a frame for $L^2(\mathcal{R})$. Let $\rho(t)$ be defined by

$$\hat{\rho}(\gamma) = \frac{1}{2}|\gamma|\hat{\psi}(\gamma). \tag{10.21}$$

Suppose that for each $\theta \in [0, 2\pi)$,

$$R_\theta f(\theta, s) = \sum_{j,k} c_{j,k}(\theta)\, \psi_{j,k}(s), \tag{10.22}$$

for some coefficients $c_{j,k}(\theta)$. Then $\rho(t)$ is an admissible function, and

$$f(\mathbf{x}) = \sum_{j,k} 2^{-j} \int_0^{2\pi} c_{j,k}(\theta)\, \rho_{j,k}(\mathbf{x} \cdot \theta)\, d\theta. \tag{10.23}$$

The reconstruction formula in Theorem 5 directly reconstructs point-values of a function f using the wavelet coefficients of $R_\theta f$ for each θ. In [10], the authors use this formula as the basis for a local reconstruction algorithm. They observe that if ψ has compact support and sufficiently many vanishing moments, then ρ will have essentially the same support as ψ, that is, ρ will decay very rapidly outside the support of ψ (cf. Figures 10.1–10.3). Hence, for $j < 0$, and for $\mathbf{x}$ and θ fixed, $c_{j,k}(\theta)$ can be computed accurately from $R_\theta f(s)$ for s in a small interval around $\mathbf{x} \cdot \theta$, i.e., from projections of f on lines through a small disk centered at $\mathbf{x}$. Using now

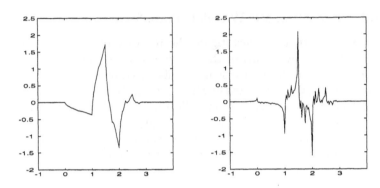

Figure 10.1
Left: the Daubechies 4 coefficient wavelet $\psi(t)$; Right: the corresponding function $\rho(t)$ given by (10.21).

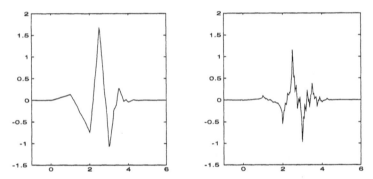

Figure 10.2
Left: the Daubechies 6 coefficient wavelet $\psi(t)$; Right: the corresponding function $\rho(t)$ given by (10.21).

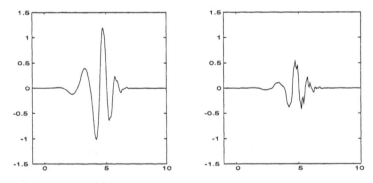

Figure 10.3
Left: the Daubechies 10 coefficient wavelet $\psi(t)$; Right: the corresponding function $\rho(t)$ given by (10.21).

(10.23), reconstruction of the fine-scale features of f at $\mathbf{x}$ (where "fine scale" refers to coefficients with $j < 0$), is possible using only local projections. To reconstruct the large-scale features of f near $\mathbf{x}$, it was noted in [10] that for $j \geq 0$, and all k, $c_{j,k}(\theta)$ is essentially bandlimited in θ, and hence can be accurately estimated from its samples on a sparse set of angles. In this way, the large-scale features of f near $\mathbf{x}$ can be recovered from a small set of global measurements, and local recovery is achieved with a significant reduction in exposure. For more details, see [10] and [11].

Numerical examples of functions $\rho(t)$ corresponding to different wavelets $\psi(t)$ are shown in Figures 10.1, 10.2, and 10.3. Note that the essential support of the $\rho(t)$ are not much larger than the support of the corresponding $\psi(t)$. This is due to the fact that the wavelets have vanishing moments and indicates why wavelets have been effective in local tomography algorithms.

Next, suppose that φ, $\mathring{\varphi}$, ψ, and $\mathring{\psi}$ are the scaling function, dual scaling function, wavelet, and dual wavelet for a wavelet basis generated by some multiresolution analysis. The standard construction for a corresponding separable wavelet basis in two dimensions is to form the functions,

$$
\begin{aligned}
\Phi(\mathbf{x}) &= \varphi(x_1)\varphi(x_2), & \Psi^2(\mathbf{x}) &= \psi(x_1)\varphi(x_2), \\
\Psi^1(\mathbf{x}) &= \varphi(x_1)\psi(x_2), & \Psi^3(\mathbf{x}) &= \psi(x_1)\psi(x_2),
\end{aligned}
\tag{10.24}
$$

and the dual functions,

$$
\begin{aligned}
\mathring{\Phi}(\mathbf{x}) &= \mathring{\varphi}(x_1)\mathring{\varphi}(x_2), & \mathring{\Psi}^2(\mathbf{x}) &= \mathring{\psi}(x_1)\mathring{\varphi}(x_2), \\
\mathring{\Psi}^1(\mathbf{x}) &= \mathring{\varphi}(x_1)\mathring{\psi}(x_2), & \mathring{\Psi}^3(\mathbf{x}) &= \mathring{\psi}(x_1)\mathring{\psi}(x_2).
\end{aligned}
\tag{10.25}
$$

Then an arbitrary function $f(\mathbf{x})$ can be written as,

$$
f(\mathbf{x}) = \sum_{j,k} \sum_{i=1}^{3} \langle f, \Psi^i_{j,k} \rangle \, \mathring{\Psi}^i_{j,k} = \sum_{j,k} \sum_{i=1}^{3} \langle f, \mathring{\Psi}^i_{j,k} \rangle \, \Psi^i_{j,k},
$$

or as

$$
f(\mathbf{x}) = \sum_{k \in \mathbb{Z}^2} \langle f, \Phi_{J,k} \rangle \, \mathring{\Phi}_{J,k} + \sum_{j=-\infty}^{J} \sum_{k \in \mathbb{Z}^2} \sum_{i=1}^{3} \langle f, \Psi^i_{j,k} \rangle \, \mathring{\Psi}^i_{j,k}
$$

$$= \sum_{k \in \mathcal{Z}^2} \langle f, \overset{\circ}{\Phi}_{J,k} \rangle \, \Phi_{J,k} + \sum_{j=-\infty}^{J} \sum_{k \in \mathcal{Z}^2} \sum_{i=1}^{3} \langle f, \overset{\circ}{\Psi}^i_{j,k} \rangle \, \Psi^i_{j,k},$$

where

$$\Phi_{j,k}(\mathbf{x}) = \varphi_{j,k_1}(x_1)\varphi_{j,k_2}(x_2), \qquad \Psi^2_{j,k}(\mathbf{x}) = \psi_{j,k_1}(x_1)\varphi_{j,k_2}(x_2),$$

$$\Psi^1_{j,k}(\mathbf{x}) = \varphi_{j,k_1}(x_1)\psi_{j,k_2}(x_2), \qquad \Psi^3_{j,k}(\mathbf{x}) = \psi_{j,k_1}(x_1)\psi_{j,k_2}(x_2),$$

and

$$\overset{\circ}{\Phi}_{j,k}(\mathbf{x}) = \overset{\circ}{\varphi}_{j,k_1}(x_1)\overset{\circ}{\varphi}_{j,k_2}(x_2), \qquad \overset{\circ}{\Psi}^2_{j,k}(\mathbf{x}) = \overset{\circ}{\psi}_{j,k_1}(x_1)\overset{\circ}{\varphi}_{j,k_2}(x_2),$$

$$\overset{\circ}{\Psi}^1_{j,k}(\mathbf{x}) = \overset{\circ}{\varphi}_{j,k_1}(x_1)\overset{\circ}{\psi}_{j,k_2}(x_2), \qquad \overset{\circ}{\Psi}^3_{j,k}(\mathbf{x}) = \overset{\circ}{\psi}_{j,k_1}(x_1)\overset{\circ}{\psi}_{j,k_2}(x_2).$$

THEOREM 6

Given φ, $\overset{\circ}{\varphi}$, ψ, and $\overset{\circ}{\psi}$ from a wavelet multiresolution analysis, and with Φ, $\overset{\circ}{\Phi}$, Ψ^i, and $\overset{\circ}{\Psi}^i$, $i = 1, 2, 3$, defined by (10.24) and (10.25), define for each $\theta \in [0, 2\pi)$ the functions $\sigma_\theta(t)$, and $\rho^i_\theta(t)$, $i = 1, 2, 3$, by

$$\widehat{\sigma_\theta}(\gamma) = \tfrac{1}{2}|\gamma|\hat{\varphi}(\gamma \cos \theta)\hat{\varphi}(\gamma \sin \theta), \qquad \widehat{\rho^2_\theta}(\gamma) = \tfrac{1}{2}|\gamma|\hat{\psi}(\gamma \cos \theta)\hat{\varphi}(\gamma \sin \theta),$$

$$\widehat{\rho^1_\theta}(\gamma) = \tfrac{1}{2}|\gamma|\hat{\varphi}(\gamma \cos \theta)\hat{\psi}(\gamma \sin \theta), \qquad \widehat{\rho^3_\theta}(\gamma) = \tfrac{1}{2}|\gamma|\hat{\psi}(\gamma \cos \theta)\hat{\psi}(\gamma \sin \theta),$$

and the functions $\overset{\circ}{\sigma}_\theta(t)$, and $\overset{\circ}{\rho}^i_\theta(t)$, by

$$\widehat{\overset{\circ}{\sigma}_\theta}(\gamma) = \tfrac{1}{2}|\gamma|\widehat{\overset{\circ}{\varphi}}(\gamma \cos \theta)\widehat{\overset{\circ}{\varphi}}(\gamma \sin \theta), \qquad \widehat{\overset{\circ}{\rho}^2_\theta}(\gamma) = \tfrac{1}{2}|\gamma|\widehat{\overset{\circ}{\psi}}(\gamma \cos \theta)\widehat{\overset{\circ}{\varphi}}(\gamma \sin \theta),$$

$$\widehat{\overset{\circ}{\rho}^1_\theta}(\gamma) = \tfrac{1}{2}|\gamma|\widehat{\overset{\circ}{\varphi}}(\gamma \cos \theta)\widehat{\overset{\circ}{\psi}}(\gamma \sin \theta), \qquad \widehat{\overset{\circ}{\rho}^3_\theta}(\gamma) = \tfrac{1}{2}|\gamma|\widehat{\overset{\circ}{\psi}}(\gamma \cos \theta)\widehat{\overset{\circ}{\psi}}(\gamma \sin \theta).$$

Then,

$$\langle f, \Phi_{j,k} \rangle = 2^{-j/2} \int_0^{2\pi} (W_{\sigma_\theta} R_\theta f)(2^j, 2^j(k \cdot \theta)) \, d\theta, \tag{10.26}$$

$$\langle f, \Psi^i_{j,k} \rangle = 2^{-j/2} \int_0^{2\pi} (W_{\rho^i_\theta} R_\theta f)(2^j, 2^j(k \cdot \theta)) \, d\theta, \tag{10.27}$$

$$\langle f, \overset{\circ}{\Phi}_{j,k} \rangle = 2^{-j/2} \int_0^{2\pi} (W_{\overset{\circ}{\sigma}_\theta} R_\theta f)(2^j, 2^j(k \cdot \theta)) \, d\theta, \tag{10.28}$$

and

$$\langle f, \mathring{\Psi}^i_{j,k} \rangle = 2^{-j/2} \int_0^{2\pi} (W_{\mathring{\rho}^i_\theta} R_\theta f)(2^j, 2^j(k \cdot \theta)) \, d\theta, \qquad (10.29)$$

for $i = 1, 2, 3$.

Theorem 6 shows how the wavelet coefficients of a function f can be recovered from backprojecting the wavelet transform of $R_\theta f$ at each angle θ. Formulas similar to these were used in [9] as the basis for a local tomography algorithm. Specifically, the authors proposed recovery of the function $f_0(\mathbf{x})$ by the formula

$$\begin{aligned} f_0 &= \sum_{k \in \mathcal{Z}^2} \langle f, \Phi_{0,k} \rangle \, \mathring{\Phi}_{0,k} \\ &= \sum_{k \in \mathcal{Z}^2} \langle f, \Phi_{J,k} \rangle \, \mathring{\Phi}_{J,k} + \sum_{j=1}^J \sum_{k \in \mathcal{Z}^2} \sum_{i=1}^3 \langle f, \Psi^i_{j,k} \rangle \, \mathring{\Psi}^i_{j,k}. \end{aligned} \qquad (10.30)$$

In this formula, $j = 0$ represents the finest resolution recoverable, and $J > 0$ is a fixed resolution representing the coarsest scale that one wishes to compute. The sum over k is in practice always finite and depends on the support of f.

The fundamental observation is that if the wavelet ψ has compact support and sufficiently many vanishing moments, then the functions ρ^i_θ, $\theta \in [0, 2\pi)$, $i = 1, 2, 3$, will have essentially the same radius of support as the two-dimensional wavelets Ψ^i (cf. Figures 10.4–10.6). Hence, given $j = 1, \ldots,$ J, and k fixed, $\langle f, \Psi^i_{j,k} \rangle$ can be computed accurately from $R_\theta f(s)$ with $\theta \in [0, 2\pi)$ and s in an interval of radius $2^j T$ around $2^j k \cdot \theta$, where T is the radius of the essential support of $\Psi^i_{0,0}$. Note that these values of $R_\theta f$ are just the projections of f on lines through a disk of radius $2^j T$ centered at $2^j k$. Note also that the radius of this disk becomes larger as j increases to J. Hence the localization is better at finer scales and poorer at coarser scales.

Now, given $\mathbf{x}$, the coefficients $\langle f, \Psi^i_{j,k} \rangle$ where $2^j k$ is within a distance $2^j T'$ of $\mathbf{x}$, where T' is the radius of the essential support of $\mathring{\Psi}^i_{0,0}$, can be used to recover the features of f near $\mathbf{x}$ at scale j by using only local projections, where again the localization becomes worse for larger j. The authors in [9] use (10.27) for larger j but use a sparse sampling in θ to compute the right-hand side. This is justified since the coarser scale wavelets $\Psi^i_{j,k}$ are essentially bandlimited to a disk of radius $2^{-j}\Omega$ about the origin, where Ω is the essential bandlimit of $\Psi^i_{0,0}$. Finally, $\langle f, \Phi_{J,k} \rangle$ is computed from the full set of projections at $\theta = 0$. The resulting sampling geometry is very similar to that of [10], with a comparable savings in exposure.

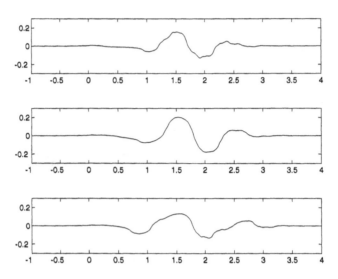

Figure 10.4
Graph of $\rho_\theta^1(t)$ defined in Theorem 6, where $\psi(t)$ and $\varphi(t)$ are the
Daubechies 4 coefficient wavelet and scaling functions supported
in $[0,3]$. From top: $\theta = 15°$, $\theta = 30°$, and $\theta = 45°$.

In [26], the authors make the surprising observation that in some cases,
given a scaling function φ with compact support, the functions σ_θ have
essentially the same radius of support as the two-dimensional scaling function Φ. This phenomenon is related to the number of vanishing moments
of the scaling function. Specifically, if $\hat{\varphi}^{(j)}(0) = 0$ for $j = 1, \ldots, K$ for K
sufficiently large, then σ_θ will have very rapid decay. Scaling functions with
vanishing moments have been called "coiflets" by Daubechies (Section 8.2
of [8]). Symmetric scaling filters related to coiflets (see [3], Section 8.3.2 of
[8]) have been used in [26] as the basis for a local tomography algorithm.
In this algorithm, formula (10.30) is used with $J = 1$. Since σ_θ and ρ_θ^i have
about the same support radius as Φ and Ψ^i for each θ, full recovery of f_0
at $\mathbf{x}$ is achievable in practice from projections on lines through a disk of
radius $2T$ centered at $\mathbf{x}$. In discretized images, this extra radius is about
12 pixels. The savings in exposure in this algorithm is significantly greater
than that in [10] or [9].

Numerical examples of $\rho_\theta^1(t)$ for various wavelet and scaling function
pairs, and for various angles θ, are shown in Figures 10.4, 10.5, and 10.6.
Note that the essential support of the $\rho_\theta^1(t)$ is very close to the support
of the corresponding wavelet and scaling function. In Figure 10.7, the
wavelet transform of a test image is reconstructed directly from the Radon
transform data.

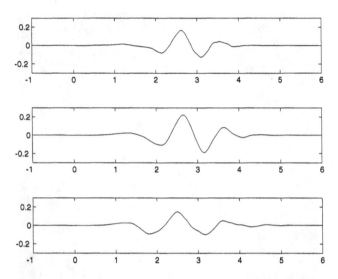

Figure 10.5
Graph of $\rho_\theta^1(t)$ defined in Theorem 6, where $\psi(t)$ and $\varphi(t)$ are the Daubechies 6 coefficient wavelet and scaling functions supported in $[0,5]$. From top: $\theta = 15°$, $\theta = 30°$, and $\theta = 45°$.

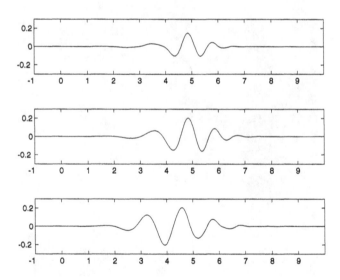

Figure 10.6
Graph of $\rho_\theta^1(t)$ defined in Theorem 6, where $\psi(t)$ and $\varphi(t)$ are the Daubechies 10 coefficient wavelet and scaling functions supported in $[0,9]$. From top: $\theta = 15°$, $\theta = 30°$, and $\theta = 45°$.

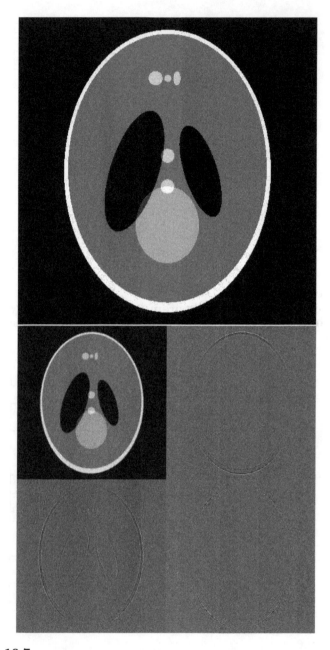

Figure 10.7
Top: Shepp-Logan head phantom. Bottom: Wavelet transform of
Shepp-Logan phantom computed directly from the Radon trans-
form data.

10.5   Wavelet Localization of the Radon Transform

As described in Section 10.3.1, the inversion of the Radon transform is not local in even dimensions because the Riesz potential operator I^{1-n} does not preserve compact support if n is even. However, as pointed out in Section 10.3.2, it is true that $I^{1-n}f$ will have rapid decay if f has vanishing moments. Since all wavelets have at least one vanishing moment, this suggests that the wavelet transform of f can be recovered locally from local projections via any of the formulas presented in Section 10.4. The degree of localization depends on how rapidly the Riesz potential of the wavelets decays.

In this section, explicit decay estimates are derived for $I^{1-n}\psi$ in terms of the number of vanishing moments of ψ. In particular, we have the following theorem.

THEOREM 7
Suppose that n is even, and that the function $h(t)$ satisfies the following.

(a)   *$h(t)$ is compactly supported,*

(b)   *$\int_{-\infty}^{\infty} t^j h(t)\, dt = 0$, for $j = 0, 1, \ldots, m$, for some $m \geq 0$,*

(c)   *$\int_{-\infty}^{\infty} |\gamma^j \hat{h}^{(k)}(\gamma)|\, d\gamma < \infty$, for $j = 0, 1, \ldots, m$, and $k = 0, 1, \ldots, n + m - 1$, and*

(d)   *$\int_{-\infty}^{\infty} |\gamma^j \hat{h}^{(k)}(\gamma)|^2\, d\gamma < \infty$, for $j = 0, 1, \ldots, m$, and $k = 0, 1, \ldots, n + m - 1$.*

Then

$$I^{1-n}h(t) = o(|t|^{-n-m+1}), \quad |t| \to \infty, \tag{10.31}$$

and

$$t^{n+m-1} I^{1-n}h(t) \in L^2(\mathcal{R}). \tag{10.32}$$

Equation (10.31) gives a pointwise bound on the growth of $I^{1-n}h(t)$ for large values of t. Equation (10.32) gives an average decay estimate and says that the energy of $I^{1-n}h(t)$ is very small away from the origin. These estimates give a solid mathematical justification for the observed decay in Figures 10.1–10.6.

In Figure 10.8, we show the edge picture of the central portion of the Shepp-Logan head phantom computed using only local projections. The original image is 512 × 512 pixels in size, and the local edge data was computed using only those projections on lines passing within 45 ($\approx$ 32 ×

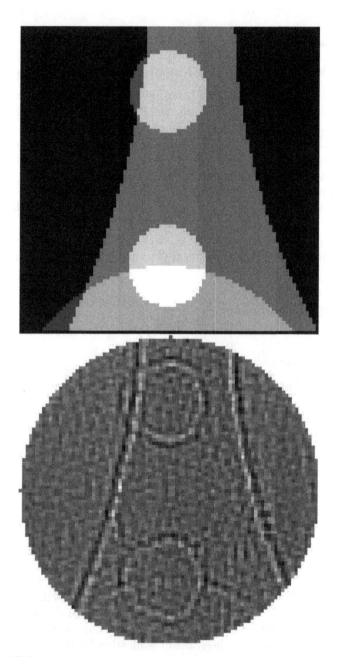

Figure 10.8
Top: The central 91×91 pixel region of the Shepp–Logan phantom. Bottom: Local edge picture of Shepp-Logan head phantom, computed using projections on lines passing through the central disk of diameter 91 pixels.

$\sqrt{2}$) pixels of the center. The image was computed using the portion of the separable wavelet transform given by (10.27) with $j = 1$, where the wavelet filters are from Table II, p. 209 of [3].

10.6 Conclusions

In this paper, we have presented a collection of wavelet-based reconstruction formulas for the Radon transform. Our goal has been to show that, because of the translation and dilation invariance of the Radon transform, and because of the nature of the Radon transform inversion formula, the wavelet transform and its variants are natural tools for Radon inversion.

One application of these observations is to localized tomography. It has been shown in this paper that using wavelets that have a large number of vanishing moments leads to inversion formulas that are approximately local in even dimensions. This observation has been used in several places, specifically [9–11], and [26], as the basis for local inversion algorithms from reduced data. The algorithms described in [10, 11], and [9] are not true local tomography algorithms in that they require full measurements at a sparse set of angles. The algorithm described in [26] uses only local measurements plus a small margin, to invert the Radon transform in the region of interest. In this sense, the latter algorithm is more closely related to Λ-tomography.

If one is interested not only in inverting the tomographic data, but also in doing some processing of the data, the convenient intertwining of various multiscale transforms with the Radon transform, and with Radon transform inversion means that this can effectively be done in the Radon domain. This can result in considerable savings in time and computations, not only because the step of reconstructing the image is eliminated, but also because most of the calculations can be done locally using only local measurements.

10.7 Appendix: Proofs of Theorems

Proof of Theorem 1: First observe that

$$\widehat{\rho_\theta^\gamma}(\gamma) = \frac{1}{2}|\gamma|^{n-1}\widehat{R_\theta\psi}^\vee(\gamma),$$

so that

$$\rho_\theta^\vee(t) = \frac{1}{2} I^{1-n} R_\theta \psi^\vee(t).$$

Hence

$$(R^\# \rho_\theta^\vee)(\mathbf{x}) = \frac{1}{2} R^\# I^{1-n} R_\theta \psi^\vee(\mathbf{x}) = \psi^\vee(\mathbf{x}).$$

Next note that

$$(D_a \rho_\theta^\vee)^\wedge(\gamma) = a^{1/2} \widehat{\rho_\theta^\vee}(a\gamma) = \frac{1}{2} a^{1/2} |a\gamma|^{n-1} \widehat{R_\theta \psi^\vee}(a\gamma)$$

$$= \frac{1}{2} a^{n-(1/2)} |\gamma|^{n-1} \widehat{\psi^\vee}(a\gamma\theta)$$

$$= \frac{1}{2} a^{n-(1/2)} |\gamma|^{n-1} a^{-n/2} a^{n/2} \widehat{\psi^\vee}(a\gamma\theta)$$

$$= \frac{1}{2} a^{(1-n)/2} |\gamma|^{n-1} (R_\theta D_a \psi^\vee)^\wedge(\gamma).$$

Hence

$$(R^\# D_a \rho_\theta^\vee)(\mathbf{x}) = a^{(n-1)/2} \frac{1}{2} R^\# I^{1-n} R_\theta (D_a \psi^\vee)(\mathbf{x}) = a^{(n-1)/2} D_a \psi^\vee(\mathbf{x}).$$

Now, by (10.3),

$$(W_\psi f)(a, \mathbf{b}) = f * D_a \psi^\vee(\mathbf{b}) = a^{(1-n)/2} (f * R^\# D_a \rho_\theta^\vee)(\mathbf{b})$$

$$= a^{(1-n)/2} R^\# (R_\theta f * D_a \rho_\theta^\vee)(\mathbf{b})$$

$$= a^{(1-n)/2} \int_{S^{n-1}} (W_{\rho_\theta} R_\theta f)(a, \mathbf{b} \cdot \theta) \, d\theta.$$

This is (10.12).

Now, in order to verify that ρ_θ is actually a wavelet for each $\theta \in S^{n-1}$, note that

$$\int_{-\infty}^{\infty} \frac{|\widehat{\rho_\theta}(\gamma)|^2}{|\gamma|}\, d\gamma$$

$$\text{(10.33)}$$

$$= \frac{1}{4}\int_{-\infty}^{\infty} |\gamma|^{2n-3}|\widehat{\psi^1}(\gamma\theta_1)|^2|\widehat{\psi^2}(\gamma\theta_2)|^2 \cdots |\widehat{\psi^n}(\gamma\theta_n)|^2\, d\gamma.$$

Now, suppose that $\theta_i = 0$ for some i. Then since ψ^i is admissible, $\widehat{\psi^i}(0) = 0$, and the right-hand side of (10.33) vanishes so that $\rho_\theta \equiv 0$. If $\theta_i \neq 0$ for all i, then

$$\int_{-\infty}^{\infty} \frac{|\widehat{\rho_\theta}(\gamma)|^2}{|\gamma|}\, d\gamma$$

$$\leq \frac{1}{4}\int_{|\gamma|\leq 1} |\widehat{\psi^1}(\gamma\theta_1)|^2|\widehat{\psi^2}(\gamma\theta_2)|^2 \cdots |\widehat{\psi^n}(\gamma\theta_n)|^2\, d\gamma$$

$$+ \frac{1}{4}\int_{|\gamma|>1} |\gamma|^{-3}|\gamma\widehat{\psi^1}(\gamma\theta_1)|^2|\gamma\widehat{\psi^2}(\gamma\theta_2)|^2 \cdots |\gamma\widehat{\psi^n}(\gamma\theta_n)|^2\, d\gamma$$

$$\leq \frac{1}{4}(C_1 C_2 \cdots C_n)^2 + \frac{1}{2}\left(\frac{C_1}{|\theta_1|}\frac{C_2}{|\theta_2|}\cdots\frac{C_3}{|\theta_3|}\right)^2 \int_{|\gamma|>1} \frac{1}{|\gamma|^3}\, d\gamma < \infty. \quad \square$$

Proof of Theorem 2:   First observe that for $\gamma \in \hat{\mathcal{R}}$,

$$\hat{\rho}(\gamma) = \frac{1}{2}|\gamma|^{n-1}\hat{\psi}(\gamma\theta) = \frac{1}{2}|\gamma|^{n-1}\widehat{R_\theta\psi}(\gamma),$$

for each $\theta \in S^{n-1}$, so that

$$\rho(t) = \frac{1}{2}I^{1-n}R_\theta\psi(t).$$

Hence, defining $\rho(\theta, t) = \rho(t)$ for each θ,

$$(R^\#\rho)(\mathbf{x}) = \frac{1}{2}R^\# I^{1-n}R_\theta\psi(\mathbf{x}) = \psi(\mathbf{x}).$$

Therefore, applying (10.3) as in Theorem 1, (10.15) follows.

To verify that ψ is a wavelet, note that by (10.13),

$$\int_0^\infty \frac{|\hat\psi(r)|^2}{r}\,dr = 2\int_0^\infty \frac{r^{2-2n}|\hat\rho(r)|^2}{r}\,dr = 2\int_0^\infty \frac{|\hat\rho(r)|^2}{r^{2n-1}}\,dr < \infty. \quad \square$$

Proof of Theorem 3: Note that by the definition of G, $R^\# \rho = G$, and that G is radial. Also, since $\lim_{\gamma\to 0}|\gamma|^{-1}\hat\rho(\gamma) = 1/2$, $\hat G(0) = 1$ or $\iint_{\mathcal{R}^2} G(\mathbf{x})\,d\mathbf{x} = 1$.

Now, for any function $s(\theta,t)$,

$$\frac{\partial}{\partial x_1} R^\# s(\mathbf{x}) = \frac{\partial}{\partial x_1}\int_0^{2\pi} s(\theta, x_1\cos\theta + x_2\sin\theta)\,d\theta$$

$$= \int_0^{2\pi} \frac{\partial}{\partial x_1} s(\theta, x_1\cos\theta + x_2\sin\theta)\,d\theta$$

$$= \int_0^{2\pi} \cos\theta\,\frac{\partial}{\partial t} s(\theta, x_1\cos\theta + x_2\sin\theta)\,d\theta$$

$$= R^\#(\cos\theta\,\frac{\partial}{\partial t} s(\theta,t))(\mathbf{x}).$$

Similarly,

$$\frac{\partial}{\partial x_2} R^\# s(\mathbf{x}) = R^\#(\sin\theta\,\frac{\partial}{\partial t} s(\theta,t))(\mathbf{x}).$$

Therefore, applying (10.3),

$$(W_{\psi^1} f)(2^j, \mathbf{x}) = f * D_{2^j}(\psi^1)^\vee(\mathbf{x}) = f * D_{2^j}\left(\frac{\partial}{\partial x_1} G\right)^\vee(\mathbf{x})$$

$$= f * D_{2^j}\left(\frac{\partial}{\partial x_1} R^\# \rho\right)^\vee(\mathbf{x})$$

$$= 2^{-j}\left(f * \left[\frac{\partial}{\partial x_1} D_{2^j} R^\# \rho\right]^\vee\right)(\mathbf{x})$$

$$= 2^{-j/2}\left(f * \left[\frac{\partial}{\partial x_1} R^\# D_{2^j}\rho\right]^\vee\right)(\mathbf{x})$$

$$= 2^{-j/2} \left(f * R^{\#}(\cos\theta \, \frac{d}{dt} D_{2^j} \rho)^{\vee} \right)(\mathbf{x})$$

$$= 2^{j/2} \left(f * R^{\#}(\cos\theta \, D_{2^j} \frac{d\rho}{dt})^{\vee} \right)(\mathbf{x})$$

$$= 2^{j/2} R^{\#} \left(R_{\theta} f * \cos\theta \, (D_{2^j} \frac{d\rho}{dt})^{\vee} \right)(\mathbf{x})$$

$$= 2^{j/2} \int_0^{2\pi} \cos\theta \, (R_{\theta} f * D_{2^j} \left[\frac{d\rho}{dt} \right]^{\vee})(\mathbf{x} \cdot \theta) \, d\theta$$

$$= 2^{j/2} \int_0^{2\pi} \cos\theta \, (W_{d\rho/dt} R_{\theta} f)(2^j, \mathbf{x} \cdot \theta) \, d\theta.$$

Similarly, $(W_{\psi^2} f)(2^j, \mathbf{x}) = 2^{j/2} \int_0^{2\pi} \sin\theta \, (W_{d\rho/dt} R_{\theta} f)(2^j, \mathbf{x} \cdot \theta) \, d\theta.$ $\square$

Proof of Theorem 4: Since the continuous wavelet transform is linear in the analyzing wavelet, we may write,

$$(W_{\psi^\beta} f)(2^j, \mathbf{x}) = (W_{\cos\beta \, \psi^1} f)(2^j, \mathbf{x}) + (W_{\sin\beta \, \psi^2} f)(2^j, \mathbf{x})$$

$$= \cos\beta \, (W_{\psi^1} f)(2^j, \mathbf{x}) + \sin\beta \, (W_{\psi^2} f)(2^j, \mathbf{x})$$

$$= 2^{j/2} \int_0^{2\pi} (\cos\beta \cos\theta + \sin\beta \sin\theta)(W_{d\rho/dt} R_{\theta} f)(2^j, \mathbf{x} \cdot \theta) \, d\theta$$

$$= 2^{j/2} \int_0^{2\pi} \cos(\beta - \theta)(W_{d\rho/dt} R_{\theta} f)(2^j, \mathbf{x} \cdot \theta) \, d\theta. \quad \square$$

Proof of Theorem 5: Assuming sufficient smoothness and decay on $f(\mathbf{x})$, it follows from the basic theory of frames and bases that (10.22) holds for some coefficients $c_{j,k}(\theta)$.

Now, formally applying the Radon transform inversion formula (10.7), with $n = 2$ and $\alpha = 0$, we obtain

$$f(\mathbf{x}) = \frac{1}{2} \int_0^{2\pi} I^{-1} R_{\theta} f(\mathbf{x} \cdot \theta) \, d\theta = \sum_{j,k} \int_0^{2\pi} c_{j,k}(\theta) \frac{1}{2} I^{-1} \psi_{j,k}(\mathbf{x} \cdot \theta) \, d\theta.$$

Finally, note that

$$\frac{1}{2}(I^{-1}\psi_{j,k})^{\wedge}(\gamma) = \frac{1}{2}|\gamma|\widehat{\psi_{j,k}}(\gamma) = \frac{1}{2}|\gamma|\,e^{-2\pi i\gamma(2^j k)}\,2^{j/2}\hat{\psi}(2^j\gamma)$$

$$= \frac{1}{2}2^{-j}\,e^{-2\pi i\gamma(2^j k)}\,2^{j/2}|2^j\gamma|\hat{\psi}(2^j\gamma)$$

$$= 2^{-j}e^{-2\pi i\gamma(2^j k)}\,2^{j/2}\hat{\rho}(2^j\gamma) = 2^{-j}\widehat{\rho_{j,k}}(\gamma).$$

Therefore, (10.23) holds. □

Proof of Theorem 6: Let us first consider Equation (10.26). By the definition of $\sigma_\theta(t)$, it follows that $R^{\#}\sigma_\theta(\mathbf{x}) = \Phi(\mathbf{x})$. Also, recall that for any function $s(\theta,t) = s_\theta(t)$, $R^{\#}(D_{2^j}s_\theta)(\mathbf{x}) = 2^{j/2}D_{2^j}R^{\#}s_\theta(\mathbf{x})$. Therefore, applying (10.3),

$$\langle f, \Phi_{j,k}\rangle = f * D_{2^j}\Phi^{\vee}(2^j k_1, 2^j k_2) = f * D_{2^j}(R^{\#}\sigma_\theta^{\vee})(2^j k_1, 2^j k_2)$$

$$= 2^{-j/2}(f * (R^{\#}D_{2^j}\sigma_\theta^{\vee}))(2^j k_1, 2^j k_2)$$

$$= 2^{-j/2}R^{\#}(R_\theta f * D_{2^j}\sigma_\theta^{\vee})(2^j k_1, 2^j k_2)$$

$$= 2^{-j/2}\int_0^{2\pi}(R_\theta f * D_{2^j}\sigma_\theta^{\vee})(2^j(k_1\cos\theta + k_2\sin\theta))\,d\theta$$

$$= 2^{-j/2}\int_0^{2\pi}(W_{\sigma_\theta}R_\theta f)(2^j, 2^j(k\cdot\theta))\,d\theta.$$

Equations (10.27)–(10.29) follow similarly. □

In order to prove Theorem 7, we require the following Lemma.

LEMMA 1
Suppose that n is even and that the function h(t) satisfies the following.

(a) *$h(t)$ is compactly supported, and*

(b) *$\int_{-\infty}^{\infty}t^j h(t)\,dt = 0$, for $j = 0, 1, \ldots, m$, for some $m \geq 0$.*

Then the function $|\gamma|^{n-1}\hat{h}(\gamma)$ has $n+m-1$ continuous derivatives over $\mathcal{R}$.

Proof of Lemma 1: Note first that restricted to $(0, \infty)$, $|\gamma|\hat{h}(\gamma)$ is infinitely differentiable since $\hat{h}$ is analytic and $|\gamma|^{n-1}$ is infinitely differentiable for all $\gamma \in (0, \infty)$. The same holds for the interval $(-\infty, 0)$. Therefore, it is sufficient to show that

$$\lim_{\gamma \to 0+} \frac{d^k}{d\gamma^k}(|\gamma|^{n-1}\hat{h}(\gamma)) = \lim_{\gamma \to 0-} \frac{d^k}{d\gamma^k}(|\gamma|^{n-1}\hat{h}(\gamma)), \qquad (10.34)$$

for $k = 0, 1, \ldots, n + m - 1$.

To see that this is true, let $k \leq n - 1$. If $\gamma \in (0, \infty)$, then by Leibnitz rule,

$$\frac{d^k}{d\gamma^k}(|\gamma|^{n-1}\hat{h}(\gamma)) = \frac{d^k}{d\gamma^k}(\gamma^{n-1}\hat{h}(\gamma))$$

$$= \sum_{\ell=0}^{k} \binom{k}{\ell} \frac{(n-1)!}{(n-1-\ell)!} \gamma^{n-1-\ell} \frac{d^{k-\ell}}{d\gamma^{k-\ell}}\hat{h}(\gamma),$$

and if $\gamma \in (-\infty, 0)$, then

$$\frac{d^k}{d\gamma^k}(|\gamma|^{n-1}\hat{h}(\gamma)) = -\sum_{\ell=0}^{k} \binom{k}{\ell} \frac{(n-1)!}{(n-1-\ell)!} \gamma^{n-1-\ell} \frac{d^{k-\ell}}{d\gamma^{k-\ell}}\hat{h}(\gamma).$$

Therefore, if $k < n - 1$, then clearly,

$$\lim_{\gamma \to 0+} \frac{d^k}{d\gamma^k}(|\gamma|^{n-1}\hat{h}(\gamma)) = \lim_{\gamma \to 0-} \frac{d^k}{d\gamma^k}(|\gamma|^{n-1}\hat{h}(\gamma)) = 0,$$

and if $k = n - 1$, then

$$\lim_{\gamma \to 0+} \frac{d^k}{d\gamma^k}(|\gamma|^{n-1}\hat{h}(\gamma)) = \lim_{\gamma \to 0+}(n-1)!\hat{h}(\gamma) = 0,$$

and

$$\lim_{\gamma \to 0-} \frac{d^k}{d\gamma^k}(|\gamma|^{n-1}\hat{h}(\gamma)) = \lim_{\gamma \to 0-} -(n-1)!\hat{h}(\gamma) = 0,$$

by (b).

If $n - 1 < k \leq n + m - 1$, then for any $\gamma \neq 0$, $(d^k/d\gamma^k)(|\gamma|^{n-1}\hat{h}(\gamma))$ has the form

$$\sum_{\ell=0}^{n-1} c_\ell \gamma^\ell \, \hat{h}^{(\ell+k-n+1)}(\gamma),$$

for some constants c_ℓ. Now, if $\ell > 0$, then

$$\lim_{\gamma \to 0+} \gamma^\ell \, \hat{h}^{(\ell+k-n+1)}(\gamma) = \lim_{\gamma \to 0-} \gamma^\ell \, \hat{h}^{(\ell+k-n+1)}(\gamma) = 0,$$

and if $\ell = 0$, then $\ell + k - n + 1 = k - n + 1 \leq m$ so that by (b)

$$\lim_{\gamma \to 0+} \hat{h}^{(\ell+k-n+1)}(\gamma) = \lim_{\gamma \to 0-} \hat{h}^{(\ell+k-n+1)}(\gamma) = 0. \quad \square$$

Now, we are able to prove Theorem 7.

Proof of Theorem 7:   By (a), (b), and Lemma 1, the function

$$(I^{1-n}h)^\wedge(\gamma) = |\gamma|^{n-1}\hat{h}(\gamma),$$

has $n + m - 1$ continuous derivatives.

By (c),

$$\frac{d^k}{d\gamma^k}(|\gamma|^{n-1}\hat{h}(\gamma)) \in L^1(\mathcal{R}),$$

for $k = 0, 1, \ldots, n + m - 1$, so that its inverse Fourier transform,

$$(2\pi i t)^{n+m-1} \, I^{1-n}h(t),$$

is bounded and continuous on $\mathcal{R}$, and vanishes at $\pm\infty$. Therefore, (10.31) holds.

By (d),

$$\frac{d^k}{d\gamma^k}(|\gamma|^{n-1}\hat{h}(\gamma)) \in L^2(\mathcal{R}),$$

for $k = 0, 1, \ldots, n + m - 1$, so that its inverse Fourier transform,

$$(2\pi i t)^{n+m-1} \, I^{1-n}h(t),$$

is in $L^2(\mathcal{R})$. Therefore, (10.32) holds. $\quad \square$

10.8   Acknowledgments

The authors wish to thank Farrokh Rashid-Farrokhi for providing the pictures used in this paper. Also, the second author wishes to thank Prof.

KuoJuey Ray Liu of the Institute for Systems Research at the University of Maryland for providing support during the completion of the last phases of this paper. Berenstein's work was supported by NSF.

References

[1] A. Aldroubi and M. Unser. Families of wavelet transforms in connection with Shannon's sampling theory and the Gabor transform. In *Wavelets: A Tutorial in Theory and Applications*, C. Chui, editor, 509–528. Academic Press, San Diego, CA, 1992.

[2] A. Aldroubi and M. Unser. Families of multiresolution and wavelet spaces with optimal properties. *Numer. Funct. Anal. Optimiz.*, 14(5):417–446, 1993.

[3] M. Antonini, M. Barlaud, P. Mathieu, and I. Daubechies. Image coding using wavelet transform. *IEEE Trans. Image Process.*, 1(2): 205–220, 1992.

[4] C. Berenstein and D. Walnut. Local inversion of the Radon transform in even dimensions using wavelets. In *75 Years of Radon Transform*, S. Gindikin and P. Michor, editors, 45–69. International Press, Cambridge, MA, 1994.

[5] J. Boman and E. T. Quinto. Support theorems for real-analytic Radon transforms. *Duke J. Math.*, 55:943–948, 1987.

[6] C. K. Chui. *An Introduction to Wavelets*. Academic Press, New York, 1992.

[7] S. Deans. *The Radon Transform and Some of its Applications*. John Wiley & Sons, New York, 1983.

[8] I. Daubechies. *Ten Lectures on Wavelets (CBMS–NSF Conference Series in Applied Mathematics, 61)*. SIAM, Philadelphia, 1992.

[9] A. Delaney and Y. Bresler. Multiresolution tomographic reconstruction using wavelets. *IEEE Trans. Image Process.*, 4(3), 1995.

[10] J. DeStefano and T. Olson. Wavelet localization of the Radon transform. *IEEE Trans. Signal Process.*, 42(8): 2055–2067, 1994.

[11] T. Olson. Optimal time-frequency projections for localized tomography. *Ann. Biomed. Eng.* To appear.

[12] A. Faridani, D. Finch, E. Ritman, and K. Smith. Local tomography II. *SIAM J. Appl. Math.*, submitted.

[13] A. Faridani, F. Keinert, F. Natterer, E. Ritman, and K. Smith. Local and global tomography. In *Signal Processing*, IMA Vol. Math. Appl., Vol. 23, Springer-Verlag, New York, 1990, 241–255.

[14] A. Faridani, E. Ritman, and K. Smith. Local tomography. *SIAM J. Appl. Math.* 52(2): 459–484, 1992.

[15] A. Faridani, E. Ritman, and K. Smith. Examples of local tomography. *SIAM J. Appl. Math.* 52(4): 1193–1198, 1992.

[16] W. Freeman, and E. Adelson. The design and use of steerable filters. *IEEE Trans. PAMI*, 13(9): 891–906, 1991.

[17] J.-P. Guédon and M. Unser. Least squares and spline filtered back-projections. Preprint.

[18] P. Kuchment, K. Lancaster, and L. Magilezskaya. On the structure of local tomography. *Inverse Problems.* To appear.

[19] P. Maass. The interior Radon transform. *SIAM J. Appl. Math.*, 52(3): 710–724, 1992.

[20] S. Mallat and W. Hwang. Singularity detection and processing with wavelets. *IEEE Trans. Inf. Theory (Special Issue on Wavelet Transforms and Multiresolution Signal Analysis)*, 38(2): 617–643, 1992.

[21] S. Mallat and S. Zhong. Wavelet transform maxima and multiscale edges. In *Wavelets and Their Applications*, M. B. Ruskai et al., editors, 67–104. Jones and Bartlett Publishers, 1992.

[22] F. Natterer. *The Mathematics of Computerized Tomography.* John Wiley & Sons, New York, 1986.

[23] F. Peyrin, M. Zarin, and R. Goutte. Multiscale reconstruction of tomographic images. In *Proc. IEEE-SP Int. Symp. Time-Frequency Time-Scale Analysis.* 1992.

[24] A. Ramm and A. Zaslavsky. Singularities of the Radon transform. *Bull. AMS*, 25(1): 109–115, 1993.

[25] A. Ramm and A. Zaslavsky. Reconstructing singularities of a function from its Radon transform. *Trans. AMS.* To appear.

[26] F. Rashid-Farrokhi, K. J. R. Liu, C. Berenstein, and D. Walnut. Localized wavelet based computerized tomography. *Proc. ICIP95.* Washington, DC, October 1995.

[27] E. Simoncelli, W. Freeman, E. Adelson, and D. Heeger. Shiftable multiscale transforms. *IEEE Trans. Inf. Theory (Special Issue on Wavelet Transforms and Multiresolution Signal Analysis)*, 38(2): 587–607, 1992.

[28] E. T. Quinto. Singularities of the X-ray transform and limited data tomography in $\mathcal{R}^2$ and $\mathcal{R}^3$. *SIAM J. Math. Anal.*, 24: 1215–1225, 1993.

[29] M. Unser and A. Aldroubi. Polynomial splines and wavelets—a signal processing perspective. In *Wavelets: A Tutorial in Theory and Applications*, C. Chui, editor, 543–601. Academic Press, San Diego, CA, 1992.

[30] M. Unser and A. Aldroubi. Multiresolution image registration procedure using spline pyramids. In *Mathematical Imaging: Wavelet Applications in Signal and Image Processing*, Vol. 2034, A. F. Laine, editor, 160–170. SPIE—The International Society for Optical Engineering, Bellingham, WA, 1993.

[31] D. Walnut. Applications of Gabor and wavelet expansions to the Radon transform. In *Probabilistic and Stochastic Methods in Analysis, with Applications*, J. Byrnes et al., editors, 187–205. Kluwer Academic Publishers, Boston, 1992.

[32] D. Walnut. Local inversion of the Radon transform in the plane using wavelets. In *Proc. SPIE's Int. Symp. Optics, Imaging, and Instrumentation.* San Diego, July 1993.

[33] M. Holschneider. Inverse Radon transforms. *Inverse Problems*, 7:853–861, 1991.

[34] A. I. Katsevich and A. S. Ramm. New methods for finding values of the jumps of a function from its local tomographic data. *Inverse Problems*, 11:1005–1024, 1995.

11

Optimal Time-Frequency Projections for Localized Tomography

Tim Olson

Department of Mathematics and Computer Science, Dartmouth College, Hanover, NH

Abstract   An algorithm for recovering a function from essentially localized values of its Radon transform and sparse nonlocal values was outlined in [12]. That algorithm utilized the time-frequency properties of wavelets, coupled with the range theorems for the Radon transform to essentially localize the dependence of the Radon transform. In this chapter we utilize alternative time-frequency projections which were introduced by Coifman and Meyer in [4]. We present evidence that these bases are optimal according to our criterion for localized tomography. These bases require significantly less data than the wavelet bases which were used in [12]. Finally we present numerical results supporting this work.

11.1   Introduction

11.1.1   Historical Notes

Computerized tomography (CT) refers to the recovery of a two-dimensional density $f(x, y)$ from the one-dimensional line integrals of that density at different angles and locations. Medical CT scanners, for instance, reconstruct the two-dimensional densities of slices of the body, from one-dimensional X-rays or line integrals. The theoretical basis for CT is the

Radon transform. The Radon transform was first introduced by J. Radon in 1917 [14]. Little computational attention was given to it until the advent of computers enabled the fast evaluation of Fourier transforms and their corresponding convolutions. A. M. Cormack investigated many of the numerical issues involved in computerized tomography and built the first CT machine in the 1960s. In the late 1960s, a group led by Murray Eden of the NIH constructed the first CT machine for imaging biomedical specimens. The NIH was not interested in the idea, however, and denied their application for further development funds. G. N. Hounsfield built the first CT machine to image the human brain in the early 1970s, and for their efforts Cormack and Hounsfield were awarded the 1979 Nobel prize in medicine.

Tomography is useful in a number of settings. This is due to the fact that the absorption of a electromagnetic beam directed along a line through an object can be used to measure the line integral of the density of that object, noninvasively. The electromagnetic beams can consist of an electron beam, as in an electron microscope, or an X-ray as in the standard X-ray CT machines. The Radon transform is now a mainstay of medical imaging as well as many other remote imaging sciences, such as electron microscopy.

In two dimensions, however, the inversion or reconstruction formula for the Radon transform is globally dependent upon the line integrals of the object function f [11]. In many situations, a physician may only be interested in images of a very local area of the body. One would prefer to expose only that local portion of the patient's body to radiation. Spinal injuries seem to be the most obvious and common example of this type of situation. The physician is generally not interested in anything but the spinal column, and therefore one would like to minimize the amount of radiation which passes through the heart, lungs, and other organs. Given that approximately 30–40% of CT scans at hospitals without MRI scanners are spinal scans, a serious reduction in the amount of radiation in spinal scans would be significant.

The nonlocality of the Radon transform, however, forces standard reconstruction techniques to completely irradiate all of the two-dimensional slices of the body which intersect with the region of interest. We have illustrated this problem in Figure 11.1.

While understanding and controlling the nonlocality of the Radon transform may allow us to reduce the amount of radiation in X-ray CT, understanding the nonlocality of the Radon transform may also be important for the sake of understanding a variety of imaging situations, when there is a limited amount of data available.

11.1.2   Prior Work

There have been a number of attempts to alleviate the problems associated with the nonlocality of the Radon transform. Although local values

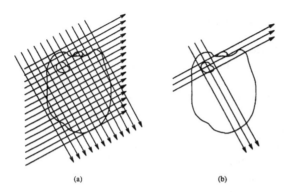

(a)   (b)

Figure 11.1
The nonlocal and local tomographic data problems are illustrated
above. In the nonlocal problem (a), we gather line integrals along
all of the lines passing through the object. In practice this would
be done along hundreds of lines, with hundreds of angles. In
(b), we illustrate the reduction in radiation exposure offered by
local tomography data acquisition. Thus local tomographic reconstruction would use data from the same number of angles as
with ordinary tomography, but would only use the data from lines
which pass through the region of interest.

are not even uniquely determined by local integrals over hyperplanes, it
has been proven that the elements which are not uniquely determined do
not vary wildly on the interior of the region of interest [7, 10, 11]. While
this is true, these results are asymptotic in nature, and do not really apply
to a very localized region [12]. The question of how much additional data
must be gathered in order to utilize this type of approach has been further
studied by Berenstein and Walnut, who found bounds on the amount that
one would have to increase the radius of the localized region in order to
guarantee an approximation to a fixed resolution ϵ, in the interior of the
region [2, 3].

A recent approach which has shown great promise was introduced by
Faridani, Smith, and co-workers [7, 8]. This approach does not reconstruct
the density function f, but rather another function $\Lambda f - \mu\Lambda^{-1}f$, which is
similar to the original function in many ways. This approach is well adapted
for edge detection but it is not designed to recover the original density of
the image.

It has been noted that a rough estimate of the global properties of the
Radon transform would be sufficient to obtain a reliable reconstruction of a
local region [11]. This is the foundation for our algorithm. We reconstruct
a low-resolution approximation to the global properties of the Radon transform through efficient sparse sampling. This global low resolution estimate
allows us to produce a true reconstruction in the region of interest, from
essentially localized measurements.

11.1.3   Organization

In the next section we explicitly outline the goals of this chapter. In Section 11.3, we outline the background which is necessary to understand the algorithm presented. In Section 11.4, we review the standard reconstruction techniques for doing tomographic reconstruction and outline the source of the nonlocal dependence of the reconstructions. We introduce our algorithm to essentially localize the reconstruction process in Section 11.5, and present numerical results in Section 11.6. We show that this algorithm is optimal in Section 11.7, and present our final conclusions in Section 11.8. The Appendix contains sections on error analysis and background material on the bases of Coifman and Meyer.

11.2   Algorithmic Goals

The goal of this chapter is not to reconstruct the local values of f from local values of the Radon transform. The goal of this chapter is to develop a stable algorithm that will reconstruct local values of f from local values of the Radon transform, together with sparsely sampled nonlocal values of the Radon transform. Thus when we refer to essentially localized data, we are referring to the line integrals which pass through the region of interest, and a small number of line integrals which do not pass through the region of interest.

We emphasize here that reconstruction of a density from only the line integrals which pass through a restricted region of the density is not possible [11], and therefore one must either regularize the reconstruction or gather more data. Our approach is to gather enough data so that a well-conditioned, true reconstruction of the density can be made, rather than reconstructing an altered version of the function.

11.3   Background

11.3.1   The Radon Transform

We will review some of the basic properties of the Radon transform. For details and proofs, we recommend [11]. By S^1 we are simply referring to the one sphere or the unit circle, i.e., $S^1 = \{\vec{\theta} = (\cos\theta, \sin\theta)\}$, where we have abused the notation by referring to θ as the angle generated by $\vec{\theta}$ and

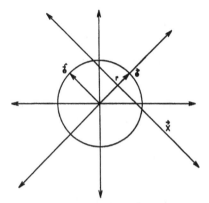

Figure 11.2
The mathematical notation of the Radon transform is illustrated above. The elements of S_1 are merely vectors that start at the origin and end on the unit circle. The notation $\vec{\theta}^{\perp}$ stands for the vector that is perpendicular to $\vec{\theta}$. Putting this together we see that the line integral $R_f(\theta, r) = \int f(r\vec{\theta} + t\vec{\theta}^{\perp})\, dt$ is taken along the illustrated line at a distance r from the origin. If $\vec{x}$ is a point along that line, then we can realize this same line integral by the formula $R_f(\theta, \vec{x} \cdot \vec{\theta}) = \int f(\vec{x} + t\vec{\theta}^{\perp})\, dt$ because $r = \vec{x} \cdot \vec{\theta}$.

the x-axis. For an illustration see Figure 11.2. Throughout we will use the notation F_1 and F_2 to denote the Fourier transform on $L^2(\mathbb{R})$ and $L^2(\mathbb{R}^2)$, respectively, defined by

$$F_1(g)(\omega) \equiv \hat{g}(\omega) = \frac{1}{\sqrt{2\pi}} \int_{\mathbb{R}} g(t) e^{-i\omega t}\, dt$$

and

$$F_2(g)(u, v) \equiv \hat{g}(u, v) = (2\pi)^{-3/2} \iint_{\mathbb{R}^2} g(x, y) e^{-i(xu + yv)}\, dx\, dy. \qquad (11.1)$$

The reader who is not well versed in the mathematical aspects of the Fourier transform should not become frightened at this point. The spaces $L^2(\mathbb{R})$ and $L^2(\mathbb{R}^2)$ merely represent one- and two-dimensional functions with finite energy, i.e.,

$$\int |f(x)|^2\, dx < \infty.$$

Since all real objects have a finite amount of energy, a rigorous understanding of these spaces is not necessary for the purposes of this chapter.

The Radon transform of a function $f : \mathbb{R}^2 \to \mathbb{R}$ is defined by

$$R_f(\vec{\theta}, r) = \int_{\mathbb{R}} f(r\vec{\theta} + t\vec{\theta}^{\perp})\, dt. \tag{11.2}$$

It follows that $R_f(\vec{\theta}, \vec{\theta} \cdot \vec{x})$ is the line integral of f through $\vec{x} \in \mathbb{R}^2$ and perpendicular to $\vec{\theta}$. This is illustrated in Figure 11.2.

The Interior Radon Transform   The interior Radon transform is the restriction of the Radon transform given by

$$R_f(\vec{\theta}, t) \to R_f(\vec{\theta}, t)\mathcal{X}_{[-a,a]}(t), \tag{11.3}$$

where $|a| < 1$. Thus, instead of knowing $R_f(\vec{\theta}, t)$ for all t one only knows $R_f(\vec{\theta}, t)$ for $t \in [-a, a]$. One can view this as the restriction of the Radon transform to lines that pass through a circle of radius a about the origin, which we will subsequently refer to as the (local) region of interest. This is the situation illustrated in Figure 11.1(b). Notice that the localized region need not be at the center of the object, but rather can be anywhere within the support of the object. We apply the mathematical formulation given above, by assuming that the center of the region of interest is the center of our object.

The operator $R : f \to R_f(\vec{\theta}, \vec{\theta} \cdot \vec{x})$ has been extensively studied in many contexts, and an excellent overview of the literature may be found in [11]. A detailed study of the singular value decomposition of the interior Radon transform, Equation 11.3, can be found in [9, 10]. The results of [9, 10] confirm those in [11], and suggest that the problem of local reconstruction is not severely ill-conditioned, when the inversion is done modulo the nullspace. The singular values $\sigma_{m,l}$ of the operator, which are doubly indexed due to the spherical harmonics used in the construction, behave like $O(m^{-1/2})$ for l fixed, $O(m^{-1/4})$ for $m = l$, and $O(l^{-1/2})$ for fixed m [10].

We assume throughout that we are trying to recover a density function $f : \mathbb{R}^2 \to \mathbb{R}$ which has support in B_1, where B_1 is the unit disc centered at the origin in $\mathbb{R}^2$. Moreover, we will view the Radon transform $R_f(\vec{\theta}, t)$ as an element of either the weighted Chebyshev space

$$L^2(S^1 \times [-1, 1], dx \times (1 - t^2)^{-1/2} dt)$$

or as elements of L^2 with the usual inner product. We will use the notation $\| \cdot \|_{2,w}$ for the norm in the weighted space, and $\| \cdot \|_2$ for the norm in L^2 with the usual inner product. Once again, a detailed understanding of these spaces is not necessary to understand the algorithm of interest in this chapter.

The Range of the Radon Transform   We will make use of the following theorem characterizing the range of the Radon transform, which can be found in [11].

THEOREM 1

The Radon transform of a function $f \in L^2(\mathbb{R})$, which is denoted by

$$R_f(\vec{\theta}, t) \in L^2\left[S^1 \times [-1, 1]\right]$$

can be represented in the form

$$R_f(\vec{\theta}, t) = (1 - t^2)^{-1/2} \sum_{l=0}^{\infty} T_l(t) h_l(\theta) \tag{11.4}$$

where the $T_l(t)$ are Chebyshev polynomials of the first kind,

$$h_l(\vec{\theta}) = \sum_{n \in H_l} a_{l,n} e^{in\theta}$$

and $H_l = \{-l, -l+2, \ldots, l-2, l\}$.

One can interpret this theorem by realizing that when viewed as a function of $\vec{\theta}$, for fixed ω, $\hat{f}(\omega\vec{\theta})$ will be essentially bandlimited with bandlimit ω. Thus, the angular bandlimit in polar coordinates is tied to the radial variable ω. The derivation of this result depends upon the fact that the Fourier transform of a weighted Chebyshev polynomial is a Bessel function [11].

The useful concept behind this Theorem is that if you have an object which is zero outside of a circle of radius 1, then the low frequency components can be completely determined from only a few sample points. Thus, for ω_1 small, the values of the Fourier transform of f along a circle of radius ω_1, or $\hat{f}(\omega_1\vec{\theta})$, can be determined for every $\vec{\theta}$ from only a few sample values $\hat{f}(\omega_1\vec{\theta}_i)$. If ω_2 is twice as large as ω_1, then it will take twice as many values $\hat{f}(\omega_2\vec{\theta}_i)$ to determine $\hat{f}(\omega_2\vec{\theta}_i)$ for every $\vec{\theta}$. This is illustrated in Figure 11.3.

The Sinogram   Often in tomography one refers to the sinogram. The sinogram is a discrete sampling of the Radon transform. Each row of the sinogram contains the line integrals of f at a fixed angle, i.e., $R_f(\vec{\theta}, r)$ for $\vec{\theta}$ fixed. Different rows correspond to different, equally spaced angles. An illustration of a sinogram, and our sampling schemes in the sinogram, is given in Figure 11.9.

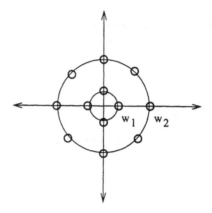

Figure 11.3
The Range characterization implies the fundamental properties
of the Radon transform which allow us to localize the dependence
of the reconstruction process on the data. We illustrate this by
noting that the Fourier transform of $\hat{f}(\omega\vec{\theta})$ will be very smooth,
or band-limited on the interior circle of radius ω_1, but will not
necessarily be as smooth on the circle of radius ω_2. This fundamental fact allows us to determine the function $\hat{f}(\omega_1\vec{\theta})$ with a
small number of measurements. We need more measurements to
adequately sample $\hat{f}(\omega_2\vec{\theta})$, and this is illustrated by the increased
number of circled sample points.

It will be important to use the sinogram to visualize the reconstruction
process and isolate the difficulties of doing a localized reconstruction.

11.3.2   Basic Fourier Analysis

Smoothness and Locality   There are a couple of basic ideas from Fourier
analysis which will be needed in this chapter. The first is that a function
can be well localized if and only if its Fourier transform is smooth and has
smooth derivatives.

Mathematically, this is contained in the statement that a function f will
have n continuous derivatives in L^2, if and only if its Fourier transform is
such that

$$\int |\omega^n \hat{f}(\omega)|^2 \, d\omega < \infty.$$

Thus if $\hat{f}$ does not die out quickly enough as $\omega \to \infty$, $\omega^n \hat{f}(\omega)$ will not be
square integrable, and possibly not even bounded, and thus f will not have
an nth derivative. Similarly, a function whose derivative does not exist or
is not continuous will have a Fourier transform which dies out very slowly.

This will be important in order to understand the nonlocality of the
Radon transform.

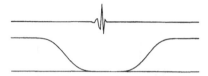

Figure 11.4
Above we illustrate a function with zero moments, the Daubechies D6 wavelet, and the absolute value of its Fourier transform. Notice that the Fourier transform is zero at the origin and essentially zero around the origin.

The Uncertainty Principle Another way to understand the locality properties of functions and their Fourier transforms is the uncertainty principle. Suppose that a function $f(t)$ is essentially supported on an interval of length Δ_t, and its Fourier transform $\hat{f}(\omega)$ is essentially supported on an interval of length Δ_ω (see [5] for specifics). Then the uncertainty principle states that

$$\Delta_t \Delta_\omega \geq 1.$$

Thus, if we want a function supported on a narrow interval in time, its Fourier transform must be supported on a wide interval in frequency. This will be the fundamental idea in optimizing the localization of our algorithm.

Zero Moments In this chapter we will refer to functions f which have n zero moments. Mathematically this means that

$$\int x^n f(x)\, dx = 0$$

for $0 \leq k \leq n - 1$. It can be shown that this is equivalent to the first $n - 1$ derivatives of the function's Fourier transform, $\hat{f}$, having zeros at the origin. This type of condition will guarantee that the function has average value 0, and moreover, it contains very little low frequency information. A function having six zero moments and its Fourier transform are illustrated in Figure 11.4.

11.4 Reconstruction Techniques

11.4.1 Fourier Reconstruction

An essential property of the Radon transform is that the one-dimensional Fourier transform of $R_f(\vec{\theta}, \vec{\theta} \cdot \vec{x})$ with respect to the variable $t \equiv \vec{\theta} \cdot \vec{x}$ is a

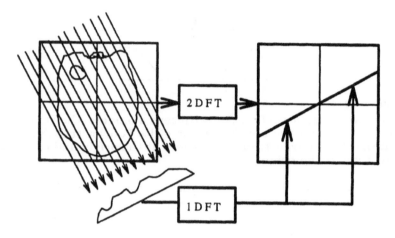

Figure 11.5
The central slice theorem is illustrated above. One can calculate
the values along the line in the two-dimensional Fourier transform (2DFT) by calculating the one-dimensional Fourier transform (1DFT) of the line integrals.

line through the two-dimensional Fourier transform of f, i.e.,

$$F_1\left(R_f(\vec{\theta}, \vec{\theta} \cdot \vec{x})\right) = F_2(f)(\omega\vec{\theta}) = \hat{f}(\omega\vec{\theta}).$$

This is often referred to as the central slice theorem, and is illustrated in
Figure 11.5.

Using this fact and a polar Fourier inversion formula, one can easily relate
the Radon transform $R_f(\vec{\theta}, \vec{\theta} \cdot \vec{x})$ to $f(\vec{x})$ through the reconstruction formula

$$f(\vec{x}) = \int_{S^1} \int_{\mathbb{R}} \hat{f}(\omega\vec{\theta})|\omega|e^{i(\vec{x}\cdot\omega\vec{\theta})} \, d\omega \, d\theta \qquad (11.5)$$

$$= \int_{S^1} \int_{\mathbb{R}} F_1\left(R_f(\vec{\theta}, \vec{\theta} \cdot \vec{x})\right)(\omega)|\omega|e^{i(\vec{x}\cdot\omega\vec{\theta})} \, d\theta.$$

From Equation 11.5 we see that the original function may be reconstructed from Fourier transforms of the line integrals, using a two-
dimensional inverse Fourier transform. One problem with this inversion
is that the Fourier transform is infamously nonlocal. Moreover, in this
setting the Fourier transform would be sampled on a radial grid and interpolation would be necessary in order to use a conventional fast Fourier
transform based on a rectangular grid.

11.4.2 Filtered Backprojection

The most common alternative to Fourier reconstruction is the commonly used reconstruction method called filtered backprojection [11]. To obtain the filtered backprojection algorithm we assume that the function f is essentially bandlimited on a circle of radius r and insert a characteristic function, or similar window, into Equation 11.5 to obtain

$$f_b(\vec{x}) = \int_{S^1} \int_{\mathbb{R}} F_1\left(R_f(\vec{\theta}, \vec{\theta} \cdot \vec{x})\right) (b(\omega)|\omega|)e^{i(\vec{x}\cdot\vec{\theta})\omega} \, d\omega \, d\theta \qquad (11.6)$$

$$= \int_{S^1} R_f(\vec{\theta}, \vec{\theta} \cdot \vec{x}) * F_1^{-1}(b(\omega)|\omega|) \, d\theta$$

$$= \int_{S^1} \int R_f(\vec{\theta}, t) F_1^{-1}(b(\omega)|\omega|)(\vec{\theta} \cdot \vec{x} - t) \, dt \, d\theta.$$

The window must be chosen to meet two criteria. First, the window should be chosen to agree with the essential bandlimit of f, so that f_b will be a good approximation to f. Second, the window also represents a mollification of the inversion of the Radon transform, which is an unbounded operator without the addition of the window [11].

The reconstruction process is then relatively simple. First, one filters the line integrals, at each angle, using the convolution filter generated by $|\omega|b(\omega)$. Then one backprojects the result, as is illustrated in Figure 11.6. This is done for every angle θ, and the result will be an accurate reconstruction of the image. A typical window $b(\omega)$ might be $b(\omega) = \mathcal{X}_{[-r,r]}(\omega)$, where r is chosen to agree with the essential bandlimit of f.

11.4.3 Nonlocality of the Radon Inversion

Nonlocal Convolution A fundamental idea in Fourier analysis is that a function f can only be supported on a localized region if its Fourier transform $\hat{f}$ is very smooth or possesses many smooth derivatives. Thus, if a function's Fourier transform is discontinuous or has a discontinuous derivative, the function can not be well localized.

The problem with the reconstruction formula of Equation 11.6 is that the inverse Fourier transform of $|\omega|b(\omega)$ will not be locally supported. This stems from the fact that $|\omega|$ is not differentiable at the origin, and the strict cutoff causes discontinuities at $\pm r$. The nonlocality of this inverse Fourier transform implies that local calculation of the convolution in Equation 11.6 will require global values of the Radon transform. The discontinuities at the endpoints can be eliminated with the choice of a suitable window, but

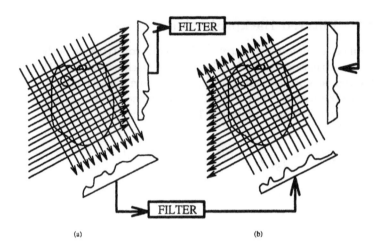

(a)   (b)

Figure 11.6
We illustrate the filtered backprojection reconstruction technique
above. In (a), we have illustrated the gathering of data from two
angles. In practice, this is generally done for several hundred
angles. The data are then filtered, and backprojected as is illustrated in (b).

the nondifferentiability at the origin can not be significantly altered without
harming the structure of the image.

   To summarize, the convolution function $|\omega|\widehat{b(\omega)}$ will not be well localized,
and therefore the filtering operation illustrated in Figure 11.6 and mathematically represented in Equation 11.6 can not be carried out with only
the values of the line integrals which pass through a given region.

Spreading of Local Basis Functions   We will consider the convolution,
or multiplication in the Fourier domain, as a filter $\mathcal{F}$, and we will write it
as a two-step process. The first is multiplication by $(i\omega)$ in the frequency
domain (or differentiation in the time domain). The second is the applica-
tion of the Hilbert transform $Hf : \hat{f}(\omega) \to \frac{1}{i}\text{sign}(\omega)\hat{f}(\omega)$. Thus the filtering
process is given by

$$\mathcal{F} : \hat{f} \to \frac{1}{i}\text{sign}(\omega)(i\omega)\hat{f}(\omega) = |\omega|\hat{f}(\omega).$$

Differentiation is local. The Hilbert transform is not, since it imposes a
discontinuity upon the Fourier transform of any function whose average
value is not zero and discontinuities on the higher derivatives which are not
zero at the origin.

   The imposition of these discontinuities at the origin in the frequency
domain will therefore spread the support of functions in the time domain.

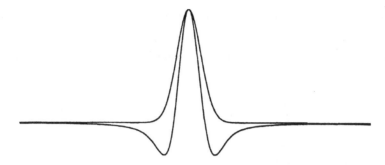

Figure 11.7
Above we illustrate the nonlocal nature of the filter in tomographic reconstruction. The upper function is a well-localized Gaussian. The lower function is the filtered version of this Gaussian. Notice that the support of the Gaussian is spread by the filter so that the filtered version has a support which is essentially three times as large as the original function.

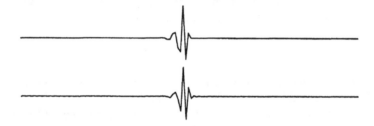

Figure 11.8
We illustrate the fact that a localized function with enough zero moments will not be spread by the filtering operation with the Daubechies D6 wavelet. At top is the Daubechies D6 wavelet, and its filtered version. The support of the filtered version is virtually unchanged.

For this reason, a local basis will not remain local after filtering. This spreading of local elements is illustrated by a Gaussian in Figure 11.7.

Local Basis Elements with Zero Moments Are Not Spread   However, the imposition of discontinuities at the origin in the frequency domain, and the subsequent spreading of the support of the function, *will not occur* if the function's Fourier transform is zero at the origin, and the function has arbitrarily many zero moments. Further, one can construct functions with only a few zero moments whose support is essentially unchanged by the Hilbert transform, as is illustrated in Figure 11.8. This property is fundamental to the use of our algorithm, as will be described below.

11.4.4   Visualization via the Sinogram

It is helpful at this time to visualize the reconstruction process using the sinogram. Recall the reconstruction formula for filtered backprojection, Equation 11.6,

$$f_b(\vec{x}) = \int_{S^1} \int R_f(\vec{\theta}, t) F_1^{-1}(b(\omega)|\omega|)(\vec{\theta} \cdot \vec{x} - t) \, dt \, d\theta. \qquad (11.7)$$

If we denote the convolution filter by $\mathcal{F}$, then we have

$$f_g(\vec{x}) = \int_{S^1} \mathcal{F}\left(R_f(\vec{\theta}, \cdot)\right)(\vec{x} \cdot \vec{\theta}) \, d\theta. \qquad (11.8)$$

Since the filter is independent of θ, the values inside the integral are the values of the sinogram, after a line-by-line filtering operation. Thus the final outcome of filtered backprojection, $f_b(\vec{x})$, where $\vec{x}$ is contained in a localized region Q, is dependent upon the values of the filtered sinogram, in a strip

$$Q' = \{\vec{y} : \vec{y} = \vec{x} \cdot \vec{\theta}, \vec{x} \in Q, \vec{\theta} \in S^1\}.$$

Therefore, in order to calculate the localized values of f_b, we must be able to calculate the values of the filtered sinogram in the strip Q'. If Q were centered at the origin, then such a strip would be illustrated by Figure 11.9 (a). The values needed to construct an off-centered reconstruction would lie in a strip such as the one in Figure 11.9 (b). If our convolution function were localized, then we could calculate these values from localized values of the sinogram. Our convolution function is not well localized, as we noted earlier, so we need values outside of this region.

In order to avoid gathering a large quantity of nonlocal information, we think of separating each line of our filtered sinogram into two components: a high frequency component $\mathcal{F}(R_f^h)$ which will have infinitely many zero moments, and a low frequency component $\mathcal{F}(R_f^l)$. We will be able to calculate the high frequency component locally, because the corresponding high frequency filter will not spread the values of functions which have many zero moments (see Figure 11.8). These local measurements are illustrated by the central strip in Figure 11.9.

The calculation of the filtered values of the low frequency component will require global measurements of the Radon transform. The range theorem for the Radon transform will allow us to calculate this low frequency component at a few angular samples of $R_f^l(\vec{\theta}_i, r)$ and then interpolate the rest of the values $R_f^l(\vec{\theta}, r)$. This is illustrated in Figure 11.9, by the complete, sparse lines in the sinogram.

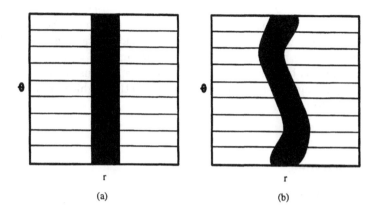

r   r

(a)   (b)

Figure 11.9
If a localized reconstruction were to be obtained for a central
region Q, then the values of the filtered sinogram would have
to be calculated on the darkened central strip illustrated in (a)
above. If a localized reconstruction of a region Q which is not
centered is desired, then values of the filtered sinogram will have
to be calculated in a region such as that illustrated in (b). The
sparse lines through the entire sinograms illustrate the sparse
nonlocal sampling which is necessary to calculate the nonlocal
low frequency components.

11.4.5 Comparison to Local Tomography

At this time let us emphasize the differences between our algorithm and
local tomography as it appears in [8]. In [8], *the only data which is gathered
is the data represented by the dark central strips* of Figure 11.9. Since the
convolution against the kernel $|\omega|b(\omega)$ cannot be computed accurately with
this data, the authors choose to calculate the convolution using the kernel
$\omega^2 b(\omega)$. Since this function is smooth at the origin, its inverse Fourier transform, which is the convolution kernel, is well localized and the convolution
can be accurately computed with limited data.

The authors of [8] conducted an extensive analysis of the properties of the
function which will be reconstructed via this process, namely, Λf, where
Λf has the Fourier transform $|\omega|\hat{f}(\omega)$. It was shown that Λf has the same
edge structure as f, and moreover, the edges are somewhat enhanced. This
type of image is desirable for detecting edges from the point of view of a
signal processer. The final judgment on whether or not it will be acceptable
to the radiologist has not been made, although these images have been used
in cardiac imaging at the Mayo clinic.

The algorithm which we are about to present *uses slightly more information* than that of [8]. This additional information is represented in Figure
11.9 by the sparse complete horizontal lines. The advantage of using this
information is that it allows us to present an image to a radiologist which is

essentially identical, on the region of interest, to the image the radiologist would see using standard algorithms and complete data. Thus we reduce radiation exposure and present the same information to the radiologist. This is important because it avoids an extensive, expensive study of radiologist performance on the "altered" reconstructions which they have not been trained to read.

11.5   Localization

11.5.1   Utilizing Functions with Zero Moments

In Section 11.4, we discussed the fact that nonlocalities in the Radon transform are induced via the filtering step in the filtered backprojection algorithm. These nonlocalities are induced if the Hilbert transform causes discontinuities in the low-order derivatives of the Fourier transforms of localized basis functions. These problems are not present when a basis function has sufficiently many zero moments. This phenomenon is due to the fact that if a function is zero at the origin, and its low-order derivatives are zero at the origin, multiplication by the sign (ω) will not cause a discontinuity in the function or in its low-order derivatives.

The algorithm presented in [12] relied on wavelets, which have zero moments, to localize the Radon transform. The finest wavelets have very well-localized support, and therefore their coefficients can be calculated from local measurements of the Radon transform. More important, the essential support of these wavelets does not spread when they are filtered in the filtered backprojection algorithm (see Figure 11.8). Thus their contribution to the final image is localized. Wavelets at coarser scales have wider support, however, and therefore one must gather additional nonlocal data in order to calculate their coefficients.

The gathering of the additional nonlocal data would have made the algorithm useless, except for the fact that the range theorems for the Radon transform specify that the bandlimits of the wavelet coefficients are essentially the same as the essential bandlimits of the wavelets [11]. Thus nonlocal data only needs to be gathered from a few angles, and the coarse wavelet coefficients can then be interpolated at the other angles.

11.5.2   How Many Frequency Windows?

It has come to our attention that we did not need to use wavelets for the algorithm. Moreover, wavelets are far from optimal. Utilizing wavelets to do the reconstruction requires the decomposition of the data into many different frequency scales, or windows. The finest scale wavelets are well localized, and therefore no interpolation is necessary, since their coefficients can be calculated locally.

The intermediate-scale wavelets, however, require additional information in order to interpolate their values. These intermediate-scale wavelets cause the algorithm presented in [12] to be suboptimal. Instead of interpolating the coefficients of these intermediate-scale wavelets, we want to combine the frequency content of these wavelets with the frequency content of the fine-scale wavelets. Since we will have a larger frequency decomposition, we should be able to construct basis functions which are even more localized in time. Therefore we will not need additional information to calculate the intermediate-scale frequency representation. Thus we want to use only one low frequency subspace, and one high frequency subspace.

Decompositions such as the one outlined above can be accomplished by utilizing a properly constructed version of the local cosine projections of Coifman and Meyer [4]. We will now outline the construction of optimal projections, according to the range theorems of the Radon transform and the constraints of the uncertainty principle.

11.5.3 High Frequency Computation

Let us concentrate on the convolution involved in filtered backprojection. We will denote the convolution filter in Equation 11.6 by $k(t) = \widehat{|\omega|b(\omega)}$. We are going to use the projections developed by Coifman and Meyer to decompose $k(t)$ into high-frequency and low-frequency components, so that we have

$$k(t) = k^h(t) + k^l(t).$$

We want to design our projection so that k^h is well localized, which will allow for localized calculation of the high frequency component of our image. If we want k^h to be well localized, the uncertainty principle dictates that its Fourier transform $\hat{k}^h$ cannot be well localized. Moreover, we also need $\hat{k}^h$ to be smooth, if k^h is to be well localized. Thus we have two constraints on $\hat{k}^h$: (1) $\hat{k}^h$ must be as smooth as possible, and (2) $\hat{k}^h$ must be as widely supported as possible.

To accomplish smoothness, we need to do two things. First of all, we need to make sure that the discontinuity of the derivative in $\hat{k} = |\omega|b(\omega)$ is contained in the low resolution component of the decomposition, k^l. Therefore we let $\hat{k}^h(\omega) = 0$ for small ω. Second, we need to make sure that $\hat{k}^h$ makes a smooth transition from 0 to $|\omega|$. This is accomplished via the construction of Coifman and Meyer. The function $\hat{k}^h(t)$ is illustrated in Figure 11.10.

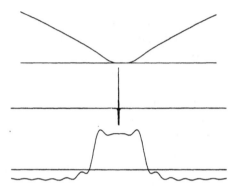

Figure 11.10
The Fourier transform $\hat{k}^h(t)$ is illustrated at the top above. It is identical to the ramp function $|\omega|$ away from the origin and the cutoff points, but is zero in a small region about the origin, and is smoothed at the cutoff points. The localized high-frequency kernel k^h is shown in the middle, and the nonlocal low-frequency kernel k^l is shown at the bottom.

We can now decompose the filtering operation into two steps,

$$R_f(\vec{\theta}, t) * k(t) = R_f(\vec{\theta}, t) * (k^l(t) + k^h(t)) \qquad (11.9)$$

$$= R_f(\vec{\theta}, t) * k^l(t) + R_f(\vec{\theta}, t) * k^h(t).$$

The advantage of this decomposition is that $k^h(t)$ is well localized, so the second integral can be computed with only information from regions such as the darkened strips of Figure 11.9.

An important final detail in constructing $\hat{k}^h(\omega)$ is that the discontinuity of the derivative of $|\omega|$ at π on $[-\pi, \pi]$ be eliminated. This can be done without altering the algorithm, by simply smoothing the endpoints of $|\omega|$.

11.5.4   Low Frequency Computation

The function $k^l(t)$ will not be well localized, however. Thus we need to estimate the second convolution in Equation 11.9, using our knowledge of the range of R_f and the construction of $k^l(t)$. We recall that k^l is the projection of k onto a low-resolution subspace, and denote this projection by P^l. At this point, we would like to claim that the convolution is merely a series of inner products against k^l, and therefore the convolution will be unaffected by functions in the orthogonal complement of P^l. This is unfortunately not true. This is because the translates of k^l are not necessarily in P^l, since P^l is not translation invariant. This clouds the issue slightly.

This argument is morally correct, however, and we can use a similar argument. The bandlimited spaces are translation invariant. Since k^l is bandlimited we can define the B_l to be the space of functions with the same bandlimit as k_l. It is now true that the functions orthogonal to B_l, or the high-frequency functions, will not affect the convolution. If we denote the bandlimiting projection by P_{B_l} it follows that

$$k^l * R_f(\vec{\theta}, t) = k^l * P_{B_l}\left(R_f(\vec{\theta}, t)\right). \tag{11.10}$$

We know that the Fourier components of $R_f(\vec{\theta}, r) = \hat{f}(\omega\vec{\theta})$ are essentially bandlimited for each fixed ω. This allows us to interpolate $P_{B_l}\left(R_f(\vec{\theta}, t)\right)$ accurately with a fixed number of samples. Interpolating the low resolution components of the Fourier transform will be equivalent to interpolating the low resolution components of the Radon transform, or sinogram. Thus we can interpolate the low resolution version of the sinogram $P_{B_l}\left(R_f(\vec{\theta}, t)\right)$ from the sparse nonlocal samples illustrated in Figure 11.9. We then compute the convolution in Equation 11.10, with sparse nonlocal samples.

11.5.5   The Algorithm

We must emphasize that we do not actually use the local cosine bases of Coifman and Meyer [4]. We need only the projections which were proposed and used to construct the bases in Coifman and Meyer [4]. We use windows such as the bell illustrated in Figure 11.14. This window will be centered at the origin of the one-dimensional Fourier transform of the line integrals $R_f(\vec{\theta}, r)$, for each angle θ. Thus the subspace associated with this window will contain the low-frequency component of the filtering kernel k. The low-frequency components of the Radon transform $R_f^l(\vec{\theta}, r)$ will then be calculated at a few angles, and interpolated to the remaining angles. The filtered version of the low-frequency component can then be calculated.

The local, high frequency component of the Radon transform $R_f(\vec{\theta}, t)$ can be measured locally, for each angle, allowing us to essentially localize the dependence of the Radon transform on the input data. We summarize the algorithm below:

1.   Gather full data $R_f(\vec{\theta}_i, r)$ at a few, evenly spaced angles.

2.   Interpolate the low-frequency component R_f^l at each angle from these sparse angular samples.

3.   Calculate the filtered values of the low-frequency component from this interpolated data.

4.   At each angle, calculate the filtered high frequencies from local mea-

surements of the Radon transform, $R_f(\vec{\theta}, r)$, where r comes from a localized strip, as in Figure 11.9.

5. Combine these high- and low-frequency components into one approximate sinogram. Use this approximate filtered sinogram and backprojection to approximate the density f.

Thus our local approximation to the sinogram will be given by

$$R_f^{l,i}(\vec{\theta}, r) * k^l + R_f^{loc}(\vec{\theta}, r) * k^h$$

where $R_f^{l,i}$ is the low frequency component of the Radon transform which has been interpolated (l, i = low, interpolated), and R_f^{loc} is the local component of the Radon transform. Filtered backprojection will then be used to construct the final image.

This algorithm will be subject to two types of error. The first will be a truncation error, from the high-frequency components which are not gathered. The second will be an aliasing error in the low-frequency components which will be due to the fact that these components are not truly bandlimited, but rather only essentially bandlimited. Mathematically we have

$$\|Err\| = \left\| R_f(\vec{\theta}, r) * k - \left(R_f^{l,i}(\vec{\theta}, r) * k^l + R_f^{loc}(\vec{\theta}, r) * k^h \right) \right\| \qquad (11.11)$$

$$= \left\| \left(R_f(\vec{\theta}, r) - R_f^{l,i}(\vec{\theta}, r) \right) * k^l + \left(R_f^l(\vec{\theta}, r) - R_f^{loc}(\vec{\theta}, r) \right) * k^h \right\|$$

$$\leq \left\| \left(R_f(\vec{\theta}, r) - R_f^{l,i}(\vec{\theta}, r) \right) * k^l \right\| + \left\| \left(R_f^l(\vec{\theta}, r) - R_f^{loc}(\vec{\theta}, r) \right) * k^h \right\|.$$

The first error is the aliasing error, from interpolating the low frequencies. The second error is the truncation error, from the high frequencies which are not calculated. These errors are analyzed in the Appendix and shown to be negligible if proper parameters are chosen.

11.6   Numerical Results

We will present two numerical examples of the algorithm. In each case, the "full" set of data consists of 256 angles with 256 samples per angle. The first example, illustrated in Figure 11.11, shows the localization on input data on the interior 32/256 or 1/8 of the Shepp-Logan phantom. For this reconstruction we used 16 full projections, and a "cushion" of 4 around the interior 32 pixels of the localized projection data, for a total of 40 line integrals in each localized projection. A detailed count reveals that this comprises a total of 20% of the data. For comparison, wavelet localized tomography required more than 40% of the data. Since 12.5% of the data is truly local, it would seem difficult to reduce this number much further, especially since even Lambda reconstructions have to gather the additional "cushion" data around the central region. One possible reduction technique would involve the interlaced sampling technique [11], although commercial utilization of this technique does not seem feasible.

The second numerical example, Figure 11.12, illustrates the reconstruction of an off-center region of the Shepp-Logan phantom. This reconstruction centers the localized region about the three small lobes in the phantom, Once again 20% of the data was utilized. At this point, we should point out that it is much easier to reconstruct a noncentered region using this algorithm than it is with wavelet-localized tomography.

11.7 Optimality

We have claimed that this algorithm is optimal. Since no algorithm is ever globally optimal we need to clarify this claim. The type of algorithm which has been presented is optimal in the class of algorithms which localize the Radon transform by using nonlocal projections to recover the low-frequency component of the image and use local information to recover the high-frequency components of the image.

Our goal is to minimize the amount of nonlocal data which is needed for our reconstruction. This data comes from two different places.

1. The number of angles at which we gather full data $R_f(\vec{\theta}, r)$. This is determined by our ability to accurately interpolate the low frequencies. We refer to this as interpolation data.

2. The amount of data, next to the central strips of localized data, illustrated in Figure 11.9, which is necessary for accurate calculation of the high-frequency convolution. This is determined by the width of the high-frequency convolution kernel. We refer to this as overlap data.

We begin by discussing the minimization of the interpolation data.

One must remember that although it is true that the essential bandlimit of $q(\vec{\theta}) = \hat{R}_f(\vec{\theta}, \omega) = f(\omega\vec{\theta})$ is proportionate to ω, for ω sufficiently large,

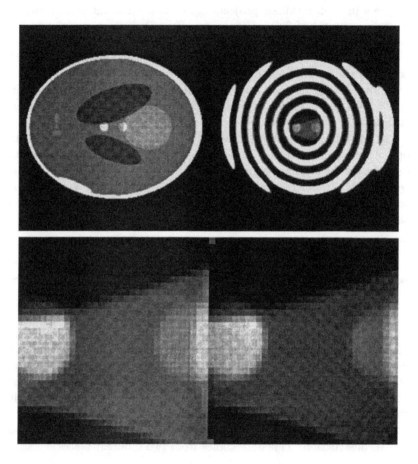

Figure 11.11

In the above numerical example, we performed a localized reconstruction on a central region, which is 1/8 the size of the total
image. The top left is the reconstruction from full data. The top
right is the reconstruction using 20% of the data. On the bottom
left is a blow-up of the interior 32 pixels of the reconstruction
from full data. On the bottom right is a blow-up of the interior
32 pixels reconstructed using 20% of the data. Note that only the
circle inscribed in this square is intended to be reconstructed accurately. As expected, there is essentially no difference between
the images in the region of interest.

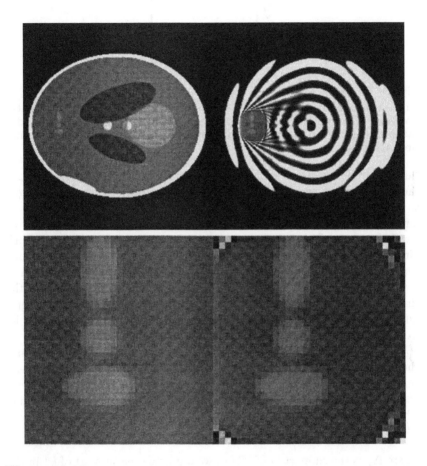

Figure 11.12

A noncentral region is reconstructed using our localized reconstruction algorithm. At the top left is the reconstruction from full data. The top right is the reconstruction using 20% of the data. On the bottom left we have a blow-up of an off-center region. On the bottom right is a blow-up of a reconstruction of this off-center region, using our algorithm and 20% of the data. In the region of interest, which is not the whole blown-up square, but rather the inscribed circle, there is essentially no difference.

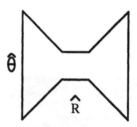

Figure 11.13
The support of the Fourier transform of $R_f(\vec{\theta}, r)$ is illustrated
above. The width of the central portion of the bow tie dic-
tates the minimum amount of nonlocal information which must
be gathered.

this fails to be true for ω arbitrarily close to zero. The Fourier transform of
the Radon transform is supported on a bow tie, rather than two triangles,
as is illustrated in Figure 11.13. Therefore there is a lower bound on the
number of projections which one must gather in order to determine the
low frequencies. This information cannot be gathered locally, because the
filter is global. Thus we choose our low-frequency window to be sufficiently
small, so that the low frequencies can be accurately interpolated from as
few projections as possible. To visualize this via Figure 11.13, realize that
the width of the center of the bow tie dictates the minimum number of
full projections $R_f(\vec{\theta}, r)$ which must be gathered to interpolate the low
frequencies.

The high frequencies can now be determined by a convolution against
the high-frequency kernel k^h. The size of the support of the high-frequency
kernel k^h determines the amount of overlap data which is needed. The size
of the essential support of k^h, Δ_t, is limited by the uncertainty principle
which states that

$$\Delta_t \Delta_\omega \geq 1,$$

where Δ_ω is the support of $\hat{k}^h$. Thus we minimize the support of k^h in time
by maximizing the support of $\hat{k}^h$ in frequency. This must be done subject
to the constraint that $\hat{k}^h(\omega)$ must be very smooth in order for k^h to be
locally supported. This requires that the discontinuity of the derivative in
$|\omega|$ be contained in $\hat{k}^l(\omega)$, and therefore $\hat{k}^h(\omega) = 0$ for $\omega \in [-\epsilon, \epsilon]$. The
quantity ϵ is picked so that the transition of $\hat{k}^h(\omega)$ from 0 to $|\omega|$ will be
smooth.

Summarizing, we have three criteria which must be met for optimality.

1. The low-resolution convolution function k^l must be sufficiently
    band- limited, so that the low-resolution information can be inter-
    polated at the optimal rate, determined by the inner region of the
    bow tie in Figure 11.13. This will minimize the interpolation data.

2. The high-resolution convolution function k^h must be as compactly supported as possible, implying via the uncertainty principle that its Fourier transform $\hat{k}^h$ must have as wide a support as is possible.

3. The function $\hat{k}^h(\omega)$ must be as smooth as possible. Thus the limit on the width of the support of $\hat{k}^h(\omega)$ is given by the fact that the discontinuity of $|\omega|$ must be contained in $\hat{k}^l(\omega)$ so that $\hat{k}^h(\omega)$ must be 0 in a region about the origin.

11.7.1 Minimization of Nonlocal Data

We have outlined the criteria which will make our algorithm optimal. We will now formalize these criteria, and show that in fact these types of projections, or at least windows of this type, are optimal.

The basic goal is simple. We want to produce a true reconstruction on the region of interest and minimize the amount of nonlocal data which we need to use. We will try to do this with as little rigor as possible, and a few basic assumptions.

For these purposes we need to define certain quantities. First, the essential supports of k^h in time and frequency will be denoted by Δ_t^h and Δ_f^h, respectively. We will assume that we are using projections which are essentially optimal with respect to the uncertainty principle, so that the uncertainty inequality in nearly met, i.e., $\Delta_t^h \Delta_f^h \approx 1$.

Denoting the essential supports of k^l by Δ_t^l and Δ_f^l, we recall that the frequency spectrum is partitioned between the high- and low-pass kernels, so that we expect Δ_f^h to increase when Δ_f^l decreases, etc.

The first source of nonlocal data will be the overlap data regions around the dark central strips. We must gather this nonlocal data in order to accurately calculate the high frequency convolution. The amount of data necessary for this calculation is equivalent to the support in time of the high frequency convolution kernel, or Δ_t^h.

The second source of nonlocal data will be the interpolation data, which must be gathered in order to interpolate the low-frequency information. This data is represented by the full lines in Figure 11.9. The essential bandwidth of this low-frequency information is essentially equivalent, via the range theorem of the Radon transform, to the bandlimit of the low-frequency kernel, Δ_f^l. Since Shannon sampling theory implies that the number of samples which are necessary to recover this information is proportional to the bandlimit of the information, the number of full lines is proportional to Δ_f^l.

Not all of this additional information is nonlocal, however. We have already accounted for gathering line integrals from $R + \Delta_t^h$ of each line, where R is the radius of the circle on which we are doing the reconstructions. Thus, if our intervals are of length 1, the additional portion which we are going to gather is $1 - (R + \Delta_t^h)$. Gathering this additional interpolation data on Δ_f^l lines yields the final nonlocal data cost function:

$$Non - Local - Data - Cost = \Delta_f^l(1 - (R + \Delta_t^h)) + \Delta_t^h$$

$$= \Delta_f^l(1 - R) + \Delta_t^h - \Delta_f^l\Delta_t^h.$$

The first two terms will be minimized as Δ_f^l approaches zero. This is because the uncertainty principle allows us to make Δ_t^h more compactly supported if Δ_f^h is more widely supported, and Δ_f^h becomes more widely supported as Δ_f^l goes to zero. The third term is more difficult to analyze, but it ends up being a second-order effect, and is negligible compared to the first two terms, in the appropriate region where Δ_t^h and Δ_f^l are very small.

Thus it would seem that our low-frequency window should be arbitrarily small. This is not quite the case, however. Since the Range characterization of the Fourier transform of the sinogram, shown in Figure 11.3, is a bow tie, and not two triangles, you cannot subsample the low frequencies below a certain threshold.

Therefore, this additional constraint says that we should make the low-frequency projection bandlimited enough to maximize our use of the range theorems. Making it any more bandlimited will not decrease the amount of interpolation data which we will need. In addition, we need to make the high-frequency window zero in a region about the origin, if the high-frequency kernel is to be free of the discontinuity in $|\omega|$ at the origin.

Thus optimality is achieved with any window below the threshold dictated by the range theorem, which causes the high-frequency kernel to be optimally well localized. In practice, it seems that fine tuning of the second portion of this criterion is not all that difficult, and an extensive analysis of the details does not seem necessary.

11.8   Conclusion

We have presented an algorithm which is optimal over this class of algorithms for localized tomography. This algorithm reduces the amount of needed radiation by a factor of 2 from wavelet localized tomography [12], without the use of interlaced sampling. When compared to conventional sampling, this algorithm reduces radiation exposure by 80% or more, when a localized region is to be imaged. We have demonstrated in [12] that an additional gain in minimization can be accomplished via the incorporation of interlaced sampling [11]. This could also be done with the algorithm presented here. This does not seem to be commercially viable, however, so its usefulness may be purely academic.

Wavelet localized tomography [12] utilized interpolations at intermediate scales, which required that localized regions of the image be centered, for reconstruction. Therefore one would have to shift the sinogram, or projections, before using the algorithm. Often this will cause one to double the size of the array in which the input projection data is stored, and create additional numerical difficulties.

The algorithm presented here only interpolates the lowest frequency information. We do not need to interpolate the intermediate frequency bands, which greatly simplifies the numerical aspects of the algorithm.

It has been pointed out that it is difficult in current commercial machines to gather localized data, in the method proposed in [12]. It is much easier to gather the type of data needed for this algorithm. One would simply use one "slow" helical fan beam scan, whose beams pass through the localized region of interest to gather the localized data. To gather the sparse nonlocal data a "fast" helical fan beam scan whose beams pass through the whole image would be utilized.

The medical community has become increasingly concerned about the possible long-term effects of radiation exposure. There are a number of situations in which a radiologist is not interested in the whole image, but rather a localized portion of the image. For these reasons, we are currently working on an alteration of this algorithm for use in current state of the art CT machines, which utilize helical fan beam scans.

Beyond the justification of radiation reduction in X-ray CT, the understanding of the nonlocality of the Radon transform allows one to better understand a variety of instances, when imaging is to be done with limited data using the Radon transform.

11.9   Appendix: Error Analysis

11.9.1   Aliasing Error Analysis

We begin with the analysis of the aliasing errors. We recall that the range characterization for the Radon transform, Equation 1, states that

$$R_f(\vec{\theta}, t) = (1 - t^2)^{-1/2} \sum_{l=0}^{\infty} T_l(t) h_l(\theta). \tag{11.12}$$

The Fourier transform of this with respect to t is given by

$$\hat{R}_f(\vec{\theta}, \omega) = \left(\frac{\pi}{2}\right)^{1/2} \sum_{l=0}^{\infty} i^{-l} J_l(\omega) h_l(\theta) \tag{11.13}$$

$$= \left(\frac{\pi}{2}\right)^{1/2} \left(\sum_{l=0}^{N-1} i^{-l} J_l(\omega) h_l(\theta) + \sum_{N}^{\infty} i^{-l} J_l(\omega) h_l(\theta) \right).$$

The first term in Equation 11.13 is bandlimited in the variable θ. Therefore we can accurately interpolate this term, with an appropriate number of samples. The second term is not bandlimited with respect to θ, and therefore this term will lead to aliasing. Thus we want to show that the second term

$$\hat{R}f(\vec{\theta}, \omega) = \left(\frac{\pi}{2}\right)^{1/2} \sum_{l=N}^{\infty} i^{-l} J_l(\omega) h_l(\theta) \tag{11.14}$$

is negligible, if ω is sufficiently small.

Since the terms h_l are the terms of the orthogonal Chebyshev coefficients in the weighted space $L_2([-1,1], (1-r^2)^{-1/2})$, it follows that

$$\sum |h_l(\theta)|^2 = \frac{2}{\pi} \left| \int_{-1}^{1} R_f(\theta, r) T_l(r) \, dr \right|^2 \leq \frac{2}{\pi} \|R_f(\theta, r)\|_{L_2}^2 .$$

Applying the Cauchy-Schwartz-Bunyakovskii inequality to Equation 11.14 we get

$$|\hat{R}f(\vec{\theta}, \omega)| \leq \|R_f(\theta, r)\|_{L_2}^2 \sum_{l=N}^{\infty} |J_l(\omega)|^2. \tag{11.15}$$

We need to use the Bessel function inequality [11, p.198]

$$0 \leq |J_l(\eta l)| \leq (2\pi l)^{-1/2} (1 - \eta^2)^{-1/4} e^{(-l/3)(1-\eta^2)^{3/2}} .$$

Since the above inequality becomes small only when $\theta < 1$, we want to consider the above inequality when ω is a fixed integer, and $l > 2\omega$. Thus $J_l(\omega) = J_l(l\frac{n}{l})$ where $n = \omega$, and $\eta \equiv n/l < 1/2$. Then Equation 11.15 becomes

$$\left| \left(\frac{\pi}{2} \right)^{1/2} \sum_{l=N}^{\infty} i^{-l} J_l(\omega) h_l(\theta) \right| \qquad (11.16)$$

$$\leq \| R_f(\theta, r) \|_{L_2}^2 \sum_{l=N}^{\infty} \left| (2\pi l)^{-1} (1 - \eta^2)^{-1/2} e^{(-l/3)(1-\eta^2)^{3/2}} \right|^2$$

$$= \| R_f(\theta, r) \|_{L_2}^2 \sum_{l=N}^{\infty} (2\pi l)^{-2} \left(1 - \left(\frac{n}{l} \right)^2 \right)^{-1} e^{(-2l/3)(1-(\frac{n}{l})^2)^{3/2}}.$$

Since $n/l < 1/2$ the above reduces to

$$\left| \left(\frac{\pi}{2} \right)^{1/2} \sum_{l=N}^{\infty} i^{-l} J_l(\omega) h_l(\theta) \right| \leq \| R_f(\theta, r) \|_{L_2}^2 \sum_{l=N}^{\infty} (2\pi l)^{-2} \frac{4}{3} e^{-\sqrt{3} l/4}. \qquad (11.17)$$

Our algorithm will therefore consist of using $2N$ projections to determine the inner N Fourier coefficients in the Radon transform. This oversampling is necessary to make the above estimates sharp. The remaining high frequencies will then be determined by local measurements of the Radon transform. The above discussion can be concluded in the following theorem.

THEOREM 2
The term which would lead to aliasing in this algorithm, is dominated by

$$\left| \left(\frac{\pi}{2} \right)^{1/2} \sum_{l=N}^{\infty} i^{-l} J_l(\omega) h_l(\theta) \right| \leq \| R_f(\theta, r) \|_{L_2}^2 \sum_{l=N}^{\infty} (2\pi l)^{-2} \frac{4}{3} e^{-\sqrt{3} l/4}. \qquad (11.18)$$

If $N = 16$, this bound is on the order of 10^{-7}, and if $N = 8$, this is 10^{-5}, both of which are acceptable.

11.9.2 Truncation Error Analysis

Truncation error will occur whenever the support of the convolution function, k^h, exceeds the range over which we have gathered data. If k^h were compactly supported, then one could simply gather enough additional data so that the truncation error would be zero. This suggests that the construction of a compactly supported k^h would be worthwhile. While this is a possibility and is very intriguing academically, we will show that this is not necessary for the numerical stability of the algorithm.

Let us write $k^h = k_s^h + k_{err}^h$, where k_s^h is the restriction of $\hat{k}$ to its essential support (which can be chosen arbitrarily). If we gather enough additional overlap data around our region of interest, then we can calculate $k_s^h(t) * R_f(\vec{\theta}, t)$ exactly. Thus our error would be dominated by

$$\left\| k^h * R_f(\vec{\theta}, t) - k_s^h(t) * R_f(\vec{\theta}, t) \right\| = \left\| k_{err}^h(t) * R_f(\vec{\theta}, t) \right\|.$$

From Figure 11.10 we can see that the term k_{err}^h, which is the portion of the high-pass kernel which is not localized around zero, appears to be very small. This is indeed the case, and we can summarize this discussion in the following.

THEOREM 3

If we gather overlap data on a region of strip of size ϵ around the local data depicted in Figure 11.9, then the truncation error of this algorithm is bounded by

$$\left| k_{err}^h(t) * R_f(\vec{\theta}, t) \right| \leq \left\| k_{err}^h(t) \right\| \left\| R_f(\vec{\theta}, t) \right\|$$

where $k_{err}^h(t) = k^h(t) \mathcal{X}_{\mathbb{R} \setminus [-\epsilon, \epsilon]}(t)$.

Even with only four extra samples included as overlap data around the data of interest, this term is dominated by 10^{-5}. Since this is below the resolution of a typical gray scale display, this is certainly acceptable.

11.10   Appendix: The Local Cosine and Sine Bases of Coifman and Meyer

Local sine and cosine bases were introduced in [4]. This work was reviewed in [1] where their connections to the construction of smooth wavelets were also discussed. For the sake of completeness, we will briefly review the construction of these bases. For a more complete discussion, we recommend either [4] or [1].

The short-time Fourier transform has long been a tool for time-frequency analysis. Typically long signals are broken up into smaller segments, with disjoint supports. The discrete Fourier transform is used to analyze these short segments separately. This approach is not entirely satisfactory, however, because the spectrum of a function f which is well localized about the origin may be spread dramatically when one considers $f\mathcal{X}_{[a,b]}$. For instance, if f is a function in $L^2(\mathbb{R})$ which corresponds to an entire function of finite exponential type, then $\hat{f}$ is compactly supported. The imposition of the characteristic function to the above function causes $\hat{f}$ to lose its compact support, and obscure the spectral analysis.

One would therefore like to construct an orthogonal projection $f \to \rho f$ with a smoother window ρ. This is impossible, however, because if this were an orthogonal projection, then $\rho^2 f = \rho f$ for all f which would imply that $\rho^2 = \rho$. This can only be the case if ρ takes on only the values 0 or 1, and thus ρ could not be continuous. This problem led Coifman and Meyer to consider projections of the type

$$Pf(x) = \rho(x)f(x) + t(x)f(-x).$$

Let us assume for now that $\rho(x) + \rho(-x) = 1$, and $\rho(x) = \rho(-x)$. It can be further shown that this is only self-adjoint if $t(x) = \overline{t(-x)}$. If these properties hold, then the condition that $P^2 f = Pf$ would reduce to

$$P^2 f = \left(\rho^2(x) + t(x)t(-x)\right) f(x) + t(x)f(-x) \tag{11.19}$$

$$= \rho(x)f(x) + t(x)f(-x) = Pf.$$

This is equivalent to $\rho(x)(1 - \rho(x)) = \rho(x)\rho(-x) = t(x)t(-x)$. Since we have assumed that t is even, this reduces to

$$t(x) = \pm\sqrt{\rho(x)\rho(-x)}. \tag{11.20}$$

Thus if ρ and t satisfy these assumptions, then

$$Pf = \rho(x)f(x) \pm \sqrt{\rho(x)\rho(-x)}\, f(x)$$

is an orthogonal projection.

We will now construct the function ρ in a manner such that ρ can be made arbitrarily smooth. First choose an arbitrarily smooth, nonnegative, even function ϕ such that $\mathrm{supp}\phi \subset [-\epsilon, \epsilon]$, which is normalized so that

$$\int_{\mathbb{R}} \phi = \frac{\pi}{2}.$$

We then define

$$\theta(x) = \int_{-\infty}^{x} \phi(t)\, dt.$$

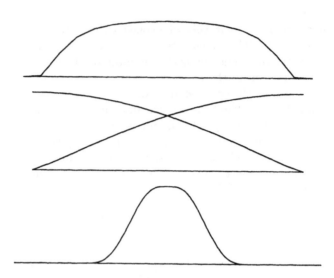

Figure 11.14
The functions involved in the construction of the local trigonometric projections are given above. At the top is the function
ϕ. In the middle we display the functions c_ϵ and s_ϵ used in the
local trigonometric construction. The bell b_I is displayed at the
bottom.

Since ϕ is even it follows that $\theta(x) + \theta(-x) = \pi/2$.

Let us define $s_\epsilon(x) = \sin\theta(x)$ and $c_\epsilon(x) = \cos\theta(x)$. It then follows from
the above that $c_\epsilon(x) = s_\epsilon(-x)$. A plot of s_ϵ and c_ϵ is given in Figure 11.14.

If we make $\rho(x) = s_\epsilon^2(x)$ we see that ρ satisfies all of the above properties.
The projection now becomes

$$Pf = s_\epsilon^2(x)f(x) \pm s_\epsilon(x)c_\epsilon(x)f(-x).$$

We have not windowed the function yet, but rather we have only cut
it off on one side. A similar translated construction in reverse order will
provide an orthogonal cutoff, with a smooth window on the right. The
only detail which must be observed is that the supports of the functions
$t(x) = s_\epsilon(x)c_\epsilon(x)$ should not intersect.

Following this procedure through, we will have a bell, given by

$$b_I(x) = s_\epsilon(x - \alpha)c_\epsilon(x - \beta),$$

which is illustrated in Figure 11.14.

This bell can then be used to realize a projection onto this localized support via the formula

$$Pf = b_I^2 f(x) \pm b_I(x)b_I(2\alpha - x)f(2\alpha - x) \pm b_I(x)b_I(2\beta - x)f(2\beta - x).$$

The choice of plus or minus in the above is then referred to as the polarity of the projection, on either the right or left, according to the support of the appropriate correction term $b_I(x)b_I(2\alpha - x)$ or $b_I(x)b_I(2\beta - x)$.

Since we need only the above projections, we will now leave the discussion of local sine and cosine bases to [4] and [1].

11.11 Acknowledgments

This work was supported in part by DARPA as administered by the AFOSR under contract AFOSR-90-0292, and ARPA, as administered by the AFOSR under contract DOD F4960-93-1-0567. The author is grateful to the Annals of Biomedical Engineering for allowing the reproduction of major portions of this work.

References

[1] Auscher, P., G. Weiss, and M. V. Wickerhauser, Local sine and cosine bases of Coifman and Meyer and the construction of smooth wavelets. In: *Wavelets, A Tutorial in Theory and Applications*, edited by C. Chui, Academic Press, New York, 237–256.

[2] D. Walnut, Local inversion of the Radon transform in even dimensions using wavelets. In: *Probabilistic and Stochastic Methods in Analysis, with Applications*, edited by J. S. Byrnes, Kluwer, Boston, 1992, 187–205.

[3] Berenstein, C. and D. Walnut, Local inversion of the Radon transform in even dimensions using wavelets. In: *Proc. Conf.: 75 Years of the Radon Transform, Vienna, Austria, 1992*, International Press, 1994, 38–58.

[4] Coifman, R. R. and Y. Meyer, Remarques sur l'analyse de fourierā fenêtre, série I, *C. R. Acad. Sci. Paris*, **312**, 259–261, 1991.

[5] Donoho, D. L. and P. B. Stark, Uncertainty principles and signal recovery, *SIAM J. Appl. Math.*, 49, 1989, 906–931.

[6] Faridani, A., E. Ritman, and K. T. Smith, Examples of Local tomography, *SIAM J. Appl. Math.*, 52, 1992, 1193–1198.

[7] Faridani, A., F. Keinert, F. Natterer, E. L. Ritman, and K. T. Smith, Local and global tomography, *Signal Processing* (IMA Vols. in Math and Appl), Vol. 23, Springer Verlag, New York, 1990, 241–255.

[8] Faridani, A., E. Ritman, and K. T. Smith, Local tomography, *SIAM J. Appl. Math.*, 52, 459–484, 1992.

[9] Louis, A. K. and A. Reider, Incomplete data problems in X-Ray computerized tomography, *Numer. Math.*, **56**, 371–383, 1989.

[10] Maass, P., The interior Radon transform, *SIAM J. Appl. Math.*, 52, 710–724, 1992.

[11] Natterer, F., *The Mathematics of Computerized Tomography*, Wiley and Sons, Stuttgart, 1986, 222 pp.

[12] Olson, T. and J. DeStefano, Wavelet localization of the Radon transform, *IEEE Trans. Signal Process.*, 2056–2067, 1994.

[13] Olson, T., "Optimal time-frequency projections for localized tomography", to appear, *Ann. of Biomed. Eng.*, Sept-Oct. 1995.

[14] Radon, J., Über die Bestimmung von Funktionen durch ihre Integralwerte längs gewisser Mannigfaltigkeiten, *Berichte Sächsishe Akademie der Wissenschaften*, Liepzig, Math.-Phys.Kl, **69**, 262–267.

12

Adapted Wavelet Techniques for Encoding Magnetic Resonance Images

Dennis M. Healy, Jr.[1] and John B. Weaver[2]

[1] *Department of Mathematics and Computer Science, Dartmouth College, Hanover, NH*
[2] *Department of Diagnostic Radiology, Dartmouth-Hitchcock Medical Center, Lebanon, NH*

Abstract   We present techniques for signal acquisition in magnetic resonance imaging (MRI) based on recent advances in adapted wavelet theory. These approaches generalize existing MRI encoding schemes, and permit flexible adaptation of encoding to particular imaging tasks.

Various figures of merit for MRI are presented, and their use in selecting a particular encoding approach is discussed. In particular, we summarize an analysis of the signal-to-noise ratios of images formed with this technique, as this is a factor of paramount importance in MRI. Other considerations discussed include imaging time and motion artifacts. Some implementation issues are presented.

An application to fast MRI is presented, in which the encoding scheme is designed to approximate the Karhunen-Loeve basis for a given class of images. The approximate basis is a local cosine basis which is much easier to implement in MRI than the actual Karhunen Loeve basis.

12.1   Introduction

This chapter presents some applications of adapted wavelet analysis in the field of magnetic resonance imaging (MRI). MRI is a relatively new noninvasive medical imaging modality which is now an essential part of diagnostic radiology, complementing older techniques like ultrasound and X-ray computed tomography (CT). MRI offers the ability to image motion, temperature effects, and chemical effects, in addition to providing excellent high-contrast imaging of soft tissues without the use of contrast agents. However, it can be limited in resolution and speed of image acquisition. Getting around these problems poses an interesting challenge in some of the ambitious application areas recently proposed for MRI, including heart imaging, joint and muscle motion studies, and functional imaging of the brain. There is a large, active research effort devoted to finding hardware and software approaches to these imaging tasks; see, for example, [3, 4, 18, 53, 57, 58, 63, 66].

We concentrate here on the impact of some of the new ideas from wavelet signal processing in the arena of signal acquisition and measurement in MRI. We should point out that there are also important research efforts devoted to the different problems of postprocessing images already obtained by a scanner; some of the other chapters of this monograph discuss techniques that would be useful for this purpose. For some approaches to postprocessing which have been considered by our research group, one might consult [27, 36, 37].

There are many techniques used to obtain MR images; all of these encode information about some object of interest in radio frequency signals generated by the stimulated precession of nuclear magnetic moments in a portion of the object. In this chapter, we shall indicate that this encoding process may be considered as the measurement of projections of functions representing various sample properties onto the elements of various simple bases. We shall examine benefits of encoding with some of the new bases provided by the recent advances in wavelet and related methods. In particular, we shall study techniques of *adapted waveform encoding*, which adapt the MR encoding scheme to a particular imaging task. Advantages of this new approach include ease of implementation, optimization of trade-offs among various imaging parameters, reduction of artifacts, and decreased imaging time.

The chapter is organized as follows. In Section 12.2, we sketch MRI techniques from the particular viewpoint of projections onto basis elements. From this perspective, Section 12.3 presents adapted waveform encoding as an extension of more traditional methods in MRI. We show that adapted waveform encoding offers a great deal of flexibility with respect to some of the important MRI imaging parameters, and present some of the considerations in choosing a basis to fit a particular imaging task. Some considerations arising in the implementation of the method are discussed. Section 12.4 presents an application of these ideas to the problem of choosing bases for fast imaging. In this approach, we take advantage of prior knowledge about statistical regularities in a particular image class in order to design encoding bases which reduce imaging times for objects in that class. Section 12.5 concludes.

12.2 Encoding in Magnetic Resonance Imaging

This section presents a thumbnail sketch of some techniques and practices of MRI which may help the reader appreciate both the unique promise and problems of this modality. We present only enough to motivate the application of wavelet and related bases for encoding diagnostically useful information about tissues. For more information, one may consult one of the many basic references describing MRI background; for example, [11, 25, 41, 55].

MRI is a noninvasive medical imaging modality which has carved out an important niche in medical imaging over the last decade or so. Some appreciation of its role in diagnostic medicine is gained by a comparison with alternatives like ultrasound and CT.

Ultrasound imaging is inexpensive and is done in real time. However, ultrasound can not be used for structures that are deep in the body or where there is air or bone around the structure of interest. Therefore, with few exceptions, ultrasound is mainly used in the abdomen and heart.

X-ray CT techniques offer excellent spatial resolution, but have very limited soft tissue contrast. Contrast in CT is determined primarily by the electron density of the materials imaged. Bone is the only tissue in the body with dramatically different electron density; soft tissues generally have very similar electron densities and atomic numbers.

MRI contrast, on the other hand, is determined by the relaxation parameters of the water in tissue; the intrinsic contrast between soft tissues in MRI is many times what it is for CT. For example, the white matter of the brain has 12% lower CT number than the gray matter [7], while white matter has a 140% higher signal than gray matter in an MRI examination [17]. Another important advantage for MRI over CT is the ability to obtain views at arbitrary positions and orientations. On the other hand, MRI is sometimes limited by its spatial resolution properties and long imaging times.

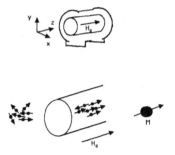

Figure 12.1
Placing a sample in the strong magnetic field $\mathbf{H}_0 = H_0\hat{\mathbf{z}}$ of the MR scanner causes a net alignment of the nuclear magnetic moments of the hydrogen nuclei of the sample. The resulting net magnetization M is manipulated to produce signal in MRI.

MR images are obtained without the ionizing radiation of CT. Instead, MRI works with the intrinsic magnetic moments of certain types of nuclei (usually hydrogen) found in the object under investigation. It is possible to stimulate these nuclear magnetic moments within the object so that they produce a radio-frequency (RF) output signal at a characteristic resonance frequency. This signal can be used to encode the information needed for imaging. The means by which this signal is evoked from the sample is the phenomenon of nuclear magnetic resonance (NMR), which we now describe.

12.2.1   Nuclear Magnetic Resonance

A typical imaging session begins by placing the sample object (such as a human subject) in a strong, homogeneous, magnetic field $\mathbf{H}_0$ inside the scanner. By convention, this field defines the z direction along the scanner axis, so that $\mathbf{H}_0 = H_0\hat{\mathbf{z}}$ with $\hat{\mathbf{z}}$ the unit vector field in the z direction.

Placing the sample in the scanner's field causes a net alignment of the magnetic moments of the hydrogen nuclei in the sample along the direction of $\mathbf{H}_0$. This allows us to work with a resultant bulk magnetization $\mathbf{M}$, created as the vector sum of the aligned nuclear magnetic moments. See Figure 12.1.

The bulk magnetization, $\mathbf{M}$, can be knocked out of alignment or "excited" with a radio-frequency electromagnetic pulse, resulting in its precession at a characteristic frequency around the external field $\mathbf{H}_0$. A sensitive coil detects a component of the resulting oscillating magnetic field and produces a signal which may be used to carry information about the properties of the sample. See Figure 12.2.

The frequency of the precession of $\mathbf{M}$ and of the resulting output signal is proportional to the strength of the external magnetic field: $f_{Larmor} = \gamma\|\mathbf{H}_0\|$. This is the natural resonant frequency of the spin system; the

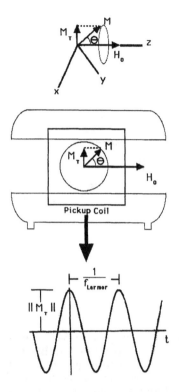

Figure 12.2
An RF excitation at the Larmor frequency may be used to tip
the magnetization **M** by angle θ away from H_0. It then begins to
precess around at the Larmor frequency. A pickup coil records
an oscillation at the Larmor frequency and with amplitude proportional to the length of M_T, the transverse component of **M**.

term "magnetic resonance" refers to the fact that the spin system absorbs
and emits radiation at the characteristic frequency f_{Larmor} determined by
the magnetic environment H_0. For hydrogen nuclei in a typical scanner
$f_{Larmor} \approx 60$ MHz (megahertz).

Properties of the sample may be inferred from the parameters of the
measured output signal. For instance, the amplitude of this signal is proportional to the number of nuclear magnetic moments contributing to the
net magnetization **M** as it precesses. This directly reflects a property of
the sample. The amplitude also depends on a user-determined parameter,
namely, how much energy is pumped into the sample by the RF excitation.

A typical sequence of operations is shown schematically in Figure 12.3.
One begins by stimulating the sample with an RF excitation signal at the
resonant frequency f_{Larmor}, and then measures the responding output signal.
The output signal generated after excitation is called the free induction

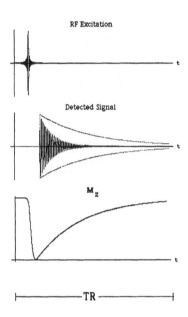

Figure 12.3
The sequence of events in a typical MR measurement is indicated
on three time lines. The sequence begins when an RF excitation
(top line) at the Larmor frequency is input to excite the spins
in the subject. These produce a decaying sinusoid (FID) signal
(middle line) at the Larmor frequency. The decay is partly caused
by the eventual realignment of the spins with the static field,
as indicated by the recovery of the longitudinal magnetization
(bottom line). This recovery determines the repetition time, TR,
which should be allowed before the spin system is queried again.
Unfortunately, signal measurements are usually unavailable for
much of this time, due to another, faster decay effect stemming
from the loss of coherence among the spins contributing to the
bulk magnetization.

decay (FID). In the absence of magnetic inhomogeneities and susceptibility
effects, the signal eventually dies off as a superposition of two types of
exponential decay, characterized by decay constants: T_1 and T_2. These
time constants are properties of the materials imaged, and may vary in
space throughout the sample.

- T_1 **decay.** Spin-lattice, or longitudinal relaxation is characterized
  by T_1. T_1 typically varies from 200 ms (milliseconds) to 800 ms.
  This decay reflects the magnetization realigning itself with the static
  magnetic field as the spins lose energy to the lattice.

- T_2 **decay.** Spin-spin, or transverse relaxation, occurs faster, with
  time constant $T_2 \approx 50$ ms in tissues. It is caused by loss of phase

coherence, or dephasing, among the precessing spins contributing to **M**, and comes from local interactions among the spins.

In cases where a given group of spins must be measured repeatedly, the T_1 parameter helps determine a required repetition time, *TR*, between successive excitations. This resting period is mandated by the necessity of waiting for the spin system to relax back towards alignment with the external magnetic field before the next excitation. *TR* can be quite long when imaging material with a long T_1 relaxation time, resulting in long imaging times.

Contributing to the difficulty of MR measurements is the fact that the usable signal generally dies away by fast T_2 decay (or faster) long before the longitudinal magnetization has recovered by the slower T_1 process. This can have the effect that much of the *TR* resting period is wasted as far as obtaining useful measurements is concerned. Later we shall discuss how this very important issue is addressed in our work.

So far, the output signal reflects properties of the sample as a whole. Imaging requires localization, i.e., the ability to determine what is contributed to the signal by a given region of the sample, and therefore permit inference about the local properties of each portion of the sample.

12.2.2 Imaging

For a sample in the uniform field $\mathbf{H}_0$, all the nuclei produce signal at the corresponding Larmor frequency after excitation. The output signal thus reflects the properties of the sample as a whole. In order to do imaging, we must somehow map the variation of some property of interest within the sample. In most examinations, we are trying to determine a map of the weighted spin density over the extent of the sample. Typically, this is accomplished by perturbing the external magnetic field so as to vary in strength across the sample. Nuclei at different positions now experience a slightly different field strength and therefore have a Larmor frequency that depends on their position.

This may be used in several ways to encode information on the RF signal so that one may map tissue properties across a region of the sample. The principal techniques are:

- Selective excitation
- Frequency, phase encoding

The measurements made with these methods may be interpreted as projections against elements of various bases. We now present the standard

MRI technique from this perspective; later we shall see how this may be generalized.

Selective Excitation

Perhaps the most straightforward approach to obtaining localized information is to collect signal from only a small region of the sample. For example, one may study sample properties near a given position by only "turning on" the spins in that portion of the sample; the resulting output signal necessarily reflects only the properties of nuclei in the activated region.

This *selective excitation* is obtained by supplying a narrowband RF excitation, which stimulates only those nuclei whose resonant frequency is near that of the excitation signal. The nuclei so selected live only in the region of the sample which experiences the corresponding magnetic field strength. Their output signal is associated only with that location. Selective excitation amounts to projection of the signal density onto a localized amplitude profile, as we now see.

The requisite variation of Larmor frequency across the sample is provided by special gradient coils in the scanner, which add to the background field H_0 a linear variation in one direction across the sample, say the z direction, while the narrowband RF excitation signal is supplied. The natural frequencies of the spins then vary linearly with z,

$$f_{Larmor} = f_{Larmor}(z) = \gamma(H_0 + G_z z),$$

where G_z is a constant reflecting the gradient of magnetic field strength in the z direction. Only nuclei in those regions corresponding to frequency components present in the RF pulse will be excited into contributing to the output signal. To first order (low tip angle approximation), the amplitude and phase of the nuclear excitations in a given plane $z = z_0$ will be proportional to the amplitude and phase of the frequency component of the RF excitation at the corresponding frequency $f_{Larmor}(z_0)$. See Figure 12.4.

For example, an idealized RF excitation pulse could be a modulated sinc function comprised of pure harmonics with amplitude 1 in a certain band and amplitude 0 outside that band. Nuclei at positions with Larmor frequencies inside the band are excited; nuclei with Larmor frequencies outside are not excited. This results in a slab of excited nuclei transverse to the z-axis, with the depth of the slab corresponding to the support of the Fourier transform of the RF excitation. The thickness of the slab can be changed by changing either the time constant of the sinc or the gradient strength. The z position of the slab can be changed by changing the center frequency of the RF pulse. More general amplitude profiles would require more complicated RF pulses with a different balance of Fourier components.

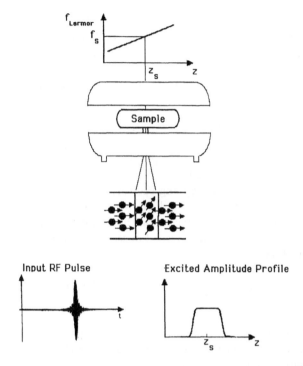

Figure 12.4
Selective excitation of a slice in the sample. A magnetic gradient is imposed along the z direction of the sample, making the resonant frequency vary linearly with position. A narrowband RF excitation tips only those nuclei whose resonant frequencies correspond to frequency components in the excitation; only these nuclei precess and produce signal. The resulting amplitude profile along the z-axis is approximated by the Fourier transform of the RF pulse.

Obtaining a precisely shaped excited amplitude profile along the z-axis can be nontrivial due to nonlinearities in the physical system; to first order, one makes the RF pulse equal to the Fourier transform of the desired amplitude profile as a function of z. See [13, 23, 32, 39, 65] for some discussions of the general excitation problem.

At the end of the RF excitation, the z gradient is turned off and the output signal is measured. The result is a sinusoidal signal obtained by summing the contributions of all the excited spins now precessing again at the common $f_{Larmor} = \gamma \|\mathbf{H}_0\|$. The amplitude contributed from spins near a given plane $z = z_0$ depends on :

- The number of spins there, $\rho(z_0)\Delta z$, where $\rho(z)$ denotes the density of nuclei along the z-axis.

- The excitation amplitude at $z = z_0$, $A(z_0)$, determined by how much RF excitation was provided to that position ($\approx$ the Fourier component of the RF pulse at frequency $\gamma(H_0 + G_z)$).

Essentially, the output signal looks like a weighted sum of the spin density:

$$S_A(t) = \int A(z)\rho(z)e^{i\gamma H_0 t}\, dz = \langle A, \rho \rangle e^{i\gamma H_0 t}. \tag{12.1}$$

If we choose a *basis* of amplitude profiles, we can reconstruct the density in z. As a simple example of the use of selective excitation encoding, suppose we were interested in mapping the variation of spin density along the z-axis of a sample. This could be done by selectively exciting a succession of slabs along the z-axis, and recording the signal strength from each slab. Assume the profiles are ideal boxcar functions partitioning the z-axis into slabs of width Δz :

$$\phi_k(z) = \begin{cases} 1 & \text{if } k\Delta z < z < (k+1)\Delta z \\ 0 & \text{otherwise.} \end{cases}$$

These correspond to sinc-like RF excitations applied with gradient G_z turned on; this gradient is turned off at the end of the RF pulse; we would then measure signals proportional to

$$S_k(t) = \langle \phi_k, \rho \rangle e^{i\gamma H_0 t}, \tag{12.2}$$

successively, for $k = 1, 2, \ldots, N$. This imaging process is represented schematically in Figure 12.5. After demodulating the Larmor frequency carrier, we have the projections of the spin density onto the elements of a boxcar basis or, equivalently, the averages of the spin density over the voxels determined by the partition of the z-axis. From this, we could reconstruct ρ up to the resolution Δz .

One could obtain the same information by selective excitation of different amplitude profiles, which can be done by using an appropriate RF excitation along a selection gradient as discussed above. In principle, any of a number of bases could be used as amplitude profiles for selective excitation encoding; one which has been considered for MRI is the Hadamard basis [11, 20, 22]. See Figure 12.6 for a depiction of the Hadamard basis as well as some other bases used for encoding. Orthogonality is obtained in the Hadamard encoding by weighting some portions of the spin system with amplitude $+1$ and other portions with amplitude -1. The physical meaning of weighting some spin regions with a negative amplitude is simply that phase of their precession is π radians ahead of those spins weighted with a positive amplitude.

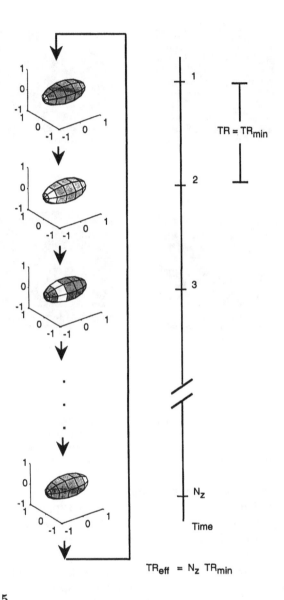

Figure 12.5
Volumetric imaging by successive excitation of slices along the z-axis. White indicates excited regions; gray regions do not produce signal. In many situations, each slice must be measured more than once. By looping through the excitations in the sequence given here, we assure that a long time passes between successive excitations of a given slice.

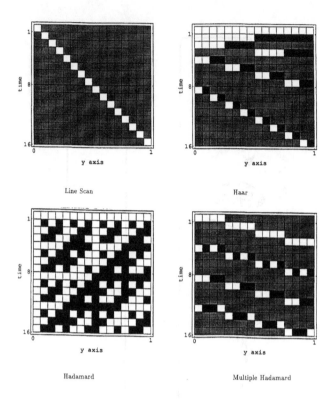

Figure 12.6
Density plots representing four orthonormal bases for encoding
an interval to a resolution of 16 pixels. Each row represents one
basis function; white represents a +1 value, black represents −1,
and gray represents 0.

The Hadamard function basis is very different from the boxcar basis in
that all of the Hadamard functions are globally supported; that is to say,
they are nonvanishing on the entire interval being encoded. This has important implications in MRI, as we shall see when we discuss the considerations
which make one basis preferable to another.

The "stack of boxcars" basis described above is commonly used in volumetric imaging to resolve the sample into slabs transverse to the z-axis, but
the variation of density with x and y in each slab is usually not constant
and remains to be mapped. This is usually done with the techniques of *fre-*
quency and phase encoding. As we shall see, these correspond to techniques
for projecting onto a Fourier basis.

Frequency Encoding

If we are interested in mapping the spin density in all three dimensions,
$\rho(x, y, z)$, we must go beyond encoding only the z-axis. This may be done as

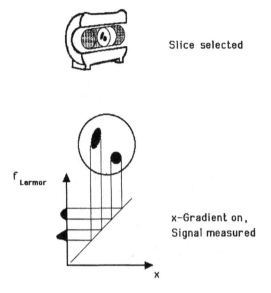

Slice selected

f_{Larmor}

x-Gradient on,
Signal measured

x

Figure 12.7
Frequency encoding the x-axis. A given slice is selectively excited, and then a magnetic gradient is imposed across the slice during signal readout and measurement. The gradient causes the Larmor frequency to vary linearly across the slice. Therefore a given frequency component of the output signal corresponds to a particular x position; its amplitude reflects the amount of precessing nuclei at that position.

follows. After selective excitation along the z-axis, as described above, the magnetic field strength is now made to vary linearly in one direction *across* the excited region, say the x direction, during the time at which output signal is being measured. The Larmor frequency in the excited region of the sample now varies linearly with x; $f_{Larmor} = f_{Larmor}(x) = \gamma(H_0 + G_x x)$, where G_x is a constant reflecting the gradient of magnetic field strength along the x direction. See Figure 12.7.

The demodulated signal output then amounts to

$$S(t) = \int dx \int dy \int dz\, \phi(z)\, \rho(x,y,z)\, e^{i\gamma G_x x t}$$

where ϕ is the amplitude profile of the selective excitation. The time samples of this signal give projections of the spin density onto the elements of a basis which look like the Fourier basis elements in the x-coordinate, constant in the y-coordinate, and have the slice profile in z:

$$S(k\Delta t) = \langle \rho, e_k \rangle$$

with

$$e_k(x, y, z) = e^{-ikx(\Delta t \gamma G_x)} \phi(z).$$

Notice this output signal gives no information about the variation of density in the y direction. It is common current practice to acquire this additional information by *phase encoding*.

Phase Encoding

In this technique one uses a magnetic gradient to build up a linear phase variation in the y direction of the excited slice, prior to frequency encoding and signal measurement. The signal output is then a modification of what we saw in the case of frequency encoding alone:

$$S_\theta(t) = \int dx \int dy \int dz \, \phi(z) \, \rho(x, y, z) \, e^{i\gamma G_x xt} \, e^{i\theta y} \qquad (12.3)$$

measured for t over a small interval of time, and θ is the constant phase gradient.

For example, in a common imaging application the profile ϕ corresponds to a thin slice near $z = z_0$. Then our signal gives us the values of the 2-D spatial Fourier transform of the spin density of that slice, $\widehat{\rho_{z_0}}(\omega_x, \omega_y)$, along one line segment through the 2-D spatial frequency plane: $\omega_x = \gamma G_x t$, $\omega_y = \theta$ for t varying over the measurement time interval.

Of course, this one signal only gives part of the information required to build up a map of the spin density within the slice. In practice, one gets more data by repeating the steps of excitation and encoding according to a specific schedule. This consists of many repetitions of the basic sequence: slice excitation, followed by phase encoding, and then finally signal measurement while frequency encoding. With each repetition, the MR scanner outputs a signal corresponding to the values along a new line of the 2-D spatial Fourier transform of the proton spin density in the slice being imaged. This is done by varying the phase gradient in the y direction from repetition to repetition. In this way, a sufficiently dense sampling of the Fourier transform of the spin density may be acquired at a rate of one line per repetition. When this is done, the spin density in the slice may be reconstructed by inverse discrete Fourier transform, up to a given resolution.

Note an important distinction between phase and frequency encoding. Frequency encoding implements the projection onto a whole range of Fourier basis elements in one signal acquisition. In a standard scanner, phase encoding usually only computes the projection onto one Fourier basis element in a given signal measurement.

12.2.3 Imaging Time and Signal-to-Noise Ratio

All imaging techniques involve a trade-off among resolution, imaging speed, and signal-to-noise ratio (SNR). SNR considerations are serious in MRI: the signals tend to be low in strength, and the primary noise source in modern scanners is thermal noise from sources other than the hardware (such as the patient), and can not be removed.

Most standard scanners can also provide only limited imaging speed. Hardware modifications can increase this, but often at the cost of resolution and contrast. This limitation can make imaging moving structures difficult, and also contributes to the rather high cost of MRI examinations.

Let us illustrate these considerations in the example of volumetric imaging which we have considered earlier. We may choose to encode a volume with a stack of N_z boxcar excitations as a basis to break the z-axis into nonoverlapping slices, as in Equation (12.2) above.

The time required to generate an image of this volume with a resolution of N_z pixels in the encoded z direction is $T_I = M_s(N_z \, TR)$ because N_z different slices must be successively excited and measured, each in a time TR. M_s is the number of times each slice must be measured; this will be more than one if the density within the slice is to be resolved with standard phase encoding; it can also take into account repetitions for signal averaging if the SNRs in the images are too low and one is forced to average images to reduce noise. In practice, M_s is almost always greater than one, i.e., each slice must be called on more than once to give a signal. The overall imaging time now depends critically on the resting time between successive excitations of a given group of spins and on the ordering of the excitations.

The resting time is an important parameter in determining signal strength and image contrast. It is typically much larger than the time for which usable signal can be measured from a given group of spins. This resting time is required to allow the precessing magnetization to realign via (slow) T_1 relaxation with the static magnetic field $\mathbf{H}_0$; otherwise, there is little signal produced by the next excitation of these spins. This is the primary obstruction to fast imaging.

The minimum possible time interval between successive signal measurements, TR_{min} is determined by hardware considerations and the particular type of contrast weighting; for a T_2 weighted image it might be around 100 ms, whereas the resting time for a given group of spins needs to be about 2500 ms.

In this situation, the ordering of the signal measurements has a critical impact on the total imaging time. We know we must obtain M_s signals from each slice, and that a relatively long resting time must be allowed to elapse between the successive excitation and signal measurements from this slice. In this case, the time difference between TR_{min} and the (order of magnitude longer) resting time need not be wasted. Other slices can be

imaged during that time, one after the other, while allowing the first slice
a sufficient recuperation interval.

This idea is indicated schematically in Figure 12.5. In this approach, the
slices in the stack along the z-axis are excited and measured sequentially,
one every TR_{min} seconds. This sequence of measurements obtains from
each slice the first of the M_s signals it must contribute. When the last
slice is finished, we return to the top of the stack and start over, obtaining
the second signal required of each slice. The loop is repeated M_s times to
obtain all the required measurements from each slice.

Suppose the number of slices along the z-axis to be imaged is N_z. Although we conduct a measurement every TR_{min} seconds, the effective resting time for a *given* slice of spins is much longer: $TR_{eff} = N_z TR_{min}$. The
effective time cost per slice is then:

$$\frac{T_I}{N_z} = TR_{min} M_s.$$

Note, however, that a single slice could not be imaged in T_I/N_z; T_I must
be used to get a batch of N_z slices.

The effective repetition time, $N_z TR_{min}$, can be made very large by dividing the sample into a large number of slices. However, this has its cost in
SNR as we shall now see. The signal in an imaging experiment is proportional to the number of spins contributing to the signal. Signal is therefore
proportional to voxel size, and so resolution is purchased at the cost of
lowered signal. The noise may be modeled as white noise within the sampled bandwidth. The larger the gradients used, the larger the bandwidth
and so the noise power. Signal strength is also determined by the timing
parameters. For example, longer TR buys more signal.

Let us examine these SNR considerations in our example. We encoded
with a stack of N_z boxcar excitations as a basis to break the z-axis into
nonoverlapping slices, as in Figure 12.5. Applying the time-sharing described above, the effective repetition time experienced by any slice is
$N_z TR_{min}$, which will be large if there are many slices. However, as the
number of slices goes up, their width decreases, and so does the signal
strength obtained from each one. This eventually becomes prohibitive.

On the other hand, we might instead encode the z-axis with amplitude
profiles from the Hadamard basis. Again we wish to resolve the z-axis into
N_z pixels of equal width, but now encode by exciting all of these pixels
at once with profiles corresponding to the elements of a Hadamard basis
on these N_z pixels; see Figure 12.8. Each Hadamard encode yields signal
from the entire sample at once, which leads to a good SNR. In fact, in some
sense the Hadamard encoding is optimal in this respect, as may be seen from
standard considerations of statistical weighing designs [56]. However, any
time-sharing possibility is precluded; since all of the spins in the sample are

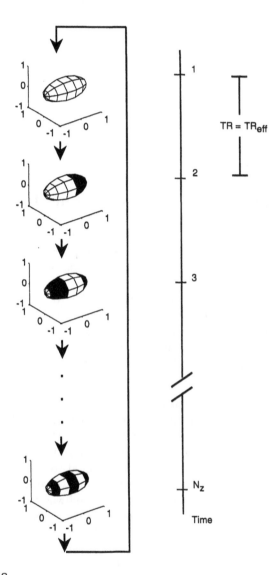

Figure 12.8
Volumetric imaging by Hadamard encoding the z-axis. Each encode excites the entire sample with an amplitude profile drawn from the Hadamard basis. White corresponds to $+1$ amplitude, black to -1. The global excitation produces good SNR, but longer imaging times than the line-scanning approach in Figure 12.4.

excited on every encode, we must wait a long TR time between successive excitations in order to get decent signal strength. In general this will force a big increase in imaging time.

These approaches represent two extremes with respect to the critical figures of merit of SNR and imaging time. The question naturally arises as to whether there is any practical way to interpolate between these two extremes. We take up this issue now.

12.3   Adapted Waveform Encoding in MRI

One may greatly expand the number of possible bases of amplitude profiles used in MR encoding by utilizing more general RF pulses and gradient sequences. Here we consider some particular bases for encoding this way, and give some criteria for choosing the basis for a given imaging situation. We will use the term *adapted waveform encoding* to refer to the measurement of projections of the spin density onto bases tailored to the imaging requirements of a particular task. In this section, we consider the advantages and disadvantages these new schemes offer over more conventional approaches to MRI, such as the volumetric slicing by encoding with the boxcar basis or Hadamard encoding described previously.

In order to make this comparison, we must describe some of the considerations of wavelet and adapted waveform encoding. We offer a discussion of some important implementation details, such as the need for bases comprised of smooth profiles. We present some important properties and figures of merit to be applied in choosing a basis suited to a particular imaging task. In particular, we summarize the results of a quantitative analysis of the signal-to-noise issues associated with adapted waveform encoding, and compare this to SNR computations for more conventional schemes. We present results concerning the tradeoff of SNR for effective repetition time, TR_{eff}, a parameter related to imaging speed and image contrast. This gives us a quantitative measure to employ in the evaluation of encoding schemes and to use in our efforts to balance the various requirements of a particular imaging task.

The tailored sequences we design through these considerations allow us to obtain useful images by accommodating a priori information about the type of scan and the particular information we are seeking. We conclude the section by sketching some possible applications of the techniques of these methods.

12.3.1 MRI Encoding with a Basis

In the last section we discussed standard MRI encoding schemes which employed boxcar or Hadamard bases for the excited amplitude profiles in selective excitation. Wavelet-encoded MRI and, more generally, adapted waveform-encoded MRI are simple variants of these techniques which address the imaging time problem and several other issues.

We may encode any given direction by selective excitation along a magnetic gradient in that direction. Each RF pulse excites the spin density with a wavelet or more general waveform-shaped excitation profile along the encoded axis. The signal produced is the inner product of the excited profile and the spin density along the encoded axis:

$$S_j(t) = \left(\int dx \int dy \int dz\, \rho(x,y,z)\psi_j(y) \right) e^{i\gamma H_0 t}. \qquad (12.4)$$

Here we have chosen to encode the y-axis with an amplitude profile given by the jth element of a basis. Any direction could be encoded in the same way. We can then reconstruct the projection of the spin density onto the encoded axis from these measurements in the usual fashion.

Note that we can frequency encode another axis with no cost in time by turning on a readout gradient in, say, the x direction during signal measurement. There are several slice selection techniques that can be used [2, 42] to additionally localize to a slice perpendicular to the z direction; this type of encoding could also be applied in 3-D imaging, using phase encoding to localize the third direction.

Example: Wavelet Encoding

In [25] we described some of the benefits associated with choosing the set of excited profiles to be an orthogonal wavelet basis. This technique has since been studied by several other research groups [48, 49].

Wavelet encoding produces an (idealized) output signal which is the wavelet transform of the spin distribution $\rho(x,y)$ measured by exciting spins with a sequence of RF pulses at correct dilations and translations:

$$S_{j,k}(t) = \int dx \int dy\, \rho(x,y)\psi_{j,k}(y)e^{i\gamma G_x x t}, \qquad (12.5)$$

with

$$\psi_{j,k}(y) = \psi\left(\frac{x}{2^j} - k\right),$$

with $(j,k) \in \mathbb{Z}^2$. Note the lack of the usual normalizing factor for the scaled wavelets. This reflects the fact that the peak amplitude of the excitation profile is limited in MRI; we can not exceed this limit at our will. In order

to obtain as much signal as possible, all scales of wavelets are normalized
to this peak amplitude, and the energy normalization is applied in the
reconstruction. This can lead to low SNRs, as we'll see in detail later;
intuitively, this is clear from the fact that amplitude profiles corresponding
to the fine-scale wavelets have localized support and so produce less signal
than coarse scale profiles which excite a larger group of spins.

Nevertheless, wavelet encoding works reasonably well in practice, and
the SNR figure of merit proves to be unduly pessimistic in many circumstances. This is because the wavelet transform tends to concentrate energy
in coefficients corresponding to edges. These features tend to remain above
the noise floor [61]; the resulting image can be very useful, particularly for
locating (oriented) edges.

In our previous work we noted the following advantages of wavelet encoding over phase encoding:

- Reduced ringing caused by partial volume effects (Gibbs ringing).

- Immunity to motion artifacts. Motion of the object over the course
  of standard Fourier based image acquisition causes small inconsistencies in the measurement of the spatial Fourier transform. Traditional Fourier transform reconstruction spreads the misregistered
  signal all the way across the image; the basis functions of the expansion are not local, so the effect of the error is global. This is
  much reduced with wavelet encoding due to the localization of the
  basis elements. See Figure 12.9.

- Novel time-sharing or scheduling possibilities for certain types of
  examinations. Since each wavelet amplitude profile excites only a
  portion of the field of view, we schedule the sequence of excitations so that successive excitations involve spatially nonoverlapping
  bands. This means that we can use a very short TR and yet any
  given spin will experience a much longer *effective TR*, TR_{eff}, between excitations.

This last result is analogous to the multislice time-sharing concept discussed at the end of Section 12.2. However, the scheduling problem in
this case is considerably more interesting because the excited regions have
varying sizes, corresponding to the various scales. Our previous work constructed optimal schedules, so that for an $N \times N$ resolution Haar wavelet-
encoded image

$$TR_{eff} = \left[\frac{N-2}{\log_2 N - 1} \right] TR,$$

was possible. We found that a speedup of about a factor of 3 was possible
for images in which it was necessary to obtain a few slices with T_1 effects

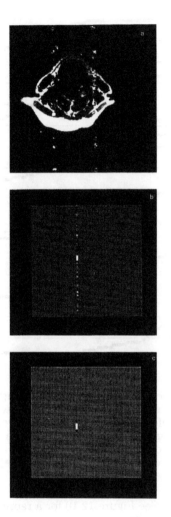

Figure 12.9
Motion artifacts in phase encoding vs. wavelet coding. (a) An axial MR image of the neck. The noisy vertical stripes through the
image are caused by the movement of the carotid arteries due to
the pulsing blood. The artifact is in the phase-encoded direction.
(b) A computer-simulated phase-encoded image of a square body
with a single bright pixel moving as the encoding is obtained.
The bright spot moves randomly from echo to echo within a 6
pixel-length radius of its initial position. The artifact generated
is in the phase-encoding direction, and occupies the entire length
of the reconstruction. (c) A computer-simulated wavelet-encoded
image of a square body with a single bright pixel moving as the
encoding is obtained, exactly as before. The artifact generated is
much smaller than the phase-encoded artifact.

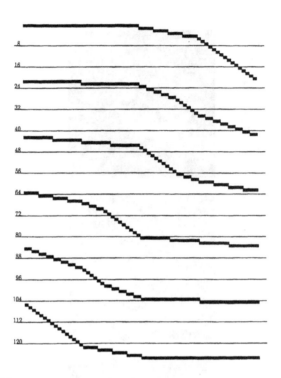

Figure 12.10
Optimal excitation schedule in Haar encoding of 128 pixels. Each
row represents one step of the encoding; a time TR_{min} elapses
between each pair of rows. The darkened region in a given row
indicates the subinterval to be excited with a Haar profile on that
encoding step. Notice that the excitations are arranged so that
a given subinterval can rest many steps between its successive
excitations.

de-emphasized [16, 25]. See Figure 12.10 for a representation of an optimal
schedule in the case $N = 128$.

We have used wavelet-encoding schemes of various types with a standard
GE Signa 1.5 T (tesla) scanner. Figure 12.11 shows an example image
produced with this method. This figure shows an actual wavelet-encoded
MR image of a calibration phantom obtained at one scale of wavelet encoding. The phantom itself is a large block of plexiglass with various other
materials (water doped with copper sulfate, air) embedded in it to produce
arrays of shapes in various sizes and orientations. This is placed in the
scanner and imaged for testing purposes. In the case of Figure 12.11, notice that wavelet encoding preferentially images edges oriented along the
wavelet-encoded direction. This feature of wavelet encoding should prove
useful in several applications, such as angiography and heart wall tracking
as described in [27, 61, 62]. We now briefly sketch another potential use.

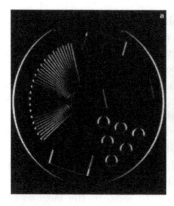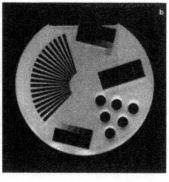

Figure 12.11
An MR calibration phantom image. (a) Image formed from only
the smallest scale of wavelet encoding. This is essentially an image
using an edge-sensitive RF pulse. No signal is produced from
homogeneous material. Signal is produced from vertical edges.
This is useful for oriented edge detection. (b) Full image of the
phantom.

Application of Wavelet Encoding in MR Phosphorus Spectroscopy

MR spectroscopy provides a method of studying physiology by providing
information about the proportions of certain important chemical species
and their distribution in the tissue of interest. In spectroscopy, the *chemical shift* of each signal provides information about the various molecules
contributing to the signal.

In particular, phosphorus spectroscopy makes use of the different chemical shifts of different phosphorus compounds to detect the relative amounts
of these compounds in a given region. This has shown great promise in
studying the metabolism of both cancer and heart disease. The physiology
of tissue can be studied by observing the phosphorus compounds such as
ADP, ATP, and inorganic phosphate [6, 52]. For example, spectroscopy
allows the pH of a tissue to be measured; pH has been linked to tissue
insult. Spectroscopy of cardiac function is particularly promising, as it is
very difficult to predict how permanent the damage to cardiac tissue will
be from the temporary loss of perfusion [44, 45].

The chemical shift is due to the slight variation of Larmor frequency
among the various phosphorus compounds. This is a consequence of the
fact that the magnetic field each phosphorus nucleus feels is the sum of
the static magnetic field of the scanner and the fields produced by the surrounding atoms. Consequently, the local Larmor frequency at the nucleus
of a phosphorus atom is affected by the particular atoms it is bonded to.
For example, the phosphorus in ATP produces three spectral peaks in the

signal that represent the three phosphates in ATP. ADP has two of the peaks but lacks the third because one phosphate is missing. As a result, a phosphorus spectrum allows the relative amounts of ATP, ADP, phospho-creatin, and inorganic phosphorus to be estimated from the relative sizes of the peaks. Changes in the relative concentrations can provide information about the damage produced by ischemia or hypoxia. The relative amount of lactate that is present can be estimated from the hydrogen spectra. Lactate is produced during glycolysis, so it reflects the oxygen supply to the tissue and is thought to cause a drop in pH.

Spectra are acquired with no gradient fields because the Larmor frequency is being used to measure small chemical shifts instead of position; i.e., frequency encoding can not be used to localize the various contributions to the spectra. This is unfortunate; localization is important because physiology changes with blood supply and tissue type. Therefore, several different methods have been devised for localizing the volume from which each spectrum is obtained [1, 33]. The signal from a small coil can be used when the coil is small enough to be sensitive to a limited volume. Alternately, a single volume can be localized by exciting the spins with a series of slice-selective RF pulses all in orthogonal planes. Another common technique is one- or two-dimensional chemical shift imaging (CSI). CSI uses phase encoding to localize the spectra. The problem here is always the balance between SNR and localization. The signal in spectroscopy is small because the amount of each chemical is relatively small and the sensitivities of phosphorus and of the elements are small compared to that of hydrogen. As a result, spatial resolution is always poor and the acquisition times are long. Hadamard encoding was developed to localize the signal while maintaining the signal-to-noise ratio in the spectra [20, 22], and still is actively pursued [10, 21].

Wavelet encoding promises improvement over other localization methods in spectroscopy. First, the effective TR can be made very long. Phosphorus spectroscopy requires T_1 effects to be relatively small so a long effective TR would be very helpful, especially considering the long T_1 of phosphorus [34]. Wavelet-encoding schemes can be designed to have a long effective TR and to offer low spectral leakage. Reduced spectral leakage is important for improving the quantitation of the spectra. Quantitation is important in applications like finding the ratios of peak sizes which are used in many applications: e.g., for measurements of the pH of the tissue. Spectral leakage is often a major source of error in the ratios. For example, when phosphorus signal from skeletal muscle in the chest wall leaks into the spectra from the myocardium, the ratios become contaminated.

Encoding with Other Bases

So far, we have mentioned three rather different sorts of bases for use in waveform encoding. First and simplest is the basis of boxcars used in multislice volumetric imaging. This is also sometimes referred to in MRI as the technique of *line scanning*. Here, one simply divides the axis to be encoded into narrow strips, and excites one strip on each repetition. Next we discussed an encoding technique in which excited profiles from the Hadamard basis were used instead of boxcar functions. This has been proposed for use in MRI by various groups [11, 20, 22]. In contrast to the boxcar basis, all of the Hadamard basis functions are globally supported on the image, and so offer a different set of advantages and disadvantages. Finally we mentioned our previous work on wavelet encoding which used the well-known Haar wavelets for simplicity of presentation.

These three bases represent very different approaches to encoding in MRI. In line scanning, the excited profiles are zero over most of the encoded interval, so that only a small band of nuclei is excited by each repetition. This can be exploited to increase the effective repetition time experienced by any group of spins and to reduce motion artifacts. However, line scanning suffers a much reduced SNR compared to Hadamard encoding. As originally proposed, wavelet encoding with Haar wavelets steered a middle ground between Hadamard encoding and line scanning, using basis elements more localized (on average) than Hadamard functions, but less so than line scanning.

Despite the obvious differences, these bases are all drawn from a common family of bases, all comprised of piecewise constant waveforms, called the Haar-Hadamard library [12]. The term *library* in this context refers to a large collection of bases linked together by some defining common feature. In the familiar case of bases for time domain signals, a given basis from a library can be interpreted as providing a particular tiling of the time-frequency plane. Some of the bases offer better localization in time at the cost of poorer localization in frequency. Some of the bases make this trade-off in a flexible fashion across the time-frequency plane. Some standard bases and their associated tilings are represented in Figure 12.12.

Beyond the three bases we have already considered, there are many others to choose from in the Haar-Hadamard library, such as the dilated multiple Hadamard basis represented in Figure 12.6. We can use the freedom to choose bases from within this library to meet certain design criteria. The variety of adapted waveform bases allow us to construct customized encoding schemes that trade SNR against other useful imaging parameters: longer TR_{eff}, reduced motion artifacts, and reduced Gibbs ringing. We may choose a basis of localized elements to prolong the TR_{eff}, or a less localized basis to increase the SNR. We may also consider compromise bases, comprised of local elements in some regions of the field of view (FOV), and of more globally supported profiles in other regions.

Just as important is the freedom to consider other libraries entirely, and in particular libraries comprised of smooth waveforms. The existence of smooth libraries proves to be essential for practical implementation of wave-

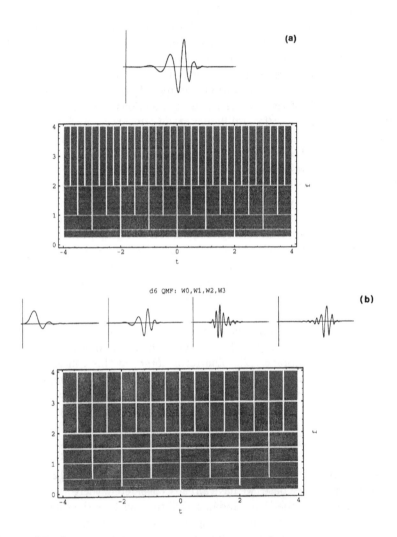

Figure 12.12
(a) Dilations and translations of a Daubechies wavelet on a dyadic grid produce an orthonormal wavelet basis corresponding to the tiling of the time-frequency plane. Note this basis offers better time resolution at high frequencies at the cost of poor frequency resolution. (b) The defining relation for this wavelet may be used to produce a family of related wavelet packets, the first four of which are shown here. Dilations and translations of these may be used to produce a wavelet packet basis with better midrange frequency resolution than the wavelet basis, as seen in the time-frequency tiling.

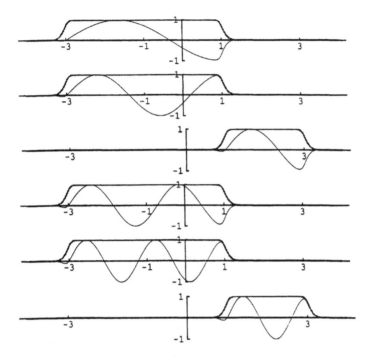

Figure 12.13
Some elements of a local cosine basis associated with a partition
of the interval $[-3, 1]$ into subintervals $[-3, -1]$ and $[-1, 1]$.

form encoding. The considerations for choosing an encoding basis from
within one of these libraries closely parallel those indicated in the case of
the Haar-Hadamard library.

An important family of smooth bases for use in adapted waveform encoding is provided by the local trigonometric library [64]. The local trigonometric bases provide something like an adaptive, orthogonal version of the
short-time Fourier transform decomposition. Given any partition of the
encoded axis into disjoint intervals, one can cut up the spin density along
that axis into pieces living (essentially) on the various intervals. An orthogonal sine or cosine basis is then employed for each interval to represent the
harmonic content of the part of the signal living on that interval. This construction limits spectral leakage by utilizing smooth cutoff windows while
nevertheless maintaining orthogonality by a clever parity construction.

Local trigonometric bases can be designed which localize the encode axis
into many short intervals, into a small number of larger intervals, or into
intervals of various sizes. This yields a whole library of different orthogonal
bases, permitting us to represent the density along the encode axis in many
different ways. One may then determine the best encoding from this set for
a particular signal, or class of signals. We will take advantage of this prop-

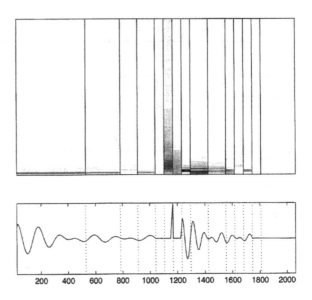

Figure 12.14
The partition determining a local cosine basis may be chosen
adaptively to give an optimal representation of a specific signal.
Here is the partition chosen for a particular test signal. Note the
use of short subintervals for transients, and longer intervals for
relatively stationary portions of the signal.

erty in Section 12.4. See Figure 12.13 for some local cosine basis elements
corresponding to a particular partition of the field of view; Figure 12.14
shows a partition corresponding to a best local cosine basis for representing
a specific signal.

We now examine more closely the process of fitting our encoding scheme
to the task at hand, and give examples of the trade-offs which can be
effected by choosing bases appropriately.

12.3.2   Figures of Merit in Adapted Waveform Encoding

Here we summarize the SNR and repetition time performance of wavelet
encoding and adapted waveform encoding relative to more standard encoding techniques in MRI. We can quantify these and obtain useful figures of
merit for use in the design of adapted waveform-encoding schemes.

SNR Analysis

We sketch quantitative average signal-to-noise results for adapted waveform encoding [61]. Suppose that the object to be imaged is encoded
by exciting a finite selection of profiles from an adapted waveform basis
$\{\psi_j \mid j = 1, \ldots, N\}$. As indicated earlier, these profiles are normalized so

that they all have the same peak amplitude. This reflects the physical constraints of the MR encoding scheme.

In our applications, the basis consists of orthogonal, but not necessarily orthonormal profiles; the procedure below can be generalized beyond this assumption. We wish to obtain the best possible reconstruction of the spin density consistent with the N projections onto the encoding basis, and to have a measure of the SNR in that reconstruction.

We may reduce the reconstruction to the one dimensional estimation problem: estimate $\rho(z)$ in $L_2[0, 1]$ from the N-vector of noisy measurements

$$\mathbf{m} = \mathcal{W}_N\rho + \mathbf{n}, \quad \mathcal{W}_N\rho = \begin{pmatrix} \langle \psi_1, \rho \rangle \\ \vdots \\ \langle \psi_N, \rho \rangle \end{pmatrix}, \tag{12.6}$$

with $\mathbf{n}$ a Gaussian random vector of known covariance R modeling the noise in the measurement process.

A simple and standard procedure is provided by the Gauss-Markoff least squares estimate (the same as the maximum likelihood estimate in this case); namely, the reconstruction estimate $\hat{\rho}$ is chosen to minimize the expected squared error functional $\mathrm{E}\left(\|\rho - \hat{\rho}\|^2\right)$ [30, 38]. This error has both a random and deterministic component: even if the noise were not present we could not expect our estimator to make up for the information about ρ which is lost by taking only finitely many measurements with $\mathcal{W}_N$.

We therefore consider estimates (reconstructions) which lie in the subspace that we do have information about; that is, we restrict our attention to minimum bias estimators. Further, we shall consider only *linear* estimators $\hat{\rho} = L\mathbf{m}$ defined by linear operators L chosen such that the bias $\mathrm{E}(\hat{\rho} - \rho)$ is as small as possible in energy.

If we assume independent identically distributed errors, $R = \sigma^2 I$, it is easy to show that the estimator has a simple form: $\hat{\rho} = \mathcal{W}_N^+\mathbf{m}$, where $\mathcal{W}_N^+$ denotes the pseudo-inverse of the operator $\mathcal{W}_N$ [8, 47]. Further, in our applications, the basis of excited profiles ψ_j may usually be taken to be orthogonal, though not always orthonormal. In this case, one easily verifies that:

$$\hat{\rho} = \sum_{l=1}^{N} \frac{m_l}{\|\psi_l\|^2} \psi_l. \tag{12.7}$$

The mean squared error has a bias term, reflecting the incomplete measurements, and a variance term given by

$$\mathrm{Trace}\left(\mathcal{W}_N^+ \sigma^2 (\mathcal{W}_N^+)^*\right) = \sigma^2 \, \mathrm{Trace}\,(\mathcal{W}_N^* \mathcal{W}_N)^+ = \sigma^2 \sum_{l=1}^{N} \frac{1}{\|\psi_l\|^2}. \tag{12.8}$$

We may use this latter figure of merit to compare the signal-to-noise performance of the image reconstructions associated to the different members of a class of encoding schemes $\{\mathcal{W}_N\}$ so long as they all share the same bias properties. For example, line scanning, Haar encoding, and Hadamard encoding for a given number of pixels will all have the same bias, as will any other scheme from the Haar-Hadamard library, but they will have very different variance behaviors. Alternately, we could encode with a basis from a library of smooth wavelet packets, such as the one depicted in Figure 12.12. Again, it is possible to show that all bases in this library have the same bias when reconstructions in terms of these bases are truncated at a fixed scale. Therefore the best basis is again determined by comparing variance behavior.

For a simple illustration, we consider the signal-to-noise comparison of line scanning, Haar wavelet encoding, and Hadamard encoding, all of which have been previously proposed for MRI. While these profiles are not as practical as smoother libraries, they do give a simple illustration of results that generalize without much trouble to smoother libraries.

This class of examples is nice in that the encoding may be viewed as a discrete problem, by replacing the continuous spin density with step function approximants. The analysis of the noise then reduces to the well-studied field of weighing designs [11, 56]. As it is easy to see, the operator $\mathcal{W}_N$ is replaced by a matrix W_N, the design matrix of the encoding scheme. Design matrices for some of the standard examples of encoding schemes considered in this chapter can be found in Figure 12.6. The values in the matrices are restricted to $+1$, 0, and -1; this reflects the fact that the encoded profiles are normalized by peak amplitude rather than by total energy.

A comparison of the scaling properties of signal-to-noise with the number of voxels for these three basic encoding schemes is given in Figure 12.15. Hadamard encoding has about the same signal-to-noise performance as phase encoding, and Haar encoding has SNR performance analogous to encoding with other wavelet-based schemes. Note that Hadamard encoding is optimal for this measure of signal-to-noise, line scanning is very poor, and wavelet encoding is intermediate. Similar considerations and results similar to those of the previous example apply to the case of smooth waveforms.

There are limitations on the interpretation of this type of SNR measure in the particular case of wavelet encoding, as we now indicate. We shall see that the location of an edge in wavelet encoding can be done with reasonable SNR, due to the localization of the energy of the edge in the wavelet transform domain. In contrast, the signal from an edge in the phase-encoded Fourier transform domain is dispersed. Therefore, while wavelet encoding suffers a drop in average SNR compared to phase encoding, the localization of the signal partially compensates for the loss in SNR at an edge.

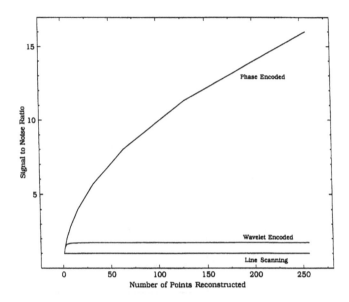

Figure 12.15
Signal-to-noise curves for line scan, Haar, and phase or Hadamard encoding. SNR curve normalized to that of line scanning.

We can see this property of wavelet encoding by means of a simple example. In Figure 12.16 we contrast the phase-encoded and wavelet-encoded data produced by a one-pixel impulse in the object being imaged. The phase encoding produces data which is the Fourier transform of the impulse; its energy is spread out over the entire possible domain of the phase-encoded data, as represented by the DFT in the picture. On the other hand, wavelet encoding produces data which is an (un-normalized) wavelet transform of the impulse, and so is concentrated at one position in each scale.

One consequence of the lack of energy normalization is that the energy of the coefficients of the wavelet-encoded impulse is smaller than the original impulse energy. This is in contrast to phase encoding, which preserves the impulse energy. So we see again that the poor average SNR for wavelet encoding comes from the constraints of MRI which prevent us from normalizing the energy of the finer scale wavelets. In fact, the total energy in each scale of the wavelet encoding of the impulse drops relative to the total energy of the background noise at that scale. However, when encoding the impulse, that energy is concentrated at one position in each scale; therefore the *amplitude* of the corresponding coefficient does not drop with scale. In fact, the amplitude of any nonvanishing coefficient in the wavelet-encoded representation of the impulse is the same as the amplitude of the coefficients in its phase encoding.

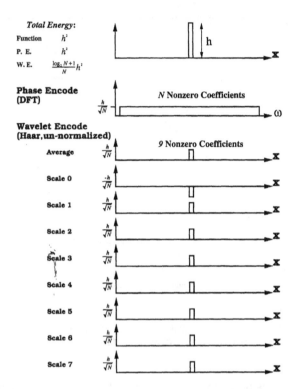

Figure 12.16
A comparison of phase (Fourier) encoding (P.E.) with wavelet
encoding (W.E.) of an impulse. W.E. concentrates the energy
of the impulse energy at a given position throughout the scales,
whereas P.E. disperses the energy over the entire range of frequencies. The concentration of energy in W.E. makes edge localization better than one might expect from the average SNR
calculations.

On the other hand, the standard deviation of the noise contribution is
the same at any position in either phase encoding or wavelet encoding. This
shows that in this case the wavelet-encoded representation of the impulse
sticks out above the noise just as well as the phase-encoded representation
does.

We have found that this sort of phenomenon enables us to pick out fine-
scale structures of interest out of the noise by means of postprocessing techniques like those presented in [27]. Further discussion of this phenomenon
may be found in [61].

Scheduling, Imaging Time, and Motion Artifacts
From the perspective of average SNR alone, there is no reason to choose
anything other than basis functions with the largest possible support. This
would suggest using only phase encoding or Hadamard encoding.

However, in many cases the true situation is much more interesting; there are, in fact, powerful reasons for using more localized basis elements, as we have indicated in our previous work on wavelet encoding. It is desirable to quantify some of the benefits and detriments of localized bases, in order to design compromise bases that perform well for given imaging schemes. We can then choose bases which strike the correct balance between localized profiles and global profiles. In practice, we always choose the optimal basis from a library of smooth bases whose functions can be localized in space as well as in spatial frequency, the latter determining the RF pulse length as discussed a bit later.

Localized encoding has many benefits, including the reduction of artifacts caused by motion or undersampling effects. For example, in phase-encoded images, any motion at a localized position can cause a serious global motion artifact in the phase-encoded direction. A slight variation of a portion of the image from one signal to the next causes slight errors in the measurement of the Fourier coefficients by phase encoding. These errors are spread in reconstruction, due to the global nature of the Fourier basis elements. This is much reduced in wavelet encoding, for example. An example of this was seen in Figure 12.9. We have found that this feature may be of use in a cardiac edge tracking application [27].

Another important figure of merit is contrast per unit imaging time; the ratio TR_{eff}/TR has direct bearing on this. As we have seen in the case of wavelet encoding, we may schedule localized excitations in such a way that a given region of the sample is allowed to rest for many repetition times TR while other, remote portions of the sample are queried.

The solution of the excitation scheduling problem is an interesting combinatorial result in the case of wavelets and wavelet packets, and has been partially solved [16, 25]. For smooth wavelets, the problem is complicated by the overlap of the wavelets at a given scale. Nevertheless, some simple schedules may be obtained for smooth libraries. These schedules may be constructed to obtain a good TR_{eff}/TR ratio whenever the basis elements are well localized. It is particularly easy to deal with local trigonometric bases, which may be chosen subordinate to any particular partition of the field of view and have a constant overlap.

12.3.3   Choosing a Basis for Encoding

The ratio TR_{eff}/TR is a useful figure of merit for several MRI applications, such as spectroscopy, described earlier. Using this and the previously described SNR calculations to quantify image noise, we may try to jointly optimize these over the bases of a given library.

For example, as originally proposed, wavelet encoding used the largest scale scaling function and $\log_2 N$ wavelet scales to encode N pixels. Half of the excited profiles correspond to wavelets of a very small size (two pixels), leading to the SNR problems we discussed above. Alternately, the SNR can be increased by using an encoding basis in which the smallest excitation is larger than in wavelet encoding. The easiest way to do that is to use sequency rather than scale to encode the fine details. For example, one can obtain better SNR without losing too much of the benefit of localized support by dividing the FOV into subregions and Hadamard encoding the subregions. A density matrix for one of these bases may be found in Figure 12.6

Figure 12.17 presents the SNR and TR_{eff} curves for some of these Haar-Hadamard wavelet packet bases. Note how these curves interpolate between those given earlier for line scan, Haar encoding, and Hadamard encoding. This permits the tradeoff of these two parameters, which is an important degree of freedom in some applications.

Other choices of adapted bases in encoding may be made in other situations. For instance, note that the localization of artifacts in the reconstructed image due to localized object motion can be accomplished without the poor SNR of line scanning and wavelet encoding. This may be done by using localized basis elements in the vicinity of the moving region and more global elements elsewhere.

Explicit analysis of signal to noise and TR_{eff} generalizes in a fairly straightforward manner to smooth bases. As we now see, these are actually of great practical interest in MRI due to implementation considerations.

12.3.4   Implementation of Adapted Waveform Encoding

From the implementation point of view, a disadvantage of the Haar-Hadamard library is the fact that all of its functions have discontinuities, or equivalently, poor localization in the frequency domain. This greatly increases the duration of the RF pulse required to produce these shaped excited profiles, which can cause great difficulties. In fact, our simulations for Haar wavelet encoding required RF pulses as long as 20 ms [62]; RF pulses commonly used in MRI are 3 ms to 8 ms long. Longer RF pulses can cause significant difficulties in MRI. The RF power amplifier and the gradient amplifiers are usually not built to withstand long pulses. The echo time is necessarily lengthened by long RF pulses; long echo times produce necessarily T_2 weighted images, which is often undesirable, and long echo times eliminate signal from spins that decay swiftly. More important, the excited profile is degraded by the T_2^* decay during the RF pulse; the decay could be compensated for if all the spins experienced the same decay, but images will always have spins with many decay rates. This implies that the excited profiles obtained with long RF pulses are always degraded, which is unpleasant since wavelet encoding depends on accurate excited profiles. Many techniques have been employed to reduce the RF pulse length required to obtain a given profile [31, 50] and to generate more accurate

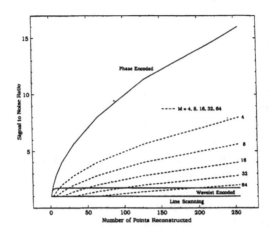

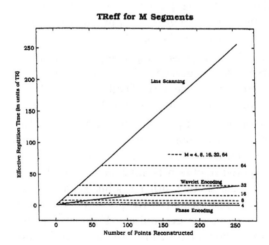

Figure 12.17
SNR and TR_{eff} results for one family of Haar-Hadamard wavelet
packet bases obtained by Hadamard encoding M segments of the
FOV.

excited profiles [13, 23, 39, 54, 65]. Hadamard encoding faces the same problems [20, 22, 54]: long RF pulses and the resulting inaccurate excited profiles. Some of the pulse-shaping techniques developed for Hadamard encoding may mitigate the long RF problem.

However, there is a simpler alternative to Haar-Hadamard encoding available in the smooth wavelet packet libraries associated with the wide variety of smooth wavelet bases that have been discovered [12, 14, 15, 40, 46]. Alternately, we may use the local trigonometric libraries of Coifman and Meyer [12]. These smooth libraries offer many of the same useful features as the Haar-Hadamard library, such as localization, and obviate the RF problems, as they provide good localization simultaneously in the space and spatial frequency domains. As indicated above, the localization in the frequency domain corresponds to shorter RF pulses.

Given the desired excited profile for use in waveform encoding, we can estimate the length of the RF pulse required to make it. A common approach is to linearize the actual procedure which requires solving the Bloch equations [5] governing the dynamics of the magnetization. The linearization, corresponding to low tip angles, gives a Fourier transform relationship between the excited profile and the RF pulse. For example, with the first-order approximation, the RF pulse used to generate a boxcar excited profile is given by a sinc in time. This first approximation can then be improved by various iterative schemes if desired.

We compared the RF pulse length required by wavelet encoding with several smoother wavelet bases to the the requirements of the Haar basis. For this study, we present one of the Daubechies family of wavelets, [14, 15], the Battle-Lemarié wavelet [40], and the Meyer wavelet [46].

We begin with the low tip angle approximation of the Bloch equations described earlier. This approximation is used to estimate the length of the RF pulse required to excite an accurate wavelet profile. The time scale is that required to obtain 1-mm resolution with magnetic gradients of 10 mT/m (milliTesla/meter); other resolutions and times can be obtained by simple scaling. The estimated RF pulse was cut off at different lengths to produce a set of shorter RF pulses. These shorter RF pulses were put through an inverse Fourier transform to estimate the resulting solutions of the Bloch equations, and the error in the estimate of the excited profile was calculated. The RMS and maximum errors are plotted vs. RF pulse length in Figure 12.18.

This leads us to conclude that adapted waveform encoding can be implemented with very short RF pulses. With 10 mT/m magnetic gradients, one mm resolution can be obtained with RF pulses approximately 3 ms long [60]. Wavelet encoding, and by extension, adapted waveform encoding is therefore not limited by long RF pulses and may be a good replacement for phase encoding.

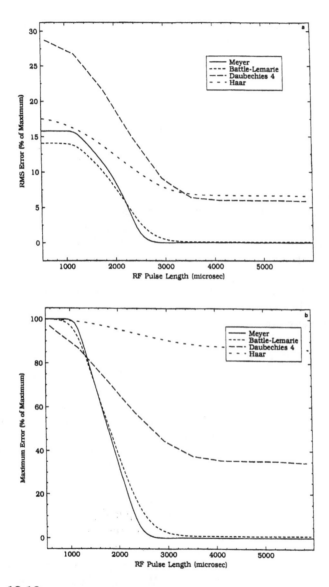

Figure 12.18
RMS and peak errors in various wavelet excited profiles as a
function of RF pulse length. The smoother wavelets can be more
accurately excited with short RF pulses.

12.4   Encoding with Joint Best Bases for Reduced Imaging Times

There are several applications where adaptive waveform encoding could be productive. In the last section, we sketched a possible application in phosphorus spectroscopy; in [27], we discussed an approach to adaptive imaging of the heart with some early experimental results. At this point, we present a different application, in fast MR imaging. The goal here is to exploit statistical regularities among the elements of a class of images in order to find bases which efficiently encode those images. The point of this is a reduction in the time required to obtain MR images of a new object, given that we know it belongs to the given class.

As already mentioned, long imaging times can be a major drawback of MRI. Depending on the contrast in the images, acquisition with a standard scanner requires from a second or two to half an hour. A great deal of research effort has been devoted to faster imaging, motivated by the promise of many new and exciting applications like cardiac imaging and functional imaging of the brain. The latter permits one to study evolving activity in areas of the brain during memory and motor tasks. This is an application with diagnostic potential as well as research interest. For example, knowing which parts of the brain are used in certain motor tasks helps minimize damage from neurosurgery. Localizing the parts of the brain involved in cognitive tasks (such as memorization of word lists) may help identify and develop treatments for Alzheimer's patients and patients with schizophrenia.

Recent MRI techniques such as gradient echo imaging [24], echo planar imaging [43], RARE [29], and BURST [28] produce images faster by increasing the rate at which data is acquired. There are limitations to these techniques: the image contrast can be adversely affected and expensive hardware modifications are required for some. There have also been a few techniques that attempt to reduce imaging times by using a priori information to reduce the amount of data required [9, 26, 35, 51, 67].

This section describes and analyzes fast imaging methods of the latter type. We try to reduce the number of encode steps required to image objects from a certain class of images by encoding with waveforms adapted to the covariance structure of that class. We need to find bases which capture most of the variability of the given class within the first few basis elements. More specifically, we are interested in parsimonious representations in this basis, in the sense that truncated image expansions should have minimal expected mean square error. A natural choice would be the Karhunen-Loeve basis, which has precisely this characteristic property [19]. A schematic representation of this is given in Figure 12.19.

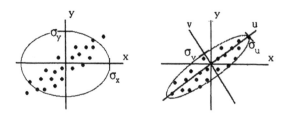

Figure 12.19
Schematic representation of K-L coordinates. Left: A class of signals (with two samples each) have high variance in each (standard) coordinate. Right: In a different coordinate system, the variance of the same class of signals is concentrated mainly on the first coordinate. These are the K-L coordinates.

We start by examining the advantages and disadvantages of using a Karhunen-Loeve (K-L) basis derived from a training set of images to reduce the number of encodes required for an MR image of a new object. We evaluate the expected error as a function of the number of encodes and consider two implementation problems: reduced SNR in the images and smoothing of the K-L functions due to RF pulse length restrictions. To get around these technical problems, we propose the use of joint best bases [64] derived from the local trigonometric library as an approximation to the K-L basis. These bases approach the rate-distortion characteristic achieved by the K-L basis, but they are easier to use in MRI and can be applied with existing methods for fast acquisition.

12.4.1 Adapted Waveform Encoding with K-L Bases

Cao and Levin [9] considered the problem of finding an optimum set of phase encodes to estimate the first elements of the Karhunen-Loeve (K-L) basis from a training set of related images. This reduced set of phase encodes was used to acquire an approximate image of a new object with a reduced data set. They also suggested that the direct measurement of the K-L coefficients could improve the performance of their technique. The first elements of the K-L basis have also been used by Zientara, Panych, and Jolesz to estimate changes over time in the repeated acquisitions of a given subject [67].

We have studied the feasibility of direct measurement of the K-L coefficients by selective excitation of K-L basis functions in adaptive waveform encoding. We took a typical set of images and measured the mean squared error in the reconstruction of a test image as a function of the number of K-L coefficients used. This approach shares the technical limitations of any adapted waveform encoding as discussed in the last section. In particular, the accuracy of the profiles excited by the selective RF pulses is limited by the length of the RF pulse. This makes excitation of the K-L basis functions difficult and of limited accuracy. In addition, the SNR of the images acquired with the K-L basis suffers compared to that in standard images. The reduction in SNR may be understood from the analysis of the previous section.

Karhunen-Loeve Basis from Training Images

For this study, we collected a number of clinical MR images for use as training and test data. We used images from a number of standard image classes; each class is a collection of trans-axial head images taken at a given level; see Figure 12.20. All images came from daily clinical studies using a standard scan. Only studies with no gross pathology were used.

Nine typical head images were chosen from each image class; the T_2 weighted images from eight of these studies were extracted and used as the training set for the K-L expansion corresponding to that class. The ninth was used as a test image to measure the error in reconstruction as a function of the truncation of the K-L data.

The eight images of the head used to generate the (empirical) K-L basis for each class were chosen to reflect the variation in positioning and in anatomy likely to be seen in clinical practice. Of course, a much larger data set would be required to generate a basis for the variety of pathology seen in clinical practice.

The training matrix, X, contains the eight normalized training images as 256×256 submatrices,

$$X = \begin{pmatrix} I_1 \\ \dots \\ \vdots \\ \dots \\ I_8 \end{pmatrix}.$$

Each image formed a set of 256 rows in the 2048×256 image matrix. X can also be viewed as a collection of 2048 vectors; each vector represents a line in the image that will be encoded with the K-L basis. The K-L basis vectors are the eigenvectors of XX^t. The eigenvectors are ordered so the associated eigenvalues decrease in size.

The K-L profiles $\{\psi_j\}_{j=1}^{256}$ obtained by this process for a given image class are used as amplitude profiles in MRI for imaging test objects from that same class. The profiles are excited by a selective RF pulse in the y direction; the acquired data are frequency encoded in the x direction to produce signal as described in Section 12.3. All the lines in the frequency-encoded direction are acquired at once and all are amplitude scaled with the same K-L basis vector. One frequency-encoded data string is acquired for each excitation; the inverse Fourier transform of the data string is a single K-L coefficient for all the lines in the image.

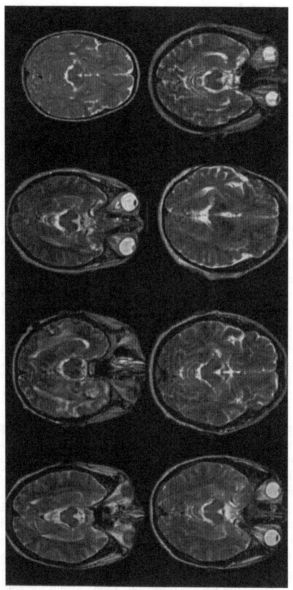

Figure 12.20
Training images from one of the class of head studies.

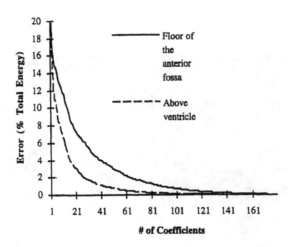

Figure 12.21
Error energy as a function of the number of coefficients used in K-L encoding of test images from the best and worst image classes.

The form of the sample covariance matrix reflects the fact that one of the two dimensions in a slice can be efficiently frequency encoded in MRI, so we are only concerned with the covariance in the second dimension. We are essentially performing a one-dimensional principal component analysis.

We applied this process in simulation to a number of the standard image classes described above. The error in the estimates of test images for the various classes were computed as functions of the number of coefficients. Figure 12.21 plots the error energy as a percentage of the total energy in the image for the best and worst classes. For the test image of the class of head images taken at level 14, where the image plane is superior to the ventricles, the error energy is below 1% with 45 coefficients and below 0.5% with 62 coefficients. For all image planes, the error energy is below 1% with 100 coefficients and below 0.5% with 127 coefficients. The error in the expansion of the image in the K-L basis is dominated by how closely the training set matches the image being acquired. The variation in the training set should be large enough to include all the variation likely to be encountered in practice. Therefore, the practical training set should be relatively large, which can lead to poor convergence. However, better convergence can be obtained by weighting the images and recalculating another K-L basis after each acquisition. Images from the training set that are like the acquired image should have greater weight than those that are unlike it. An iterative adaptive process results. For more details, see [59]. This process yields improved results for large, diverse training sets. For the small training sets we considered, the process only yields a 1 to 2% decrease in RMS error over the first eight coefficients.

Implementation of Karhunen-Loeve Encoding

The methods presented in Section 12.3.2 show that SNR in images acquired with a K-L basis is lower than in conventionally acquired images, even if a complete set of encodes are used. Recall that the reduction is caused by the inability to excite energy-normalized basis vectors combined with the presence of additive noise of fixed power. Because the amplitude profiles are not normalized, each projection of the spin density onto a profile must be multiplied by the appropriate factor for use in the reconstruction. The noise contribution in each measurement is multiplied by the same factor, leading to a reduction in the SNR.

As we have seen, an amplitude profile which excites the magnetization across the entire slice in the transverse plane has better SNR than localized excitations of the magnetization. The more localized the basis function, the larger the reduction in SNR. We saw that the complex exponential basis functions used in conventional imaging have optimum SNR, while wavelet bases are more localized, leading to a lower average SNR performance. The K-L bases are between the two; the reduction in SNR we have seen for K-L bases averages to a factor of around three and a half.

The second implementation factor that should be considered is the length of RF pulses required for exciting basis functions with discontinuities. As seen in Section 12.3.4, the profile excited by an RF pulse is approximately the Fourier transform of that RF pulse. Therefore, long RF pulses with wide bandwidths are required to excite profiles with sharp edges. The K-L basis functions we have seen have many sharp edges, instead of tight localization, as seen in Figure 12.22. In practice, the edges of these basis functions will not be present in the function actually excited, due to limitations on RF pulse length. These bandlimited profiles increase the error in the reconstructed test images significantly.

12.4.2 Approximate K-L Bases

An alternative to the K-L basis has been proposed by Wickerhauser [64]. In this paradigm, the K-L basis for a given class of signals on an interval is approximated from a large collection of simple bases: in our case, the local trigonometric library associated with a family of partitions of the interval. This approximation method utilizes a fast search over a tree-structured library of possible bases to quickly find the basis which best approximates the K-L basis with respect to a certain cost function. In the MRI application, the approximate basis turns out to be much easier to work with than the actual K-L basis.

For the approximate K-L transform, we seek a basis from our library which minimizes the volume of the variance ellipsoid for the ensemble of signals represented in that basis. This equals the product of the diagonal elements in the autocovariance matrix of the signal coefficients with respect

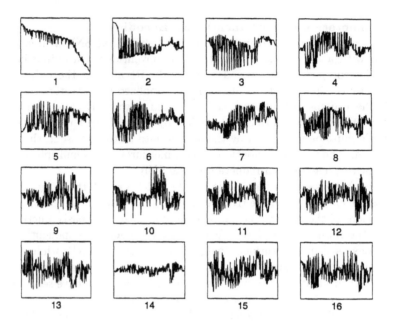

Figure 12.22
The first 16 K-L basis elements obtained from one of the image classes. Note the extremely rough profiles.

to the basis. The best basis search itself uses the variance of the coefficients to evaluate a suitable cost function, namely, the sum of the logs of the variances. This cost function is additive with respect to the partition of the interval. That is, the cost of a basis associated with a partition of an interval into two subintervals equals the sum of the costs of the bases for each subinterval separately [64].

Each basis of the local trigonometric library corresponds to a particular partition of the interval on which the signals live. Given a specified partition (the search partition) of the domain into a power of two number of subintervals, a fast binary tree searching strategy exists for finding a best partition (basis) from a collection of subpartitions of the search partition. With our student Doug Warner, we have considered a more general tree searching strategy to find a best partition over the entire collection of subpartitions of the search partition. In Figure 12.23 (a) we show such a tree where the search partition splits the domain into four subintervals.

A particular partition of the interval corresponds to a path from the root to a leaf. The first vertex below the root in one of these paths shows the position of the left-most point of the corresponding partition as a solid vertical line. Similarly the nth vertex shows the position of the nth partition point. The dashed lines indicate the positions of possible partition points, whose inclusion remains to be decided at a particular level of the search.

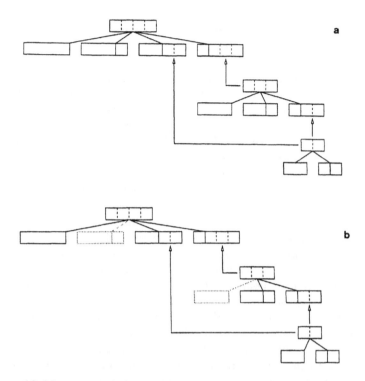

Figure 12.23
Dynamic programming search for best subpartition of a 4-interval search partition. (a) Starting with the smallest, right-most sub-problems, we use their solutions repeatedly in solving the larger subproblems. (b) Reducing the search tree to a set of "dyadic" subpartitions.

To find the best partition, we search for a path which minimizes the spec-ified information cost function. The first row below the root of the tree in Figure 12.23 (a) shows the four possible positions for the left-most partition point. The two vertices on the left of the first row correspond to the triv-ial partition and to a partition comprised of two subintervals, respectively. These partitions are completely specified at this level. The two vertices on the right of this row have additional possible partition points and require some further decisions about whether to include or exclude these points. In each of these cases we need only know the best splitting of the subinterval containing those candidate partition points, because of the additivity of the cost function. In other words, we can reduce to the subproblems of find-ing a best partition for the right-most subintervals containing two or three partition points. Then we can take those best partitions together with the indicated left-most partition point to make a list of four partitions, with at least one of them a best partition. Now we just evaluate the cost function on the basis corresponding to each of these partitions and take the one with minimal cost as our best basis.

In practice, we solve the smallest subproblems first and use those solutions in solving the larger subproblems. In terms of the tree, we start at the lower right and work our way up to the root. We begin with the choice of the best partition of the interval of length 2, shown as the tree of size 2 in the lower right. There are only two choices, so we compute their costs and choose the winner. Using this result for the best partition for length 2, we need only consider three possibilities for the best partition of length 3. When this is settled, we can use the best partitions for length 2 and 3 subintervals to get the costs of the four remaining possibilities for partitioning the whole interval, and finally choose the best.

This applies in general, and we use the subproblems of size $1, \ldots, n$ to solve the subproblem of size $n + 1$. The search complexity is $O(N^3)$ where N is the maximum possible number of partition points; that is, the size of the search partition. By eliminating some of the possibilities for positions of left-most partition points, faster searches are possible. As an example, one may restrict the search to partitions whose intervals contain a power of two of the intervals from the original search partition. In this case, the search complexity reduces to $O(N^2)$. The vertices and edges which this removes are shown ghosted out in Figure 12.23 (b). One may further reduce this to the binary tree method by requiring that the midpoint of certain subintervals occur in any nonempty partition.

12.4.3   Approximate Karhunen-Loeve Encoding

We have explored the use of approximate K-L bases chosen from a library of localized trigonometric bases, as discussed in above. Encoding with local trigonometric bases sidesteps some of the technical limitations associated with K-L encoding. In particular, the basis functions have a simple envelope with a linear phase. This offers two big advantages. First, the basis functions do not have sharp discontinuities, so they can be accurately excited with simple, short RF pulses. Second, the linear phase can be obtained with phase-encoding gradients. This allows the same techniques developed to reduce the number of excitations in phase encoding to be applied. In particular, several phases across the same envelope could be acquired from one excitation with the RARE technique [29].

The joint best basis algorithms discussed previously can be used on the training images to obtain a localized trigonometric basis that approximates the performance of the K-L basis. The joint best basis search is applied to the 2048 rows from the 8 images contained in the training matrix X. The interval to be encoded is initially partitioned into 16 intervals of equal length; the resulting collection of local cosine bases is searched by the dynamic programming algorithm outlined above. The result is a local cosine

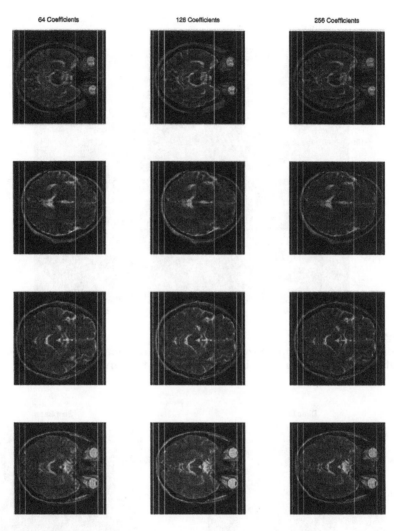

Figure 12.24
Some images from the training set and their reconstructions from reduced approximate K-L data sets. The approximate K-L partition lines are superimposed. The approximate K-L basis elements are local cosine functions associated with this partition.

basis associated with a particular of partition of the encoding axis, shown in Figure 12.24 superimposed over the training images. A density plot of the basis elements is shown in Figure 12.25. This basis effectively diagonalizes the sample covariance as shown in Figure 12.26, which compares the covariance of the training matrix in its original form (Dirac basis) to the covariance in the best basis.

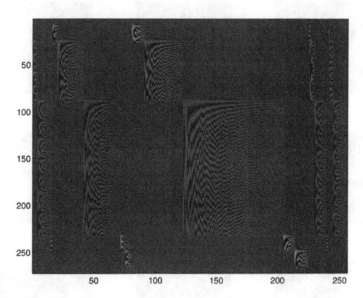

Figure 12.25
Density plot of approximate K-L basis of local cosine functions
obtained as a joint best basis for one of the image classes.

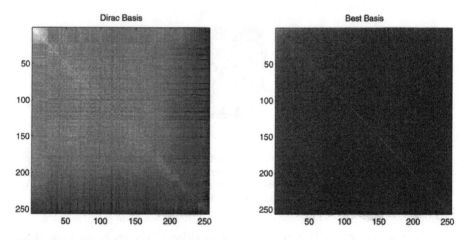

Figure 12.26
Covariance matrix of the original data (images in Dirac basis)
and of the transformed data (images expanded in approximate
K-L basis).

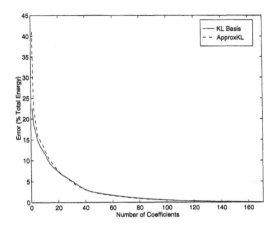

Figure 12.27
Comparison of error energy as a function of the number of coefficients used in approximate K-L encoding and K-L encoding for a test image from one of the image classes.

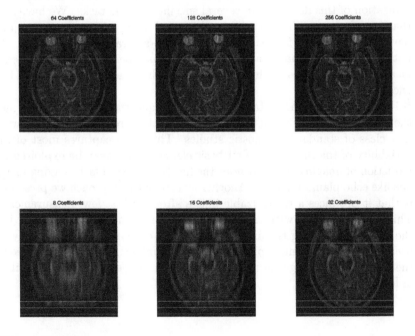

Figure 12.28
A sequence of reconstructions of a test image using approximate K-L encoding.

For our purposes, the important property is that the best basis concentrates the variance of the training set quite well into its first few components. This means that an average test image can be encoded with a reduced data set. Figure 12.27 shows the error energy vs. the number of encodes for a test image with respect to the approximate K-L basis and the K-L basis itself. This is also illustrated in Figure 12.28 by a sequence of reconstructions of one of the images from the ensemble. This suggests an application of our technique to progressive imaging for scout images.

12.5   Conclusions

We have presented applications of wavelet and related transforms to various problems of image acquisition in magnetic resonance imaging.

Magnetic resonance imaging is a very flexible modality; the images produced in this modality depend critically on the values of many parameters. We have presented adapted waveform encoding as a tool for the intelligent utilization of this flexibility in several specific imaging tasks. We have seen that waveform encoding can be implemented with existing scanners, and have analyzed its performance with regard to several figures of merit. We noted several performance advantages which may be attributed to the edge localization properties of the wavelet bases which can be employed in this encoding technique.

Finally, a particular instance of the technique was presented, in which the encoding basis was chosen to reflect statistical regularities in a particular class of standard diagnostic studies. This basis captures most of the variability of the class in the first basis elements. This can be exploited for reduction of imaging times without the hardware cost of fast imaging methods like echo planar imaging. Another feature of the approach we presented is that it produces a recognizable image after the first few measurements. This image is refined with each additional measurement. The operator has the option of stopping the process at any level of refinement, which may be useful for scout imaging applications. The technique may also be applied to the detection of changes in repeated scans of a single subject, as described in [67].

12.6 Acknowledgments

We would like to thank our student Doug Warner for his excellent Matlab code and for generating some very nice figures.

References

[1] Aue, W. P. Localization methods for in vivo nuclear magnetic resonance spectroscopy. *Rev. Magn. Reson. Med.* 1:21–72, 1986.

[2] Aue, W. P., S. Muller, T. A. Cross, and Seelig. Volume selective excitation: a novel approach to topical NMR. *J. Magn. Reson.* 56:350–354, 1984.

[3] Axel, L. and L. Dougherty. Heart wall motion: improved method of spatial modulation of magnetization for MR Imaging. *Radiology* 172:349–350, 1989.

[4] J. W. Belliveau, B. R. Rosen, H. L. Kantor et. al. Functional cerebral imaging by susceptibility—contrast NMR. *Magn. Reson. Med.* 14:538, 1990.

[5] Bloch, F. Nuclear induction. *Phys. Rev.* 70:460, 1946.

[6] Bore, P. J. Principles and applications of phosphorus magnetic resonance spectroscopy. In *Magnetic Resonance Annual*, H. Y. Kressel, ed. Raven Press, New York, 1985, 45–69.

[7] R. A. Brooks, G. DiChiro, and M. R. Keller, Explanation of cerebral white-gray contrast in computed tomography. *J. Comput. Assist. Tomogr.* 4:489–491, 1980.

[8] Catlin, D. *Estimation, Control, and the Discrete Kalman Filter.* Springer-Verlag, New York, 1989, 274 pp.

[9] Cao, Y. and D. Levin. Feature recognizing MRI. *Magn. Reson. Med.* 30:305–317, 1993.

[10] Chen, P. and O. Nalcioglu. 3-D multi-voxel NMR spectroscopy by Hadamard encoding. *Proc. Soc. Magn. Reson. Med.*, Berlin, August 1992, p. 3824.

[11] Cho, Z. H., O. Nalcioglu, and H. W. Park. Methods and algorithms for Fourier-transform nuclear magnetic resonance tomography. *J. Opt. Soc. Am.* 4:923–932, 1987.

[12] Coifman, R. R. and M. V. Wickerhauser. Entropy based algorithms for best basis selection. *IEEE Trans. Inf. Theory.* 38:713–718, 1992

[13] Conolly, S., D. Nishimura, and A. Macovski. Optimal control solutions to the magnetic resonance selective excitation problem. *IEEE Trans. Med. Imaging* MI-5(2):106–115, 1986.

[14] Daubechies, I. The wavelet transform, time-frequency localization, and signal analysis. *IEEE Trans. Inf. Theory.* 36:961–1005, 1990.

[15] Daubechies, I. Orthonormal bases of compactly supported wavelets. *Commun. Pure Applied Math.* 41:909–996, 1988

[16] Driscoll, J. R., D. M. Healy, and G. Isaak. Scheduling dyadic intervals. To appear in *Discrete Applied Mathematics*, 1995

[17] R. T. Droege, S. N. Wiencer, M. S. Rzeszotarski, G. N. Holland, and I. R. Young. Nuclear magnetic resonance: a gray scale model for head images. *Radiology* 148:763–771, 1983.

[18] Ferrari, V. A., J. A. C. Lima, L. Axel, C. M. Kramer, M. R. Llaneras, L. C. Palmon, B. Tallant, and N. Reichek. Regional changes in segmental rigid body motion and deformation after myocardial infarction by magnetic resonance tissue tagging. *Proc. Soc. Magn. Reson. in Med.*, Berlin, August 1992, p. 16.

[19] Fukunaga, K. *Statistical Pattern Recognition*, 2nd edition Academic Press, Boston, 1990.

[20] Goelman, G. and J. S. Leigh. B1-insensitive Hadamard spectroscopic imaging technique. *J. Magn. Reson.* 91:93–101, 1991.

[21] Goelman, G. and J. S. Leigh. The use of high order Hadamard matrices for metabolic maps. *Proc. Soc. of Magn. Reson. Med.*, Berlin, August 1992, p. 3823.

[22] Goelman, G., V. H. Subramanian, and J. S. Leigh. Transverse Hadamard spectroscopic imaging technique. *J. Magn. Reson.* 89:437–454, 1990.

[23] Grunbaum, F. A. and A. Hasenfeld. An exploration of the invertibility of the Bloch transform. *Inverse Problems* 2:75–81, 1986.

[24] Haase, A., J. Frahm, W. Hanicke, and K. Merboldtt. *J. Magn. Reson.* 67:258, 1986.

[25] Healy, D. M. and J. B. Weaver. Two applications of wavelet transforms in MR imaging. *IEEE Trans. Inf. Theory* 38:840–860, 1992.

[26] Healy, D., T. Olson, and J. Weaver. Reduced motion artifacts in medical imaging by adaptive spatio-temporal reconstruction. To appear in *Numerical Algorithms*, 1995.

[27] Healy, D. M., J. Lu, and J. B. Weaver. Two applications of wavelets and related techniques in medical imaging. *Ann. Biomed. Eng.* To appear, 1995.

[28] Heid, O., M. Deimling, and W. Huk. *Magn. Reson. Med.* 29:280, 1993.

[29] Hennig, J., A. Nauerth, and H. Friedburg. *Magn. Reson. Med.* 3:823, 1986.

[30] S. M. Kay, M. S. *Fundamentals of Statistical Signal Processing.* Prentice Hall, Englewood Cliffs, NJ, 1993, 595 pp.

[31] Kooijman, H. Short low power self-refocussing pulse. *Proc. Soc. Magn. Reson. Med.*, San Francisco, August 1991, p. 685.

[32] Korin, H. W., J. P. Felmlee, R. L. Ehman, and S. J. Riederer. Adaptive technique for three-dimensional MR imaging of moving structures. *Radiology* 177:217-221, 1990.

[33] Lenkinski, R. E. *Clinical MR Spectroscopy, Syllabus: Special Course.* RNSA Publications, 1990, 279 pp.

[34] Li, S. J., G. Y. Jin, and J. E. Mooulder. Effects of local irradiation on spin-lattice relaxation time of phosphate metabolites in mouse tumors monitored by 31-P magnetic resonance spectroscopy. *Magn. Reson. Med.* 23(2) 302–310, 1992.

[35] Liang, Z. and P. Lauterbur. *IEEE Trans. Med. Imaging* 10:132, 1991.

[36] Lu, J., D. M. Healy Jr, and J. B. Weaver. Contrast enhancement of medical images using multiscale edge representation. *Optic. Eng.* 33:2151–2161.

[37] Lu, J., J. B. Weaver, and D. M. Healy Jr. Noise reduction with multiscale edge representation and perceptual criteria. *Proc. IEEE-SP Int. Symp. Time-Frequency and Time-Scale Analysis*, Victoria, B.C., Oct. 1992, pp. 555–558.

[38] Luenberger, D. G. *Optimization by Vector Space Methods.* Wiley, New York, 1969, 326 pp.

[39] Lurie, D. J. A systematic design procedure for selective pulses in NMR imaging. *Magn. Res. Imaging* 3:235–243, 1985.

[40] Mallat, S. Multiresolution approximation and wavelets. *Trans. AMS*, 135:69–88, 1989.

[41] Mansfield, P. and P. G. Morris. *NMR Imaging in Biomedicine*, Academic Press, San Diego, 1982, 354 pp.

[42] Mansfield, P., A. A. Maudsley, and T. Baines. Fast scan proton density by NMR. *J. Phys.* E9, 271–278, 1976.

[43] Mansfield, P. and I. Pykett. *J. Magn. Reson.* 29:355, 1978.

[44] Massie, B., G. G. Schwartz, J. Garcia, S. Steinman, M. W. Weiner, and J. Wisneski. Changes in energy phosphates with increased left ventricular workload represent "demand ischemia". *Proc. Soc. Magn. Reson. Med.* Berlin, August 1992, p. 343.

[45] Menon, R. S., K. Hendrich, X. Hu, and K. Ugurbil. 31P NMR spectroscopy of the human heart at 4T: detection of uncontaminated cardiac spectra and differentiation of subepicardium and subendocardium. *Proc. Soc. Magn. Reson. Med.*, Berlin, August 1992, p. 342.

[46] Meyer, Y. Principe d'incertitude, bases hilbertiennes, et algebres d'operateurs. In *Semin. Bourbaki, 1985/86, exposes 651–668.* Societe Mathematique de France, Paris, 1987, 209–223.

[47] Nashed, M. Z. (ed). *Generalized Inverses and Applications: Proceedings of an Advanced Seminar.* Academic Press, New York, 1976, 1054 pp.

[48] Panych, L. P., P. D. Jakab, and F. A. Jolesz. An implementation of wavelet encoded magnetic resonance imaging. *J. Magn. Reson. Imaging* 3:649–655, 1993.

[49] Peters, R. D. and M. L. Wood. Practical Considerations for implementation of wavelet encoding. *Proc. Soc. Magn. Reson. Med.*, New York, August 1993, p. 1212.

[50] Pauly, J., S. Conolly, D. Nishimura, and A. Macovski. Slice-selective excitation for very short T2 species. *Proc. Soc. Magn. Reson. Med.*, San Francisco, August 1991, p. 28.

[51] Pike, G., J. Fredrickson, G. Glover, and D. Enzmann. Dynamic susceptibility contrast imaging using a gradient-echo sequence. *Abstr. Soc. Magn. Reson. Med., 11th Annu. Meet.* 1992, 1131.

[52] Radda, G., P. J. Bore, and B. J. Rajagopalan. Clinical aspects of 31-P NMR spectroscopy. *Br. Med. Bull.* 40:155–159, 1984.

[53] Shellock, F., J. Mink, and J. Fox. Patellofemoral joint: kinematic MR imaging to assess tracking abnormalities. *Radiology* 168:551, 1988.

[54] Shinnar, M. and J. S. Leigh. Frequency response of soft pulses. *J. Magn. Reson.* 75:502–505, 1987.

[55] Slichter, C. P. *Principles of Magnetic Resonance.* Springer-Verlag, New York, 1980, 397 pp.

[56] Sloane, N. J. A. Hadamard and other discrete transforms in spectroscopy. In *Fourier, Hadamard, and Hilbert transforms in Chemistry*, A. G. Marshall, ed. Plenum, New York, 1982, pp. 45–67.

[57] Turner, R., D. LeBihan, C. T. W. Moonen, D. Despres, and J. Frank. Echo-planar time course MRI of cat brain oxygenation changes. *Magn. Reson. Med.* 22:159, 1991.

[58] Villringer, A., B. R. Rosen, J. W. Belliveau et al. Dynamic imaging with lanthanide chelates in normal brain: contrast due to magnetic susceptibility effects. *Magn. Reson. Med.* 6:164, 1988.

[59] Weaver, J. B. and D. M. Healy. *Proc. IEEE Int. Conf. Image Process.*, III-35. Austin, 1994.

[60] Weaver, J. B., D. M. Healy, Jr., D. Crean, and Y. Xu. Wavelet encoding with smooth wavelets: short RF pulses. *Proc. Soc. Magn. Reson. Med.*, Berlin, August 1992, p. 4264.

[61] Weaver, J. B. and D. M. Healy, Jr. Signal to noise ratios and effective repitition times for wavelet and adapted wavelet encoding. *J. Magn. Reson., Ser. A* 113:1–10, 1995.

[62] Weaver, J. B., Y. Xu, D. M. Healy, and J. R. Driscoll. Wavelet encoded MR imaging. *Magn. Reson. Med.* 24:275–287, 1992.

[63] V. Wedeen. Magnetic resonance imaging of myocardial kinematics: a technique to detect, localize and quantify the strain rates of the active human myocardium. *Magn. Reson. Med.* 27:52, 1992.

[64] Wickerhauser, M. *Adapted Wavelet Analysis from Theory to Software.* A. K. Peters, Wellesley, MA. 1994.

[65] Yagle, A. E. Inversion of the Bloch transform in magnetic resonance imaging using asymmetric two-component inverse scattering. *Inverse Problems* 6:131–151, 1990.

[66] Zerhouni, E. A., D. M. Parish, W. J. Rodgers, A. Yang, and E. P. Shapiro. Human heart tagging with MR imaging—a method for non-invasive assessment of myocardial motion. *Radiology* 169:59–63, 1988.

[67] Zientara, G., L. Panych, and F. A. Jolesz. *Magn. Reson. Med.* 32:268, 1994.

Part III

Wavelets and Biomedical Signal Processing

13

Sleep Images Using the Wavelet Transform to Process Polysomnographic Signals

Richard Sartene, Laurent Poupard, Jean-Louis Bernard, and Jean-Christophe Wallet

Laboratoire d'Explorations Fonctionnelles Respiratoires Hôpital Robert Ballanger
AULNAY/BOIS FRANCE
Laboratoire de Physique Théorique (IPN) Université Paris-Sud ORSAY FRANCE

13.1   Introduction

In the past few years, substantial attention has been given to the study of the sleep apnea syndrome and similar or related syndromes such as snoring and sudden infant death syndrome [14]. This attention has led to the development of new methods of investigation and multidisciplinary involvement (pneumology, neurology, cardiology, endocrinology, psychiatry, pediatrics, pharmacology).

The whole range of these research works, particularly the pathophysiologic ones, evidently proves that the wake-sleep alternation relies on the complex interaction of the neurological, humoral, and homeostatic systems. The mechanisms that control the vigilance states are still largely unknown.

On the one hand, all the vegetative (respiratory, cardiovascular, homeo-thermic) functions are influenced by the wake-sleep alternation. On the other hand, the main vital functions can in turn affect the variations of vigilance state. The most significant example is the hyperventilation which follows an apneic episode and can induce a microarousal.

Three clinical notions can be related to the study of sleep:

a. Sleep is a multidisciplinary field. The main physiological systems come into play and interact with each other.

b. The activity of these systems corresponds to continuous rhythms or oscillations which undergo frequency and amplitude modulations due to intersystem interactions. Relevant frequency ranges corre-sponding to the various biological oscillations are large: 1 to 40 Hz for EEG, 0.15 to 0.25 Hz for respiratory centers, 1 to 2 Hz for heart sine rhythm system, and 0.1 to 0.015 Hz for chemical regulation and autonomous neural system oscillations.

c. Sleep appears as a continuous process rather than as a mere parti-tion in several discrete states, particularly in drowsiness or in the deep sleep.

Spectral analysis based on the Fourier transform provides quantitative information on the frequency content of the electrophysiological signals dur-ing the (quasi-)stationary sleep episodes, but it leaves out event timing. For instance, this does not allow the detection and the identification of (patho-) physiological events (sleep, heart rate, blood pressure disorders, apneas, ...). These characteristics show immediately that time-frequency analysis methods are an absolutely necessary tool to the study of sleep.

Any method which tends to be really efficient with this investigation has to comply with three criteria:

• To give access to the timing of events;

• To make the analysis possible on a time scale adaptable to the user's needs, viz., one second to account for time-localized phenomena, one minute for autonomous regulation mechanisms, one hour for a sleep cycle duration;

• To provide quantitative data about the interactions between the dif-ferent physiological (neurological, cardiovascular, respiratory) sys-tems through characteristic modulations induced by these interac-tions in amplitude and in frequency.

Analysis by wavelet transform, a time-scale analysis method, satisfies these three criteria simultaneously. It turns out to be one of the preferential tools in the analysis of polysomnographic signals representing these activities.

More generally, biomedical signals are particularly rich in dynamic, time-related data, very often nonstationary, partly disturbed by noise and artifact. They can easily be submitted to the time-frequency and time-scale methods. Various instances of this were shown at the International IEEE-SP Symposium held in Philadelphia in October 1994 [13] and the IEEE-EMBS Symposium held in Baltimore in November 1994 [1]. We can cite QRS complex analysis among the electrocardiographic signals, transient spikes detection in the electroencephalogram of epileptic patients, the analysis of electromyographic activity of the uterus, and the analysis of heart rate variability. In this review, our objective is to provide examples of the wavelet process in research on sleep. We want to show physiologists and physicians the value of the new methods which, at least theoretically, overcome some of the limitations of the traditional frequency or time-domain analyses (visual scorage or sequential analysis of amplitudes).

13.2 Sleep Polygraphy

13.2.1 Signals

Polygraphy is a rather extensive method of investigation of the main physiological functions during sleep, especially neuro-cardio-respiratory ones. This requires a simultaneous recording of a great number of signals, through various techniques. Neurophysiological signals (EEG, EOG, EMG) make a definition of sleep quality and quantity possible. Respiratory signals (spirometry, rib cage, and abdominal movements) make it possible to measure ventilation and to define respiratory patterns. Cardiovascular signals (EKG, blood pressure, peripheral saturation in oxygen) make it possible to know the consequences of sleep troubles.

The electro-encephalogram (EEG) (Figure 13.1)

The electroencephalogram is the main signal used to define sleep stages. It is collected by using AgCl electrodes attached to the scalp with collodion. The electrodes are set according to an international convention [6]. The signal collected before amplification has an amplitude of 10 to 100 μV and a frequency range of 0.5 to 40 Hz. It is not stationary. It is usually described with the following frequency bands [10]:

- below 4 Hz (δ band);
- from 4 to 8 Hz (θ band);

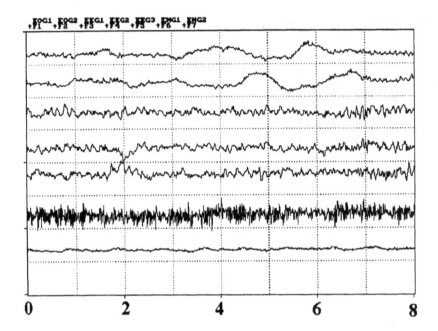

Figure 13.1
Electrophysiologic tracings. From top to bottom, we have, respectively, represented two EOGs (right and left), three EEGs
(F_Z-C_Z, C_Z-P_Z, P_Z-T_4), and two EMGs (chin and left leg). They
are sampled at a 100 Hz frequency. The slow eye movements
show that the subject is in a light sleep stage (I).

- from 8 to 12 Hz (α band);
- above 12 Hz (the high rhythm β band).

The electro-oculogram (EOG)

This signal can separate some sleep stages. It is collected with two pairs
of electrodes set up between the eye's external canthus and the nasion.
The electrodes record potential variations (from 20 to 250 μV) caused by
movements of the eyeballs.

The electromyogram (EMG)

The EMG is used to assess the average muscular tone and obtain a more
precise recognition of the sleep stages. This is collected through electrodes
stuck on either side of the chin. Its frequency range is 10 to 1000 Hz and
its amplitude is only a few μV. Other EMGs can be examined with the use
of superficial electrodes such as the diaphragm EMG and the leg muscle
EMG.

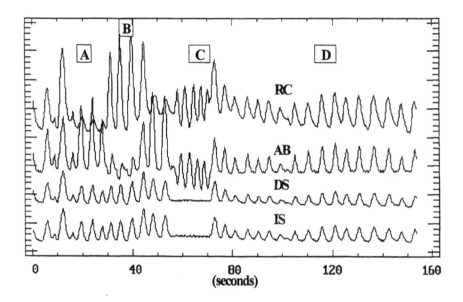

Figure 13.2
An example of Indirect Spirometry. We have represented the cross-sectional area changes of ribcage (RC) and abdomen (AB), the direct spirometry measured at the mouth (DS), and the indirect spirometry (IS) obtained after an adequate calibration of RC and AB. Note the excellent correspondence between direct and indirect spirometry whatever the respiratory modes are (A: predominant abdomen, B: predominant thorax, C: isovolumes maneuvers, D: quiet breathing).

Respiratory signals (Figure 13.2)

The usual methods in closed circuit (spirometry, pneumotachography) have restraints because the patient has to remain connected with a nose-mouth mask. One of the drawbacks is that it alters the spontaneous respiratory pattern (lower frequency, greater tidal volume). Thus, it is preferable to use measurement of respiratory movements.

The respiratory mechanical system is a two-degree of freedom system (rib cage and abdomen) for a subject in a stable posture (such as supine). In this case, two simultaneous and continuous signals are sufficient to reconstruct an indirect spirometry with an available accuracy. The most commonly used device is the RESPITRACE*, which measures self-inductance changes within a wire sewn to a belt encircling each respiratory compartment [11]. For our part, we use a technique that is two times more accurate, with a residual error under 5%. This technique consists in measuring dynamic changes in cross-sectional areas of the rib cage and of the abdomen [12].

The subject is placed within an external homogeneous magnetic field.

$$B = B_0 \cos 2\pi f t \quad (B_0 = 10^{-7} \text{ Tesla}, f = 10^5 \text{ Hz})$$

The device measures the induced voltage during respiration $e = d\phi/dt$ where ϕ is the magnetic flux embraced in the belt.

Cardiovascular signals

1. *Oxygen saturation* (SaO2) is measured by a transcutaneous method. The captor is set up on a finger surface. This principle is based on the measuring of wavelength absorption variation in the infra red band between oxyhemoglobin and desoxyhemoglobin. The apparatus is available and commercialized under the name NELLCOR®

2. *ECG* measures cardiac electric activity recorded through skin electrodes.

3. *Blood pressure*: Noninvasive continuous measurement of blood pressure is made through a peripheral sensor FINAPRES® (Ohm-eda) set up on a finger with a cuff which contains an infra-red photoplethysmographic element [7]. The measure is based upon the principle of a constant equilibrium of arterial volume with requires the equality between external applied pressure (P_b) and arterial pressure (P_a). The transmural pressure $P_{tm} = P_a - P_b$ is permanently maintained to a null level.

13.2.2   Sleep Architecture (Figure 13.3)

The usual classification refers to the classical criteria of Rechtschaffen and Kales [10], which state precisely the respective proportion of the various EEG activities. In addition to EEG recordings, eye movements (EOG) and muscular (EMG) electric activities are generally recorded. With these various measures the different types of sleep can be divided into two main categories:

- the slow sleep (NREM);

- the rapid-eye-movement sleep (REM).

In the normal subject, the NREM is divided into four different stages of increasing depth, defined by the following electrophysiological criteria:

- When the subject is completely awake, the electric activity recorded is shaped as a desynchronized mixture of several frequencies among which the most predominant waves have high frequencies (above 15 Hz) and low amplitude.

- When the subject is in relaxed state with closed eyes (active wake), the graph displays a different rhythm made up of regular oscillations called α rhythm (8 to 12 Hz), the amplitude of which is about 50 μV.

- Drowsiness, stage I: when settling, rhythm amplitude decreases and is replaced by lower amplitude waves, called θ waves (4 to 8 Hz), with lower and irregular frequencies. This episode can last for a few minutes and it generally goes along with a reduction of the EMG amplitude.

- Stage II: EEG is marked by episodes called spindles, i.e., bursts (14 to 18 Hz) which occur four or five times in a minute, with K complexes, high amplitude deviations preceding some spindles. The EMG amplitude decreases once more (muscular relaxation).

- Deep sleep, stages III and IV: in the first part of the night, stage II is followed by stage III, in which sleep can be characterized by slow waves with rather high amplitude, called δ waves (1 to 4 Hz). The muscles continue relaxing, which induces a decrease in EMG amplitude. This eventually leads to stage IV, defined by a continuous train of high amplitude waves and a disappearance of eye movements.

Stages I to IV are parts of slow sleep.

In the first part of the night, the subject who has fallen asleep normally goes through all the stages in about 1 hour, and has a quick return to stage II. Then a transition towards a completely different stage occurs. The EEG shows rapid, low amplitude activity similar to the wake state, except that the muscles are fully relaxed; hence the apparent contradiction between this muscular state and electroencephalographic activity. Because of this apparent contradiction, this stage is called paradoxical sleep (REM). Under the eyelids, the eyes have rapid movements. During these REM episodes, the main alterations of the body position are observed, together with physiological changes (variable heart rate; irregular, even rapid breathing).

In the normal subject, the night sleep includes several cycles with a progressive transition from light slow sleep to deep slow sleep and paradoxical sleep. These cycles last about 90 to 110 minutes, and they recur about three to five times a night. In the beginning, these cycles are shorter and slow wave sleep represents a greater part, whereas the REM is typically more frequent in the last cycles of the night. The first REM episode is shorter and lasts only for 5 or 6 min, whereas the last one preceding the awakening can be about 45 min long.

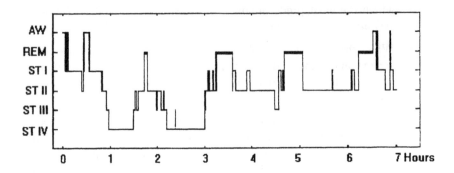

Figure 13.3
Hypnogram of a normal subject. Each EEG sequence of 30 s or
1 min is coded according to its visual dominant frequency. EMG
and EOG are used as additional coders.

The sleep indices which have been taken into account are:

- The drowsiness latency (10 to 20 min), which is the time interval
  between the light switching off and the onset of stage II or confirmed
  sleep (appearance of the first spindle);

- The total sleeping time (TST), waking time excluded.

Various parameters can be added, such as the number of awakenings,
the number of stage changes, and the ratio of the various stages related to
TST, which is approximately 5% in stage I, 50% in stage II, 25% in stages
III and IV, and 20% in REM.

To assess sleep, one must check the visual reading of the EEG for a
sequential analysis (30 s or 1 min), with a stage scorage according to the
predominant frequency of the EEG, using EMG and EOG as supplementary
coders.

This sequential analysis leads to the construction of the hypnogram (Figure 13.3). This hypnogram is already a time-frequency graphical representation, as the coding is made according to a visual frequency analysis.

13.2.3   Sleep and Cardiorespiratory Activity [5, 9]

Various studies have been carried out since 1960, thanks to modern investigations and the international classification of sleep stages. This enables us
to study precisely hemodynamic changes evolution during sleep. In general,
a decrease in blood pressure related to the depth of sleep can be measured
with either invasive or noninvasive methods in normal subjects. These
decreases are about 5 to 10% of the reference values when the subject is
awake. During REM, there is a slight rise of the blood pressure towards

the reference values. Nonetheless rapid and transient increases in blood pressure can be observed, together with phasic activities of REM (rapid eye movements).

Heart rate tends to decrease gradually during slow sleep, especially in deep slow sleep, with low level variability. Whereas in REM, heart rate as well as blood pressure are submitted to wide fluctuations (10 to 20 bpm) which correspond to accelerations followed by slowing down in each phasic event. In a normal subject, some transient rhythm troubles such as atrioventricular block or sine pause up to a few seconds can happen.

Blood pressure modulations are observed during awakening and light sleep as well. These circulatory changes settle mostly in the 0.15 to 0.30 Hz frequency band, which corresponds to the basic respiratory frequency (10 to 18 cycles per minute). They are called sinusal respiratory arrhythmia (more intense in children).

The development of spectral analysis methods (fast Fourier transform) has permitted the identification of other bands: a medium frequency band (MF) band of 0.1 to 0.05 Hz, and a low frequency band (LF) of 0.05 to 0.015 Hz. These frequency bands correspond to periodical activities generally linked to the autonomous nervous system activity (sympathetic, parasympathetic, thermoregulation). There are no experimental quantitative data in these frequency bands in normal subjects.

Breathing is a periodical and automatic physiological phenomenon, and its features can be voluntarily or involuntarily modified by internal or external conditions in the system.

The respiratory centers driving this command belong to different areas in the cerebral truncus (reticular formation) and build an anatomical complex with facilitating or inhibiting interconnections. These different groups, constituting the respiratory centers, receive afferencies from the tenth pair of cranial nerves (pneumogastric nerves, including sympathetic and parasympathetic fibers). Respiratory center stimulation induces a contraction of the respiratory muscles (the intercostal muscles and the diaphragm).

Normal resting subjects inhale in each breath a volume of a few hundred millimeters (about 400 ml) called tidal volume (V_T). The minute ventilation ($\dot{V}_{min}$) corresponding to a breathing rate of 0.25 Hz (15 min^{-1}) is 6 l/min.

One considers that breathing is regulated by two mechanisms, at least during the waking state:

a. The automatic control regulates the arterial O_2 and CO_2 partial pressure by integrating in the cerebral truncus the data provided by central (pH and CO_2 sensitive) and peripheral (O_2 sensitive) chemoreceptors. All these data provide an appropriate command to the respiratory muscles.

b. Voluntary or comportmental control which implies cortical front

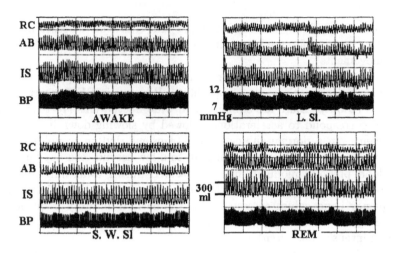

Figure 13.4
Cardio-respiratory recordings in a normal subject during sleep.
We have represented the ribcage (RC) and the abdominal (AB)
movements recorded with a noninvasive method [12], recon-
structed or indirect spirometry (IS) and the finger arterial pres-
sure monitored by the Finapres*. Four sleep stages are repre-
sented (awake, light sleep (L Sl), slow wave sleep (SW Sl), and
REM). The time scale is 30 s. See text for explanations.

structures and which enable the subject to adapt his own breathing.
It becomes evident that the respiratory system cannot be considered as a single one but rather as a part of an integrated neuro-
cardio-respiratory system. One must also note that all humoral
stimulations (physical changes linked to blood pressure and chemical
changes of circulating blood) will also have an effect on respiratory
centers. Consequently, all the elements regulating blood pressure
and heart rate will be implied in ventilation regulation.

The ventilation-sleep relation has been intensively studied, particularly in
the last 20 years, and especially in the field of respiratory pathologies. In the
adult normal subject, the most constant point which has been made is that
minute ventilation decreases at least by 10% during slow sleep (compared
to wake-ventilation). Respiratory pattern could also change according to
sleep stages. Periodic breathing is a nonuniversal feature of light slow sleep
(stages I to II); it consists of successive cycles (30 to 60 s) in which tidal
volume may increase, thus leading to an apnea. This modulation varies
according to the subject age; it is common in children and elderly subjects,
moderate with young adults, but frequent in altitude.

Regular breathing (tidal volume and frequency) is the most commonly
observed respiratory mode deep slow sleep (Figure 13.4).

During REM, breathing is generally described as more rapid and more irregular during eye movement episodes, with a mean and with a standard deviation of the respiratory frequency wider than those observed during deep sleep. These respiratory fluctuations are also associated with heart rate and blood pressure fluctuations.

13.3 The Wavelet Transform—Practical Use

13.3.1 Practical Considerations

In the following applications, we exclusively used the continuous one-dimensional wavelet transform, which is particularly suitable for polysomnogram issues.

The mother wavelet $\Psi(t)$ that we have used is the Morlet-Grossman wavelet defined by [3, 4, 8]:

$$\Psi(t) = e^{i\omega_0 t} e^{-t^2/2} \tag{13.1}$$

Notice that these wavelets are not strictly "admissible" (since they verify $\hat{\Psi}(0) > 0$). In practical (numerical) applications, however, ω_0 is usually chosen to be large enough ($\omega_0 \geq 5.5$), so that $\hat{\Psi}(0) < 10^{-33}$ and $\Psi_{(a,b)}(t)$ can be considered as numerically "admissible". Heuristically, we can illustrate this wavelet transform behavior as a local spectral analysis method. For a simple sine function $f(t) = e^{i\omega t}$, the wavelet transform modulus is locally maximum for $a = \omega_0/\omega$. Note that a, the scale parameter, appears proportional to the inverse of a frequency.

When $a > 1$ and increases, the width of the wavelet $\Psi_{(a,b)}(t)$ increases, such that the frequency resolution increases. When $a < 1$ and decreases, the interval over which the wavelet $\Psi_{(a,b)}(t)$ is nonzero is more closely tightened around the point b, thus increasing temporal resolution, at the expense of frequency resolution.

The uncertainty principle which rules the limitation of localization at any frequency in space time is expressed by

$$\Delta t \cdot \Delta f \geq \frac{2}{\pi},$$

where Δt and Δf represent temporal and frequency deviations from a baseline. In the case of a Gaussian function, Δt is chosen equal to $2a$, so

$$\Delta f \geq \frac{2}{2\pi a} = \frac{2f}{\omega_0}.$$

The uncertainty relationship becomes

$$\frac{\Delta f}{f} \geq \frac{2}{\omega_0}.$$

In practice, variation range of the parameter a is chosen by the user according to the interesting frequency domain of the signal. The interval $[a_{\min}, a_{\max}]$ is cut up according to an appropriate number of dilations such as

$$\frac{\Delta a}{a} = \frac{\Delta f}{f} = \text{constant},$$

where Δa represents the interval between two successive sequences of a. The choice of ω_0 defines the minimum number of dilations (without any overlapping).

For the EEG signal analyzed in the frequency range [1 to 20 Hz] according 80 dilations and for $\omega_0 = 5.5$, we get $\Delta t(1 \text{ Hz}) \geq 1.8$ sec and $\Delta t(20 \text{ Hz}) \geq 0.09$ sec.

The wavelet transform permits us to extract the modulation laws (AM/FM) of a signal. If the physical signal has the form: $f(t) = A(t)\cos\alpha(t)$, we can show, that the wavelet transform is given by:

$$\left[(W_\Psi f)(a,b) = \frac{1}{2}A(b)e^{(i\alpha(b))} \overline{\hat{\Psi}}(a\alpha'(b)) + \cdots \right] \tag{13.2}$$

where (...) are nonessential corrective terms. The ridge of the wavelet transform is a privileged curve defined as the locus of points (b,a) where the modulus of the wavelet transform is maximum. In the case of Morlet wavelets, the ridge is defined by the points (b,a) for which $a = \omega_0/\alpha'(t)$. Thus, its determination allows us to obtain $\alpha(t)$, then $A(t)$ from Equation (13.2).

Concerning polysomnographic signals, calculation of the wavelet transform was continuously realized for all recorded signals (7 to 8 hours), with a specific tuning for each signal.

EEG: the signal was sampled at a 100 Hz and compressed at 50 Hz frequency; it was decomposed in wavelets in the [1 to 20 Hz] frequency range, using 80 dilations.

Blood pressure: the signal was sampled at a 10-Hz frequency and decomposed in wavelets in the [0.5 to 2 Hz] frequency range around the basic heart frequency (~ 1 Hz), using 200 dilations for extraction of the modulation laws.

Respiration: signals were sampled at a 10-Hz frequency, split in wavelets in the [0.1 to 0.6-Hz] frequency range, around the basic respiratory frequency (~ 0.25 Hz), according 100 dilations.

The execution speed was excellent. For instance, the phase and the modulus calculation of the wavelet transform for $1024 * 200$ points, by using 30 dilations, requires 10 s on a SUNSPARC classic work station. The software (TECLET*) was realized by Science & Tec.* It works in a UNIX environment. It contains two independent parts. The numeric part is written in the C language and the graphic part (windows, menu) works with the XWINDOWS* MOTIF* environment.

13.3.2   Validation of the Modulation Laws (FM-AM)

One of the main interests of the wavelet transform is to detect nontrivial modulation laws due to weak interactions. It is the case of the blood pressure signal where various regulating mechanisms induced simultaneously an amplitude modulation (AM) of a few mmHg for a global amplitude of 50 mmHg and a frequency modulation (FM) (0.1 Hz) less than 10% of the basic heart frequency (~ 1 Hz). To justify the use of the wavelet transform for those estimation tasks, we evaluated potential errors introduced by this method to extract the FM (first example) and the AM (second example).

Frequency modulation (FM)

We consider a sine function ($f_0 = 1$ Hz, amplitude 50 mV), sampled at a 10 Hz frequency. This signal is modulated in frequency by another sine function ($f_1 = 0.25$ Hz, amplitude 0.1 Hz). Thus, the theoretical modulation is equivalent to the experimental one, which is observed in the blood pressure signal. Its analytical expression is: $s_1(t) = 50 \sin(2\pi f_0 t + (0.4 \sin 2\pi f_1 t))$.

Figure 13.5 shows the results obtained by applying the wavelet transform to this signal (panel A). We find an AM (panel C) which is a modulation of the power spectral density ($2500 = 50^2$). This spurious modulation is weak (< 1 mV, i.e., 2% of $s_1(t)$ amplitude) and varies at twice the frequency of f_1. So it can be suppressed by the reconstruction procedure. We find again (panel D) the FM of the fundamental frequency ($f_0 = 1$ Hz) at a

---

*SCIENCE & TEC, Moulin Saint Melaine Route de Rouen, 14130 Pont L'Eveque (France).

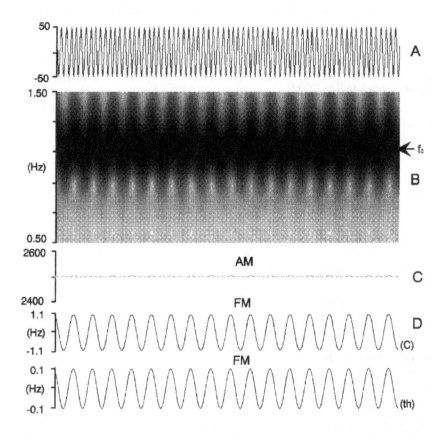

Figure 13.5
Application of the wavelet transform to a frequency modulated
signal. $s_1(t) = 50\sin(2\pi f_0 t + (0.4\sin 2\pi f_1 t))$, with $f_0 = 1$ **Hz** and
$f_1 = 0.1$ **Hz**. A: the analyzed signal; B: the modulus image; C:
the calculated AM; D: comparison between the calculated (c) FM
and the theoretical (th) FM.

frequency $f_1 = 0.25$ Hz and with an amplitude of 0.088 Hz, which must be compared to the imposed amplitude (0.1 Hz). The difference has the same order of magnitude as the frequency resolution (0.01 Hz); it can be decreased by increasing the number of dilations (200) or by increasing the studied frequency range [0.5 to 2.5 Hz].

Amplitude modulation (AM)

We consider a sine function ($f_0 = 1$ Hz, amplitude 50 mV) sampled at a 50 Hz frequency. This signal is modulated in amplitude by two sine components defined, respectively, by $f_1 = 0.25$ Hz, amplitude = 2 mV and by $f_2 = 0.025$ Hz, amplitude = 5 mV. f_1 and f_2 correspond, respectively, to the HF and LF physiological regulations. We associate with them two additive terms, at the same frequencies, in order to be closest to physiological reality. The analytical expression of the test signal is:

$$s_2(t) = [(50 + 2\sin 2\pi f_1 t + 5\sin 2\pi f_2 t)\sin 2\pi f_0 t]$$

$$+ [\sin 2\pi f_1 t] + [2.5\sin 2\pi f_2 t].$$

Figure 13.6 represents the power spectrum of $s_2(t)$.

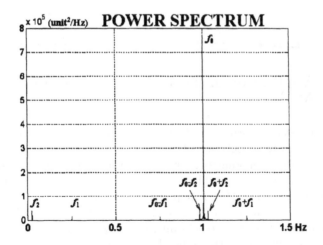

Figure 13.6
Power spectrum of an amplitude modulated signal. $s_2(t) = [(50 + 2\sin 2\pi f_1 t + 5\sin 2\pi f_2 t)\sin 2\pi f_0 t] + [\sin 2\pi f_1 t] + [2.5\sin 2\pi f_2 t]$. **It is easy to find the central frequency f_0, the lateral components $f_0 \pm f_1$ and $f_0 \pm f_2$ introduced by the amplitude modulation, and the two isolated components (f_1, f_2) due to the additive terms.**

Figure 13.7 represents the image of the wavelet transform modulus (panel A); we find three different frequency components (f_0, f_1, f_2). By using the reconstruction procedure, we find the specific signal associated to each frequency. The first one (around f_0) gives the signal modulated in amplitude (without additive terms) with a good accuracy (error $< 0.2\%$). The second and third ones (around f_1 and f_2) represents additive signals (errors less than, respectively, 5% and 0.1%). They highlight the energy conservation law in time and frequency spaces (Plancherel equality). Panel C shows the modulation laws extraction; we do not observe any FM. The measured fundamental frequency f_0 is 0.995 Hz slightly different of 1 Hz (frequential resolution is 0.007 Hz). The AM is in fact a modulation of the power spectral density; it oscillates around 2600 $(51)^2$, with a maximum equal to 3200 $(56.7)^2$ and a minimum equal to 2000 $(44.7)^2$. The modulation ratio is 6/51 as compared to the imposed ratio 7/50. Such results are quite satisfactory, if we consider that experimental errors on blood pressure variations (5 mmHg) are 0.5–1 mmHg.

To obtain the specific AM (at f_1 and f_2), we again apply the reconstruction procedure to the global modulation (panel D). We get calibrated signals, but the square root of the ratio of their maxima gives the ratio of their respective contribution: $740/120 = 6.17$, as compared to the imposed ratio $(5/2)^2 = 6.25$.

13.4 Application of the Wavelet Transform to the EEG Analysis

The wavelet transform of the EEG signal will provide a spectral decomposition in which representation of temporal dynamics is maintained. Figure 13.8 represents the modulus of the EEG wavelet transform in a normal subject in the time/frequency plane. The left panel represents an awakened period during 1 min. The right panel shows a deep sleep period. On this image, values of the modulus are coded with gray levels. During awakening, the energy is distributed in all frequency components α, θ, δ with a slight preponderance in the α band. During deep sleep, energy remains concentrated in the δ component (slow wave sleep), with a great temporal stability.

The main interest in visualizing the modulus of the wavelet transform is to provide a better global visualization of the information.

From the wavelet transform of the EEG, we can define instantaneous

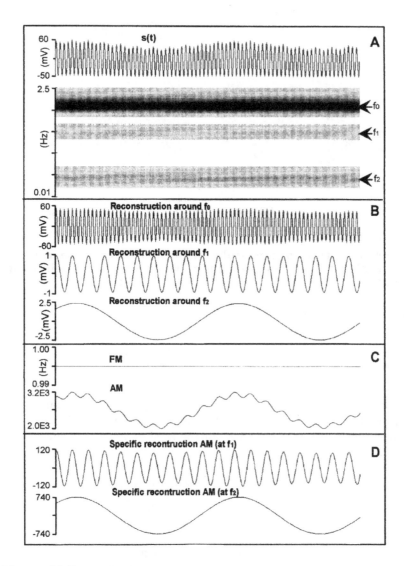

Figure 13.7
Application of the wavelet transform to an amplitude-modulated signal $(s_2(t))$. A: the analyzed signal with the image of its wavelet transform. B: the reconstructed signals around f_0, f_1, f_2. C: the calculated FM and AM. D: the specific reconstructed AM (at f_1 and f_2).

E.E.G SPECTRA

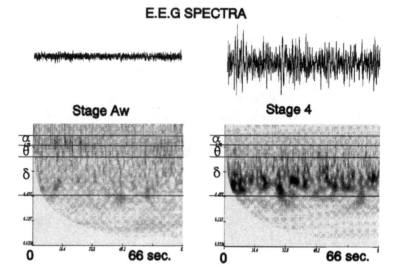

Figure 13.8
The wavelet transform modulus of an EEG signal in a normal subject while awake (left panel) and during deep sleep (right panel). Values of the modulus are coded with gray levels.

spectral energies. They are given by

$$E^m_{[f_0,f_1]}(b) = \int_{f_1}^{f_0} \frac{|(W_\Psi f)\,(a,b)|^2}{a}\, da \qquad (13.3)$$

where $(W_\Psi f)\,(a,b)$ is the wavelet transform of the EEG signal $f(t)$ and $[f_0, f_1]$ is the frequency domain corresponding to the different α, θ, δ components defined in Section 13.2. In the same manner, we can define an instantaneous mean frequency:

$$f^m_{[f_0,f_1]}(t) = \frac{\int_{f_1}^{f_0} \frac{|(W_\Psi f)(a,b)|^2 f_a}{a}\, da}{E^m_{[f_0,f_1]}(t)} \qquad (13.4)$$

where $f_a = \frac{\omega_0}{2\pi a}$ is the instantaneous "local frequency".

Figure 13.9 gives a representation of these different variables in the normal subject whose hypnogram is given in Figure 13.3. From the top to the bottom, we see the EEG signal, the instantaneous $E_\alpha(t)$, $E_\theta(t)$, $E_\delta(t)$ and the mean frequency $f^m_{[f_0,f_1]}(t)$. The corresponding hypnogram is also given for illustrative purpose. It is evident that this hypnogram is a rustic representation, although useful for a clinician, but it does not permit one to describe precisely the dynamics of electroencephalographic activity. Behavior of the mean frequency $f^m_{[f_0,f_1]}(t)$ shows a progressive sliding towards

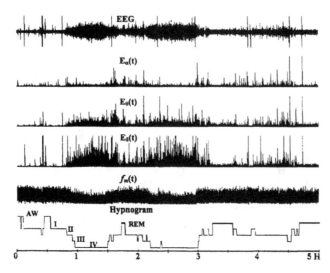

Figure 13.9
Representation of the different instantaneous energies extracted from an EEG signal, in a normal subject during a complete night. The EEG signal (C_Z-P_Z) is sampled at 50 Hz frequency.

low frequencies (characteristics of deep sleep) with some transient fluctuations. In the same manner, $E_\delta(t)$ increases progressively when the subject arrives in deep sleep. This progression is common to all normal subjects. Figure 13.10 represents the evolution of $\langle E_\delta(t)\rangle/\langle E_\alpha(t)\rangle$ in relation with the different sleep stages; it shows that this parameter can be chosen as an index of sleep depth [2].

Notice that such an analysis could also have been done via the short time Fourier transform.

The next picture, Figure 13.11, shows an enlargement of a 5 min period of time in REM. Apparently, we don't observe any special event in the EEG, but the instantaneous $E_\alpha(t)$ shows microarousals (dreams?) during this paradoxical sleep. These short periods of time are correlated with irregular breathing.

The principal application of the wavelet transform, in the processing of EEG signals, is the determination as well as the description of events localized in time. Figure 13.12 shows an obstructive apnea period in a patient with sleep apnea. We have represented respiratory movements of the thorax and abdomen (measured noninvasively by a respiratory area flux meter [12]) and the simultaneous different energies derived from EEG tracings and calculated by the wavelet transform. Forty seconds are shown beginning during obstructive inspiratory efforts and following airway opening (arrow). During obstructed inspiratory efforts, thoracic and abdominal movements are 180 degrees out of phase (paradoxical) and the simultane-

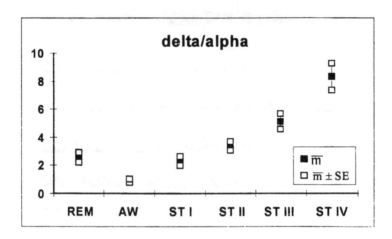

Figure 13.10
Evolution of $\langle E_\delta(t)/E_\alpha(t) \rangle$ with the different sleep stages, in a group of 10 normal subjects. Quantities between brackets represent temporal means (5 min) calculated during the different sleep stages considered as neurogically stable [16].

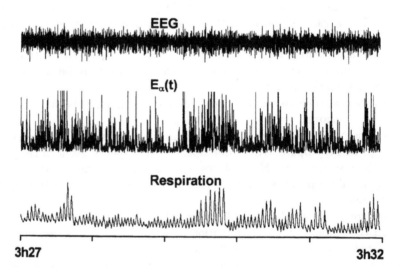

Figure 13.11
Representation of a short period of time (5 min) during REM sleep (subject represented in Figure 13.9). We observe some prominent fluctuations in the α band corresponding partially with an irregular breathing.

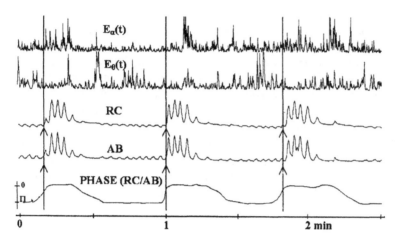

Figure 13.12
Representation of an obstructive apnea period in a patient with sleep apnea. See text for descriptions and explications. Note that the use of the Morlet-Grossman wavelets allows us to obtain the phase relation between the ribcage (RC) and abdomen (AB) signals.

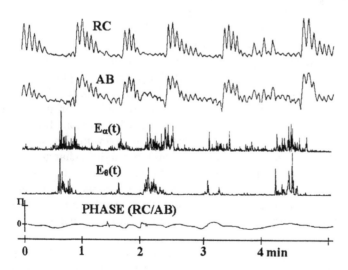

Figure 13.13
Representation of a central apnea/hypopnea period.

ous $E_\theta(t)$ shows the character of the patient's sleep during this obstructive phase. After airway opening (arrow), pulmonary ventilation resumes and respiratory movements are in phase. Shortly after pulmonary ventilation recurs, (within a few seconds), there is a sharp rise in $E_\alpha(t)$, which is not in synchrony with $E_\theta(t)$, corresponding to an "event" known as a microarousal (brief waking EEG). In this individual, the electroencephalographic arousal is secondary to the reoccurrence of breathing, following the apnea and corresponding to an arousal. Time resolution was 0.1 s in this analysis, and frequency resolution 1 Hz.

Figure 13.13 shows a central apnea hypopnea period in another patient. The same tracings are represented. In this case we cannot clearly distinguish the asleep periods from the awake ones. However the sharp rises in $E_\alpha(t)$ precedes the reoccurrence of breathing.

13.5   Using the Wavelet Transform to Analyze Cardiorespiratory Variations

Figure 13.14 shows the application of the wavelet transform to cardiorespiratory signals in a normal subject reclining during sleep (stage I). The left panel shows finger arterial pressure (OHMEDA-FINAPRES*) monitored continuously over a period of a few minutes with decomposition into wavelets. There is a clear concentration of energy in the frequency domain around 1 Hz, corresponding to the fundamental frequency of cardiac contraction. This heart rhythm is evidently modulated. We observe equally a significant component around 0.3 Hz (HF). The right panel shows the simultaneous respiratory signal whose main power is centered around 0.3 Hz in common with arterial pressure. This additive band around 0.3 Hz corresponds to the mechanical cardio-respiratory interaction. Indeed, for each breathing cycle, intrathoracic pressure swings (a few mmHg) induce arterial pressure variations. These changes of pressure induce changes of the heart frequency via the rapid parasympathetic pathway which acts on the sine node (baroreflex). There are also components in the low frequency (LF) domain (0.03 Hz) which are common to both the cardiac and respiratory signals; they correspond to the slow regulation mechanisms.

The fundamental frequency component centered around 1 Hz (basic heart rate) gives rise to a clear ridge in the wavelet transform. It permits one to extract the modulation laws (AM and FM) induced by the mechanisms evoked in Section 13.2.3.

Figure 13.15 represents these modulation laws in the same normal subject during the same sleep stage. It is possible to reconstruct the specific

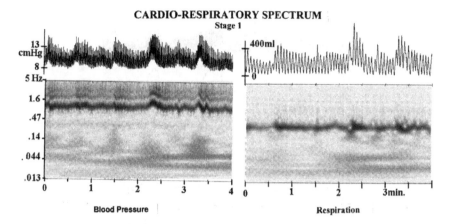

Figure 13.14
Cardio-respiratory signal processings in a normal subject during light sleep (see text for explanations).

contributions due to respiratory regulation (HF) and slow regulation (LF) in amplitude as well as in frequency. We suggest that the LF rhythm, which modulates the amplitude of respiration, the heart frequency, and the blood pressure fluctuations reflects the presence of a network common to cardiovascular and respiratory systems.

Figure 13.16 shows these AM and FM in the HF (respiratory) domain. We easily visualize that the AM and FM are nearly in opposite phase, with a delay which remains smaller than one cardiac beat. This delay expresses a correct activity of the physical regulation of the arterial pressure (baroreflex).

More generally, we show with this method that the baroreflex sensitivity is not modified by the depth of sleep in normal subjects [2].

13.6 Advantage of the Wavelet Transform to Study the Interaction Between Two Systems

Interaction studies between two systems are a particularly suitable field for application of the wavelet transform. For instance, ventilatory instabilities may occur with changes in O_2 and CO_2 and result in variable ventilation periodicites, depending on sleep stage and on the particular sensitivity of the individual. Thus, normal subjects show oscillations in ventilation in sleep stages I and II and REM, which are, in general, more prominent with increasing age. Patients with sleep apnea, of course, show marked

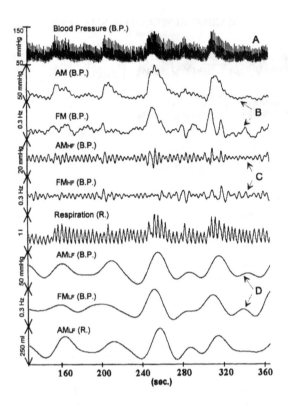

Figure 13.15
Extraction and reconstruction of the different modulation laws
(AM and FM) in the same normal subject during light sleep.
A: The blood pressure. B: The global modulation (AM, FM) of
the blood pressure. C: The specific modulation (AM, FM) of
the blood pressure at the respiratory frequency. D: The specific
modulation (AM, FM) of the blood pressure in the LF band.

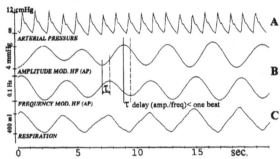

Figure 13.16
Representation of the specific HF modulation laws (AM and FM)
in the same normal subject.

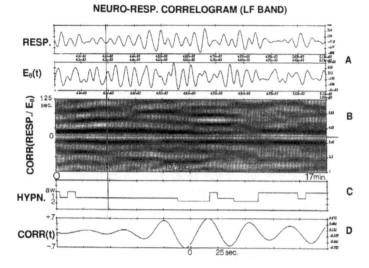

Figure 13.17
Neuro-Respiratory correlogram in the LF band in a patient with sleep apnea. Represented are: A: The modulation laws (AM) for both the ventilation and the θ energy (the scale of time is 102 seconds). B: The sliding cross-correlation function between the respiratory and $E_\theta(t)$ amplitude modulations (see text for explanations). C: The hypnogram, its analysis time-scale (30 s) is not well suited to study this dynamic process (alternance Aw $\leftrightarrow$ light sleep). D: The cross-correlation function at the time t, calculated for 126 seconds.

periodicities of ventilation. If we want to examine temporal relations between ventilatory oscillations and oscillations in state of arousal in such apneic patients, we can use the wavelet transform. It provides simultaneous information concerning ventilation and neurologic activity, in a common scale of time (20–50 seconds for the following example). The delay between ventilatory and neurologic activity is then obtained by analysis of the cross-correlation function.

Figure 13.17 illustrates this idea. The modulation laws (AM) for both ventilation and theta energy have been extracted from the corresponding wavelet transforms. Evolution of their sliding cross-correlation function is given in relation with time. The latter can be described by an alternance (corr = -1) and black (corr = $+1$) bands. This synthetic representation shows that the two systems are in general strongly correlated during the whole period of instabilities (continuous transient sequences awake $\leftrightarrow$ stages I-II). The negative correlation value is permanent and significant; it indicates that during hypoventilation the patient sleeps ($E_\theta(t)$ increases) and during hyperventilation, the patient is awake ($E_\theta(t)$ decreases) from a neurological point of view. We suggest that the 0.05 to 0.02 Hz rhythm, which modulates the amplitude of respiration, reflects the presence of the brain stem network, common to cardiovascular and respiratory systems.

13.7   Conclusion-Perspectives

In general, physicians are interested in conventional variables (systolic pressure, diastolic pressure, heart rate, respiratory frequency, tidal volume, ...) which correspond to temporal means during (quasi) stationary periods of time. However, the physiological reality is more complex and always includes a dynamic aspect which has to be taken into account, especially during as long a period of time as sleep. Notice that the representative signals of the different physiological systems provide the richest information during periods of transition (nonstationary).

Wavelet transforms are a new class of powerful signal analysis techniques which have been attracting increasing attention, especially in biomedical problems. Like spectral analysis, wavelet analysis divides a signal into simpler constituent signals. Unlike spectral analysis, these constituents are not assumed to be sinusoidal, nor are they assumed to be of infinite length. Consequently the wavelet transform yields information from both the time and frequency domain. In this paper, we have not tried to identify the time/frequency-scale method that is the most appropriate to study a given problem. Rather, our objective was to introduce sleep researchers to some basic principles and illustrations of wavelet analysis, and to outline its applications to typical polysomnogram issues.

All applications or illustrations were realized with the continuous Morlet-Grossmann wavelets which offer the possibility of using the modulus and the phase. This method offers interesting perspectives:

- Automated analysis of electroencephalographic activity: it permits quantifying the instantaneous conventional energies $E_\alpha(t)$, $E_\theta(t)$, $E_\delta(t)$ which are necessary to define the sleep stages. Moreover, it would allow detection and analysis of transient phenomena occurring at different scales of time from 20–30 s (typically duration of a recorded page) to less than 1 s (spindles occurring during stage II, K complexes, spikes, bursting events) and consequently, to refine the automated analysis.

- Extraction of the AM-FM laws. In its filtering and reconstruction procedure, the wavelet transform permits us to preserve causality relations, for instance, the phase relation between AM and FM. So, it provides in the HF (respiratory) band, a noninvasive monitoring of the baroreflex sensitivity. This method could be particularly useful in clinical exploration of subjects or patients submitted to special constraints (anesthesiology, intensive care unit, acceleration, ...).

13.8 Acknowledgments

We are very grateful to H. Amiel and M. Mathieu for the realization of polygraphies and C. Dartus and N. Lellouche for the realization of the manuscript. This work was supported by a DRET grant (N°93-341).

References

[1] A. Aldroubi and M. Unser. Workshop on wavelets in medicine and biology. In *Proc. 16th Annu. Int. Conf. IEEE-EMBS*, 1994, 1a–33a.

[2] J. L. Bernard. Acquisition et traitement des données polysomnographiques. Caracterisation des états neuro-cardio-respiratoires pendant le sommeil de l'homme normal. In *Thesis University Paris XII*, 1995.

[3] A. Grossmann and J. Morlet. Decomposition of Hardy functions into square integrable wavelets of constant shape. *SIAM J. Math. Anal.*, 15:723–736, 1984.

[4] A. Grossmann, J. Morlet, and T. Paul. Transforms associated to square integrable representations. General results. *J. Math. Phys.*, 26:2473–2479, 1985.

[5] C. Guilleminault. State of the art: sleep and control of breathing. *Chest*, 73:2935–2953, 1978.

[6] H. H. Jasper. The ten twenty electrode system of the International Federation. *Electroencephalograph. Clin. Neurophysiol.*, 10:371–375, 1958.

[7] T. Kurki, N. T. Smith, N. Head, H. Dec-Silver, and A. Quinn. Non invasive continuous blood pressure measurement from the finger: optimal measurement conditions and factors affecting reliability. *J. Clin. Monitor.*, 3:6–13, 1987.

[8] Y. Meyer, *Les ondelettes—Algorithmes et applications.* Armand Colin Ed, Paris, 1992.

[9] E. A. Phillipson and G. Bowes. Control of breathing during sleep. In *Handbook of Physiology*, Section 3: the Respiratory System, Vol. II, 1987, 649–687.

[10] A. Rechtschaffen and A. Kales. A manual of standardized terminology techniques and scoring systems for sleep stages of human subjects. *Brain Information Service/Brain Research Institute, UCLA*, 1968.

[11] J. D. Sackner, A. J. Nixon, B. Davis, N. Atkins, and M. A. Sackner. Non invasive measurement of ventilation during exercise using a respiratory inductive plethysmograph. *Am. Rev. Resp. Dis.*, 122:867–871, 1980.

[12] R. Sartene, P. Martinot-Lagarde, M. Mathieu, A. Vincent, M. Goldman, and G. Durand. Respiratory cross-sectional area-flux measurements of the human chest wall. *J. Appl. Physiol.*, 68:1605–1614, 1990.

[13] N. V. Thakor and D. L. Sherman. Biomedical problems in time frequency scale analysis. New challenges. In *Proc. IEEE-SP Int Symp. Time-Frequency and Time-Scale Analysis*, 1994, 536–588.

[14] M. J. Thorpy. *International Classification of Sleep Disorders. Diagnostic and Coding Manual.* Diagnostic Classification Steering Committee, American Sleep Disorders Association, Rochester, MN, 1990

14

Estimating the Fractal Exponent of Point Processes in Biological Systems Using Wavelet- and Fourier-Transform Methods

Malvin C. Teich,[1,2,3] Conor Heneghan,[1,3] Steven B. Lowen,[3] and Robert G. Turcott[3,4]

[1] *Department of Electrical, Computer & Systems Engineering, Boston University, Boston;*
[2] *Department of Biomedical Engineering, Boston University, Boston;*
[3] *Department of Electrical Engineering, Columbia University, New York;*
[4] *School of Medicine, Stanford University, Palo Alto, California.*

14.1 Introduction

Some random phenomena occur at discrete times or locations, with the individual events largely identical, such as the detection of particles from radioactive decay. A stochastic point process [8] is a mathematical construction which represents these events as random points in a space. Such a process may be called fractal when a number of the relevant statistics of the point process exhibit scaling with related scaling exponents, indicating that the represented phenomenon contains clusters of points over all (or a relatively large set of) time or length scales. In this chapter, we consider point processes on a line, which model a variety of observed phenomena in the biological sciences.

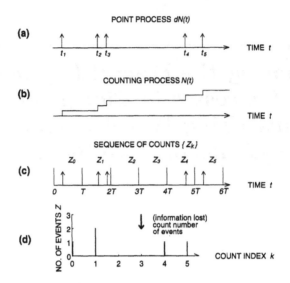

Figure 14.1
Representations of a point process. (a) The events are represented by a sequence of idealized impulses, occurring at times t_k, and forming a stochastic point process $dN(t)$. For convenience of analysis, several alternative representations of the point process are used. (b) The counting process $N(t)$. At every event occurrence the value of $N(t)$ augments by unity. (c) The sequence of counts $\{Z_k\}$, a discrete-time, nonnegative integer-valued stochastic process, is formed from the point process by recording the number of events in successive counting windows of length T. (d) The sequence of counts $\{Z_k\}$ can be conveniently described in terms of a count index k. Information is lost because the precise times of event occurrences within each counting window are eliminated in this representation. Correlations in the discrete-time sequence $\{Z_k\}$ can be readily interpreted in terms of real time.

14.1.1 Mathematical Descriptions of Stochastic Point Processes

Figure 14.1 shows several representations that are useful in the analysis of point processes. Figure 14.1(a) demonstrates the modeling of a point process as a series of impulses occurring at specified times t_k. Since these impulses have vanishing width, they are most rigorously defined as the derivative of a well-defined counting process $N(t)$ (Figure 14.1[b]), a monotonically increasing function of t, that augments by unity when an event occurs. Accordingly, the point process itself is properly written as $dN(t)$, since it is only strictly defined within the context of an integral.

The point process is completely described by the set of event times $\{t_k\}$, or equivalently by the set of interevent intervals. However, the sequence of counts depicted in Figure 14.1(c) also contains much information about the process. Here the time axis is divided into equally sized contiguous counting windows of length T seconds to produce a sequence of counts $\{Z_k\}$, where $Z_k = N[(k+1)T] - N[kT]$ denotes the number of events in the kth window. As illustrated in Figure 14.1(d), this sequence forms a discrete-time random process of nonnegative integers. In general, information is lost in forming the sequence of counts, although for a regular point process the amount lost can be made arbitrarily small by reducing the size of the counting window T. An attractive feature of this representation is that it preserves the correspondence between the discrete time axis of the counting process $\{Z_k\}$ and the absolute "real" time axis of the underlying point process. Within the process of counts $\{Z_k\}$, the elements Z_k and Z_{k+n} refer to the number of counts in windows separated by precisely $T(n-1)$ seconds, so that correlation in the process $\{Z_k\}$ is readily associated with correlation in the underlying point process $dN(t)$.

14.1.2 Fractal Stochastic Point Processes (FSPPs) Exhibit Scaling

The characterization of a stochastic process involves a complete description of all possible joint probabilities of the various events occurring in the process. Different statistics provide complementary views of the process; no single statistic can in general describe a stochastic process completely. We call a stochastic point process *fractal* if it exhibits scaling in many of its statistics. Such scaling leads naturally to power-law behavior, as demonstrated in the following. Consider a statistic f which depends continuously on the scale x over which measurements are taken. Suppose changing the scale by a factor a effectively multiplies the statistic by some other factor $g(a)$, related to the factor but independent of the scale:

$$f(ax) = g(a)f(x). \tag{14.1}$$

The only nontrivial solution of this scaling equation is

$$f(x) = bg(x) \quad \text{with } g(x) = x^c \tag{14.2}$$

for some constants b and c [22, 26]. Thus, statistics with power-law forms are closely related to this concept of a fractal.

For example, consider a commonly encountered first-order statistic for a stochastic point process, the interevent interval histogram (IIH). This estimates the interevent-interval probability density function (IIPDF) $p(t)$ by computing the relative frequency of occurrence of interevent intervals as a function of interval size. This measure highlights the behavior of the times between adjacent events, but reveals none of the information contained in the relationships among these times, such as correlation between adjacent time intervals. For a fully fractal point process, the IIPDF follows the form of Equation 14.2, so that $p(t) \sim t^c$ over a certain range of t, where $c < -1$.

A number of statistics may be used to describe an FSPP, and each statistic which scales will, in general, have a different scaling exponent c. Each of these exponents can be simply related to a more general parameter α, the fractal exponent, where the exact relation between these two exponents will depend upon the statistic in question. For example, the exponent c of the IIPDF defined above can be related to the fractal exponent α by $c = -(1 + \alpha)$.

The fractal exponent α defined above is also related to the more commonly encountered Hurst exponent H [24, 29]. The relationship is ambiguous, however, since some authors [11–13, 24, 41] use the formula $\alpha = 2H + 1$ for all values of α, while others [5] use $\alpha = 2H - 1$ for $\alpha < 1$ to restrict H to the range $(0, 1)$. In this chapter, we avoid this confusion by considering α directly instead of H.

14.1.3 The Standard Fractal Renewal Process

Comparing existing methods of estimating the fractal exponent of point processes with techniques based on wavelets requires a benchmark fractal stochastic point process. Perhaps the most easily described FSPP is the standard fractal renewal process (SFRP) [7, 18, 19, 20, 23]; we focus on this process because of its relative ease of analysis, its simple and straightforward simulation, and its usefulness in describing a variety of real-world processes.

For the SFRP, the times between adjacent events are independent random variables t drawn from the same fractal probability distribution. In particular, the IIPDF $p(t)$ decays essentially as a power law; we illustrate this with a particular form with abrupt cutoffs

$$p(t) = \frac{\alpha}{A^{-\alpha} - B^{-\alpha}} \begin{cases} t^{-(\alpha+1)} & \text{for } 0 < A < t < B \\ 0 & \text{otherwise,} \end{cases} \tag{14.3}$$

with α the fractal exponent and A and B cutoff parameters. The SFRP exhibits fractal behavior over timescales lying between A and B. This process is fully fractal: it exhibits scaling both in the IIPDF and in the second-order statistics that we discuss in Section 14.2.

14.1.4   Examples of Fractal Stochastic Point Processes in Nature

Many phenomena are readily represented by FSPPs or by functions derived from them. We provide several examples drawn from the biological sciences. We have carried out similar analyses for physical phenomena such as trapping in semiconductors [18, 19] and noise and traffic in communication systems [27].

Biological Ion-Channel Openings

Ion channels reside in cell membranes, permitting ions to diffuse in or out [28]. These channels are usually specific to a particular ion, or group of related ions, and block the passage of other kinds of ions. Further, most channels have gates, and thus the channels may be either open or closed. In many instances, intermediate conduction states are not observed. Some ion channels may be modeled by a two-state Markov process [10], with one state representing the open channel and the other representing the closed channel. This model generates exponentially distributed dwell times in both states, which are, in fact, sometimes observed. However, many ion channels exhibit independent power-law-distributed closed times between open times of negligible duration [17] and are well described by an SFRP [20, 21, 30].

Auditory-Nerve-Fiber Action Potentials

Many biological neurons transmit information by means of action potentials, which are localized regions of depolarization traveling down the length of an axon. Action potentials on a given axon are brief and largely identical events, so their reception at another neuron (or at a recording electrode) may be well represented by a point process. FSPPs have been shown to describe the action potentials in primary auditory nerve fibers in a number of species [16, 30, 31, 33, 34]. Over short timescales, nonfractal stochastic point processes prove adequate for representing such nerve spikes, but over long timescales (typically greater than one second) fractal behavior becomes evident. Furthermore, estimators of the rate of the process converge more slowly than for nonfractal processes, displaying fluctuations which decrease as a power-law function of the time used to estimate the rate [32]. With the inclusion of the refractory effects of nerve fibers, an FSPP model can be shown to provide an excellent approximation for modeling the behavior of nerve spikes in auditory fibers in several species over all time scales and for a broad variety of statistical measures [16, 21, 31, 33, 34]; only four parameters are required. This process may well arise from superpositions of fractal ion channel transitions in inner ear sensory cells, as described briefly in the section on biological ion channel openings [20, 21].

Visual-System Action Potentials

As with auditory nerve fibers, some neurons in the visual system transmit information by means of action potentials, and FSPPs provide suitable models for describing the behavior of these neurons [36]. The gamma renewal process, which is nonfractal, has proved to be a useful model for some of these processes over short timescales [37]. However, nerve spike trains recorded from both cat retinal ganglion cell and lateral geniculate nucleus neurons, like those recorded from primary auditory neurons, exhibit fractal behavior over timescales greater than one second, as will become apparent in Section 14.2. This necessitates the use of an FSPP model for these neural spike trains as well [36]. Similar fractal behavior has already been demonstrated for cat striate cortex neurons [35] and for an insect visual interneuron [39].

Human Heartbeat Times

The sequence of human heartbeats exhibits considerable variability over time and among individuals, both in the short-term and the long-term patterns of the beats. These effects can be studied by focusing on the times of maximum contraction, thus forming a point process of heartbeats. A particular FSPP, with an integrate-and-reset (rather than a Poisson) substrate, has been constructed and shown to successfully describe these events [38, 40]. In many respects the heartbeat process resembles the process formed by peripheral auditory and visual system action potentials. Over short timescales, nonfractal point processes provide suitable models for the pattern of times between contractions; for times longer than roughly 10 s, only fractal models suffice. Further, parameters of the FSPP used to model the data may have applicability for the diagnosis of various disease states [40].

14.2　Methods of Estimating the Fractal Exponent of Fractal Point Processes

As the examples described above illustrate, many natural phenomena are amenable to modeling by FSPPs. The value of the fractal exponent α can often provide important information regarding the nature of an underlying process, and can also serve as a useful classification tool (as indicated in the subsection pertaining to the human heartbeat above). Accordingly, it is desirable to estimate α reliably [29], although this task is often confounded by a variety of issues [6] (see [22] for a detailed discussion).

Here we briefly review some of the techniques used for estimating α. We show how two of these, the Fano and Allan factors, can be generalized as wavelet-based measures. To illustrate these techniques, we apply them to a train of action potentials recorded from a lateral geniculate nucleus (LGN) relay neuron in the cat visual system. There are 24,285 events in this particular spike train, with an average interevent interval of 0.132 s, comprising a total duration of 3225 s [36].

14.2.1 Coincidence Rate

The first measure we consider is the coincidence rate (CR). The CR measures the correlations between pairs of events with a specified time delay between them, regardless of intervening events, and is related to the autocorrelation function used with continuous processes. The CR is defined as

$$G(\tau) \equiv \lim_{\Delta \to 0} \frac{\Pr\{\mathcal{E}[0, \Delta] \text{ and } \mathcal{E}[\tau, \tau + \Delta]\}}{\Delta^2}, \qquad (14.4)$$

where $\mathcal{E}[s, t]$ denotes the occurrence of at least one event of the point process in the interval $[s, t)$. For an ideal fractal point process the coincidence rate assumes the form [22]

$$G(\tau) = \lambda\delta(\tau) + \lambda^2 \left[1 + (|\tau|/\tau_0)^{\alpha-1}\right], \qquad (14.5)$$

where λ is the mean rate of the process, $\delta(\tau)$ denotes the Dirac delta function, τ_0 is a fractal onset time constant, and $0 < \alpha < 1$ is the fractal exponent.

The coincidence rate can be directly estimated from its definition. However, in practice the CR is a noisy measure, since its definition essentially involves a double derivative. Furthermore, for FSPPs typical of physical and biological systems, the CR exceeds its asymptotic value λ^2 at $\tau \to \infty$ by only a small fraction at any practical value of τ, so that determining the fractal exponent with this small excess presents serious difficulties. Therefore we do not specifically apply this measure to the LGN data, although the formal definition of coincidence rate plays a useful role in developing other, more reliable measures.

14.2.2 Power Spectral Density

The power spectral density (PSD) is a familiar and well-established measure for continuous-time processes. For point processes, the PSD and the CR introduced above form a Fourier transform pair, much like the PSD and the autocorrelation function do for continuous-time processes. The PSD provides a measure of how the power in a process is concentrated in various frequency bands. For a fractal point process, the PSD assumes the form

$$S(\omega) = \lambda \left[1 + (\omega/\omega_0)^{-\alpha} \right], \tag{14.6}$$

for relevant time and frequency ranges, where λ is the mean rate of events and ω_0 is a cutoff frequency.

The PSD of a point process can be estimated with the periodogram (PG) $S_N(\omega)$ of the sequence of counts, rather than from the point process itself [25]. This method introduces a bias at higher frequencies, since the fine time resolution information is lost as a result of the minimum-count window size. Nevertheless, since estimation of the fractal exponent principally involves lower frequencies where this bias is negligible, and employing the sequence of counts permits the use of vastly more efficient fast Fourier transform methods, we use this technique in this chapter. Alternate definitions of the PSD for point processes (and thus for the PG used to estimate them) exist; for example, a different PSD may be obtained from the real-valued discrete-time sequence of the interevent intervals. However, features in this PSD cannot be interpreted in terms of temporal frequency [40].

Figure 14.2 displays the PG for the visual system LGN data calculated using the count-based approach. (Throughout the text of this chapter we employ radian frequency ω [radians per unit time] to simplify the analysis, while figures are plotted in common frequency $f = \omega/2\pi$ [cycles per unit time] in accordance with common usage.) For low frequencies, the PG decays as $1/\omega^\alpha$, as expected for a fractal point process. Fitting a straight line (shown as dotted) to the doubly logarithmic plot of the PG, over the range from 0.002 Hz to 1 Hz, provides an estimate $\alpha \approx 0.67$. Similar results obtain for the other LGN and retinal ganglion cells (RGC) data sets that we have examined [36].

14.2.3   Fano Factor

Another useful measure of correlation over different timescales is provided by the Fano factor (FF), which is the variance of the number of events in a specified counting time T divided by the mean number of events in that counting time. In terms of the sequence of counts illustrated in Figure 14.1(c), the Fano factor is simply the variance of $\{Z_k\}$ divided by the mean of $\{Z_k\}$, i.e.,

$$F(T) \equiv \frac{\mathrm{E}[Z_k^2] - \mathrm{E}^2[Z_k]}{\mathrm{E}[Z_k]}. \tag{14.7}$$

The FF generally varies as a function of counting time T. The exception is the homogeneous Poisson point process (HPP), which is important as a benchmark in point process theory, just as the Gaussian is in the theory of continuous stochastic processes. For an HPP, the variance-to-mean ratio is always unity for any counting time T. Any deviation from unity in the

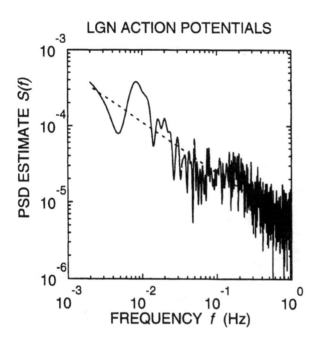

Figure 14.2
Doubly logarithmic plot of the count-based periodogram vs. frequency for the point process representing a nerve spike train recorded at the output of a visual-system relay neuron in the lateral geniculate nucleus (LGN) of the cat (solid curve). No external stimulus was present. The data segment analyzed here consists of **24,285** events with an average interevent time of **0.132** s, comprising a total duration of **3225** s. Over long timescales (low frequencies), the curve can be fit by a straight line (dotted) of slope **−0.67**, representing fractal behavior. This linear best fit to the data was calculated over the region from **0.002 Hz to 1 Hz**.

value of $F(T)$ therefore indicates that the point process in question is not Poisson in nature. An excess above unity reveals that a sequence is "less ordered" than an HPP, while values below unity signify sequences which are "more ordered". For an FSPP, the FF can be shown to vary as $\sim T^\alpha$ for long counting times provided $0 < \alpha < 1$; therefore a straight-line fit to an estimate of $F(T)$ vs. T on a doubly logarithmic plot can also be used to estimate the fractal exponent.

Figure 14.3 shows the estimated FF curve for the same data set as shown in Figure 14.2. For counting times T greater than approximately 0.5 s, this curve behaves essentially as $\sim T^\alpha$. The estimated value is $\alpha = 0.65$ (dotted line), closely agreeing with the value obtained from the PG. Similar estimated FF curves emerge not only for other LGN data sets, but also from spike trains recorded from retinal ganglion cells [36].

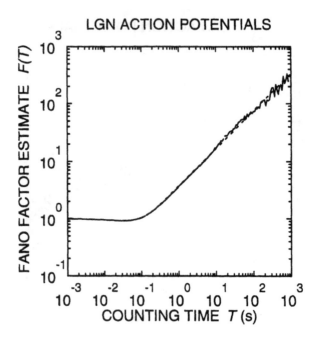

Figure 14.3
Doubly logarithmic plot of the Fano factor estimate vs. counting time, for the same spike train as used for Figure 14.2 (solid curve). Over long timescales, the curve can be fit by a straight line (dotted) of slope 0.65, representing fractal behavior with a similar exponent to that obtained from the PSD. This linear best fit to the data was calculated over the region from 0.3 s to 1000 s.

14.2.4 Allan Factor

The Allan variance, as opposed to the ordinary variance, is defined in terms of the variability of *successive* counts [3, 4]. In analogy with the Fano factor (FF), we define the Allan factor (AF) for the sequence of counts shown in Fig. 14.1 as

$$A(T) \equiv \frac{E\left[(Z_{k+1} - Z_k)^2\right]}{2E[Z_k]}. \qquad (14.8)$$

As for the FF, the value of the Allan factor for the HPP is unity. For an FSPP, the AF also varies as $\sim T^\alpha$ for long counting times with $0 < \alpha < 3$; therefore a straight line fit of an estimate of $A(T)$ vs. T on a doubly logarithmic plot yields yet another estimate of the fractal exponent.

Figure 14.4 shows the estimated Allan factor curve for the same data set as shown in Figures 14.2 and 14.3. This measure appears to be considerably "rougher" than the FF, which is typical of the data sets we have analyzed.

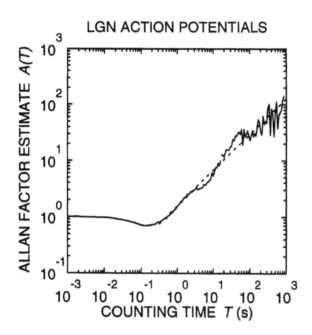

Figure 14.4
Doubly logarithmic plot of the Allan factor estimate vs. counting time, for the same spike train as used for Figures 14.2 and 14.3 (solid curve). Over long timescales, the curve can be fit by a straight line (dotted) of slope 0.64, representing fractal behavior with a similar exponent to that obtained from the PSD and the FF. This linear best fit to the data was calculated over the region from 0.3 s to 1000 s.

Nevertheless it is clear that for counting times T greater than approximately 0.5 s, its behavior can also be approximated as $\sim T^{\alpha}$. To estimate the value of α, a straight line fit to the doubly logarithmic plot of the estimate of $A(T)$ vs. counting time T was provided. The value of $\alpha = 0.64$ obtained agrees well with the values calculated using the PSD and FF. AF curves for other LGN and RGC data sets we have examined appear similar to this one.

14.2.5 Haar-Basis Representation of the Fano and Allan Factors

The Fano and Allan factors can be expressed as special cases of more general measures based on the statistics of the wavelet- and scaling-coefficient sequences of stochastic point processes. In this section, we outline the relation between the FF and AF on the one hand, and the wavelet- and scaling-coefficient-based measures on the other. In particular, we show that these measures coincide for the special case of the Haar wavelet basis.

Scaling and Wavelet Coefficients for a Point Process

We first define the scaling and wavelet coefficients for the point process $dN(t)$. In analogy with the continuous-time definitions of these coefficients provided in Chapter 1, we define the scaling and wavelet coefficients of the point process as

$$(S_\varphi N)(a, k) = c[a, k] \equiv a^{-1/2} \int_{-\infty}^{+\infty} \overline{\varphi(u/a - k)} \, dN(u), \qquad (14.9)$$

and

$$(W_\psi N)(a, k) = d[a, k] \equiv a^{-1/2} \int_{-\infty}^{+\infty} \overline{\psi(u/a - k)} \, dN(u), \qquad (14.10)$$

where $\varphi(t)$ and $\psi(t)$ are the scaling and wavelet functions, respectively, and a is a real-valued scale factor by which the scaling and wavelet functions are dilated. The quantities $c[a, k]$ and $d[a, k]$ are notational conveniences for $(S_\varphi N)(a, k)$ and $(W_\psi N)(a, k)$, respectively. The overbar denotes complex conjugation.

The Haar Basis

The Haar basis plays a central role in uniting the Fano and Allan factors with their corresponding wavelet-based measures. As shown in Chapter 1, the scaling function for the Haar basis is defined as

$$\varphi_H(t) = \begin{cases} 1 & \text{for } 0 \le t < 1 \\ 0 & \text{otherwise} \end{cases} \qquad (14.11)$$

while the wavelet function is defined as

$$\psi_H(t) = \begin{cases} 1 & \text{for } 0 \le t < 1/2 \\ -1 & \text{for } 1/2 \le t < 1 \\ 0 & \text{otherwise.} \end{cases} \qquad (14.12)$$

Figures 14.5(a) and (b) display these functions.

Haar-Basis Scaling and Wavelet Coefficients

For the special case of the Haar wavelet basis introduced above, the integrals in Equations 14.9 and 14.10 are easily evaluated in terms of the counting process $N(t)$ as

$$c[a, k; \text{Haar}] = a^{-1/2} \{N(ka + a) - N(ka)\} \qquad (14.13)$$

HAAR-BASIS SCALING FUNCTION   HAAR-BASIS WAVELET FUNCTION

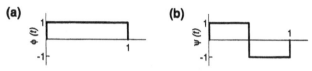

HAAR-BASIS SCALING COEFFICIENTS

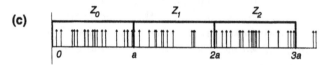

HAAR-BASIS WAVELET COEFFICIENTS

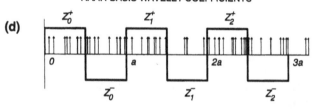

Figure 14.5
Determining the scaling and wavelet coefficients of a point process using the Haar basis. (a) The scaling function for the Haar basis, defined over the domain $[0, 1]$. (b) The wavelet function for the Haar basis, defined over the domain $[0, 1]$. (c) Using sequences of counts to evaluate the scaling coefficients for a point process $dN(t)$. In keeping with the notation of Figure 14.1(c), Z_k denotes the number of events, starting at time ka, and contained within a Haar wavelet that has been scaled by a. The scaling coefficient $c[a, k; \text{Haar}]$ is equal to $a^{-1/2}Z_k$. (d) Using sequences of counts to evaluate the wavelet coefficients for the same point process. The quantity Z_k^+ denotes the number of events, starting at time ka, during the positive portion of a Haar wavelet function (scaled by a); Z_k^- denotes the number of events during the negative half of the same Haar wavelet function. The wavelet coefficient $d[a, k; \text{Haar}]$ is equal to $a^{-1/2}(Z_k^+ - Z_k^-)$.

and

$$d[a, k; \text{Haar}] = a^{-1/2} \{[N(ka + a/2) - N(ka)] \tag{14.14}$$

$$-[N(ka + a) - N(ka + a/2)]\},$$

where the notation $c[a, k; \text{Haar}]$ and $d[a, k; \text{Haar}]$ explicitly indicates that these scaling and wavelet coefficients are obtained using the Haar basis.

Figures 14.5(c) and (d) show graphically how the Haar-basis scaling and wavelet coefficients are calculated by windowing the original data set. The quantities Z_k, Z_k^+, and Z_k^- represent numbers of events contained beneath (or above) their associated rectangular windows. The unitless scale factor a is numerically equal to the duration of the counting window in seconds (which was the T used in the original definition of the FF and AF). The Haar-basis scaling and wavelet coefficients are therefore readily written in terms of the quantities

$$c[a, k; \text{Haar}] = a^{-1/2} Z_k \tag{14.15}$$

and

$$d[a, k; \text{Haar}] = a^{-1/2} \left(Z_k^+ - Z_k^- \right). \tag{14.16}$$

The connection proceeds by observing that the FF for a scale factor a (or a counting time T) is equal to the variance-to-mean ratio (FF) for counting windows of that duration. Considering the definition of the FF (Equation 14.7) in the context of Figures 14.5(c) and (d), we have

$$F(a) = \frac{E\left[Z_k^2\right] - E^2\left[Z_k\right]}{E\left[Z_k\right]}. \tag{14.17}$$

Since $c[a, k; \text{Haar}] = a^{-1/2} Z_k$, the FF may be represented purely in terms of the Haar-basis scaling coefficients:

$$F(a) = a^{1/2} \left(\frac{E\left\{c^2[a, k; \text{Haar}]\right\} - E^2\left\{c[a, k; \text{Haar}]\right\}}{E\left\{c[a, k; \text{Haar}]\right\}} \right). \tag{14.18}$$

Similarly, the AF can be expressed in terms of Z_k, Z_k^+, and Z_k^- as

$$A(a/2) = \frac{E\left[\left(Z_k^+ - Z_k^-\right)^2\right]}{2E\left[Z_k^+\right]}, \tag{14.19}$$

which can be rewritten in terms of the scaling and wavelet coefficients as

$$A(a/2) = a^{1/2} \left(\frac{\mathrm{E}\left\{d^2[a, k; \mathrm{Haar}]\right\}}{\mathrm{E}\left\{c[a, k; \mathrm{Haar}]\right\}} \right). \tag{14.20}$$

The argument $a/2$ for $A(\cdot)$ reflects the fact that the counting windows in Figure 14.5(d) are half the length of the counting windows in Figure 14.5(c).

Equations 14.18 and 14.20 therefore demonstrate that, for the special case of the Haar basis, the scaling and wavelet coefficients of a point process provide a means of estimating the fractal exponent of an FSPP.

14.2.6 Wavelet-Based Fano and Allan Factors

Aside from the Haar basis, other wavelet bases may be employed for estimating α. The results are the wavelet Fano factor (WFF) and wavelet Allan factor (WAF), which are generalizations of the Fano and Allan factors respectively:

$$F_W(a) \equiv a^{1/2} \left(\frac{\mathrm{E}\left\{|c[a, k]|^2\right\} - \mathrm{E}^2\left\{|c[a, k]|\right\}}{\mathrm{E}\left\{|c[a, k]|\right\}} \right) \tag{14.21}$$

$$A_W(a) \equiv a^{1/2} \left(\frac{\mathrm{E}\left\{|d[a, k]|^2\right\}}{\mathrm{E}\left\{|c[a, k]|\right\}} \right), \tag{14.22}$$

where, by using the absolute value of the scaling and wavelet coefficients, we permit the use of complex-valued scaling and wavelet functions. Equation 14.22, defined here as the wavelet Allan factor (WAF), was first proposed as a measure by Flandrin and Abry [1, 2, 13, 14], who called it the wavelet Fano factor. More recently, they also considered a measure similar to $F_W(a)$ [1]. We have defined $A_W(a)$ to coincide with $A(a/2)$ for the special case of the Haar basis, to avoid a superfluous factor of 2 in the definition of the WAF.

These measures permit the estimation of the fractal exponent of an FSPP. To demonstrate this, we first calculate the expected values of $|c[a, k]|$, $|c[a, k]|^2$, and $|d[a, k]|^2$, employing the coincidence rate $G(\tau)$ of a fractal point process defined in Equation 14.5, and the scaling and wavelet functions $\varphi(t)$ and $\psi(t)$, respectively. The expected value of $|c[a, k]|$ is

$$\mathrm{E}\left\{|c[a, k]|\right\} = a^{-1/2} \left| \int_{-\infty}^{+\infty} \overline{\varphi(t/a - k)} \, \mathrm{E}[dN(t)] \right| \tag{14.23}$$

$$= a^{-1/2} \left| \int_{-\infty}^{+\infty} \overline{\varphi(t/a - k)} \, \lambda \, dt \right|$$

$$= \lambda a^{1/2} \left| \int_{-\infty}^{+\infty} \overline{\varphi(z)} \, dz \right|$$

$$= \lambda a^{1/2},$$

since $E[dN(t)] = \lambda \, dt$ by definition, with λ the mean rate of the point process. Note that we have chosen the scaling function to be normalized to unit area.

The expected value of $|c[a, k]|^2$ is readily calculated as

$$E\left\{ |c[a, k]|^2 \right\} \tag{14.24}$$

$$= a^{-1} \int_{-\infty}^{+\infty} \int_{-\infty}^{+\infty} \varphi(t/a - k)\overline{\varphi(u/a - k)} \, E[dN(t) \, dN(u)]$$

$$= a^{-1} \int_{-\infty}^{+\infty} \int_{-\infty}^{+\infty} \varphi(t/a - k)\overline{\varphi(u/a - k)} \, G(t - u) \, dt \, du,$$

where $G(t)$ is the coincidence rate for the process. By using the substitutions $y \equiv u/a - b$ and $z \equiv (t - u)/a$, for a stationary point process we obtain

$$E\left\{ |c[a, k]|^2 \right\} = a \int_{-\infty}^{+\infty} (S_\varphi \varphi)(1, z) G(za) \, dz, \tag{14.25}$$

where

$$(S_\varphi \varphi)(1, z) \equiv \int_{-\infty}^{+\infty} \varphi(y)\overline{\varphi(y - z)} \, dy \tag{14.26}$$

is the continuous scaling transform of the scaling function itself, at unit scale. Similarly, the expected value of $|d[a, k]|^2$ can be calculated as

$$E\left\{ |d[a, k]|^2 \right\} = a \int_{-\infty}^{+\infty} (W_\psi \psi)(1, z) G(za) \, dz, \tag{14.27}$$

with

$$(W_\psi \psi)(1, z) = \int_{-\infty}^{+\infty} \psi(y)\overline{\psi(y - z)} \, dy \tag{14.28}$$

the continuous wavelet transform of the wavelet function $\psi(t)$.

For an ideal FSPP, the CR assumes the form given in Equation 14.5; substituting this into Equation 14.25 yields for the scaling coefficients

$$E\left\{|c[a, k]|^2\right\} = a \int_{-\infty}^{+\infty} (S_\varphi \varphi)(1, z) \lambda \delta(az) \, dz \tag{14.29}$$

$$+ \lambda^2 a \int_{-\infty}^{+\infty} (S_\varphi \varphi)(1, z) \, dz$$

$$+ \lambda^2 a \int_{-\infty}^{+\infty} (S_\varphi \varphi)(1, z)(a/\tau_0)^{\alpha-1} |z|^{\alpha-1} \, dz$$

$$= a(\lambda/a)(S_\varphi \varphi)(1, 0) + \lambda^2 a$$

$$+ \lambda^2 a^\alpha \tau_0^{1-\alpha} \int_{-\infty}^{+\infty} (S_\varphi \varphi)(1, z) |z|^{\alpha-1} \, dz$$

$$= \lambda + \lambda^2 a + \lambda^2 a^\alpha \tau_0^{1-\alpha} \int_{-\infty}^{+\infty} (S_\varphi \varphi)(1, z) |z|^{\alpha-1} \, dz,$$

where we have used the identity $\int_{-\infty}^{+\infty} (S_\varphi \varphi)(1, z) \, dz = 1$ appropriate for a scaling function of unit area, and we have also normalized the scaling function to have unit energy, so that $(S_\varphi \varphi)(1, 0) = 1$. (The scaling function $\varphi(t)$ may be defined to have both unity area and unity energy. For unnormalized scaling functions, the results are qualitatively the same, although notationally more cumbersome.)

In a similar manner, the expected value of the absolute square of the wavelet coefficients for the fractal point process is calculated to be

$$E\left\{|d[a, k]|^2\right\} = a \int_{-\infty}^{+\infty} (W_\psi \psi)(1, z) \lambda \delta(az) \, dz \tag{14.30}$$

$$+ \lambda^2 a \int_{-\infty}^{+\infty} (W_\psi \psi)(1, z) \, dz$$

$$+ \lambda^2 a \int_{-\infty}^{+\infty} (W_\psi \psi)(1, z)(a/\tau_0)^{\alpha-1} |z|^{\alpha-1} \, dz$$

$$= a(\lambda/a)(W_\psi \psi)(1, 0) + \lambda^2 a \cdot 0$$

$$+\lambda^2 a^\alpha \tau_0^{1-\alpha} \int_{-\infty}^{+\infty} (W_\psi\psi)(1,z)|z|^{\alpha-1}\,dz$$

$$= \lambda + \lambda^2 a^\alpha \tau_0^{1-\alpha} \int_{-\infty}^{+\infty} (W_\psi\psi)(1,z)|z|^{\alpha-1}\,dz,$$

where this time we invoke the identities $\int_{-\infty}^{+\infty}(W_\psi\psi)(1,z)\,dz = 0$ for any admissible wavelet, and $(W_\psi\psi)(1,0) = 1$, since the scaling and wavelet functions have equal energy.

Using Equations 14.23 and 14.29 for a FSPP, the WFF defined in Equation 14.21 becomes

$$F_W(a) = a^{1/2}\left(\frac{\lambda + \lambda^2 a + \lambda^2 a^\alpha \tau_0^{1-\alpha}\int_{-\infty}^{+\infty}(S_\varphi\varphi)(1,z)|z|^{\alpha-1}\,dz - \lambda^2 a}{\lambda a^{1/2}}\right)$$

$$= 1 + \frac{\alpha(\alpha+1)}{2}\left(\frac{a}{a_0}\right)^\alpha \int_{-\infty}^{+\infty}(S_\varphi\varphi)(1,z)|z|^{\alpha-1}\,dz, \qquad (14.31)$$

where we implicitly define a_0 by the relation

$$2\lambda a_0^\alpha = \alpha(\alpha-1)\tau_0^{\alpha-1} \qquad (14.32)$$

for notational convenience [22]. The integral in Equation 14.31 depends on the scaling function φ and on the fractal exponent α, but not on the scale a; thus it does not affect the overall power-law behavior of $F_W(a)$. For large values of a, the wavelet Fano factor increases essentially as $\sim a^\alpha$. Accordingly, the fractal exponent can be readily estimated from the slope of the straight-line region on a doubly logarithmic plot of an estimate of $F_W(a)$ vs. scale a.

Similarly, the wavelet Allan factor for a fractal point process follows the form

$$A_W(a) = 1 + \frac{\alpha(\alpha+1)}{2}\left(\frac{a}{a_0}\right)^\alpha \int_{-\infty}^{+\infty}(W_\psi\psi)(1,z)|z|^{\alpha-1}\,dz, \qquad (14.33)$$

with the integral in Equation 14.33 also independent of a, so that the fractal exponent α may also be estimated from the slope of the straight-line region on a doubly logarithmic plot of an estimate of $A_W(a)$ vs. scale a.

The integrals given in Equations 14.9 and 14.10 for the scaling and wavelet coefficients can be numerically approximated for a point process by

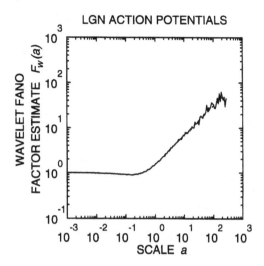

Figure 14.6
Doubly logarithmic plot of the wavelet Fano factor estimate
vs. scale a, for the same spike train as used for Figures 14.2,
14.3, and 14.4 (solid curve). The Daubechies four-tap scaling
and wavelet functions were used to calculate the estimated WFF.
The prototype wavelet function was taken to be of duration 1 s
for scale $a = 1$. Over long timescales, the curve can be fit by a
straight line (dotted) of slope 0.65, representing fractal behavior
with a similar exponent to that obtained from the PSD, FF, and
AF. This linear best fit to the data was calculated over the region
from 1 to 250.

using a summation in conjunction with well-sampled versions of the scaling and wavelet functions. Figure 14.6 shows the estimates of the wavelet
Fano factor calculated in this manner for the same data set as shown in
Figures 14.2, 14.3, and 14.4 (Daubechies four-tap scaling and wavelet functions [9] were used in this implementation). The prototype wavelet was set
to have a duration of 1 second at scale $a = 1$. For scales a greater than
approximately 1, the estimate of the WFF behaves essentially as $\sim a^{\alpha}$. To
estimate the value of α, a straight-line fit to the doubly logarithmic plot of
this estimated $F_W(a)$ vs. a was provided. The resulting value is $\alpha = 0.65$
(dotted line), closely agreeing with the value obtained from the PSD, FF,
and AF.

Figure 14.7 shows the estimate of the wavelet Allan factor calculated for
the same data set as shown in Figures 14.2–14.6. For scales a greater than
approximately 5, this estimate behaves essentially as $\sim a^{\alpha}$, though like the
estimated Allan factor shown in Figure 14.4, it is rough in appearance.
As before, to estimate the value of α, a straight-line fit to the doubly
logarithmic plot of the estimated $F_W(a)$ vs. a was provided, resulting in a
value of $\alpha = 0.62$ (dotted line). Thus all five methods for estimating the

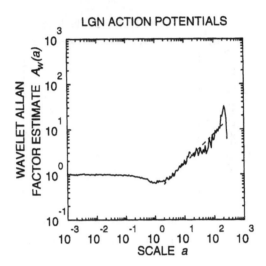

Figure 14.7
Doubly logarithmic plot of the wavelet Allan factor estimate
vs. time, for the same spike train as used for Figures 14.2, 14.3,
14.4, and 14.6. The same wavelet basis was used as in Figure
14.6. Over long timescales, the curve can be fit by a straight line
(dotted) of slope 0.62, representing fractal behavior with a similar exponent to that of the PSD, FF, AF, and WFF. This linear
best fit to the data was calculated over the region from 1 to 250.

fractal exponent, the PSD, FF, AF, WFF, and WAF, yield values in close
agreement.

14.3   Comparison of the Estimation Properties of Ex-
isting Techniques and Wavelet-Based Techniques

The question naturally arises: does this agreement extend to arbitrary
data sets, and if not, which technique provides the most reliable estimate
of the fractal exponent α?

To address this issue we undertook a systematic examination of the bias
and variance of each of these estimators. We simulated 50 runs of an SFRP
at each of three different input values of α: $\alpha = 0.2$, 0.5, and 0.8. Each
simulation was chosen to be 10^5 seconds long with an expected interevent
time of 1.0 s. The PSD, FF, AF, WFF, and WAF were estimated for each
of the 150 simulations, and the fractal exponents were in turn estimated
from these statistics by using straight-line fits over a fixed region of each
of the 750 individual doubly logarithmic curves. The means and standard

Table 14.1

Performance summary of the five fractal-exponent estimators described in Section 14.2 (PSD, FF, AF, WFF, and WAF) when applied to 50 independent realizations of an SFRP for each of three values of the fractal exponent α (0.2, 0.5, and 0.8).

	Theoretical Fractal Exponent		
	0.2	0.5	0.8
PSD	0.332 ± 0.014	0.480 ± 0.017	0.603 ± 0.012
FF	0.313 ± 0.065	0.425 ± 0.081	0.591 ± 0.075
AF	0.337 ± 0.034	0.482 ± 0.055	0.645 ± 0.041
WFF	0.322 ± 0.068	0.424 ± 0.084	0.607 ± 0.069
WAF	0.332 ± 0.025	0.482 ± 0.034	0.614 ± 0.034

Note: For each measure, the mean value $\pm$ the standard deviation is presented. The estimates were obtained over the following frequency and time ranges: PSD: 0.001–0.1 Hz; FF and AF: 5–1000 s; WFF and WAF: 25–2500. For the WFF and the WAF, the range refers to the value of the scale factor a used to dilate the mother scaling and wavelet functions.

deviations of these fractal exponent estimates are listed in Table 14.1 and presented graphically in Figure 14.8(a). The ranges over which the estimates were obtained are indicated in the table caption.

Figure 14.8(a) reveals at a glance that all of the measures perform quite poorly for $\alpha = 0.2$ and $\alpha = 0.8$. The observed bias towards the value 0.5 also emerges when estimating the fractal exponent of a superposition of SFRPs (Figure 8 of [22]). This bias is not fully understood; part undoubtedly stems from the necessity for finite data-length simulations, and part arises from the need for imposing cutoffs in the simulation of the SFRP (A and B in Equation 14.3). In fact, the simulation process itself may be inherently biased. The simulations shown here follow the techniques used in [22], where the IIPDF was chosen to have a power-law decay with an exponent of $\alpha - 3$; this yielded physiologically plausible simulations of neural spike trains. Changing this exponent to $-(\alpha + 1)$ somewhat reduced the bias in the estimate of α, but the resulting simulations no longer resembled neuronal behavior. However, this reduction in the bias does support the claim that the bias may in large part stem from simulation effects.

Therefore we focus instead on the relative differences between fractal exponent estimates obtained through wavelet-based measures and those obtained from the PSD, FF, and AF, and in particular on the means and standard deviations provided in Table 14.1 and Figure 14.8(a). The means do not show a significant difference; employing the PSD, AF, and WAF yields estimated mean values of α within 0.04 of each other, with the values corresponding to the *FF* and *WFF* only slightly farther apart. However,

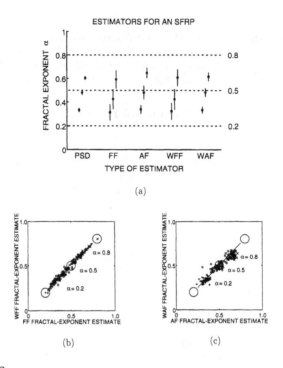

(a)

(b)   (c)

Figure 14.8

Performance summary of the five estimators considered in this chapter (PSD, FF, AF, WFF, and WAF). (a) Graphical representation of the data presented in Table 14.1. The mean values of 50 estimates for the fractal exponent of the SFRP, for each of the three different values of α, are marked by dots. The ± 1-SD regions are indicated by the vertical lines projecting from each dot. All of the estimates show strong bias for $\alpha = 0.2$ and $\alpha = 0.8$; only the measures employing the FF and WFF are significantly biased for $\alpha = 0.5$. From the perspective of the variance of the estimator, the PSD-based method is best (least variance), with the AF and WAF achieving nearly as low a variance, and the FF and WFF exhibiting the worst performance. (b) Relation between the WFF- and the FF-based estimates. The estimated value of α using the WFF is plotted against the estimated value from the FF; the correlation coefficient is 0.99. This consistency is gratifying, since the two measures are essentially the same, differing only in the change of wavelet basis from the Daubechies four-tap (for the WFF) to the Haar basis (for the FF). Both estimators show strong bias for $\alpha = 0.2$ and $\alpha = 0.8$, and have a high variance (see Table 14.1 for numerical values). (c) Relation between the WAF- and the AF-based estimates. The estimated value of α using the WAF is plotted against the estimated value from the AF; these are highly correlated, for the same reason as in (b), with a correlation coefficient of 0.95. Both estimators show strong bias for $\alpha = 0.2$ and $\alpha = 0.8$, but have a moderately low variance (see Table 14.1 for numerical values).

Figure 14.8(a) clearly shows that the standard deviations using the FF and WFF methods are significantly greater than those for the other measures, and this will be further explored in Section 14.4.

We now turn to the correlation between the estimates provided by the FF/WFF and AF/WAF pairs. A positive correlation is to be anticipated, since we have shown theoretically how the WFF and WAF are generalizations of the FF and AF, respectively. Figure 14.8(b) shows a scatter plot of the 150 estimates of α obtained from the FF and the WFF. The centers of the three large circles correspond to zero error in estimating the fractal exponent for the three values of α used to simulate the process, and the lines connecting the circles indicates where the two estimates coincide. Since the estimate pairs are strongly clustered along these lines, they are strongly correlated, confirming that the WFF is indeed closely related to the FF; the correlation coefficient is 0.99. Figure 14.8(c) shows a similar scatter plot obtained from the AF and the WAF. Again the estimate pairs are strongly clustered along the 45° line, indicating that they are strongly correlated, and that the WAF is closely related to the AF. For this pair the correlation coefficient assumes a value of 0.95. Though the estimates of the WFF and WAF displayed in Figure 14.8 are specifically calculated using a Daubechies four-tap wavelet basis, we have determined that the results do not vary significantly for different wavelet bases [15]; there tends to be a slight increase in the variance of the estimators as the number of vanishing moments of the wavelet increases—see Section 14.4.

14.4 Discussion

An interesting feature that emerges from the SFRP simulations summarized in Figure 14.8 is the consistently lower variances in fractal-exponent estimation exhibited when using AF- and WAF-based methods in comparison with those of the FF and WFF. Flandrin and Abry [1, 2, 12–14] suggested that this might relate to the behavior of the Fourier transforms of the scaling and wavelet functions. To investigate this supposition, we recast Equations 14.25 and 14.27 from time-domain integrals into frequency-domain ones. Thus, Equation 14.25 becomes

$$E\left\{|c[a,k]|^2\right\} = a \int_{-\infty}^{+\infty} (S_\varphi \varphi)(1, z) G(za)\, dz \tag{14.34}$$

$$= \int_{-\infty}^{+\infty} (S_\varphi \varphi)(1, z/a) G(z)\, dz$$

$$= \int_{-\infty}^{+\infty} \left[\int_{-\infty}^{+\infty} \varphi(y)\overline{\varphi(y - z/a)}dy \right] G(z)\, dz$$

$$= \frac{1}{2\pi} \int_{-\infty}^{+\infty} \int_{-\infty}^{+\infty} |\hat{\varphi}(\omega)|^2 \exp(i\omega z/a) G(z)\, d\omega\, dz$$

$$= \frac{1}{2\pi} \int_{-\infty}^{+\infty} |\hat{\varphi}(\omega)|^2 S(\omega/a)\, d\omega$$

$$= \frac{1}{2\pi} a \int_{-\infty}^{+\infty} |\hat{\varphi}(\omega a)|^2 S(\omega)\, d\omega,$$

where $\hat{\varphi}(\omega)$ is the Fourier transform of $\varphi(t)$, and

$$S(\omega) = \int_{-\infty}^{+\infty} G(z) \exp(-i\omega z)\, dz \tag{14.35}$$

is the PSD of the point process, as defined in Section 14.2.2. Similarly, Equation 14.27 may be expressed as

$$\mathrm{E}\left\{|d[a, k]^2|\right\} = \frac{1}{2\pi} \int_{-\infty}^{+\infty} \left|\hat{\psi}(\omega)\right|^2 S(\omega/a)\, d\omega \tag{14.36}$$

$$= \frac{a}{2\pi} \int_{-\infty}^{+\infty} \left|\hat{\psi}(\omega a)\right|^2 S(\omega)\, d\omega.$$

The forms of the integrals in Equations 14.34 and 14.36 provide some insight into the relative performances of the five fractal exponent estimators studied. For an FSPP, the PSD follows the form of Equation 14.6 and diverges at low frequencies. Any practical FSPP will have cutoff frequencies, however, beyond which the fractal scaling no longer holds, and the PSD will therefore assume some finite value at low frequencies. Fractal processes naturally exhibit fluctuations on all frequency scales, with the lowest frequencies displaying the largest fluctuations, in proportion to the PSD. Therefore the low-frequency asymptote of a PSD estimate can fluctuate widely among different simulations of the same FSPP. By definition, $|\hat{\varphi}(0)| = 1$ and is continuous at $\omega = 0$, so that the integral in Equation 14.34 does not converge for a fractal point process with $0 < \alpha < 1$ and therefore explicitly depends on the low frequency asymptote. Thus $\mathrm{E}\left\{|c[a, k]|^2\right\}$ depends directly on this fluctuating quantity, and the estimate of the FF and

WFF should exhibit the largest variance. Indeed, estimates of individual FF and WFF plots for the SFRP simulations used in this chapter exhibit wide fluctuations from run to run. Although each individual estimated FF or WFF curve appears smooth, overlays of these plots show a wide range of slopes for the same starting value of the fractal exponent α, therefore yielding wide variation in the estimates of α.

The Fourier transforms of wavelet functions, however, attain a value of zero for zero frequency, and are also continuous at this point. Therefore the behavior of the integrand in Equation 14.36 near the origin for an FSPP depends on both the divergence in the PSD and the tendency of $|\hat{\psi}(\omega)|$ to go to zero. The behavior of $|\hat{\psi}(\omega)|$ near the origin may be described by the number of vanishing moments R of the wavelet, defined as the largest integer R for which

$$\int_{-\infty}^{+\infty} t^R \psi(t)\, dt = 0.$$

For a wavelet $\psi(t)$ with R vanishing moments, the magnitude of its Fourier transform $|\hat{\psi}(\omega)|$ varies as $\sim \omega^{R+\epsilon}$ for $\omega \to 0$, where $0 < \epsilon \le 1$. Therefore, the integral in Equation 14.36 converges without a low-frequency asymptote for any $\alpha < 1 + 2R$. The Haar basis has $R = 0$ exactly; for our simulations $\alpha < 1$, so $\mathrm{E}\left\{|d[a,k]|^2\right\}$ does not depend on the fluctuating low-frequency asymptote, and estimates of the AF should exhibit lower variance than those of the FF and WFF. In fact, for the Haar basis $|\hat{\psi}(\omega)|$ varies as $\sim \omega^1$ so that the Allan factor converges for $\alpha < 3$. For the Daubechies four-tap wavelet that we have used, $R = 2$, so that the cutoffs do not greatly affect the integral for $\alpha < 5$. We expect estimates of the WAF to exhibit similar variance to those of the AF, since in our simulations we employ fractal exponents in the range $0 < \alpha < 1$. The WAF should prove more useful than the AF for FSPPs with $\alpha > 3$. In contrast to the FF and the WFF, individual AF and WAF estimates exhibit somewhat smaller fluctuations from plot to plot. These Allan-based estimates appear somewhat more ragged than those of the FF and WAF, but slopes for these plots in fact show less variation, and yield estimates of α with somewhat less variance.

Finally, we expect the PG to have the lowest variance of all, since it depends on all frequencies and thus deemphasizes the effect of the low-frequency fluctuations. Simulations validate this reasoning. Individual PG plots indeed exhibit the widest variation of all, yet the estimates of the fractal exponent α exhibit the least variance of the five measures studied. For the values of α we have chosen, the wavelet-based measures exhibit similar performance to those of their Haar-basis counterparts. In short, the Allan-based methods outperform those based on Fano factors, and the PG yields the best performance of all.

14.5   Conclusion

We have defined two wavelet-based measures for estimating the fractal exponent of a point process: the wavelet Fano factor and wavelet Allan factor. These arise as natural generalizations of two simple count-based measures: the Fano factor and Allan factor, respectively. We have shown that, at least for the standard fractal renewal process, the wavelet-based techniques reveal their Fano- and Allan-factor origins by exhibiting similar biases and variances. The AF and the WAF outperform the FF and the WFF for the SFRP, apparently because of the increased number of vanishing moments in the frequency domain of wavelet functions compared to scaling functions. Carrying this argument further, one might expect that the WAF would outperform the AF for wavelet bases with at least one vanishing moment. SFRP simulations reveal that this does not happen, however, indicating that the addition of further vanishing moments is offset by the effective widening of the support of the wavelet basis, leading to fewer independent values of wavelet and scaling coefficients for a given finite data set [15]. Still, the fractal-exponent estimation properties of the power spectral density, a Fourier-transform based method, appear to surpass the other methods investigated, at least for this simulation of the SFRP; other types of FSPPs, or even other variations of the SFRP, might well yield different results. Thus wavelet-based measures can be fruitfully added to our armament of techniques for estimating the fractal exponent of an FSPP.

14.6   Acknowledgments

This work was supported by the Office of Naval Research under grant N00014-92-J-1251, by the Joint Services Electronics Program through the Columbia Radiation Laboratory, and by the Whitaker Foundation under Grant No. CU01455801. The authors are grateful to Patrice Abry (École Normale Supérieure de Lyon), Patrick Flandrin (École Normale Supérieure de Lyon), and Cormac Herley (Hewlett-Packard Laboratories) for valuable discussions. E. Kaplan and T. Ozaki of Rockefeller University kindly provided us with the visual-system spike trains used as examples in this chapter.

References

[1] P. Abry, Transformées en ondelettes: Analyses multirésolution et signaux de presion en turbulence, Doctoral thesis, Université Claude Bernard—Lyon I, France (1994).

[2] P. Abry and P. Flandrin, Wavelet-based Fano factor for long-range dependent point processes, *Proc. 16th Annu. Int. Conf. IEEE Eng. Med. Biol. Soc.* (Baltimore, MD, 1994), pp. 1330–1331.

[3] D. W. Allan, Statistics of atomic frequency standards, *Proc. IEEE* **54**, 221–230 (1966).

[4] J. A. Barnes and D. W. Allan, A statistical model of flicker noise, *Proc. IEEE* **54**, 176–178 (1966).

[5] R. J. Barton and H. V. Poor, Signal detection in fractional Gaussian noise, *IEEE Trans. Inform. Theory* **34**, 943–959 (1988).

[6] J. Beran, Statistical methods for data with long-range dependence, *Stat. Sci.* **7**, 404–427 (1992).

[7] J. M. Berger and B. B. Mandelbrot, A new model for the clustering of errors on telephone circuits, *IBM J. Res. Dev.* **7**, 224–236 (1963).

[8] D. R. Cox and V. Isham, *Point Processes* (Chapman and Hall, London, 1980).

[9] I. Daubechies, Orthonormal bases of compactly supported wavelets, *Commun. Pure Appl. Math.* **41**, 909–996 (1988).

[10] L. J. DeFelice and A. Isaac, Chaotic states in a random world: relationship between the nonlinear differential equations of excitability and the stochastic properties of ion channels, *J. Stat. Phys.* **70**, 339–354 (1993).

[11] P. Flandrin, On the spectrum of fractional Brownian motions, *IEEE Trans. Inf. Theory* **35**, 197–199 (1989).

[12] P. Flandrin, Wavelet analysis and synthesis of fractional Brownian motion, *IEEE Trans. Inf. Theory* **38**, 910–917 (1992).

[13] P. Flandrin, Time-scale analyses and self-similar stochastic processes, *Proc. NATO Adv. Study Inst. Wavelets and Their Applications* (Il Ciocco, Italy, 1992).

[14] P. Flandrin and P. Abry, Tracking long-range dependencies with wavelets, *Proc. 1994 IEEE-IMS Workshop Inf. Stat.* (Alexandria, VA, 1994), p. 54.

[15] C. Heneghan, S. B. Lowen, and M. C. Teich, Wavelet analysis for estimating the fractal properties of neural firing patterns, *Proc. Computational Neurosci.*, 1995.

[16] A. H. Kumar and D. H. Johnson, Analyzing and modeling fractal intensity point processes, *J. Acoust. Soc. Am.* **93**, 3365–3373 (1993).

[17] L. S. Liebovitch and T. I. Tóth, Using fractals to understand the opening and closing of ion channels, *Ann. Biomed. Eng.* **18**, 177–194 (1990).

[18] S. B. Lowen and M. C. Teich, Fractal renewal processes as a model of charge transport in amorphous semiconductors, *Phys. Rev. B* **46**, 1816–1819 (1992).

[19] S. B. Lowen and M. C. Teich, Fractal renewal processes generate $1/f$ noise, *Phys. Rev. E* **47**, 992–1001 (1993).

[20] S. B. Lowen and M. C. Teich, Fractal renewal processes, *IEEE Trans. Inf. Theory* **39**, 1669–1671 (1993).

[21] S. B. Lowen and M. C. Teich, Fractal auditory-nerve firing patterns may derive from fractal switching in sensory hair-cell ion channels, in *Noise in Physical Systems and $1/f$ Fluctuations* (AIP Conference Proceedings **285**), eds. P. H. Handel and A. L. Chung (American Institute of Physics, New York, 1993), pp. 781–784.

[22] S. B. Lowen and M. C. Teich, Estimation and simulation of fractal stochastic point processes, *Fractals* **3**, 183–210 (1995).

[23] B. B. Mandelbrot, Self-similar error clusters in communication systems and the concept of conditional stationarity, *IEEE Trans. Commun. Tech.* **13**, 71–90 (1965).

[24] B. B. Mandelbrot, *The Fractal Geometry of Nature* (W. H. Freeman, New York, 1983).

[25] K. Matsuo, B. E. A. Saleh, and M. C. Teich, Cascaded Poisson processes, *J. Math. Phys.* **23**, 2353–2364 (1982).

[26] W. Rudin, *Principles of Mathematical Analysis*, 3rd ed. (McGraw Hill, New York, 1976), p. 197.

[27] B. K. Ryu and S. B. Lowen, Modeling self-similar traffic with the fractal-shot-noise-driven Poisson process, Cent. for Telecomm. Res., Tech. Rep. 392-94-39 (Columbia University, New York, 1994).

[28] B. Sakmann and E. Neher, *Single-Channel Recording* (Plenum, New York, 1983).

[29] H. E. Schepers, J. H. G. M. van Beek, and J. B. Bassingthwaighte, Four methods to estimate the fractal dimension from self-affine signals, *IEEE Eng. Med. Biol. Mag.* **11**, 57–64 (1992).

[30] M. C. Teich, Fractal character of the auditory neural spike train, *IEEE Trans. Biomed. Eng.* **36**, 150–160 (1989).

[31] M. C. Teich, R. G. Turcott, and S. B. Lowen, The fractal doubly stochastic Poisson point process as a model for the cochlear neural spike train, in *The Mechanics and Biophysics of Hearing (Lecture Notes in Biomathematics, Vol. 87)*, eds. P. Dallos, C. D. Geisler, J. W. Matthews, M. A. Ruggero, and C. R. Steele (Springer-Verlag, New York, 1990), pp. 354–361.

[32] M. C. Teich, D. H. Johnson, A. R. Kumar, and R. G. Turcott, Rate fluctuations and fractional power-law noise recorded from cells in the lower auditory pathway of the cat, *Hear. Res.* **46**, 41–52 (1990).

[33] M. C. Teich, Fractal neuronal firing patterns, in *Single Neuron Computation*, eds. T. McKenna, J. Davis, and S. Zornetzer (Academic, Boston, 1992), pp. 589–625.

[34] M. C. Teich and S. B. Lowen, Fractal patterns in auditory nerve-spike trains, *IEEE Eng. Med. Biol. Mag.* **13**, 197–202 (1994).

[35] M. C. Teich, R. G. Turcott, and R. M. Siegel, Variability and long-duration correlation in the sequence of action potentials in cat striate-cortex neurons, submitted to *IEEE Eng. Med. Biol. Mag.*, 1996.

[36] M. C. Teich, C. Heneghan, S. B. Lowen, T. Ozaki, and E. Kaplan, Fractal character of the neural spike train in the visual system of the cat, submitted to *J. Opt. Soc. Am. A*, 1996.

[37] J. B. Troy and J. G. Robson, Steady discharges of X and Y retinal ganglion cells of cat under photopic illuminance, *Visual Neurosci.* **9**, 535–553 (1992).

[38] R. G. Turcott and M. C. Teich, Long-duration correlation and attractor topology of the heartbeat rate differ for healthy patients and those with heart failure, *Proc. SPIE* **2036** (*Chaos in Biology and Medicine*), 22–39 (1993).

[39] R. G. Turcott, P. D. R. Barker, and M. C. Teich, Long-duration correlation in the sequence of action potentials in an insect visual interneuron, *J. Stat. Comput. Simul.* **52**, 253–271 (1995).

[40] R. G. Turcott and M. C. Teich, Fractal character of the electrocardiogram: Distinguishing heart-failure and normal patients, *Ann. Biomed. Eng.* **24**, No. 2, 269–293 (1996).

[41] G. W. Wornell and A. V. Oppenheim, Estimation of fractal signals from noisy measurements using wavelets, *IEEE Trans. Sig. Process.* **40**, 611–623 (1992).

15

Point Processes, Long-Range Dependence and Wavelets

Patrice Abry and Patrick Flandrin

Ecole Normale Supérieure de Lyon, Laboratoire de physique, CNRS URA 1325, LYON, France

---

15.1 Motivation: Point Processes, Long-Range Dependence and Wavelets

15.1.1 Long-Range Dependence

Phenomena that exhibit long-range dependence characteristics have been found to exist in many different areas, such as physics [27], geology [1], communications [25] and of course, biology [36, 23]. The long-range dependence phenomenon can be defined as or related to a power-law decrease of the autocorrelation function γ_f, of a time series f, for large lags t. It is, in turn, connected to a power-law behavior of the power spectral density (PSD) $\hat{\gamma}_f$

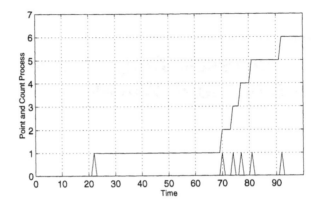

Figure 15.1
Point and count processes. A collection of events, a point process,
can either be modeled as a list of impulses located at times where
events occur or as a count process, the first being the derivative
of the second.

for frequencies close to the null frequency [24][1]

$$\left.\begin{array}{ll} \gamma_f(t) \sim t^{-H}, & t \to +\infty \\[2mm] \hat{\gamma}_f(\omega) \sim \omega^{-\alpha}, & \omega \to 0 \end{array}\right\} \tag{15.1}$$

This mostly means that the data $f(t)$ remain strongly correlated over very
large scales of time (or space) and therefore that the systems which produce them present long-memory behaviors. Long-range dependence is also
intimately connected to a self-similar, or a fractal, or a scale-invariance
property of the data. It has, therefore, mainly been associated to processes
like the fractional Brownian motion (fBm), which is known to present such
characteristics, $B_H(t)$ [31].

15.1.2   Point Processes

In many situations, actual data can efficiently be modeled as a collection
of isolated events, that is, as a point process. This is notably the case
in numerous biomedical applications (see, for instance, [29, 36]). In the
last section, we present the analysis of such a point process made of a
spiketrain of discharges recorded from auditory neurons responding to an
acoustic stimulus. One usually describes a point process through its *count
process* $N(t)$, defined as the number of events occurring between time 0

---

[1]It is commonly accepted that the definition for long-range dependence lies in the diver-
gence of the sum of the autocorrelation function [12]: $\int \gamma_f(t)\, dt = +\infty$.

and t [34] (see Figure 15.1). The derivative of $N(t)$, hereafter labeled $s(t)$, consists in a collection of pulses located at the times of event-occurrences:

$$s(t) = \sum_k \delta(t - t_k).$$

Signals basically consisting in a collection of events yet can not always simply be modeled by this sum of delta functions; they often, rather, are (nonlinearly) filtered versions of such functions.

15.1.3 Long-Range Dependent Point Processes

In some situations where long-range dependence arises, the data are better described as point processes, rather than as a continuous-time processes, like the fBm. For these event-built processes, the long-range dependence property also implies that some second-order statistics (like the variance of the count process, for instance) exhibit a power-law behavior.

15.1.4 Fano Factor

The exponents of the power-laws, whatever the statistics (spectrum, correlation, variance, ...) are the most meaningful parameters characterizing the long-range dependence phenomenon. Estimating them accurately is therefore an important issue. The standard classical tool to perform such an estimation is the so-called Fano factor [15, 22] which measures, over windows of size T, some amounts of variance in the point process. For long-range dependent point processes, such a quantity displays a power-law behavior whose exponent can be used to estimate the dependence parameter.

15.1.5 Wavelet Analysis

The scope of this chapter is to show that the Fano factor can be understood through multiresolution analysis and therefore to propose a timescale-based generalization of this tool. It will be explained how and why this wavelet analysis of long-range dependent point processes provides us with a more versatile and powerful estimator of the long-range dependence parameter [6, 20]. The fact that wavelet analysis is a particularly relevant tool for the study of continuous time long-range dependent processes like fBm has been widely evidenced in the literature [18, 16, 32]. We will underline here how the multiresolution analysis provides us with a unified framework to study both types (point or continuous-time) of processes and we will relate this point of view to $1/f$ processes dedicated spectral analysis [7, 8].

15.2   The Standard Fano Factor

15.2.1   Some Definitions

To study the statistics of point processes, one commonly makes use of the Fano factor, which is defined, for a given time lag T, as the ratio of the variance of the count process to its mean value:

$$F(T) = \frac{\text{var}\,(N(T))}{\mathcal{E}(N(T))},$$

where $\mathcal{E}$ and var stand for the expectation and the variance, respectively. What is actually measured by such a ratio will become clear with the study of the following examples.

15.2.2   Poisson Process: Theme and Variations

The Poisson process plays, for point processes, the reference role the white Gaussian noise does for continuous time random processes. It will, therefore, be used as a starting point; most results regarding the wavelet-based Fano factor can, yet, be transposed to other types of point processes.

Let us assume that the intensity $\lambda(t)$ of the Poisson process is a random second-order stationary process, whose mean and autocovariance function read $\varepsilon_\lambda = \mathcal{E}(\lambda(t))$ and $\gamma_\lambda(t) = \mathcal{E}_\lambda\,(\lambda(u)\lambda(u+t)) - \varepsilon_\lambda^2$. The corresponding Poisson process defined as

$$\left. \begin{aligned} p_\lambda\,(N(T) = n) &= \frac{(\Lambda(T))^n}{n!}\,\exp(\Lambda(T)) \\[2mm] \Lambda(T) &= \int_0^T \lambda(t)\,dt \end{aligned} \right\} \tag{15.2}$$

is also a stationary process [34], whose color (spectral behavior) is that of $\lambda(t)$. One can easily compute its mean and variance:

$$\left. \begin{aligned} \mathcal{E}_{\lambda,P}\,(N(T)) &= \varepsilon_\lambda T \\[2mm] \mathcal{E}_{\lambda,P}\,(N(T)^2) &= \varepsilon_\lambda T + \varepsilon_\lambda^2 T^2 + 2\int_0^T (T-t)\gamma_\lambda(t)\,dt \end{aligned} \right\} \tag{15.3}$$

where the double index $\mathcal{E}_{\lambda,P}$ stands for the doubly stochastic nature of the process: expectation is computed both on the point process and on the set of trials of λ. For such processes, the Fano factor takes the following closed form:

$$
\left.
\begin{aligned}
F(T) &= 1 + \frac{2}{\varepsilon_\lambda T} \int_0^T (T - t)\,\gamma_\lambda(t)\,dt \\[2mm]
&= 1 + \frac{1}{\varepsilon_\lambda} \int \mathrm{sinc}^2(\omega)\,\hat{\gamma}_\lambda\left(\frac{\omega}{T}\right) d\omega
\end{aligned}
\right\}
\tag{15.4}
$$

For the standard Poisson process (SPP: $\lambda = \mathrm{const}$, $\gamma_\lambda(t) \equiv 0$), the Fano factor no longer depends on the duration of observation T:

$$
\forall T,\; F_{\mathrm{SPP}}(T) = 1.
$$

Any departure from unity will denote an extra amount of variance, and therefore, of complexity or richness of information, compared to the SPP. This is due to the time variability of the intensity $\lambda(t)$ itself and to its autocorrelation property more specifically. From the above equation, it is obvious that for durations of observation T much larger than the typical correlation length, the Fano factor reaches a limit value that no longer depends on T: one does not learn any more on the process by increasing T. For instance, in the simple case when $\lambda(t)$ is a white noise (of mean ε_λ and variance σ_λ^2), $F(T)$ is slightly above 1 ($F(T) = 1 + 2\sigma_\lambda^2/\varepsilon_\lambda$) but does not depend on T.

15.2.3 A Long-Dependent Poisson Process

To induce long-range dependence in a point process, a simple idea [22] consists in introducing an intensity process $\lambda(t)$ that possesses such a property. The fractional Gaussian noise (fGn) $G_{H,\delta}(t)$, defined as the increment process of the fBm:

$$
G_{H,\delta}(t) = \frac{1}{\delta}(B_H(t + \delta) - B_H(t))),
$$

whose autocorrelation reads

$$
\gamma_\lambda(\tau) = \sigma^2 H(2H - 1)\tau^{2H-2}, \quad \forall \tau \gg \delta
$$

fulfills this condition and is therefore a candidate[2] for $\lambda(t)$. The resulting point process, called fractal Poisson process (FPP), also presents long-range

---

[2]The variations of H, which for the fBm range from 0 to 1, must be restricted to 1/2 to 1 to insure the existence of the variance of the process.

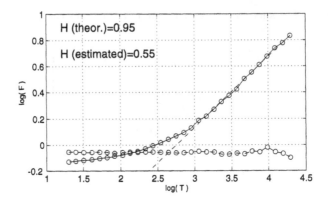

Figure 15.2
**Standard Fano factor. The standard Fano factor computed on a
FPP shows the long-range dependence phenomenon but provides
a poor estimation of the long-range dependence parameter.**

dependence characteristics. Whereas first-order statistics would not enable
us to discriminate a FPP from a SPP, the power-law behavior of the Fano
factor, which is basically a second-order statistic, gives a clear evidence of
this phenomenon:

$$F_{\mathrm{FPP}}(T) = 1 + \frac{\sigma^2}{\varepsilon_\lambda}\, T^{2H-1}, \quad H > \frac{1}{2}. \tag{15.5}$$

15.2.4   Main Limitations

As previously mentioned, it is an important issue to estimate the power-
law exponent defining the long-range dependence phenomenon. This can,
for example, be done through the correct estimation the Fano factor. It
is now well known [12] that statistics estimation is a difficult task because
of the data being strongly dependent on each other over very large scales
of time. Although first-order statistics remains correctly estimated by the
sample estimator, the use of the standard simple estimator for second-
order statistics is inappropriate, insofar as it provides a strongly biased
estimation undergoing high variance. Therefore, even though the use of
such estimators could enable the discrimination between classical and long-
range dependent processes, it would provide a *bad* estimation of the long-
dependent parameter. Figure 15.2 shows the behavior of a Fano factor
computed on a FPP and the resulting estimation of H. More sophisticated
estimators [12] have been designed to overcome this difficulty, among which
one of the oldest is the *Allan variance* [11], to which we will come back later
and whose recommendation is to estimate the variance of a long-dependent

process with the quantity:

$$V_A(t) = \frac{1}{2T^2} \mathcal{E}\left[\left(\int_t^{t+T} s(t)\,dt - \int_{t-T}^t s(t)\,dt\right)^2\right]. \qquad (15.6)$$

Whereas most of these estimators operate in the time domain, we propose to tackle this estimation problem for long-range dependent processes by designing a timescale-based estimator in the wavelet coefficients domain.

From a more practical point of view, this classical Fano factor is awkward to use because of technical difficulties. Actual data are generally not naturally simple collections of pulses, but rather consist in (linearly or not) filtered versions of point processes or could also be corrupted by additive noise. This implies a preprocessing step before one could actually make use of the Fano factor of the count process to estimate the long-range dependence parameter. Moreover, trends may exist in the intensity process $\lambda(t)$ driving the point process, which, superimposed upon the long dependence phenomenon, result in some nonstationary behavior and tend to prevent performing a correct estimation of the power-law exponent. We will see, in the next section, how the wavelet-based Fano factor enables us to overcome such drawbacks.

15.3   The Wavelet-Based Fano Factor

15.3.1   The Multiresolution Point of View

Some Definitions

Let us first recall the notations and definitions proposed in chapters 1 and 2. The coefficients of a discrete (or nonredundant) wavelet transform, performed with a mother-wavelet labeled ψ^0 read:

$$(W\psi^0 f)(2^j, k2^j) = \langle \psi^0_{j,k}, f\rangle, \qquad (15.7)$$

where f is the analyzed signal and $\psi^0_{j,k}(t) = 2^{-j/2}\psi^0(2^{-j}t - k)$ are the dilated to scale j and translated to time $2^j k$ templates of the mother wavelet (see Chapter 1, for complete definitions). By analogy, we propose to define by

$$(V\phi^0 f)(2^j, k2^j) = \langle \phi^0_{j,k}, f\rangle \qquad (15.8)$$

the approximation coefficients, which result from the inner product between the analyzed signal and templates of the scaling function ϕ^0, from which

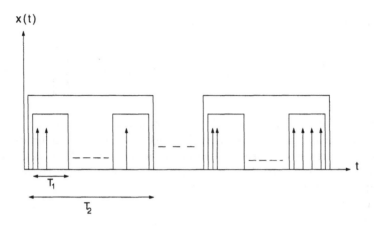

Figure 15.3
Fano factor and multiresolution analysis. Increasing the duration
of observation T used to measure the variability of the process,
in the standard Fano factor, is equivalent to performing a change
of scale in a multiresolution analysis.

the chosen multiresolution is generated and the mother wavelet designed.
Moreover, like the wavelet coefficients, the approximation coefficients can
be obtained as the output of a fast Mallat-type algorithm (see Chapter 2
and [30]). We also recall the definition of the number of vanishing moments
(hereafter labeled $\mathcal{N}$) of the analyzing wavelet ψ^0.

$$k = 0, 1, \ldots, \mathcal{N} - 1, \quad \int t^k \psi^0(t)\, dt = 0. \tag{15.9}$$

This parameter is of particular interest since it controls the behavior of the
Fourier transform $\hat{\psi}^0$ of ψ^0 at the origin,

$$\omega \to 0, \quad \hat{\psi}^0(\omega) \simeq \omega^{\mathcal{N}}$$

This parameter can be chosen when selecting or designing a multiresolution
analysis. With orthogonal wavelets, like the Daubechies's, $\mathcal{N}$ is closely
related to the regularity of the multiresolution analysis [14, 30].

The Wavelet-Based Fano Factor

Basically, the Fano factor compares measurements of variance made over
different scales of time T. Increasing T *naturally* amounts to performing
a multiresolution analysis of the point process. This is sketched on Figure
15.3.

Therefore, we proposed to design a multiresolution-based version of such a tool [6, 20, 19], which we call the wavelet-based Fano factor:

$$WF(j) = 2^{j/2} \frac{\mathcal{E}\left\{\left((W\psi^0 s)(2^j, k2^j)\right)^2\right\}}{\mathcal{E}\left\{(W\phi^0 s)(2^j, k2^j)\right\}}. \tag{15.10}$$

Compared to the former definition, the above equation evidences the key ideas underlying the design of the wavelet-based Fano factor: the rectangular analyzing window (which underlies the definition of the count process) and the increase of the duration of observation T are replaced by the wavelet and the change of scaling factor 2^j, respectively. Note that s still stands for the derivative of the count process, but the above definition can be applied without any preprocessing to any filtered version of a point process.

More on Poisson Point Processes

Let us show through examples that this new Fano factor also captures the excess of variability in the process. For the Poisson processes previously described, it is not difficult to obtain the following results:

$$\left.\begin{aligned}
\mathcal{E}_{\lambda,P}\left\{(W\phi^0 s)(2^j, k2^j)\right\} &= 2^{j/2}\varepsilon_\lambda \\
\mathcal{E}_{\lambda,P}\left\{(W\psi^0 s)(2^j, k2^j)\right\} &= 0 \\
\mathcal{E}_{\lambda,P}\left\{\left((W\phi^0 s)(2^j, k2^j)\right)^2\right\} &= \varepsilon_\lambda + \varepsilon_\lambda^2 2^j + \int \hat{\gamma}_\lambda(\omega) 2^j \left|\hat{\phi}_0(2^j\omega)\right|^2 d\omega \\
\mathcal{E}_{\lambda,P}\left\{\left((W\psi^0 s)(2^j, k2^j)\right)^2\right\} &= \varepsilon_\lambda + \int \hat{\gamma}_\lambda(\omega) 2^j \left|\hat{\psi}_0(2^j\omega)\right|^2 d\omega
\end{aligned}\right\} \tag{15.11}$$

Both wavelets and scaling functions are assumed to be of unit energy[3]. The wavelet-based Fano factor, which reads,

$$WF(j) = 1 + \frac{1}{\varepsilon_\lambda} \int \hat{\gamma}_\lambda(\omega) 2^j \left|\hat{\psi}^0(2^j\omega)\right|^2 d\omega \tag{15.12}$$

also measures the excess of variance in a point process due to its doubly stochastic nature. Again (see Equation (15.4)), it depends on the correlation properties of the intensity process. For the particular case of a SPP, the scale dependence, of course, naturally disappears $WF_{SPP}(j) = 1$.

---

[3]Although these conditions are automatically satisfied for orthonormal wavelets, they require particular attention when designing and using semi- or bi-orthogonal wavelets; see [3]

15.3.2   Unbiased Estimation of the Long Range-Dependence Parameter: A Key Feature

Unbiased Estimation

To show how and why this new Fano factor designed from multiresolution analysis quantities enables a relevant estimation of the long-range dependence parameter, we will again make use of the example of the fractal point process (FPP). The intensity $\lambda(t)$ being a long-dependent process implies a power-law behavior for $\hat{\gamma}_\lambda(\omega)$. For instance, for the fGn, one has[4]

$$\hat{\gamma}_\lambda(\omega) = \Delta(H)\sigma^2|\omega|^{1-2H}.$$

A simple change of variable in the above equation shows that the wavelet-based Fano factor takes the following closed form,

$$WF_{FPP}(j) = 1 + \frac{\sigma^2}{\varepsilon_\lambda}2^{j(2H-1)}\Delta(H)\int|\omega|^{1-2H}\left|\hat{\psi}^0(\omega)\right|^2 d\omega. \qquad (15.13)$$

This clearly indicates that there exists a range of (large) scales for which WF almost behaves as a power-law of scales,

$$WF_{FPP}(j) \simeq 2^{j(2H-1)}f(H).$$

The multiplicative constant $f(H)$, not being scale dependent, enables us to perform an **unbiased estimation** of the long-range parameter (H, for the FPP, for instance) through the simple use of a linear fit in a $(j, \log_2(WF(j)))$ plot (see Figure 15.4).

Number of Vanishing Moments

Moreover, let us notice that this correct estimation will be available only if the integral term $\int|\omega|^{1-2H}|\hat{\psi}^0(\omega)|^2 d\omega$ on the right-hand side of the above equation exists. This implies that the number of vanishing moments $\mathcal{N}$ of the analyzing wavelet and the long-range dependence exponent must satisfy the following inequality:

$$\mathcal{N} > H - 1. \qquad (15.14)$$

As further detailed, the number of vanishing moments $\mathcal{N}$ is of importance as far as the variance of the estimation is concerned, yet, one already sees from the above result that it has to be tuned to the value of the power-law exponent to insure an unbiased estimation of the long-range dependent

---

[4]$\Delta(H) = GA(2H)\sin(\frac{\pi}{2}(2H-1))(2\pi)^{2H-2}$ where GA stands for the Eulerian gamma function.

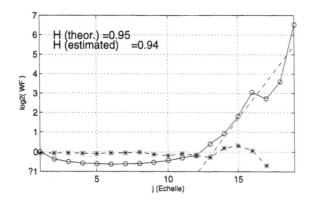

Figure 15.4
Wavelet-based Fano factor. The wavelet-based Fano factor, estimated on a FPP, clearly evidences the long-range dependence phenomenon and enables an efficient estimation of H. The horizontal (dashed + stars) curve corresponds to the wavelet-based Fano factor estimated on a standard Poisson process, showing the absence of the long-range dependence phenomenon.

parameter. The use of this degree of freedom is made effective in the wavelet-based Fano factor, by the fact that the multiresolution analysis framework permits control of $\mathcal{N}$ while designing the wavelet (see, for instance, [9, 14, 30, 33], and also Chapter 1). Particularly, $\mathcal{N}$ can be increased to estimate larger long-range dependence parameters.

Other Point Process Models

Though extensively presented on the FPP, the wavelet-based Fano factor can indeed be used to study the fractal exponent of any other long-range dependent point processes. It can, for instance, be applied to the fractal renewal process proposed in [28] or to the Pareto process [35], in which the long-range dependence phenomenon is caused by the replacement of the exponential (Poisson) probability density functions for the interarrivals law by a power-law function. The wavelet-based Fano factor can also be applied without any preprocessing to any filtered point process [2]. In the fractal shot noise [26], for instance, a standard Poisson process is used as the input of a power-law shaped filter $g(t) = t^{-\beta}$, $0 < A < t < B < +\infty$. In the resulting process $f(t) = \sum_i (t - t_i)^{-\beta}$, the long-range dependence arises from the complex shape of the impulse response used to filter simply distributed events, whereas, in the SPP, it was induced through simply shaped but complexly distributed events. In any case, the wavelet-based Fano factor provides us with a relevant estimation (see Figure 15.5) of the long-range dependence parameter provided that some Equation (15.14)-like technical condition is fulfilled.

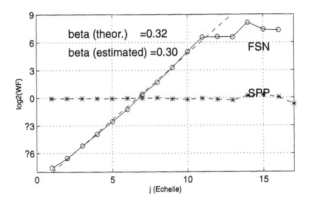

Figure 15.5
Wavelet-based Fano factor. The wavelet-based Fano factor, estimated on a fractal-shot noise (FSN), clearly evidences the long-
range dependence phenomenon and enables an efficient estimation of the parameter β. The horizontal (dashed + stars) curve
corresponds to the wavelet-based Fano factor estimated on a standard Poisson process, showing the absence of the long-range dependence phenomenon.

15.3.3   Reduction of the Range of the Dependence: Another Key Feature

Correlation in the Wavelet Domain

The standard Fano factor performs a poor estimation of the long-range
dependence exponent, mainly because it relies on the classical variance
estimator which does not suit the data being strongly dependent. In the
wavelet coefficients space of representation, on the contrary, we already
saw that we can obtain an unbiased estimation. Let us now allow a larger
part to the variance on this estimation. The correlation between wavelet
coefficients located at a given chosen scale reads[5]:

$$\mathcal{E}\left\{\left(W\psi^0 f\right)(2^j, k2^j)\,\overline{\left(W\psi^0 f\right)(2^j, k'2^j)}\right\}$$

$$= \int \gamma_f(u)\,\gamma_{\psi^0}\left(2^{-j}u + k' - k\right)du \qquad (15.15)$$

$$= \int \hat{\gamma}_f(\omega)2^j\left|\hat{\psi}^0(2^j\omega)\right|^2 \exp\left(-\imath 2\pi 2^j\omega(k'-k)\right)d\omega$$

---

[5]$\overline{x}$ stands for the complex conjugate.

where $\hat{\gamma}_{\psi^0}$ is the autocorrelation function of the mother wavelet. Because the Fourier transform of the mother wavelet is power-law shaped at the origin and the wavelets at scale j are obtained from the mother wavelet by the dilation operation, their Fourier transforms satisfy,

$$\lim_{\omega \to 0} \psi^0(2^j \omega) \simeq 2^{jN} \omega^N.$$

Moreover, since for long-range dependent processes, $\hat{\gamma}_f(\omega) \simeq |\omega|^{-\alpha}$ (for the FPP, for instance, $\hat{\gamma}_s(\omega) \sim \hat{\gamma}_\lambda(\omega) \simeq |\omega|^{-(2H-1)}$, see last section), one gets:

$$\lim_{\omega \to 0} \hat{\gamma}_s(\omega) |\hat{\psi}^0(2^j \omega)|^2 \simeq \omega^{2N-\alpha}$$

(15.16)

$$\lim_{|k'-k| \to +\infty} \mathcal{E}\left\{ (W\psi^0 s)\,(2^j, k2^j)\,\overline{(W\psi^0 s)\,(2^j, k'2^j)} \right\} \simeq |k' - k|^{\alpha - 2N - 1}$$

which shows that the range of the correlation of the transformed data has been significantly shortened compared to that of the original ones. This result was first stated in [18]. Note that this reduction of the range of the correlation is not a trivial effect. Often, indeed, the convolution of a signal with a (low-pass) analyzing waveform results in an enlarging of its correlation duration. Therefore, it is both the wavelets being band-pass analyzing functions and the wavelet basis being obtained from the dilation operator $\hat{\psi}^0\left(2^j \omega\right) \sim \hat{\psi}^0(\omega) \sim \omega^N$, $\omega \to 0$, that enable this reduction of correlation. Moreover, the higher the number of vanishing moments N, the shorter the range of dependence of the data.

A Simple Estimator for the Wavelet-Based Fano Factor

This quasi-decorrelation achieved in the wavelet coefficient space has an important practical consequence: it allows one to use the standard quantity $\sum_k |(W\psi^0 s)(2^j, k2^j)|^2$ as an efficient variance estimator. One can, hence, use the following quantity as a relevant estimator for the wavelet-based Fano factor:

$$\widetilde{WF}_1(j) = \frac{\sum_{k=1}^{N_j} \left((W\psi^0 s)(2^j, k2^j)\right)^2}{\sum_{k=1}^{N_j} \left((V\phi^0 s)(2^j, k2^j)\right)}, \tag{15.17}$$

where $N_j = 2^{-j} N_0$ is the number of coefficients at scale j. We have shown [7, 8] that, assuming that one precisely knows the range of scales over which the power-law behavior is valid, the power-law exponent can be estimated without bias. Moreover, under the quasi-decorrelation assumption, a closed form for the variance of the estimation for this parameter can be derived that shows that the a minimum variance estimation is achieved (i.e., the Cramér-Rao lower bound is attained).

15.3.4   Fano Factor, Allan Variance and Wavelets

Another Multiresolution-Based Fano Factor

Let us now try to point out some other connections between the standard and the wavelet-based Fano factor. One could have imagined defining a multiresolution-based Fano factor *WFA* by:

$$WFA(j) = 2^{j/2} \frac{\text{var}\left\{(V\phi^0 s)(2^j, k2^j)\right\}}{\mathcal{E}\left\{(V\phi^0 s)(2^j, k2^j)\right\}},$$

in which the rectangular box is replaced by the scaling function ϕ^0 rather than by the wavelet ψ^0 itself. Such a quantity also theoretically measures the excess of the variance of a point process; indeed, for Poisson processes, it yields

$$WFA(j) = 1 + \frac{1}{\varepsilon_\lambda} \int \hat{\gamma}_\lambda(\omega) \, 2^j \big|\hat{\phi}_0(2^j \omega)\big|^2 d\omega. \tag{15.18}$$

Note that this equation is strictly equivalent to Equation (15.4) with $T = 2^j$.

The Haar Multiresolution and the Allan Variance

Now, if we restrict ourselves to the Haar multiresolution,[6] the scaling function is itself a rectangular box and therefore, computing this multiresolution-based Fano factor simply amounts to evaluate the standard Fano factor:

$$WFA_{Haar}(j) \equiv F(T = 2^j).$$

It is, then, of course, subject to the same drawbacks as the standard Fano factor as far as estimation is concerned. On the contrary, in definition (15.10), the excess of variability of the process is measured through the variance of the wavelet coefficients rather than through that of the approximation ones. With the Haar wavelet, it amounts to computing a Fano factor based on the Allan variance, which is known to be much better adapted to long-term dependencies an estimator,

$$WF_{Haar}(j) \equiv F_{Allan}(T = 2^j).$$

This relationship between the Haar wavelet transform and the Allan variance was first noted in [17]. It explains why this latter has often been described as an estimator that suits long-range dependent processes. We

---

[6]For the Haar multiresolution, the scaling function equals 1 within 0 and 1 and 0 elsewhere: $\phi_H(t) = \chi_{[0,1]}(t)$, whereas a mother wavelet reads $\psi_H(t) = \chi_{[1/2,1]}(t) - \chi_{[0,1/2]}(t)$; see Chapter 1 or [33].

can therefore present the wavelet-based Fano factor *WF* as a generalization of the standard tool, insofar as it depends on an extra parameter: the number of vanishing moments $\mathcal{N}$ of the analyzing wavelets ψ^0, the importance of which has been strongly emphasized in the two previous sections.

The Standard Fano Factor: A Poor Estimator

These formal connections give a clear insight on the origin of the poor performance of the standard Fano factor for long-range parameter estimation purpose. More precisely, for long-range dependent point processes (like the FPP), *WFA* takes the following form:

$$WF_{FPP}(j) = 1 + \frac{\sigma^2}{\varepsilon_\lambda} 2^{j(2H-1)} \Delta(H) \int |\omega|^{1-2H} |\hat{\phi}^0(\omega)|^2 d\omega,$$

which also theoretically enables an estimation of the long-range parameter. This performance will, yet, be obtained only if the integral term $\int |\omega|^{1-2H} |\hat{\phi}^0(\omega)|^2 d\omega$ exists. Since the scaling function is a low-pass function ($\omega \to 0$, $\hat{\phi}^0(\omega) = 1$), it implies that the range of existence of the long-range parameter must be restricted to $0 < H < 1$, for the FPP. Moreover, the range of the correlation of the approximation coefficients is of the same order as that of the original data, since the convolution with the (low-pass) scaling function (see Equation (15.18) or equivalently Equation (15.4)) does not bring any reduction of correlation. This prevents the use of summation over time as a relevant estimator of the quantity $\mathcal{E}\{((V\phi^0 s)(2^j, k2^j))^2\}$, involved in the definition of *WFA* and therefore of the standard Fano factor.

15.3.5 Choosing the Number of Vanishing Moments $\mathcal{N}$

A Practical Bias-Variance Trade-Off

Choosing $\mathcal{N}$ is of practical importance since it must be tuned both to allow an unbiased estimation and to reduce the range of correlation of the data and therefore the variance of estimation. From an experimental point of view, one observes that, to obtain an unbiased estimation, $\mathcal{N}$ is to be chosen slightly above the value predicted by the bias-inequality (of the type of Equation (15.14)). There is no point in satisfying this condition too largely. It is, indeed, sufficient to insure an efficient decorrelation of the wavelet coefficients. Increasing $\mathcal{N}$ above this limit does not substantially improve the estimation and even turns out to be a drawback. Let us indeed recall that the number of available coefficients at scale j, $N_j = 2^{-j}N_0$ (where N_0 is the size of the data), decreases while scale increases. Moreover, the number of coefficients corrupted by border effects is, in most cases, roughly proportional to the number of vanishing moments. This means that, for a given size of data, the increase of $\mathcal{N}$ results in a decrease of the number of coefficients that can be involved in the estimation, and therefore in an increase of the variance estimation. There is, therefore, a trade-off in the choice of $\mathcal{N}$. We, again, emphasize that $\mathcal{N}$ is a free parameter in the wavelet design; it can be precisely and easily set to any chosen value.

Trends and Nonstationarity

One of the main difficulties encountered with actual data is that the estimation of the long-range dependent parameter may be altered by some nonstationary behavior. Since the estimator, indeed, relies on a time-marginal (i.e., a summation along time), it will be strongly affected by nonstationarities, which may have various origins. With the FPP model, for instance, one could imagine that the long-range dependent parameter H is itself time-dependent. This interesting case, under current investigations, needs more work. One can imagine a less unfavorable situation in which the long-range dependence parameter remains constant with time but where a trend $p(t)$ is superimposed to the fractal nature of the intensity process,

$$\lambda(t) = \lambda_0 + FGN_H(t) + p(t).$$

Because of this trend, the standard Fano factor will give a poor estimation of H. On the contrary, provided that the trend has a smooth enough behavior, it will be canceled by the wavelet-based Fano factor and, therefore, will not alter the estimation. More precisely, if $p(t)$ is a polynomial of degree N, then the *WF* will be blind to the trend, provided that

$$\mathcal{N} > N - 1.$$

For cases in which trends exist, increasing $\mathcal{N}$ until the estimation stops varying is an easy way to get rid of them to perform a good estimation of the long-range dependent parameter.

15.4   Practical Issues: More on the Various Wavelet Transforms

Up to now, we have only considered a wavelet Fano factor that is based on a discrete wavelet transform, but one could imagine designing another one relying on the continuous wavelet transform (see Chapter 1, for definition and differences between both transforms). Let us examine the benefits and the drawbacks.

Computational Issues

Let us first note that analyzing long-dependence phenomena often means the processing of large amounts of data. Therefore, the possibility of performing the discrete wavelet decomposition through a fast pyramidal Mallat-type algorithm (see Chapter 2 or references [14, 30] for details) is of major importance. This great advantage is lost when using any non-redundant transform (i.e., transforms that compute coefficients on a grid whose density is higher than that of the dyadic grid $(2^j, 2^j k)$) (see Chapter 2, for comparison of computational costs).

Dyadic or Continuous Time?

The main quality one recognizes in the continuous wavelet transform is the time-shift invariance, achieved thanks to a time-sampling rate which does not depend on scale as is the case for the dyadic grid. For the Fano factor estimation, on the other hand, we are interested in computing the time-marginal of the transform $\sum_k |(W\psi^0 x)(2^j, k2^j)|^2$ for which time-shift invariance is not crucial. Moreover, with strongly-dependent data, the coefficients of the continuous transform that are neighbors in time (i.e., whose time lag is smaller than the typical wavelet duration) will remain strongly correlated. Therefore, the computation of the summation $\sum_k |(W\psi^0 f)(2^j, k)|^2$ will not provide any substantial reduction of variance compared to $\sum_k |(W\psi^0 f)(2^j, k2^j)|^2$ and hence will not improve significantly the long-dependence parameter estimation, in spite of a computation cost that has been drastically increased. These statements cannot easily be made more precise by analytic computation but are strongly supported by numerical simulations. The homogeneous quasi-continuous time sampling of the timescale plan is useless as far as the Fano factor for long-dependent processes is concerned.

Dyadic or Continuous Scales?

From another point of view, there is no reason why the dyadic sampling of the scale axis should fit actual data. Specifically, when the scale-invariant behavior only exists over a finite range of scales — this is the case both in theoretical models (like the shot noise, for instance) and in actual data (as in turbulence, for instance [8]) — one may have only a small number of points to perform the linear fit for the long-dependence parameter estimation. On the contrary, the continuous wavelet transform would enable a quasi-continuous sampling of the scale axis. However, as previously mentioned, the continuous transform suffers from a high computational cost and produces a useless quasi-continuous time sampling. This is why we proposed [8, 4] the use of a redundant wavelet transform that preserves the decimation by a factor of 2 of the number of coefficients at each octave but allows as fine a sampling of the scale axis as desired. The design of this transform relies strongly on the spirit of the multiresolution analysis; its key idea is to use simultaneously, within a single chosen multiresolution, M mother wavelets where M is the number of scales to be inserted in a single octave, the M wavelets being nondyadic dilated versions of a starting pattern:

$$\psi_m(t) = 2^{-m/2M} \psi^0(2^{-m/M}t), \quad m = 0, 1, \ldots, M - 1.$$

Moreover, wavelet approximation and design techniques such as those developed in [3] allowed us to use the multiresolution analysis tool to propose a Mallat-type pyramidal algorithm that performs a fast computation of the wavelet coefficients on this specific grid. This approach preserves a dyadic scale-dependent time-sampling while enabling a finer scale sampling.

Orthonormal Wavelet Transform?

Performing a nonredundant (or discrete) wavelet transform does not necessarily imply the use of an orthonormal basis of wavelets. One can also choose semi- or bi-orthogonal bases of wavelets (for definitions see Chapter 1 or [9, 13, 21]). For the Fano factor, all the results stated above hold for any of the three versions of the discrete wavelet transform. From a practical point of view, they all give relevant estimations of the Fano factor. The use of semi- or bi-orthogonal transforms requires paying some attention to a couple of technical questions. First, such wavelets are not unit energy by construction, as is the case for orthonormal ones. One, therefore, has to perform a normalization step, which can be done easily within the multiresolution framework (see [3]). Second, a proper use of the fast pyramidal algorithm to compute a discrete wavelet transform requires performing a preliminary initialization step (that technically consists in projecting the analyzed data into the first multiresolution space labeled V_0; see Chapter 1 or [14]). We proposed in [5] a simple way to perform an excellent approximation of the initialization.[7] Whereas it is useless with orthonormal wavelets, this projection step is compulsory with non-orthogonal ones; it would, otherwise, result in a biased Fano factor.

15.5   Fano Factor and Spectral Estimation: A Unified Point of View

The wavelet-based Fano factor provides an efficient means of analyzing the long-dependence phenomenon. This is another illustration, with point

---

[7]Another general initialization procedure has been explicitly described in [10, 37]

processes, of the intimate relation between multiresolution (or timescale) analysis and self-similar (or fractal) properties of the signal, which has been previously described in the wavelet decomposition of the continuous time-fractional Brownian motion [17, 32]. We will now try to show that the basic ingredients that enable an efficient study of the long-range dependencies in both continuous-time and point-like processes are identical.

Since long-range dependence is related to a power-law behavior of the variance of the count process, it is no surprise that the essential element in the Fano factor is a second-order quantity $\sum_k (W\psi^0 f)(2^j, k2^j)^2$. More precisely, taking the expectation of this quantity:

$$\mathcal{E}\left((W\psi^0 f)(2^j, k2^j)^2\right) = \int \hat{\gamma}_f(\omega) 2^j \hat{\psi}^0(2^j \omega) \, d\omega$$

shows that computing the summation over time $\sum_k (W\psi^0 f)(2^j, k2^j)^2$ basically amounts to performing an estimation of the spectrum of the analyzed signal around the frequency $2^{-j}\omega_0$ within a band of width $\Delta\omega = \omega_0/Q_0$ (where ω_0 and Q_0 stand for the central frequency of the basic wavelet ψ^0 and its quality factor, respectively). Therefore, the Fano factor mainly produces a constant-Q (or constant relative frequency bandwidth) spectral estimation of the analyzed point process. This quantity $\sum_k (W\psi^0 f)(2^j, k2^j)^2$, of course, can efficiently be used to perform the spectral estimation of a continuous time process as well. More generally, the use of time-marginals of timescale distributions to design spectral estimators has been studied in detail in [2, 7, 8] where their adequacy for scale-invariant processes or $1/|\omega|^\alpha$ processes has been stressed. We briefly recall that the standard Welch spectrum estimator, which consists in averaging the square modulus of Fourier transform of successive sections of the data, can be read as the time-marginal of the short-time Fourier transform (see Chapter 1). It is therefore a time-frequency (or constant bandwidth) based spectrum estimator. We have shown [2, 7, 8] that, when applied to $1/|\omega|^\alpha$ processes, it produces biased estimations of the long-range dependence parameter. On the contrary, the timescale (or constant relative bandwith) based spectrum estimator yields an unbiased and minimum variance estimation of this parameter. Hence, whatever the nature of the process (continuous time, like the fBm or point-based, like the FPP), the fundamental ingredient to estimate the long-range dependent parameter lies in the use of the sum $\sum_k (W\psi^0 f)(2^j, k2^j)^2$: i.e., the use of a bandpass mother function and of the dilation operator to produce the wavelet basis of analysis.

To make this connection more explicit, we can, for instance, examine (quasi-continuous time point) processes obtained from the mixing of FPP with a fractal shot-noise. Such processes, provided that H and β satisfy some conditions, remain stationary and their spectrum is given by:

$$\hat{\gamma}_f(\omega) = (\varepsilon_\lambda + \hat{\gamma}_\lambda(\omega)) \, |G(\omega)|^2,$$

(where $G(\omega)$ is the Fourier transform of the filtering function g (see Section 15.3.2)) which highlights the diversity of the origin of the long-dependence phenomenon: it can either result from a complex distribution of simply shaped events (FPP, $\hat{\gamma}_\lambda(\omega) \sim \omega^{-\alpha}$) or from simply distributed events of complex shape FSN, $G(\omega) \sim \omega^{-\beta}$). The Fano factor essentially reads (this was first established in [19]),

$$WF(j) \simeq \int \left[(\varepsilon_\lambda + \hat{\gamma}_\lambda(\omega)) \, |G(\omega)|^2 \right] 2^j \left| \hat{\psi}^0(2^j \omega) \right|^2 d\omega$$

$$= \mathcal{E}\left((W\psi^0 f)(2^j, k2^j)^2 \right)$$

and shows that the long dependence phenomenon for both continuous time signals and point processes (or any filtered versions of point processes) can be efficiently studied through the quantity: $\sum_k (W\psi^0 f)(2^j, k2^j)^2$.

15.6   An Example: Spiketrain of an Auditory-Nerve Response

We are now going to present the use of the wavelet-based Fano factor on actual data. They consist in a spiketrain of discharges recorded from auditory neurons responding to an acoustic stimulus (made of a pure tone). Measurements consist of the time intervals (in second, time quantization is 50 microseconds) between successive action potentials (about 127,000). The data consequently do not constitute a sampled analog waveform and are often modeled as point processes. The experiment has been carried out on an anesthetized cat's auditory-nerve fiber, at the Eaton Peabody Laboratory (EPL) of the Massachusetts Eye and Ear Infirmary, by Bertrand Delgutte and Peter Cariani, who are gratefully acknowledged for sharing their data. We also thank O. Kelly from ECE, Rice University for his help in handling the data and for very fruitful discussions.

The wavelet-based Fano factor has been applied to such point processes where long-range dependencies are likely to exist. The length of the data allowed us to perform an analysis for scales ranging from 1 to 2^{22} by octaves, without being disturbed by border effects. We used the standard Daubechies wavelets. Changing the regularity of the wavelet does not make

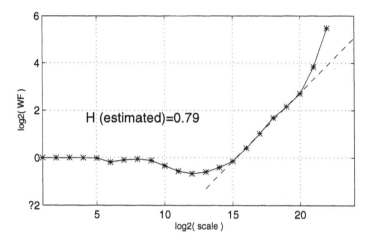

Figure 15.6
Wavelet-based Fano factor on auditory nerve fiber. Log-log plot
of the wavelet-based Fano factor measured on a spiketrain of discharges recorded from neurons responding to an acoustic stimulus. The straight line at larger scales clearly evidences the existence of the long-range dependence phenomenon. This tool allows
moreover an unbiased estimation of the long-range dependence
parameter. This plot involved the dyadic wavelet transform with
a *Daubechies2* wavelet (four taps).

significant practical differences. The resulting wavelet-based Fano factor is
plotted in Figure 15.6. This plot recalls that of Figure 15.4 presenting
the wavelet-based Fano factor for a simulated fractal Poisson process. It
suggests that a FPP model could efficiently describe the data. This wavelet-
based Fano factor remains constant to one for the smaller scales, evidencing
an absence of correlation for short ranges of time. The drop (between scales
2^{10} to 2^{15}) also exists in numerical simulations and is not fully understood.
At the largest scales (2^{15} to 2^{20}), a power-law behavior (straight line in a
log-log plot) is clearly seen, revealing the existence of the long-range dependence phenomenon over 6 octaves (that is one decade and a half). In actual
times, it means that this phenomenon exists for time lags ranging from 1.5 s
to 60 s. These are only rough estimations of these lower and upper bounds
since the dyadic division of the scale axis does not allow more accurate
estimations. The good statistical properties of the wavelet-based Fano factor estimator enables an accurate estimation of the long-range dependence
parameter:

$$\tilde{H} = 0.79$$

Although the precise value of the H parameter can not be fully interpreted,
it is believed that tools allowing accurate estimations may help to give
meaning to this measurement.

15.7   Conclusion

We have shown how the definition of a wavelet-based Fano factor enables an efficient analysis of long-range dependence in point processes. We also made explicit its connection to this spectral estimation dedicated to $1/f$ processes. This tool is currently being successfully applied in various domains such as physics, geology, telecommunications, and biology. Some theoretical work to connect this wavelet-based tool to other ones dedicated to fractal properties remains to be done. It is also an important issue to adapt this tool to long-range dependent processes whose second-order statistics are infinite or whose long-range dependence parameter changes with time.

References

[1] In Foufoula and A. R. Kumar, editors, *Wavelet Transforms in Geophysics*, Academic Press, New York, 1994, 26–38.

[2] P. Abry. *Transformées en ondelettes — Analyses multirésolution et signaux de pression en turbulence*. Doctoral thesis, Ecole Normale Supérieure de Lyon et Université Claude-Bernard Lyon I, Lyon, France, 1994.

[3] P. Abry and A. Aldroubi. Designing multiresolution analysis-type wavelets and their fast algorithms. *To appear in J. Fourier Anal. Appl.*

[4] P. Abry, E. Chassande-Mottin, and P. Flandrin. Algorithmes rapides pour la décomposition en ondelettes continue. Application à l'implantation de la réallocation du scalogramme. In *Quinzième Colloque GRETSI*, Septembre 1995.

[5] P. Abry and P. Flandrin. On the initialization of the discrete wavelet transform. *IEEE Signal Process. Lett.*, 1(2):32–34, 1994.

[6] P.Abry and P. Flandrin. Wavelet-based Fano factor for long-range dependent point processes. In *Proc. 16th Annu. Int. Conf. IEEE—Eng. Med. Biol. Soc.*, pages 1330–1331, Baltimore, MD, November 1994.

[7] P. Abry, P. Gonçalvès, and P. Flandrin. Wavelet-based spectral analysis of $1/f$ processes. In *IEEE Int. Conf. Acoust., Speech and Signal Process. ICASSP-93*, pages III.237–III.240, Minneapolis, MN, 1993.

[8] P. Abry, P. Gonçalvès, and P. Flandrin. Wavelets, spectrum analysis and $1/f$ processes. In *Wavelets and Statistics, Lecture Notes in Statistics.*, A. Antoniadis, editor, 1995.

[9] A. Aldroubi and M. Unser. Families of multiresolution and wavelet spaces with optimal properties. *Numer. Func. Anal. Opt.*, 14:417–446, 1993.

[10] A. Aldroubi, M. Unser, and M. Eden. Cardinal spline filters: stability and convergence to the ideal sinc interpolator. *Signal Processing*, 28:127–138, 1992.

[11] D. W. Allan. Statistics of atomic frequency standards. In *Proc. IEEE*, 54, 221–230, 1966.

[12] J. Beran. Statistical methods for data with long-range dependence. *Stat. Sci.*, 7(4):404–427, 1992.

[13] A. Cohen, I. Daubechies, and J.C. Fauveau. Biorthogonal bases of compactly supported wavelets. *Commun. Pure Appl. Math.*, 45:485–560, 92.

[14] I. Daubechies. *Ten Lectures on Wavelets*. SIAM, Philadelphia, 1992.

[15] U. Fano. Ionization yield of radiations. II. the fluctuations of the numbers of ions. *Phys. Rev.*, 72(1):26–29, 1947.

[16] P. Flandrin. On the spectrum of fractional Brownian Motions. *IEEE Trans. Inf. Theory*, IT-35(1):197–199, 1989.

[17] P. Flandrin. Fractional Brownian motion and wavelets. In *Wavelets, Fractals and Fourier Transforms — New Developments and New Applications*, M. Farge, J. C. R. Hunt, and J. C. Vassilicos, editors, Oxford University Press, 1992.

[18] P. Flandrin. Wavelet analysis and synthesis of fractional Brownian motion. *IEEE Trans. Inf. Theory*, IT-38(2):910–917, 1992.

[19] P. Flandrin. Time-scale analyses and self-similar stochastic processes. In *Wavelets and Their Applications*, J. S. Byrnes, J. L. Byrnes, K. A. Hargreaves, and K. Berry, editors, pages 121–142. Kluwer Academic Publishers, Boston, 1994.

[20] P. Flandrin and P. Abry. Tracking long-range dependencies with wavelets. In *Proc. IEEE-IMS Workshop Inf. Stat.*, page 54, Alexandria, VA, November 1994.

[21] B. Jawerth and W. Sweldens. An overview of wavelet based multiresolution analyses. *SIAM Rev.*, 36:377–412, 1994.

[22] D. H. Johnson and A. R. Kumar. Modeling and analyzing fractal point processes. In *IEEE ICASSP*, pages 1353–1356, 1990.

[23] O. E. Kelly, D. H. Johnson, B. Delgutte, and P. Cariani. Fractal noise strength in auditory-nerve fiber recordings. *Submitted to J.A.S.A*, preprint, 1994.

[24] M. S. Keshner. $1/f$ noise. *Proc. IEEE*, 70(3):212–218, 1982.

[25] W. E. Leland, M. S. Taqqu, W. Willinger, and D. V. Wilson. On the self-similar nature of ethernet traffic. *IEEE/ACM Trans Networking*, 2(1):1–15, 1994.

[26] S. B. Lowen and M. C. Teich. Power-law shot noise. *IEEE Trans. Inf. Theory*, 36(6):1302–1318, 1990.

[27] S. B. Lowen and M. C. Teich. Fractal renewal processes as a model of charge transport in amorphous semiconductors. *Phys. Rev. B*, 46(3):1816–1819, 1992.

[28] S. B. Lowen and M. C. Teich. Fractal renewal process. *IEEE Trans. Inf. Theory*, 39(5):1669–1671, 1993.

[29] S. B. Lowen and M. C. Teich. Estimation and simulation of fractal stochastic point processes. *Fractals*, 3(1):183–210, 1995.

[30] S. Mallat. A theory for multiresolution signal decomposition: The wavelet representation. *IEEE Trans. Pattern Anal. Mach. Intell.*, II(7):674–693, 1989.

[31] B. B. Mandelbrot and J. W. van Ness. Fractional Brownian motions, fractional noises and applications. *SIAM Rev.*, 10(4):422–437, 1968.

[32] E. Masry. The wavelet transform of stochastic processes with stationary increments and its application to fractional Brownian motion. *IEEE Trans. Inf. Theory*, IT-39:260–264, 1993.

[33] Y. Meyer. Ondelettes et algorithmes concurrents. Hermann, 1992.

[34] D. L. Snyder and M. I. Miller. *Random Point Processes in Time and Space*, 2nd ed., Springer-Verlag, 1991.

[35] S. M. Sussman. Analysis of the Pareto model for error statistics on telephone circuits. *IEEE Trans. Commun. Syst.*, pages 213–221, 1963.

[36] M. C. Teich. Fractal character of the auditory neural spike train. *IEEE Trans. Biomed. Eng.*, 36(1):150–160, 1989.

[37] M. Unser, A. Aldroubi, and M. Eden. A family of polynomial spline wavelet transforms. *Signal Process.*, 30:141–162, 1993.

16

Continuous Wavelet Transform: ECG Recognition Based on Phase and Modulus Representations and Hidden Markov Models

Lotfi Senhadji, Laurent Thoraval, and Guy Carrault

L.T.S.I. Université de Rennes I, INSERM Rennes France

16.1   Introduction

Biomedical signals are fundamental observations for analyzing the body function and for diagnosing a wide spectrum of diseases. Information provided by bioelectric signals are generally time-varying, nonstationary, sometimes transient, and usually corrupted by noise. Fourier transform has been the unique tool to face such situations, even if the discrepancy between theoretical considerations and signal properties has been emphasized for a long time. These issues can be now nicely addressed by time-scale and time-frequency analysis.

One of the major areas where new insights can be expected is the cardiovascular domain. For diagnosis purpose, the noninvasive electrocardiogram (ECG) is of great value in clinical practice. The ECG is composed of a set of waveforms resulting from atrial and ventricular depolarization and repolarization. The first step towards ECG analysis is the inspection of P,

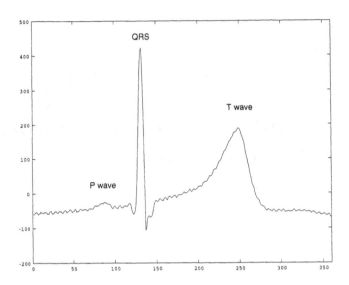

Figure 16.1
Example of a normal ECG beat.

QRS, and T waves; each one of these elementary components is a series of onset, offset, peak, valley, and inflection points (Figure 16.1). Ideally, the waves exhibit local symmetry properties with respect to a particular point (peak and inflection points locations of the considered wave). Based on these properties, one can extract significant points to study the wave shapes and heart rate variability [1].

Wavelet transforms have been applied to ECG signals for enhancing late potentials [2], reducing noise [3], QRS detection [4], normal and abnormal beat recognition [5]. The methods used in these studies were conducted through continuous wavelet transform [6], multiresolution analysis [8, 9] and dyadic wavelet transform [10]. In this chapter the continuous wavelet transform (CWT), based on a complex analyzing function, is applied to characterize local symmetry of signals, and it is used for ECG arrhythmia analysis. The first part of this chapter is more theoretical. The behavior of CWT square modulus of a regular signal $f(t)$ when the scale parameter goes to zero is studied. For a signal with local symmetry properties, the phase behavior of its CWT is also examined. These results are then extended, under some conditions, to signal without local symmetries. The second part is more experimental and numerical examples on simulated data illustrate the mathematical results. Finally, the use of these properties is considered in automatic ECG recognition and identification by means of hidden Markov models (HMMs). The presentation emphasizes how a suitable parameter vector, corresponding to the input observation sequence of the Markov chain, can be built and applied.

16.2 Properties of Square Modulus and Phase

With the same notations used in the first chapter of the book, the continuous wavelet transform (CWT) of a signal f belonging to $L^2(\mathbb{R})$ is defined by :

$$(W_\Psi f)(a,b) = \frac{1}{\sqrt{a}} \int_{-\infty}^{+\infty} f(t) \overline{\Psi\left(\frac{t-b}{a}\right)} dt$$

where Ψ is a complex valued function with zero mean and satisfying $C_\Psi < \infty$ (see Chapter 1, Equation 1.24).

The wavelet of concern here is complex, compactly supported, hermitian (i.e., $\overline{\Psi}(t) = \Psi(-t)$), and m times continuously differentiable ($m \geq 2$). The analyzed signal $f(t)$ is real and supposed to be two times continuously differentiable.

16.2.1 Square Modulus Approximation

The square modulus of CWT of f is defined by

$$|(W_\Psi f)(a,b)|^2 = (W_\Psi f)(a,b) \overline{(W_\Psi f)(a,b)},$$

and its derivative according to the space variable b is:

$$\frac{\partial |(W_\Psi f)(a,b)|^2}{\partial b} = \frac{\partial (W_\Psi f)(a,b)}{\partial b} \overline{(W_\Psi f)(a,b)} \qquad (16.1)$$

$$+ \frac{\partial \overline{(W_\Psi f)(a,b)}}{\partial b} (W_\Psi f)(a,b)$$

One can show that Equation 16.1 is equivalent to (see Appendix 1):

$$\frac{\partial |(W_\Psi f)(a,b)|^2}{\partial b} = \frac{2}{a} \text{Re} \left(\int_{-\infty}^{+\infty} f'(t) \cdot \overline{\Psi\left(\frac{t-b}{a}\right)} dt \cdot \qquad (16.2) \right.$$

$$\left. \int_{-\infty}^{+\infty} f(t) \cdot \Psi\left(\frac{t-b}{a}\right) dt \right)$$

where Re(.) is the real part of its argument. At fine scales, the above derivative may be approximated by (see Appendix 2):

$$\frac{\partial\,|(W_\Psi f)\,(a,b)|^2}{\partial b} \approx 2a^3 f'(b) \cdot f''(b) \cdot |m_1|^2 \tag{16.3}$$

with

$$m_i = \int_{-\infty}^{+\infty} x^i \cdot \Psi(x)\,dx \quad i \in \mathbb{N}$$

According to this approximation, at fine-scale analysis, connections can be made between local extrema of $|(W_\Psi f)\,(a,b)|^2$ (as a function of the space variable) on one hand and inflection points and local extrema of f on the other hand. Local maxima (minima) of $|(W_\Psi f)\,(a,b)|^2$ are always inflection points (local extrema) of f, but local minima may be also inflection points of f. These properties are summarized in Table 16.1.

16.2.2   Phase Behavior

Based on the CWT modulus, one cannot, in general, recover the decomposed signal. The phase information is necessary to reconstruct the signal. In their pioneering work on the complex Hardy wavelet, Grossmann et al. [6-b] have indicated that phase information reveals isolated singularities (or local bursts) in a signal more accurately than does the modulus. In this section, the local behavior of the phase of CWT of signals with particular points as local extrema or inflection points is studied. We first consider the case of functions exhibiting local symmetry properties around these points, and then we extend the previous results to the case of an m times continuously differentiable function ($m \geq 2$).

Let $f(t)$ be a continuous function satisfying the following property:

$$(\exists b_0 \in \mathbb{R})\,(\exists \varepsilon > 0)\,(\forall |h| < \varepsilon)\, f(b_0 + h) = f(b_0 - h) \tag{16.4}$$

which means that f is locally symmetric with respect to the vertical axis crossing in b_0. (Note that if locally f has no oscillations, b_0 is a local extremum.)

For fine scale, $(W_\psi f)(a, b_0)$ becomes (see Appendix 3, Case (1)):

$$(W_\Psi f)\,(a, b_0) = 2\sqrt{a} \cdot \int_0^{+\infty} f(at + b_0) \cdot \mathrm{Re}(\Psi(t))\,dt. \tag{16.5}$$

Hence, when the scale parameter "a" goes to zero, $(W_\Psi f)\,(a, b_0)$ is real, and its phase is then 0 or π, according to the sign of (16.5). If f has local

Table 16.1

Summary of the properties of the CWT vs. local symmetry of the analyzed signal.

If $f(b)$ presents in b_0 a ...	... then in b_0 $\lvert (W_\Psi f)(a,b) \rvert^2$ is ...
1. Maximum $b_0^- < b_0 < b_0^+$	Minimum b_0
2. Minimum b_0	Minimum b_0
3. Inflection b_0	Maximum b_0
4. Inflection b_0	Maximum b_0
5. Inflection b_0	Minimum b_0
6. Inflection b_0	Minimum b_0

Note: For those regular shapes, local maxima of $\lvert (W_\Psi f)(a,b) \rvert^2$ point out the time locations of sharp transitions and correspond to two kinds of inflection points: (3) $f''(b_0^-) > 0$, $f''(b_0) = 0$, $f''(b_0^+) < 0$; $f'(b_0) > 0$ (4) $f''(b_0^-) < 0$, $f''(b_0) = 0$, $f''(b_0^+) > 0$; $f'(b_0) > 0$

symmetry property in b_0, then the phase of $(W_\Psi f)(a, b_0)$ is equal to 0 or π.

Suppose now that f, instead of obeying (16.4), has the following property:

$$(\exists b_0 \in \mathbb{R})\,(\exists \varepsilon > 0)\,(\forall |h| < \varepsilon)\, f(b_0 + h) = 2f(b_0) - f(b_0 - h) \qquad (16.6)$$

which indicates that f is anti-symmetric around $f(b_0)$ (if f is not locally oscillating, b_0 is a local extremum of f').

The assumption (16.6) implies the following equality at fine scales (see Appendix 3, Case (2)):

$$(W_\Psi f)(a, b_0) = -2i\sqrt{a} \int_0^{+\infty} f(at + b_0)\mathrm{Im}(\Psi(t))\,dt \qquad (16.7)$$

which means that the CWT of f in b_0 is imaginary, with constant phase equal to $\pm\pi/2$ according to the sign of (16.7). This property underlines that: if f has a local center of symmetry in b_0 then the phase of $(W_\Psi f)(a, b_0)$ is equal to $\pi/2$ or $-\pi/2$.

The observed signal may not comply with symmetry assumptions but, even so, we still want to use the CWT tools to locate peak and inflection points. Let us now suppose that f is an m times continuously differentiable function ($m \geq 2$); then, at fine resolution, $(W_\Psi f)(a, b_0)$ can be approximated by:

$$(W_\Psi f)(a, b_0) \approx \sqrt{a} \cdot \sum_{n=1}^{m} \frac{a^n}{n!}\, \overline{m_n}\, f^{(n)}(b_0) \qquad (16.8)$$

where $f^{(n)}$ denotes the nth derivative of f. Using the Fourier Transform of Ψ to express m_n, (16.8) becomes

$$(W_\Psi f)(a, b_0) \approx \sqrt{a} \cdot \sum_{n=1}^{m} \left(\frac{a}{i}\right)^n \cdot \frac{\overline{\widehat{\Psi}}^{(n)}(0)}{n!}\, f^{(n)}(b_0) \qquad (16.9)$$

Hence, at high resolution (i.e., small value of "a" or high frequency) CWT in b_0 is a linear combination of the analyzed signal derivatives. The variations of $(W_\Psi f)(a, b_0)$ across scales express the behavior of the derivatives of the signal according to the choice of the wavelet (consequently, all the moments m_n are fixed). For example, if the first moment of Ψ is null, asymptotically $f'(b_0)$ does not influence the evolution of CWT in b_0 across scales. By limiting the approximation to the second order, we get:

$$(W_\Psi f)(a, b_0) \approx -\sqrt{a^3} \cdot f'(b_0)\mathrm{Im}(m_1) \cdot i - \frac{\sqrt{a^5}}{2}\, f''(b_0)\mathrm{Re}(m_2) = \alpha i + \beta$$

where α and β are real. It is then possible to associate particular values of the phase to local extrema and inflection points. For example, if a local extremum is reached in b_0 ($f'(b_0) = 0$), the phase is equal to 0 or π, depending on the sign of β and, in the same way, a local inflection in b_0 ($f''(b_0) = 0$) is associated with phase value $-\pi/2$ or $\pi/2$, according to the sign of α.

16.3 Illustration on Signals

In this section, numerical examples on synthetic data and real ECG signals are given to illustrate the above mathematical properties. The analyzing wavelet of concern is defined by (Figure 16.2):

$$\Psi(t) = g(t) \cdot e^{2i\pi k f_0 t} \tag{16.10}$$

where

$$g(t) = \begin{cases} C \cdot (1 + \cos 2\pi f_0 t) & \text{for } |t| \le \dfrac{1}{2f_0} \\ 0 & \text{elsewhere} \end{cases} \tag{16.11}$$

The required admissibility conditions are satisfied for k integer other than -1, 0, 1, and has been set to 2. f_0 represents the normalized frequency ($0 < f_0 < 1/2$). For this wavelet, $\text{Im}(m_1)$ is positive and $\text{Re}(m_2)$ is negative.

16.3.1 Results on Simulated Data

In the following examples, $f_0 = 0.005$, the scale parameters are

$$a_i = \frac{f_0}{f_0 + i \cdot \Delta} \quad \text{with } \Delta = 0.005,\ 0 \le i \le 10.$$

Example 1
See Figure 16.3. The input signal (Figure 16.3a) behaves like

$$A_1 \text{Exp}\left(-\frac{(t - m_1)^2}{b_1}\right) + A_2(t - m_2)\text{Exp}\left(-\frac{(t - m_2)^2}{b_2}\right)$$

with $A_1 = 15$, $b_1 = 1700$, $m_1 = 250$; $A_2 = 0.3$, $b_2 = 2500$, $m_2 = 625$. The associated CWT square modulus is reported (Figure 16.3b); the frequency

increases (scale decreases) from the bottom to the top. We have reported
on the "Y" axis the parameter i in place of the scale a_i.

The local extremal values of the square modulus make it possible to
locate both the inflection points and the local extrema of the signal. This
is clearly established Figure 16.1c, which shows the contour plot of the
square modulus. Figure 16.1d depicts the phase variations between $\pm\pi$. As
the phase is unstable when the modulus is close to zero, its value is fixed
to zero when the modulus is less than a given threshold. Aligning the 0
and π crossing of the phase from low to high frequency, one can localize the
extrema of the signal, while $\pm\pi/2$ are associated to inflection points.   ▢

Example 2

See Figure 16.4. Define $f_0(t)$ by:

$$f_0(t) = \frac{1 - \mathrm{Exp}\left(-\dfrac{(t - m_1)^2}{c}\right)}{2 - \mathrm{Exp}\left(-\dfrac{(t - m_2)^2}{c}\right)}$$

where $m_1 = 250$, $m_2 = 300$, $c = 2500$. The signal used in this example is:
$f(t) = A_1 f_0(t) + A_2 f_0'(-(t + t_0))$ with $A_1 = 10000$, $A_2 = 225$ and $t_0 = 10$.
The symmetry properties do not hold in this case. However, inflection
points and local extrema of the signal still can be localized using phase and
modulus. According to the sign of β, the jump in the phase from $-\pi$ to
$+\pi$ corresponds to a local maximum in the signal and zero crossing to a
local minimum. As $\alpha > 0$, inflection point on an increasing positive slope,
corresponds to $-\pi/2$ and on a decreasing negative slope to $+\pi/2$.   ▢

Example 3

See Figure 16.5. The analyzed signal is the distribution

$$U(t) = \begin{cases} 1 & \text{if } t > t_0 \\ 0 & \text{elsewhere.} \end{cases}$$

The associated CWT may be written as:

$$(W_\Psi U)(a, b) = \sqrt{a} \int_{\frac{(t_0 - b)}{a}}^{+\infty} \overline{\Psi}(v) \, dv \qquad (16.12)$$

Denote $\widetilde{\Psi}$, the function which is null except on the support of Ψ and such
that its derivative is equal to Ψ. Then the square modulus of Equation

16.12 is equal to

$$|(W_\Psi U)(a,b)|^2 = a \left| \widetilde{\Psi} \left(\frac{t_0 - b}{a} \right) \right|^2.$$

This quantity reaches its maximal value for $b = t_0$, and $\widetilde{\Psi}(0)$ is imaginary with phase equal to $-\pi/2$ which means that CWT point out the time location of the jump in $U(t)$.

In practice, digital signal processing deals with input data obtained by analog low-pass filtering and a uniform sampling of a continuous time process. A signal like $U(t)$ is then smoothed (due to filtering) and becomes continuous at t_0 with a sharp transition (or maximal slope) at this point before the sampling procedure. WT of this sampled data behaves as for an inflection point on a positive increasing slope. ☐

16.3.2 Results on Real Data

The signal of concern is a normal ECG sampled at 360 Hz; f_0 is set to 0.001 and the scale parameters are

$$a_i = \frac{f_0}{f_0 + i \cdot \Delta} \quad \text{with } \Delta = 0.002, \ 0 \le i \le 25.$$

Example 4

See Figure 16.6. From the CWT square modulus, the QRS and T waves are well localized because of their high slope, while P waves are not clearly separated from the QRS. In this example, the CWT has been multiplied by -1 before phase calculus in order to change the zero crossing into π crossing. Because the phase is represented between $\pm\pi$, the π crossing point corresponds to a discontinuity in the gray level representation (jump from black to white color). Using the phase representation, one can localize all the elementary components of the ECG when aligning the jump in the phase across scales. It can be seen that the phase locates the characteristic components of the signal more accurately; the modulus enhances the waves that have high slope (i.e., sharp waves), mainly the QRS and T waves, but does not allow the localization of P waves because of their low amplitude. To overcome this drawback, we proposed a nonlinear transformation (NLT) [11] to get transients with an inflection point corresponding locally to a potential wave peak and to enhance the energy of the P and T waves with respect to the QRS one (Figure 16.7). Local maxima of the signal is analyzed by means of CWT to exploit its inherent ability to point out the time location of such transients. ☐

Example 5

See Figures 16.8 and 16.9. The CWT is applied to the output of NLT. The wavelet transform has been multiplied by the complex i to transform a $\pi/2$ crossing in a color jump. P, QRS, and T waves can be clearly separated with the help of the CWT square modulus; the phase map led to the same results. Moreover, each curve of constant phase $\pi/2$ varies according to the "propagation" across scales of the inflection point associated with a particular event in the signal. The energy distribution in the time-scale shows a similar behavior. □

These remarks have been exploited from the pattern recognition point of view. The so-called "fingerprints" are here defined as the curves obtained by connecting, in the timescale domain, the points of a given constant phase value. In Example 4 (resp. 5), the fingerprints associated with the phase value zero (resp. $\pi/2$)—jump from black to white color—vary according to the shape of the corresponding events (P, QRS, and T waves). Based on these remarks, a set of descriptors has been extracted from the timescale plane to characterize the elementary components of the ECG and to allow its recognition based on hidden Markov models.

16.4 Cardiac Beat Recognition Approach Based on Wavelet Transform and HMMs

Basically, hidden Markov models are doubly stochastic processes that can characterize any discrete sequence of feature vectors $\{o_t\}_{1 \le t \le T}$, derived from an input signal $f(t)$ and considered as realizations of the so-called "observable process" $\{O_t\}_{1 \le t \le T}$, by a set of multidimensional probability density functions (pdfs) whose parameters depend upon an unobservable first-order Markov state automaton or chain $\{X_t\}_{1 \le t \le T}$, the so called "hidden process". Practically, the hidden chain $\{X_t\}_{1 \le t \le T}$ models through its topology and its transition probabilities, the temporal and structural aspects of $f(t)$ while the state-dependent observation pdfs account for the probabilistic nature of the feature vectors from which they are derived. For both reasons, hidden Markov modeling is well suited to the analysis of structured random signals that are essentially segmental in nature. After designing several competing models of arrhythmias, beat classification and labeling, and/or complex rhythms, analysis can be performed based on dynamic programming techniques and the maximum likelihood criterion. The modeling techniques described here consider the observed ECG signal $f(t)$ as being equivalent to a sequence of events associated with state changes.

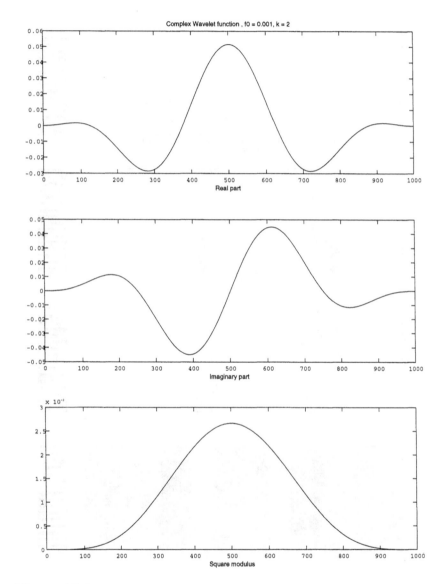

Figure 16.2
The plot of the real part, imaginary part, and square modulus of
the wavelet used.

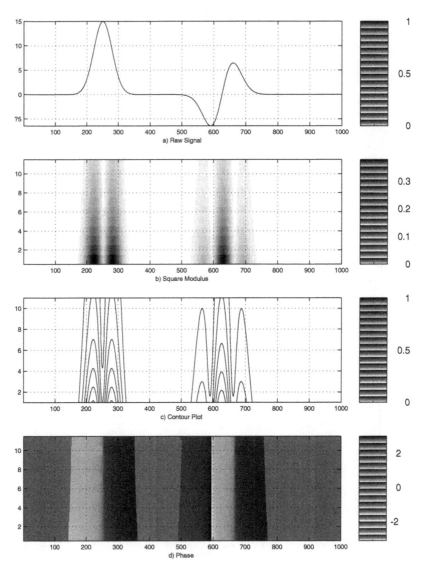

Figure 16.3
CWT of simulated data with local symmetry properties.

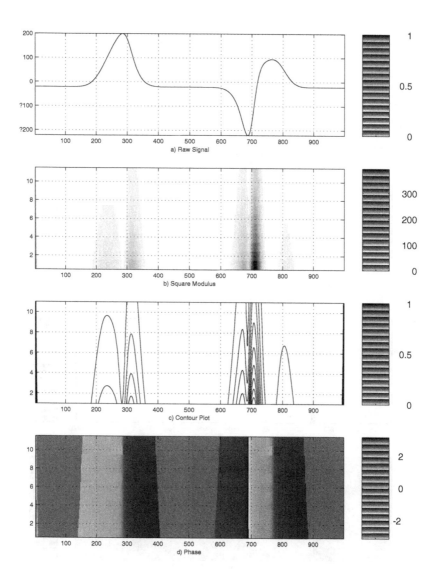

Figure 16.4
CWT of simulated data without symmetry properties.

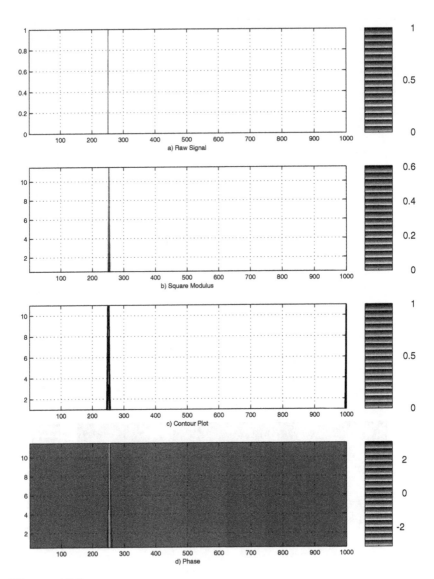

Figure 16.5
CWT of a simulated signal with a particular discontinuity.

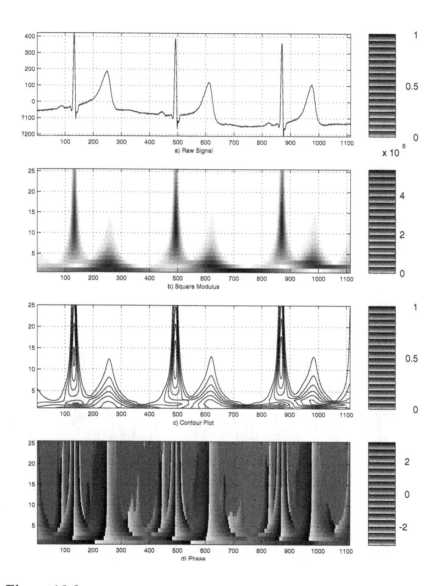

Figure 16.6
CWT of real ECG.

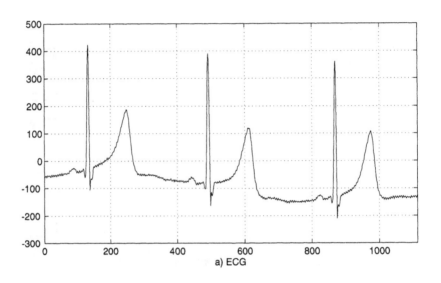

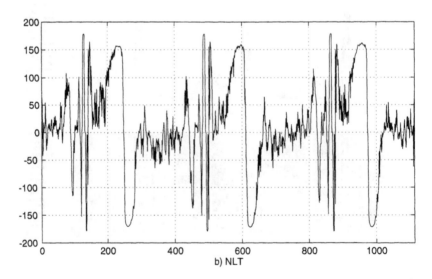

Figure 16.7
Example of the NLT procedure applied to the ECG.

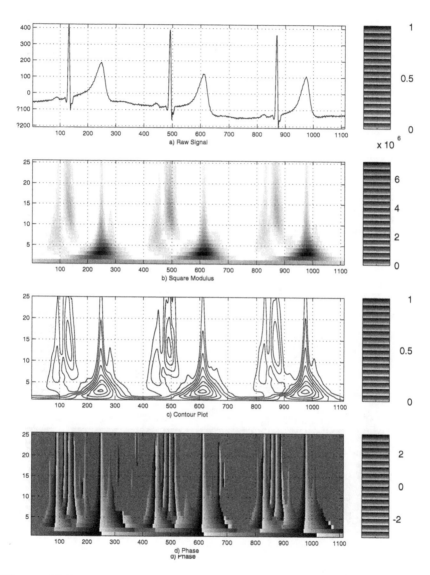

Figure 16.8
CWT performed on the NLT of the ECG.

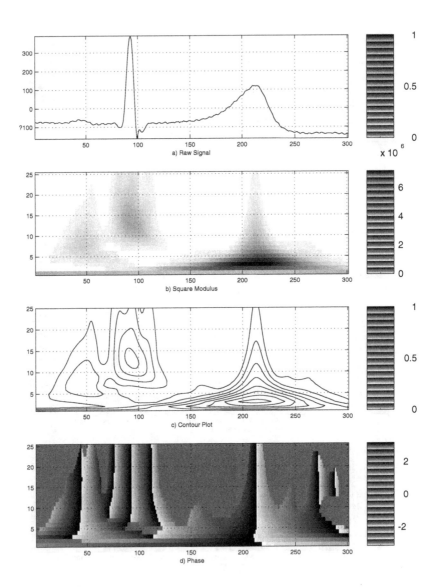

Figure 16.9
Close-up view of the second ECG beat of the Figure 16.8.

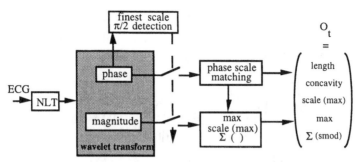

Figure 16.10
Block diagram of the data preparation procedure.

In practice, a preprocessing stage first projects the observed ECG signal $f(t)$ into a discrete sequence of feature vectors $\{o_t\}_{1 \leq t \leq T}$. Then, the likelihood of $\{o_t\}_{1 \leq t \leq T}$ is simultaneously assessed by several competing models: their respective states describe the different signal patterns that can occur in the rhythmic disorder associated with, and their topology depicts the statistical arrangement existing between them along the time axis. The objective here is to show how the wavelet transform, based on the suitable properties described previously, could be used in the ECG data preparation step (more precisely in the construction of the observation vector o_t). Markov theory is not reported here; the reader may refer to [12].

The data preparation is depicted in Figure 16.10 and relies on the extraction of shape parameters from CWT performed on the output of the NLT of the ECG. As seen before, for each elementary wave, the NLT generates transients with an inflection point corresponding locally to its dominant extremum. The ability of the CWT to focus on the edges of a signal is here of great interest. The combination NLT/WT allows enhancement of the separation between the elementary waves in the scalogram (Figure 16.9). Moreover, each fingerprint characterizes, by its length, the persistency of an event across the scales and, by its concavity, its relative time position in the signal.

For each $\pi/2$ crossing of the phase at the finest scale of decomposition and time position t, the associated fingerprint is reconstructed by an ad hoc procedure under a simple constraint of continuity; then an observation vector $\{o_t\}$ is derived. It is composed of five parameters:

- "Length": the length of the fingerprint in terms of number of associated levels of decomposition;

- "Concavity": its concavity;

- "scale (max)": the scale value, over the support of the fingerprint, where the CWT square modulus is maximum;

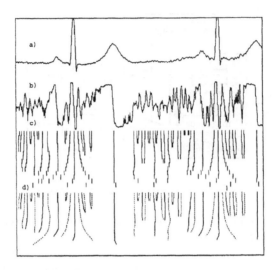

Figure 16.11
a) ECG signal, b) the corresponding NLT, c) fingerprints on the time-scale domain, d) the reconstructed fingerprints.

- the magnitude of the above maximum "max";

- the summation of all the CWT modulus on the fingerprint, "Σ(smod)".

16.5   Results

In our experiments, the phase is computed over a finite scale set in order to derive relevant fingerprints; at each $\pi/2$ crossing, the NLT is then decomposed on several levels to recover correctly the theoretical bandwidth of elementary waves. The transition probabilities of the models are set equal to consider as equiprobable the presence or the absence of inter-wave observations. The five parameters composing the observation vectors o_t are assumed to be independent. Moreover, "length", "concavity," and "scale (max)" are discrete random variables while "max" and "Σ(smod)" are Gaussian. The wave couplet durations are modeled by truncated Gaussians so that they are lower and upper bounded. All the parameters of the probability laws are initialized with a clustering of a small observations set and then refined cyclically using a modified version of the Baum-Welch's reestimation procedure [13].

Figure 16.11 depicts an ECG signal with its corresponding NLT, the fingerprints before and after reconstruction (represented on 15 levels). Thus,

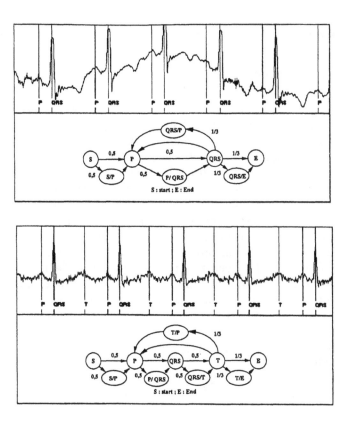

Figure 16.12
**Two examples of the structure of the Markov state chain used
to decode the corresponding observation sequence derived from
signal by data preparation stage. Vertical lines locate the elementary waves recognized by the structure.**

for each time candidate an observation vector is derived from $f(t)$. Finally,
the resulting observation serie is processed by the hidden chain depicted
in Figure 16.12. A transition between "T" and "P" states via the "T/P"
one is allowed to process successive cardiac beats. "S" and "E" states
model the onset and the end of the signal. Note that all ECG constitutive
waves are well localized and identified even when HF noise, mainly due
to the electromyography activity, is present. In our ECG recognition process, the strong nonstationarity of the signal is shaped essentially because
each wave is viewed as a unique stationary entity, rather than a locally stationary stochastic process. Although our approach is still under test, the
first results obtained show that the recognition rate is enhanced compared
to the procedure where segmentation and identification of ECG waves are
performed simultaneously by classical HMMs.

16.6　Conclusion

We have presented some properties of a complex wavelet transform. The modulus maxima and the $\pm\pi/2$ phase crossing point out the locations of sharp signal transitions, while modulus minima correspond to the "flat" segments of the signal. The results on simulated data show that phase information may be of great interest when time location of particular events of such peaks is looked for. On ECG signal, the behavior of both phase and modulus of the decomposition when the scale goes to zero allows description of the elementary components (P, QRS, T). By exploiting these properties, the Markov models, briefly presented here, can behave as a segmentation/recognition signal processing tool, achieving the numbering of all the waves (including the P ones), by probabilistically modeling the temporal structure of the observed surface ECG. The set of standard mathematical tools devoted to the use of HMMs constitutes a found theoretical basis. It must be emphasized that there is no restriction on the use of Markovian models when the physical phenomenon is only approximately Markovian. It must be said, however, that the segmentation of the observed signals may not be sufficient to identify some pathological situations, for instance, when the waves, say P and QRS, usually appearing on different time intervals, are superimposed, as in the auricular-ventricular dissociation.

16.7　Appendix

Appendix 1: Expression of CWT Square Modulus Derivative

The derivative of $(W_\Psi f)\,(a,b)$ according to the space variable b is:

$$\frac{\partial\,(W_\Psi f)\,(a,b)}{\partial b} = \frac{1}{\sqrt{a}}\int_{-\infty}^{+\infty} f(t)\cdot\overline{\frac{\partial\Psi\left(\frac{t-b}{a}\right)}{\partial b}}\,dt$$

$$= \frac{-1}{\sqrt{a^3}}\int_{-\infty}^{+\infty} f(t)\cdot\overline{\Psi'\left(\frac{t-b}{a}\right)}\,dt.$$

As Ψ is a compactly supported wavelet, using partial integration, the above quantity becomes:

$$\frac{\partial \left(W_\Psi f\right)(a, b)}{\partial b} = \frac{1}{\sqrt{a}} \int_{-\infty}^{+\infty} f'(t) \cdot \overline{\Psi \left(\frac{t-b}{a}\right)} \, dt$$

The Equation 16.1 is equivalent to

$$\frac{\partial \left|(W_\Psi f)(a, b)\right|^2}{\partial b} = 2\mathrm{Re} \left(\frac{\partial \left(W_\Psi f\right)(a, b)}{\partial b} \overline{(W_\Psi f)(a, b)}\right) ;$$

the expression of

$$\frac{\partial \left(W_\Psi f\right)(a, b)}{\partial b}$$

in this equality leads to Equation 16.2.

Appendix 2: Approximation of CWT Square Modulus Derivative

The quantity

$$\int_{-\infty}^{+\infty} U(t) \cdot \overline{\Psi \left(\frac{t-b}{a}\right)} \, dt$$

is equal to

$$a \int_{-\infty}^{+\infty} U(ax + b) \cdot \overline{\Psi(x)} \, dx.$$

Note that the last integral holds only on the support of Ψ. Assuming that U is differentiable, the above quantity can be approximated by:

$$a \int_{-\infty}^{+\infty} (U(b) + axU'(b)) \cdot \overline{\Psi(x)} \, dx = a^2 U'(b) \int_{-\infty}^{+\infty} x \cdot \overline{\Psi(x)} \, dx$$

(Ψ is zero mean) for small values of a (fine-scale analysis and then high frequencies). Assume now that f' is differentiable, one can then use this last approximation for each term in the right-hand part of Equation 16.2:

$$\int_{-\infty}^{+\infty} f'(t) \cdot \overline{\Psi \left(\frac{t-b}{a}\right)} \, dt \approx a^2 f''(b) \int_{-\infty}^{+\infty} x \cdot \overline{\Psi(x)} \, dx ;$$

$$\int_{-\infty}^{+\infty} f(t) \cdot \overline{\Psi \left(\frac{t-b}{a}\right)} \, dt \approx a^2 f'(b) \int_{-\infty}^{+\infty} x \cdot \overline{\Psi(x)} \, dx,$$

which permits obtaining Equation 16.3.

Appendix 3: Expression of $(W_{\Psi} f)\,(a, b_0)$

1. Case of: $(\exists b_0 \in \mathbb{R})\,(\exists \varepsilon > 0)\,(\forall |h| < \varepsilon)\, f(b_0 + h) = f(b_0 - h)$
   Using a change variable we obtain:

$$(W_{\Psi} f)\,(a, b_0) = \sqrt{a} \cdot \int_{-\infty}^{+\infty} f(at + b_0)\overline{\Psi(t)}\, dt$$

$$= \sqrt{a} \cdot \int_{0}^{+\infty} (f(at + b_0) + f(-at + b_0)) \cdot \operatorname{Re}(\Psi(t))\, dt.$$

As Ψ is hermitian and compactly supported, its definition domain has the form $(-\Delta/2, \Delta/2)$. Hence, for all values a such that $a\Delta/2 < \varepsilon$ we have $f(at + b_0) = f(-at + b_0)$. Based on this remark and using a simple variable change one can obtain the Equation 16.5.

2. Case of: $(\exists b_0 \in \mathbb{R})\,(\exists \varepsilon > 0)\,(\forall |h| < \varepsilon)\, f(b_0 + h) = 2f(b_0) - f(b_0 - h)$
   The same approach is adopted: for $a\Delta/2 < \varepsilon$ we use the above relation and the zero mean property of the wavelet to obtain Equation 16.6.

References

[1] P. Trahanias and E. Skordalakis. Syntactic pattern recognition of the ECG. *IEEE Trans. PAMI* 12(7), 648–657, 1990.

[2] O. Meste, H. Rix, P. Caminal, and N. V. Thakor. Detection of late potentials by means of wavelet transform. *IEEE Trans. BME* 41(7), 625–634, 1994.

[3] R. Murray, S. Kadambe, and G. F. Boudreaux-Bartels. Extensive analysis of a QRS detector based on the dyadic wavelet transform. *Proc. IEEE-Sig. Process. Int. Symp. on Time-Frequency Time-Scale Analysis*, 1994, 540–543.

[4] L. Senhadji, J. J. Bellanger, G. Carrault, and J. L. Coatrieux. Wavelet analysis of ECG signals. *Proc. IEEE-EMBS*, 1990, 811-812.

[5] L. Senhadji, J. J. Bellanger, G. Carrault, and G. F. Passariello. Comparing wavelet transforms for recognizing cardiac patterns. *IEEE-EMB Mag. Special Issue, Time-Frequency and Wavelet Analysis*, 14(2), 167–173, 1995.

[6] A. Grossmann and J. Morlet. Decomposition of hardy functions into square integrable wavelets of constant shape. *SIAM J. Math. Anal.*, 15(4), 723–736, 1984.

[7] A. Grossmann, R. K. Martinet, and J. Morlet. Reading and understanding continuous wavelet transforms. *Proc. Int. Conf. Wavelets, Time-Frequency Methods and Phase Space*, Marseille, France. J. M. Combes, et al. Eds., Inverse Problems and Theoretical Imaging, Springer-Verlag, 1989, 2–20.

[8] S. G. Mallat. A theory of multiresolution signal decomposition: the wavelet representation. *IEEE Trans. PAMI*, 11(7), 674–693, 1989.

[9] I. Daubechies. Orthonormal basis of compactly supported wavelets. *Commun. Pure Appl. Math.*, 41, 909–996, 1988.

[10] S. G. Mallat and S. Zhong. Characterization of signals from multiscale edges. *IEEE Trans. PAMI*, 14(7), 710–732, 1992.

[11] L. Thoraval. Analyse statistique de signaux ECG par modèles de Markov cachés. Ph.D. dissertation, University of Rennes I, France, July 1995.

[12] L. R. Rabiner. A tutorial on hidden Markov models and selected applications in speech recognition. *Proc. IEEE*, 77(2), 257–285,1989.

[13] L. Thoraval, G. Carrault, and J. J. Bellanger. Heart signal recognition by hidden Markov models: the ECG case. Meth. Inf. Med., 33(1), 10–14, 1994.

17

Interference Canceling in Biomedical Systems: The Mutual Wavelet Packets Approach

Mohsine Karrakchou and Murat Kunt

Signal Processing Laboratory
Swiss Federal Institute of Technology, Lausanne, Switzerland

17.1 Introduction

In recent years, the field of signal processing has witnessed the introduction of powerful new theories coming from various fields, such as the ones of time-frequency analysis, chaos, fuzzy logic and neural networks. These theories are finding their way into many different biomedical applications whose specific needs have even triggered additional innovations. In this context, we present here a monitoring problem in which the use of advanced signal processing techniques leads to significant improvements in the analysis and understanding of the underlying physiological process. The investigation of this problem has also been an incentive to develop new powerful techniques.

Our application concerns the automatic in vivo estimation of microvascular pulmonary pressure P_{mv}, for which new structures of multirate adaptive filtering based on wavelet packets have been developed in order to remove the respiratory interference. The performance of this method has been shown to be much better than classical adaptive filtering schemes and makes it possible to obtain an accurate estimate of P_{mv}.

This chapter is organized as follows: in Section 17.2, the clinical importance of measuring effective pulmonary capillary pressure is explained. The different techniques proposed in the literature are reviewed. Advantages and limitations of each of them are mentioned. Section 17.3 deals with some basics of adaptive interference canceling, while Section 17.4 exposes fundamentals of multirate adaptive filtering. In Section 17.5, the new mutual wavelet based adaptive filtering is introduced. Different implementation schemes are given for the latter structure. Algorithmic complexity is evaluated. Section 17.6 shows some experimental results obtained for the cancellation of respiratory interference in pulmonary capillary transients when using the proposed structure. Section 17.7 concludes the chapter.

17.2 Pulmonary Capillary Pressure: A Short Review

17.2.1 Clinical Relevance

The so-called adult respiratory distress syndrome (ARDS) is frequently encountered in intensive care patients. It usually arises 1 to 3 days after one or several of many associated and possibly causative conditions, such as sepsis, massive trauma, various lung infections, near drowning, or surface burns [36]. It is characterized physiologically by diffuse damage to the alveolar capillary membrane, with subsequent interstitial edema. Despite the vast amount of experimental and clinical research which has been devoted to ARDS (for review see [2, 33]), the mortality has remained high (40–70%) [15]. It has not yet been possible to successfully interrupt the chain of pathophysiological events injuring the lung, so that therapy is still largely based on supportive measures aimed at improving tissue oxygenation, such as mechanical ventilation and drug support of the cardiovascular system.

One key issue in the management of ARDS is interstitial edema of the lung. There is ample experimental evidence that interventions aiming at minimizing the accumulation of interstitial fluid improve gas exchange [41]. Recent clinical studies even suggest that control of extravascular lung water may improve the outcome [37, 43, 28].

The hallmark of ARDS is an increase in the permeability of the capillaries to both plasma protein and fluid [41, 40, 46]. The pulmonary edema occurring in this condition has been termed acute permeability edema. In permeability edema, transvascular fluid flux becomes highly sensitive to

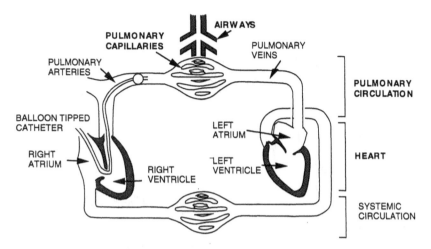

Figure 17.1
Schematic representation of the cardiopulmonary system, with a balloon-tipped catheter inserted in a pulmonary artery.

microvascular pressure P_{mv} [1]. Moreover P_{mv} has been found elevated in a variety of experimental models of lung injury; this was explained by the vasoconstriction of pulmonary veins induced by various mediators of inflammation [10, 11, 13]. These experimental results suggest that increased P_{mv} may contribute to the pulmonary edema of ARDS. In summary, acute permeability pulmonary edema is extremely sensitive to the pressure in the microvessels of the lung (P_{mv}), which may be elevated in this condition. Therefore, an essential therapeutic goal in the clinical management of ARDS is to lower P_{mv} as much as possible [35]. It is therefore important to monitor P_{mv}, the "effective" pulmonary capillary pressure, in these patients.

The arterial occlusion (AO) technique has been proposed as a convenient means for the in vivo estimation of P_{mv} [4, 12, 17, 19, 20, 56]. This technique relies on the analysis of the pressure transient observed in a pulmonary arterial branch abruptly occluded by the inflation of a Swan-Ganz catheter balloon. The sudden inflation of the balloon causes an interruption of the blood flow, yielding a sudden drop in the measured pressure. P_{mv} is then estimated from an analysis of the post–occlusion pressure transient (POPT) observed after inflating the balloon. A schematic representation of the cardiopulmonary system is given in Figure 17.1, while a typical apneic signal is shown in Figure 17.2.

Pulmonary arterial occlusion pressure (PAOP) as measured with a Swan-Ganz catheter, is widely used as an estimate of P_{mv}. In fact, PAOP estimates the pressure within the large pulmonary veins or the left atrium (P_{lv}). In order for blood to flow forward through the lungs, P_{mv} must ex-

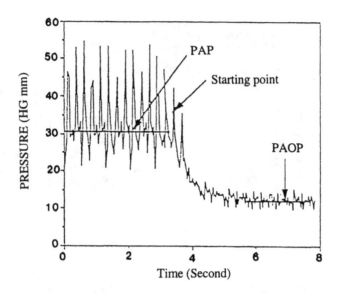

Figure 17.2
Typical signal of effective pulmonary pressure.

ceed P_{lv}. Under normal conditions, the vascular pressure gradient across
the pulmonary circulation is so small [7] that P_{mv} or PAOP are very close to
P_{lv}. Under conditions of increased pulmonary vascular resistances (PVR),
however, P_{mv} may differ considerably from PAOP because it depends on
the relative magnitudes of vascular resistances on the arterial (R_a) and on
the venous (R_v) sides of the capillary bed. Discrepancies between P_{mv}
and PAOP are expected in ARDS, because of the frequently associated
pulmonary hypertension [54]. Indeed, it is clear that elevated PVR are
intimately related to the pathogenesis of ARDS.

17.2.2   In Vivo Estimation: The Occlusion Techniques

The Double Occlusion

Given the importance of the estimation of pulmonary capillary pressure
for the diagnosis and treatment of ARDS, a considerable effort has been
devoted within the past few years to the development of simple and direct
methods to estimate P_{mv}. Indeed, the problem of measuring pulmonary
capillary pressure has been investigated in various studies [9, 22, 25, 48].
It has been shown that the clamping of arterial or venous pressures either
simultaneously or individually gives rise to transients whose analysis allows
a direct estimation of P_{mv}. When a simultaneous clamping is applied both
to the arterial and venous pressures in an isolated lung, the pressures equi-
librate to the same value which represents the value of the microvascular

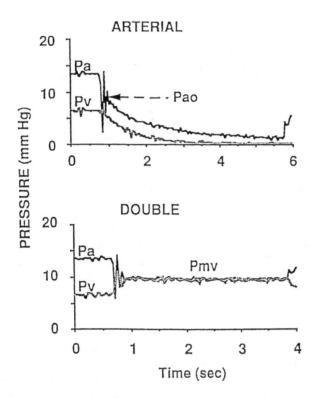

Figure 17.3
Illustration of the transients obtained either by arterial or double occlusion. Pa: lobar arterial pressure. Pv: lobar venous pressure. Pao: capillary pressure estimated from the graphical analysis of the pulmonary artery pressure transient. Pmv: microvascular pressure obtained by double occlusion

pressure. In fact, excellent agreement has been obtained when comparing this occlusion technique with the measurement obtained from gravimetric techniques in an isolated lung [9, 29]. The transients obtained when performing arterial, venous, or double occlusion are shown in Figure 17.3.

These different studies showed that the double occlusion technique represents a new and rapid way to estimate P_{mv}. This also permitted showing that most of the vascular compliance resides at the same vascular site in which the capillary filtration occurs. Also, various mathematical models have been developed from these different experiments to predict the capillary pressure and the longitudinal distribution of pulmonary vascular resistance. The simplest model and also the most widely used one is a single compartment model in which the large capillary compliance is located between arterial and venous resistances. This is illustrated in Figure 17.4. A more complicated three compartment model incorporating arterial, capil-

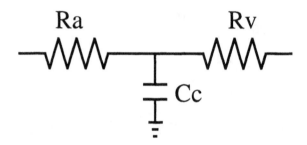

Figure 17.4
Illustration of a single compartment model.

lary, and venous compliance has been proposed by Dawson et al. [8]. This model contains four resistors in series with three capacitors in parallel. This is illustrated in Figure 17.5. The advantage of such a model is that it offers various experimental and theoretical ways through which P_{mv} can be estimated.

The Arterial Occlusion

The arterial occlusion is another way to estimate microvascular pressure. A balloon-tipped Swan-Ganz catheter is placed in the pulmonary artery. When the balloon is suddenly inflated, an abrupt interruption of flow occurs, and the pressure measured at the catheter tip drops within a few seconds to a new stationary value PAOP. The arterial occlusion technique takes advantage of the special shape of the pressure transient resulting from the sudden occlusion of a medium-sized pulmonary arterial branch. After the onset of the occlusion (starting point), there is a rapid initial drop (fast transient), and the pressure then decays exponentially to PAOP (slow transient). The point where the two transients meet is angular. It was shown from animal experimentation [20, 49] that the pressure obtained by back-extrapolation of the slow transient from the inflection point to the time of occlusion is a good estimate of P_{mv}. Several attempts to estimate P_{mv} on this principle have been made in intensive care patients. However, none of the described methods appears to be very robust nor lends itself easily to automation in an intensive care environment. The search for the inflection point by means of visual inspection, even feasible in nonpulsatile flow conditions [14, 18, 20], is subject to undocumented interobserver variation. Collee et al. [12] based their estimate of P_{mv} on the back-extrapolation to time zero (the time of occlusion) of an exponential fit to the slow part of the transient. Their estimated values, however, might be very sensitive to the choice of both inflection and occlusion points. D'Orio et al. [50] and Siegel et al. [27] modeled the transient as a sum of two exponential processes that were fitted by least-square fitting algorithms. The post-occlusion arterial

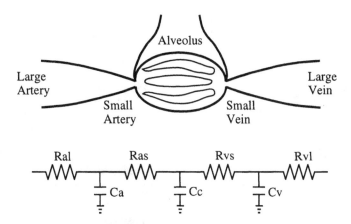

Figure 17.5
Schematic representation of the pulmonary circulation with four
resistors and three capacitors.

pressure transient is thus represented as:

$$P(t) = A_0 e^{-\alpha_0 t} + B_0 e^{-\beta_0 t} + C_0 \qquad (17.1)$$

where α_0 is the time constant of the slow exponential, β_0 is the time constant of the fast exponential, and where the time origin is assumed to be at
the occlusion point that corresponds to the inflation moment. The asymptotic value C_0 was usually assumed to be the estimation of the capillary
pressure, but has been shown to underestimate P_{mv}. The exact value of
P_{mv} has been shown to be $A_0 + C_0$. This method is now adopted, even if
some of its limitations are still to be addressed.

17.2.3 Limitations in Patients

The patient should be relaxed. He/she should be mechanically ventilated
with a properly positioned pulmonary artery catheter and the ventilation
should be held during balloon inflation. Indeed, even a slight contamination
of the transient by pressure fluctuations due to respiratory movements will
make any of the above described methods difficult to apply. An illustration of this contamination is given in Figure 17.6 where different transients
recorded in nonapneic conditions are shown. This clearly shows the difficulty of direct modeling of such transients.

Therefore, the in vivo determination of P_{mv} has so far been restricted to
paralyzed, mechanically ventilated subjects in whom the pressure transient
can be recorded during a brief (20 s) period of apnea. Although transients
heavily distorted by respiratory artifacts may be beyond the technique's

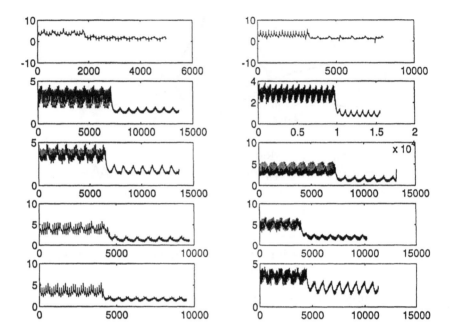

Figure 17.6
Illustration of various transients perturbed by respiratory interference.

possibilities, the practical use of the arterial occlusion technique would be greatly improved if, at least, some respiratory fluctuations could occur without compromising the estimation of P_{mv}. The purpose of this work is to cancel such a respiratory interference. The cancellation is based on adaptive filtering for which new structures based on wavelet packets are proposed.

17.3 Basics of Interference Canceling

17.3.1 Classical FIR Adaptive Filtering

Most of everyday signal processing tasks tend to be done in an unknown environment, which prevents engineers to design context-dependent filters. Since the pioneering work of Widrow and co-workers [5, 6], adaptive filtering has emerged as a powerful and intensively used tool in many applications such as control, system identification, and echo cancellation.

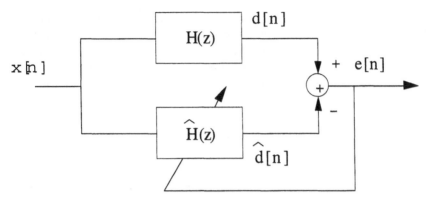

Figure 17.7
Adaptive filter configured in system identification.

The basic idea of adaptive filtering algorithms can be illustrated by the block diagram of Figure 17.7. The unknown system characterized by the transfer function $H(z)$ between the input signal $x[n]$ and the desired signal $d[n]$ has to be identified. The identification is performed using an estimate of $H(z)$, namely, $\hat{H}(z)$. The error $e[n]$ between the desired response $d[n]$ and its estimate $\hat{d}[n]$ is used by an algorithm which adjusts the coefficients of $\hat{H}(z)$ in order to minimize some function of the error.

A frequently used error criterion is the mean square error (MSE), defined as:

$$\varepsilon = E\{e^2[n]\} \tag{17.2}$$

where

$$e[n] = d[n] - \hat{d}[n] \tag{17.3}$$

Assuming that $H(z)$ can be approximated using an FIR filter, then it can be represented by an FIR filter whose impulse response is denoted by $w[n]$. The estimate of $d[n]$ can then be written as:

$$\hat{d}[n] = \sum_{i=0}^{N-1} w_i[n]\, x[n-i] = \mathbf{w}_N^T[n]\, \mathbf{x}_N[n] \tag{17.4}$$

where a bold symbol represents an N-component vector. It can be shown [47] that substituting Equations (17.4) and (17.3) in (17.2) yields the following expression of the MSE:

$$\varepsilon = E\{e^2[n]\} = \sigma_d^2 - 2\mathbf{w}_N^T[n]\, \mathbf{p}_N + \mathbf{w}_N^T[n]\, \mathbf{R}_{NN}\, \mathbf{w}_N[n] \tag{17.5}$$

where

$$\mathbf{R}_{NN} = E\left\{\mathbf{x}_N[n]\, \mathbf{x}_N^T[n]\right\}, \quad \mathbf{p}_N = E\{d[n]\, \mathbf{x}_N[n]\} \tag{17.6}$$

and σ_d^2 is the variance of the desired signal. The MSE is thus a quadratic function of the predictive filter coefficients. It can easily be shown that this performance surface is concave up and, hence, has one global minimum. The optimal filter in a Wiener sense is the one minimizing the MSE. This is obtained by differentiating Equation (17.2) with respect to the filter weights:

$$\frac{\partial \varepsilon}{\partial \mathbf{w}_N} = 0 \qquad (17.7)$$

yielding:

$$\mathbf{R}_{NN} \, \mathbf{w}_N^* = \mathbf{p}_N \qquad (17.8)$$

Equation (17.8) is called the normal equation. Although this equation is usually solvable, it is not solved as such due to the complexity of the problem. Moreover, gathering the long-term statistics of the signals may be also too time consuming. Real-world applications mostly use the famous and simple least mean square (LMS) algorithm which tries to iteratively solve this normal equation using an approximation of the long-term statistics [5, 47]. This algorithm belongs to the family of stochastic methods since it minimizes a statistical error measure.

The MSE described above is not the only criterion used. Another frequently used measure is based on the least square error. This leads to the second family of adaptive algorithms, called the exact methods, that minimize the error computed on the data themselves. These algorithms, the most well known of which being the recursive least squares (RLS) algorithm, achieve better performance than the stochastic methods at the price of a higher algorithmic complexity [47].

It should be noted that this general introduction to adaptive filtering is made in the context of system identification. The same remains valid for interference canceling. The general principle of interference canceling is the following. A first sensor receives the composite signal $x = s + n_1$ with s the signal of interest and n_1 the interference (or "noise") which is supposed to be uncorrelated with s. A second sensor receives a reference input signal $y = n_2$; n_2 is uncorrelated with s but correlated with n_1. The noise n_2 is then filtered by a filter H to produce an output as close as possible to n_1. This output is finally subtracted from $s + n_1$. This scheme is illustrated in Figure 17.8. Due to the assumptions made on the correlations of the different signals, minimizing the error power by adjusting the filter H will correspond to estimate the signal s.

While in most applications, H is supposed be linear and simple adaptive algorithms are used, there are many ways to improve the performance of such a simple scheme. Multirate adaptive filtering is one of these solutions, and is described in the next section.

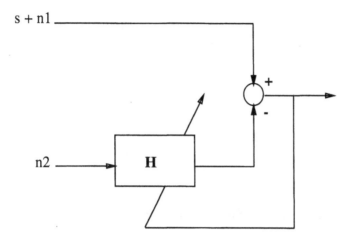

Figure 17.8
Simple diagram of the canceller.

17.4 Multirate Adaptive Filtering

FIR adaptive filtering has now been used for the last three decades in many areas, such as system identification, line enhancement, or echo cancelation. While its applications have been growing, requirements in speed and performance did as well. By now, a standard implementation of an FIR adaptive filter may not be sufficient.

The bottleneck is the order of the model to be used. Most of the processes that have to be identified or canceled are autoregressive (AR) processes. An FIR filter prescribes a moving average (MA) model for the process. Hence FIR filters should be very long in order to be efficient enough. The use of filters having one thousand coefficients is now common in echo cancelation for teleconferencing. Using such a long filter, even the fast LMS algorithm may be too time consuming.

An alternative solution that has been recently investigated is subband adaptive filtering [3, 21, 23, 53], which consists in splitting the considered signals into several frequency bands, subsampling the subband signals, and finally performing the adaptation in each of these subbands. The advantage is that the adaptation can be performed using shorter adaptive filters, which, moreover, can be adapted and operate in parallel.

Adaptive filtering is not the only signal processing area where subband decomposition proved to be particularly efficient. Signal and image compression have been using this scheme for awhile. The idea of subband decomposition is to use a filter bank composed of several bandpass filters. Each of the output signals, being bandpass signals, can now be downsam-

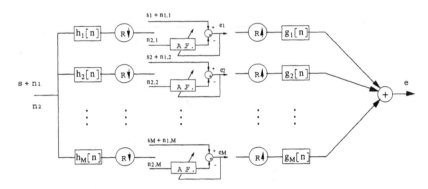

Figure 17.9
Adaptive filtering performed with an M-band filter bank.

pled according to Nyquist theorem. If the filter bank is uniform and made
up of M filters, the maximum decimation factor is equal to M. For the sake
of generality, the filter bank is not assumed to be uniform nor the subband
signals to be maximally decimated.

The advantages of such a system are that the processing can be done in
parallel and that the decimation performed on the subband signals yields
a restrained amount of data to be processed. The speed is thus dramatically increased. Once processing is done, signals can be reconstructed by
the synthesis filter bank. A careful design of the analysis and synthesis
filter banks guarantees a perfect reconstruction of the signals. An in-depth
discussion of this can be found in [51].

17.4.1   Fundamentals of Adaptive Filtering in Subbands

Subband adaptive filtering has been suggested as an alternative to classical adaptive filtering to increase computation speed and improve convergence of the adaptation process. It was first introduced by Furukawa [21]
and Kellermann [52]. A general subband echo canceler is depicted in Figure
17.9, where a noisy signal ($x = s + n_1$) composed of a desired signal s and
an interfering noise n_1 is decomposed through the analysis filter bank along
with an auxiliary noise signal $y = n_2$. The purpose of echo cancelation is
to recover the desired signal s from the noisy one using an adaptive filter.

The subband approach consists in performing the subband decomposition
of both signals yielding M pairs of sequences decimated by a factor of
R. Standard adaptive filtering can be performed in each subband before
reconstructing the sequence of output signals. Besides the usual advantages
of subband decomposition consisting in the possibility of parallel processing
and the reduction in number of data to be processed, other benefits are
achieved, namely, the reduction length of the adaptive filters and the speed
up of convergence.

However, there is one important drawback to subband adaptive filtering due to the non-ideal nature of the analysis filters. Since rejection in the stopband is not perfect, when performing one-bandpass filtering, some frequency components of the adjacent bands will be included in the output signal of that bandpass filter. The problem is that these components will be aliased at the down-sampling stage. Remedies to this situation are various. Of course, the use of sharp analysis filters will reduce this effect. Unfortunately this requires longer analysis filters. Another solution is to have a decimation factor lower than the number of subbands. Gilloire and Vetterli proposed in [3] a solution consisting in performing an additional adaptation with the reference input of the contiguous bands.

Another drawback consists in the rigid nature of the decomposition, which is totally independent of the spectral content of the signal. For instance, in the design of an adaptive notch filter or of an adaptive line enhancer, it may occur that the sinusoids of interest fall into the gap regions of the filter banks and thus may not be enhanced or canceled by the adaptive system. A signal-dependent partitioning of the frequency axis may solve the problem. This can be accomplished in the wavelet packets framework.

17.5   Wavelet Packets

The discrete wavelet transform (DWT) decomposition is a powerful tool for the processing of nonstationary signals and is closely related to subband decomposition. However, it is preferable to consider the DWT from the filter banks point of view, since the latter allows a straightforward extension to wavelet packets. Given a signal, a low-pass and high-pass (using two quadrature mirror filters), half-band filtering is performed on it, yielding two sequences. Having performed half-band filtering, one can subsample the new sequences by a factor of two following the Nyquist theorem. The process is iterated on the low-pass signal as long as needed. The corresponding filter bank has a tree structure giving the well-known octave decomposition of the frequency axis.

Wavelet packets are a generalization of the concept of wavelet transform in which arbitrary time-frequency resolution can be chosen according to the signal [38]. This will be done, of course, within the bounds of the Heisenberg uncertainty principle. The idea is to obtain an adaptive partitioning of the time-frequency plane depending on the signal of interest. This section consists in a short review of wavelet packets and a presentation of their most interesting properties. All subsequent information can be found in more detail in [34, 44].

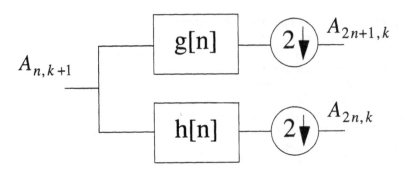

Figure 17.10
One-stage decomposition of a signal.

Let $h[n]$ and $g[n]$ be the impulse response of the two analysis filters, and let $A_{n,k+1}$ be one of the vector spaces at level $k + 1$ onto which signals are projected. The filtering operations performed by $h[n]$ and $g[n]$ split the vector space into two subspaces ($A_{2n,k}$ and $A_{2n+1,k}$). This is illustrated in Figure 17.10. It can then be shown [34] that these two subspaces are orthogonal and that $A_{n,k+1}$ is the direct sum of these two subspaces, namely:

$$A_{n,k+1} = A_{2n,k} \oplus A_{2n+1,k}. \tag{17.9}$$

Using this scheme, a tree of depth $\log L$ (where L is the length of the signal being analyzed) can be built by iterating this decomposition on each of the newly created nodes. The idea of wavelet packets is to allow any orthogonal decomposition to be performed over this entire tree, instead of choosing a rigid decomposition of a signal. The property 17.9 ensures that pruning any subtree still yields an orthonormal basis onto which the signal can be decomposed. Figure 17.11 shows the entire tree.

The tree contains several admissible bases, one of which is the wavelet basis itself. Having a large but finite library of bases, an ordering of this library can be performed with respect to some criterion. Hence it is possible to extract the best basis relatively to the criterion considered. This is known as the best basis method [34, 39, 42, 44, 55]. The basis can be any subtree of the initial entire tree, and the best basis method will yield this subtree by a pruning scheme performed on the complete tree.

17.5.1 The Best Basis Method

Let $M(x)$ be a real-valued functional on the signal sequences x_i. The purpose of the method is to find the optimal basis that minimizes this functional on the manifold of orthonormal bases. The search for the best basis is straightforward: the entire decomposition tree is spanned. A bottom-up pruning scheme is applied in which, going from leaves to the root, the values

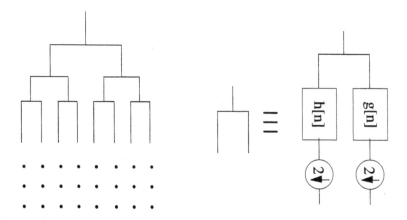

Figure 17.11
Sketch of an entire tree obtained by the wavelet packets decomposition.

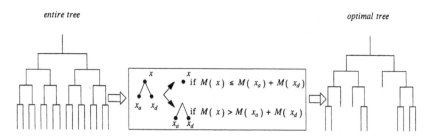

Figure 17.12
Illustration of the best basis selection principle.

of the functional on the two possible bases (the node and its two children) are compared (see Figure 17.12).

Let $A_{2n,k}$ and $A_{2n+1,k}$ be the bases chosen at level k. Let $B_{n,k+1}$ be the parent of the latter two, and let $M(B_{l,m}x)$ be the value of the functional computed on the projection of the signal x onto some basis $B_{l,m}$. The optimal basis, $A_{n,k+1}$, is going to be:

$$A_{n,k+1} = \begin{cases} B_{n,k+1} & \text{if } M(B_{n,k+1}) \leq (M(A_{2n,k}) + M(A_{2n+1,k})) \\ A_{2n,k} \oplus A_{2n+1,k} & \text{if } M(B_{n,k+1}) > (M(A_{2n,k}) + M(A_{2n+1,k})) \end{cases}$$

and it is assigned the minimum of the two functional values ($M(B_{n,k+1}x)$ and $M(A_{2n,k}x) + M(A_{2n+1,k}x)$) for further comparison.

17.6   Mutual Wavelet Packet Decomposition for Subband Adaptive Filtering

17.6.1   Introductory Comments

The purpose of this section is to obtain a nonuniform filter bank for subband decomposition that performs a signal-dependent partitioning of the frequency axis in order to overcome the intrinsic limitation of classical signal-independent subband adaptive filtering. This section shows how, using a new mutual wavelet packet scheme along with a new decomposition criterion, a nonuniform signal-dependent filter bank is obtained. Different adaptation structures are investigated, as well as their implementation and algorithmic complexity [26, 30].

17.6.2   The Mutual Wavelet Packets Decomposition

As described in Section 17.5, wavelet packets can be regarded as a powerful tool to obtain an optimal subband decomposition with respect to some criterion. This is achieved by splitting and/or merging subbands obtained by successive application of the analysis filters.

The concern here is to improve adaptive filtering. Considering Equation (17.8), this can be obtained by somehow maximizing the magnitude of either the vector $\mathbf{p}_N$ or some of its relevant components. This corresponds to maximizing some measure of the cross-correlation between the two signals considered in the adaptive process. As an illustration of the influence of the cross-correlation vector on the adaptation, consider for instance the case of two uncorrelated signals. Since the vector $\mathbf{p}_N$ will be equal to zero, the optimal filter will be zero as well. This is quite a reasonable result since there is no way to extract one signal from the other. Intuitively, maximizing the cross-correlation between the two signals will maximize their similarity and favor the performance of the adaptation. Therefore the criterion suggested in this chapter for the mutual wavelet packet decomposition is based on the maximization of the sum of the magnitude of the cross-correlation samples and is given by:

$$M(x_i[n], y_i[n]) = \sum_{k=0}^{N-1} |\varphi_{x_i y_i}[k]| \qquad (17.10)$$

where $x_i[n]$ is the signal to be filtered at a given node of the decomposition, $y_i[n]$ is the reference signal at the same node, N is the number of coefficients of the local adaptive filter within the node, and $\varphi_{xy}[k]$ is the cross-correlation sequence of $x_i[n]$ and $y_i[n]$. Each of these cross-correlation samples are estimated, as is usually done, with the biased correlation esti-

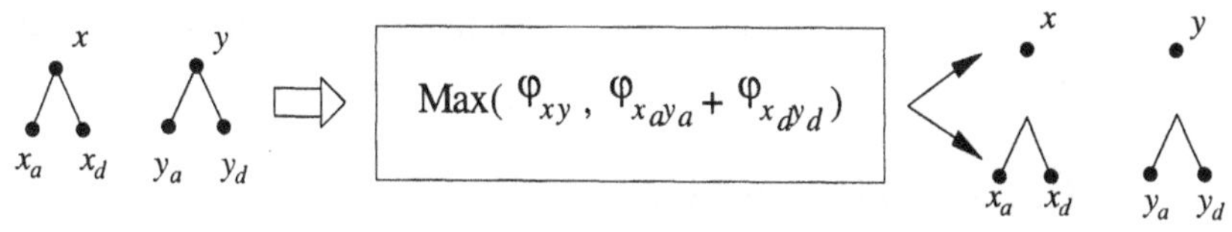

$$\text{Max}(\ \varphi_{xy}\ ,\ \varphi_{x_a y_a} + \varphi_{x_{d'} y_d}\ )$$

Figure 17.13
Illustration of the best basis selection for the mutual wavelet packets decomposition.

mate of an L-samples sequence given by:

$$\hat{\varphi}_{x_i y_i}[k] = \frac{1}{L} \sum_{n=0}^{L-1} x_i[n]\, y_i[n+k]$$

The choice of computing the criterion using N samples of the cross-correlation sequence is justified by the fact that this number corresponds to the number of components of the vector $\mathbf{p}_N$. Moreover, this could be reduced to some smaller constant when the speed of the best basis selection is of major concern. Compared to the usual wavelet packets used for signal analysis or signal compression, the mutual wavelet packets decomposition simultaneously decomposes two signals onto the same basis with respect to a common criterion, as illustrated in Figure 17.13. The best basis is thus optimal for the pair of signals instead of being adapted to only one of them.

The purpose of the method is to find the optimal basis that maximizes this functional on the manifold of orthonormal bases. The search for the best basis is performed exactly as explained for the decomposition of one signal, except that in the present case, two binary-trees will be spanned instead of one. This works as follows: the entire two decomposition trees are spanned. A bottom-up pruning scheme is applied simultaneously for both of them. When going from the leaves to the root, a correspondence is made between the nodes and the values of the functional on the two possible bases (the nodes basis and their two children basis) are compared. The optimal basis is going to be the one that maximizes the functional. The parent nodes are assigned the maximum of the two functional values for further comparisons.

Compared to standard subband adaptive filtering, the main advantage of this new scheme consists in creating a nonuniform filter bank adapted to the spectral content of the signals. The decomposition is chosen so that the signals are maximally correlated in each of the subbands, which assures a better adaptation process. The performance of this new scheme will mostly show up in the presence of structured and colored noise or interferences, where the band selection is critical. Performance in the presence of wideband signals is expected to be close to standard subband filtering since the optimal decomposition is not going to change the filter bank structure significantly.

17.6.3   Implementation Scheme

Once the best basis has been selected and the nonuniform filter bank decomposition performed, the adaptation remains to be done. Recent works in classical subband adaptive filtering [32, 45, 53] proposed different structures that differ by the adaptation criterion. The two principal structures can be applied to the mutual wavelet packet decomposition. The first one is called synthesis-independent structure and the whole adaptation process is performed in the subbands. The second one, named synthesis-dependent structure, computes its error criterion on the reconstructed error signal.

For both schemes, the size of the filter in each of the subbands is derived from the following equation given in [3]:

$$L_S = \frac{L_F}{2} + L_A \qquad (17.11)$$

where L_A is the length of the analysis filter, L_F the length of the adaptive filter used for the parent and L_S the length of the adaptive filter used for the children. At every stage of the decomposition process, when a node is split into two children, the filter lengths of the children nodes are deduced from that of their parent, according to the above equation.

Synthesis-Independent Solution

This configuration is straightforward: signals are decomposed using wavelet packets; they are filtered in their respective subbands, then reconstructed. The LMS or RLS algorithm is applied as such on each of the subband signals. Hence the error signal is a local measure within each of the subbands. This solution, depicted in Figure 17.14, will also be referred as minimization of the subband errors.

This scheme will suffer from the aliasing introduced by the nonideal characteristics of the filter bank. Due to the decomposition process, the filter bank is always maximally decimated, which creates overlapping regions in the overall frequency response of the system around the band boundaries. Moreover, this problem cannot be compensated by using any scheme similar to the one proposed by Gilloire and Vetterli in [3], since contiguous bands in this nonuniform decomposition can be sampled at different sampling rates.

17.6.4   Algorithmic Complexity

The concern of this paragraph is to evaluate the complexity of subband adaptive filtering based on mutual wavelet packet decomposition and contrast it to the complexity of a regular subband implementation.

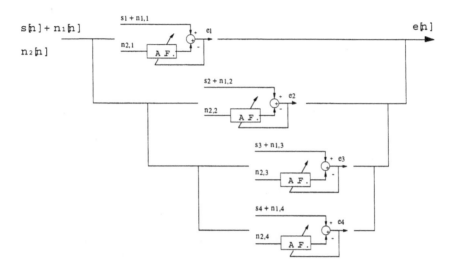

Figure 17.14
A synthesis-independent configuration.

Let L be the length of the input signals and M be the length of the analysis quadrature mirror filters used for the wavelet packet decomposition. The decomposition process is made up of filtering operations. The first stage low-pass and high-pass filters the whole signals, hence the complexity is $O(2ML)$. The second stage performs the same operation on two sequences, each half the length of the initial one, due to the subsampling by a factor of two. The complexity is thus the same ($O(2 \times 2ML/2) = O(2ML)$). Hence the complexity is the same at each level in the tree. The depth of the tree being $\log L$ [24], the overall complexity of the decomposition process is given by:

$$O(2ML \log L) \quad \text{multiplications} \tag{17.12}$$

Having performed the decomposition, the selection of the best basis has to be performed. Let $C(L)$ be the complexity of the criterion to be minimized for a L samples signal. At level k in the tree, 2^k signals of length $L/2^k$ are present. The criterion is computed exactly once for every node of the tree. Hence the complexity of the operation is given by:

$$O\left(\sum_{k=0}^{\log L} 2^k C\left(\frac{L}{2^k}\right) \right) \quad \text{multiplications.} \tag{17.13}$$

It is obvious that care should be taken in the implementation of the criterion so that this process will not be too time-consuming. The cross-

correlation criterion, for example, should be implemented using the fast
Fourier transform, which approximately yields:

$$O\left((\log L + 1)(L + 3L \log_2 L)\right) \quad \text{multiplications.} \quad (17.14)$$

The complexity of the adaptive filtering process is, of course, dependent
on the complexity of the algorithm used. What matters is the complexity
of that algorithm applied to the filter length in the largest subband, since,
at least in a hardware implementation, filtering in the subband would be
performed in parallel.

Eventually, the complexity of the reconstruction is upper bounded by the
complexity of the decomposition, since in the worst case the optimal tree
is the entire tree.

The proposed method is definitely more complex than a classical uniform
subband decomposition. For the latter, every filter (analysis and synthesis)
can operate in parallel. Hence the subband decomposition complexity is
$O(ML)$. The subband adaptation process has a complexity given by the
size of the adaptive filters in the subbands.

It is clear that the potential increase in performance of the proposed
method over regular subband adaptive filtering will be obtained at the
expense of a higher computational complexity. Despite this higher complexity, the method will prove to be worth using when filtering has to be
performed on structured noise or interferences.

17.6.5 Experimental Results

Although the methods proposed in the literature for the estimation of
P_{mv} have been validated on some animals, their use for clinical studies is
limited. In fact, strict apnea is required during the recording of the signal
to avoid respiratory artifacts. However, we have proposed a method to
suppress respiratory interference, so as to make the method more generally
applicable by overcoming the requirement of strict apnea for the in vivo
measurement of P_{mv}.

Our approach consists in using an interference canceller, where the auxiliary signal used is the right atrial pressure signal. This signal can be
recorded simultaneously with the POPT, using the same Swan-Ganz catheter. The right atrial pressure signal is well correlated with the respiratory
interference without being correlated with the pressure transient. The proposed mutual wavelet packet adaptive filtering algorithm is used for the
cancellation of respiratory interference in pulmonary capillary transients
[31]. Two respiratory periods are selected on the last part of each signal
to adapt the filters. After convergence, the filters are applied to the entire

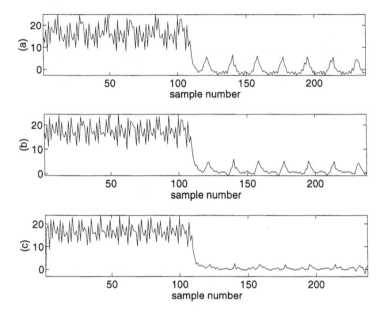

Figure 17.15
Typical result for respiratory interference canceling on the pulmonary pressure transients: (a) before interference canceling, (b) full-band implementation, (c) mutual wavelet packet scheme.

signal. This gives a measure of the average magnitude of the respiratory interference before and after cancellation.

The basic adaptive filtering scheme, performed on the original signals and denoted by full-band implementation, is compared to the mutual wavelet packet scheme. The basic analysis wavelet used for the decomposition is the D_{10} Daubechies wavelet [16].

A typical result is illustrated in Figure 17.15. It can be seen that the respiration is much more attenuated when using the mutual wavelet packet scheme. We have performed the simulations on 115 different transients recorded on different patients. In every experiment, the performance of the mutual wavelet packet scheme has been contrasted to the performance of the full-band scheme. The adaptive algorithm used in both cases is the classical least mean square algorithm. The metric used to estimate their performance is an estimate of the average magnitude of the residual error. This average magnitude has been computed on the last part of the signal where the influence of the transient is negligible. The results of these experiments are reported in Figure 17.16. It appears that the performance achieved using the mutual wavelet packets is better than that of the full-band scheme. Indeed the respiratory artifacts are more efficiently canceled in all the cases.

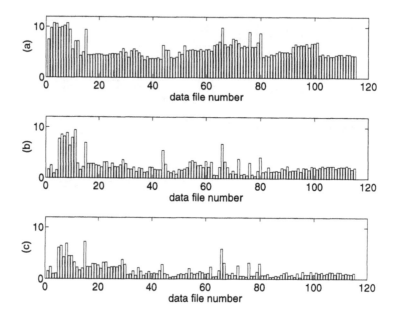

Figure 17.16
Performance comparison for interference canceling: (a) before
interference canceling; (b) full-band implementation; (c) mutual
wavelet packet scheme. For each data file, the average magnitude
of the residual error is reported.

The main advantage of the proposed method is of course an adaptive subband decomposition of the signals to be filtered, adaptively reducing the
aliasing gaps of the filter bank at the sensitive locations on the frequency
axis. To favor the adaptation process, the similarity between the signals to
be filtered has to be maximized in every subband. The application sought
being adaptive filtering — a method trying to be as independent as possible
of the environment — the decomposition process should be adaptive itself.
The mutual wavelet packet framework offers such an adaptive decomposition of the signals and proved to be advantageous.

17.7   Conclusion

In this chapter, the problem of in vivo estimation of pulmonary capillary pressure P_{mv} in intensive care units has been investigated. Multirate
adaptive filtering has been investigated and a new mutual wavelet packet
scheme has been proposed for subband adaptive filtering. Its relation to

the existing literature on the subject has been outlined. The novelty of the proposed scheme consists in the fact that it makes use of wavelet packets. In addition, and from the viewpoint of wavelet packets, this mutual wavelet packet scheme performs a decomposition of the two signals used in the adaptation process onto the same optimal basis. The basis is thus optimal for the two signals instead of being adapted to only one of them, as is usually done in the wavelet packet framework. That basis is chosen so that it favors the adaptation performance. For this reason, a new criterion based on a functional of the two signals has been introduced. The proposed criterion is to maximize the cross-correlation between the two signals considered. At the expense of a slightly higher computational complexity, the proposed mutual wavelet packet scheme reduces the aliasing drawback of regular adaptive filtering, preserving its main advantages. Two subband adaptive filtering schemes have been discussed that can minimize either a local error criterion, which is the error in the subband, or a global criterion, minimizing the reconstruction error. This mutual wavelet packet scheme has been applied to the cancelation of respiratory interference. Extremely encouraging results concerning the estimation of P_{mv} from transients perturbed by respiratory fluctuations have been obtained. It is our hope that this would significantly enhance the practicality of the pressure measurement technique.

References

[1] A. E. Taylor, J. W. Barnard, S. A. Barman, and W. Keith Adkins. Fluid Balance. In R. G. Crystal and J. B. West, eds. *The Lung: Scientific Foundations*, Raven Press, New York, 1991.

[2] A. Fein, J. P. Wiener-Kronich, M. Nieder, and M. A. Matthay. Pathophysiology of the adult respiratory distress syndrome. What have we learned from human studies? *Crit. Care Clin.*, (2), 1986.

[3] A. Gilloire and M. Vetterli. Adaptive Filtering in sub-bands. *IEEE Int. Conf. Acoustics, Speech and Signal Process. Conf.*, 1988.

[4] Audi S., C. A. Dawson, D. A. Rickaby, and J. H. Linehan. Localization of the sites of pulmonary vasomotion by use of arterial and venous occlusion. *Am. Physiol. Soc.*, 1991, 2127–2136.

[5] B. Widrow and S. D. Stearns. *Adaptive Signal Processing*. Prentice Hall, Englewood Cliffs, NJ, 1985.

[6] B. Widrow et al. Adaptive noise canceling: Principles and applications. *Proc. IEEE*, December 1975.

[7] C. A. Dawson. Pulmonary circulation. In *American Handbook of Physiology. Section 2. Respiration. Part I*. A. P. Fishman, Ed. Bethesda, 1986.

[8] C. A. Dawson, D. A. Rickaby, and J. H. Linehan. Distributions of vascular volume and compliance in the lung. *J. Appl. Physiol.*, 1988.

[9] C. A. Dawson, J. H. Linehan, and D. A. Rickaby. Pulmonary microcirculatory hemodynamics. *Ann. N. Y. Acad. Sci.*, 1982.

[10] C. E. Patterson, J. W. Barnard, J. E. Lafuze, M. T. Hull, S. J. Baldwin, and R. A Rhoades. The role of activation of neutrophils and microvascular pressure in acute pulmonary edema. *Am. Rev. Respir. Dis.*, (140), 1989.

[11] C. R. Chen, N. F. Voelkel, and S. W. Chang. PAF potentiates protamine-induces lung edema: role of pulmonary venoconstriction. *J. Appl. Physiol.*, 68:1059–1068, 1990.

[12] Collee G. G., K. E. Lynch, R. D. Hill, and W. M. Zapol. Bedside measurement of pulmonary capillary pressure in patients with acute respiratory failure. *Anesthesiology*, 66(5):614–620, 1987.

[13] D. C. Hocking, P. G. Phillips, T. J. Ferro, and A. Johnson. Mechanisms of pulmonary edema induced by tumor necrosis factor alpha. *Circulation Res.*, (67), 1990.

[14] D. K. Cope, R. C. Allison, J. L. Parmentier, J. N. Miller, and A. E. Taylor. Measurement of effective pulmonary capillary pressure using the pressure profile after pulmonary artery occlusion. *Crit. Care Med.*, 14:16–22, 1986.

[15] D. R. McCaffree. Adult respiratory distress syndrome. In *Cardiopulmonary Critical Care*, D. R. Dantzker, ed. Grune Stratton, New York, 1986.

[16] Daubechies I. Orthonormal bases of compactly supported wavelets. *Commun. Pure Appl. Math.*, 41:909–996, 1988.

[17] Dawson C. A., T. A. Bronikowski, J. H. Linehan, S. T. Haworth, and D. A. Rickaby. On the estimation of pulmonary capillary pressure from arterial occlusion. *Am. Rev. Respir. Dis.*, 140:1228–1236, 1989.

[18] F. Grimbert. Effective pulmonary capillary pressure in pulmonary edema. In *Update in Intensive Care and Emergency Medicine*. J. L. Vincent, ed. Springer, 1986.

[19] Hakim T. S., J. M. I. Maarek, and H. K. Chang. Estimation of pulmonary capillary pressure in intact dog lungs using the arterial occlusion technique. *Am. Rev. Respir. Dis.*, 140:217–224, 1989.

[20] Holloway H., M. Perry, J. Downey, J. Parker, and A. Taylor. Estimation of effective pulmonary capillary pressure in intact lungs. *Am. Physiol. Soc.*, 54:846–851, 1983.

[21] I. Furukawa. A design of canceller of broad band acoustic echo. International Teleconferencing Symposium, Tokyo, 1984.

[22] J. C. Parker, P. R. Kvietys, K. P. Ryan, and A. E. Taylor. Comparison of isogravimetric and venous occlusion capillary pressures in isolated dog lungs. *J. Appl. Physiol.*, (55), 1983.

[23] J. J. Shynk. Frequency-domain and multirate adaptive filtering. *IEEE Signal Process. Mag.*, January 1992.

[24] K. Ramchandran and M. Vetterli. Best wavelet packets in a rate-distortion sense. *IEEE Trans. Image Process.*, submitted paper 1992.

[25] K. Ryan, P. Kvietys, and J. C. Parker. Comparison of venous occlusion and isogravimetric capillary pressure in isolated dog lungs. *Physiologist*, 1980.

[26] Karrakchou M., C. van den branden Lambrecht, and M. Kunt. Mutual wavelet packets adaptive filtering for the analysis of pulmonary capillary pressure. Invited paper for the *IEEE Mag. Eng. Med. Bio. Soc.*, 1995.

[27] L. C. Siegel, R. G. Pearl, and S. L. Shafer. The longitudinal distribution of pulmonary vascular resistance during unilateral hypoxia. *Anesthesiology*, 1989.

[28] M. A. Mattay and J. P. Wiener-Kronish. Intact epithelial barrier function is critical for the resolution of alveolar edema. *Am. Rev. Respir. Dis.*, (142), 1990.

[29] M. I. Townsley, R. J. Korthuis, and B. Ripe. Validation of double vascular occlusion method for Pc in lung and skeletal muscle. *J. Appl. Physiol.*, 1986.

[30] M. Karrakchou and C. van den branden Lambrecht. New issues for the use of wavelet packets. *Workshop on Time Frequency Analysis, Lyon, France*, 1994, 26.1–26.4.

[31] M. Karrakchou and M. Kunt. Wavelet packets for interference canceling in biomedical systems. Invited paper for the Int. Conf. Artificial Neural Networks in Engineering, St. Louis, MO, November 1994, 514–518.

[32] M. Petraglia. Efficient Adaptive Filtering Structures based on Multi-rate Techniques. Ph.D. thesis, University of California at Santa Barbara, December 1991.

[33] M. R. Flick. Mechanisms of lung injury. What have we learned from experimental animal models? *Crit. Care Clin.*, (2), 1986.

[34] M. V. Wickerhauser. INRIA Lectures on Wavelet Packet Algorithms. *INRIA Lectures on Wavelet Packet Algorithms*, March 1991.

[35] N. C. Staub. The hemodynamics of pulmonary edema. *Bull. Eur. Physiopathol. Respir.*, (22), 1986.

[36] P. E. Pepe. The clinical entity of adult respiratory distress syndrome: definition, prediction and prognosis. *Crit. Care Clin.*, (2), 1986.

[37] P. R. Eisenberg, J. R Hansbrough, D. Anderson, and D. P Schuster. A prospective study of lung water measurements during patient management in intensive care unit. *Am. Rev. Respir. Dis.*, (136), 1987.

[38] P. Reynaud and B. Torresani. Paquets Continus d'Ondelettes et Décomposition Optimale. Juan-les-Pins, September 1991. 3rd Colloq. Gretsi.

[39] R. Coifman, Y. Meyer, D. Quacke, and M. Wickerhauser. Acoustic signal compression with wave packets. Wavelet Workshop. Marseilles, October 1990.

[40] R. H. Simmons. Mechanisms of lung injury. In *Cardio-Pulmonary Critical Care*. D. R. Dantzker, ed., New York, 1986.

[41] R. M. Prewitt, J. Mccarthy, and D. H. Wood. Treatment of acute low pressure pulmonary edema in dogs. *J. Clin. Invest.*, (67), 1981.

[42] R. R. Coifman and M. V. WickerHauser. Best adapted wave packet bases. 1990.

[43] R. S. Simmons, G. G. Berdine, J. J. Seidenfeld, T. J. Prihoda, G. D. Harris, J. D. Smith, T. J. Gilbert, E. Mota, and W. G. Johanson. Fluid balance and the adult respiratory distress syndrome. *Am. Rev. Respir. Dis.*, (135), 1987.

[44] R. R. Coifman and M. V. Wickerhauser. Entropy-based algorithms for best basis selection. *IEEE Trans. Inf. Theory*, 38, March 1992.

[45] S. Furui and M. M. Sondhi. *Advances in Speech Signal Processing*. Marcel Dekker, New York, 1992.

[46] S. J. Allen, R. E. Drake, J. P. Williams, G. A. Williams, and J. C. Gabel. Recent advances in pulmonary edema. *Crit. Care Med.*, 15, 1987.

[47] S. T. Alexander. *Adaptive Signal Processing.* Springer-Verlag, 1986.

[48] T. S. Hakim, C. A. Dawson, and J. H. Linehan. Hemodynamic responses of dog lung lobe to lobar venous occlusion. *J. Appl. Physiol,* (267), 1979.

[49] T. S. Hakim, R. R. J. Michel, and H. K. Chang. Partitioning of pulmonary vascular resistance in dogs by arterial and venous occlusion. *J. Appl. Physiol,* (52), 1982.

[50] V. D'Orio, J. Halleux, L. M. Rodriguez, C. Wahlen, and R. Marielle. Effects of *Escherichia Coli* endotoxin on pulmonary vascular resistance in intact dogs. *Crit. Care Med.,* (14), 1986.

[51] Vaidyanathan P. P. Multirate digital filters, filter banks, polyphase networks, and applications: a tutorial. *Proc. IEEE,* 78:56–93, 1990.

[52] W. Kellerman. Kompensation akusticher Echos in Frequenzteilbändern. Aachener Kolloquium. Aachen, FRG, 1984.

[53] W. Kellermann. Analysis and design of multirate systems for cancellation of acousticals echoes. *IEEE Int. Conf. Acoustics, Speech and Signal Process. Conf.,* 1988.

[54] W. M. Zapol and M. T. Snider. Pulmonary hypertension in severe acute respiratory failure. *New Engl. J. Med.,* (96), 1977.

[55] Y. Meyer. Méthodes temps-fréquence et méthodes temps-échelle en traitement du signal et de l'image. *INRIA Lectures on Wavelet Packet Algorithms,* March 1991.

[56] Yamada Y., M. Suzukawa, M. Chinzei, T. Chinzei, N. Kawahara, K. Suwa, and K. Numata. Phasic capillary pressure determined by arterial occlusion in intact dog lung lobes. *Am. Physiol. Soc.,* 67:2205–2211, 1989.

18

Frame Signal Processing Applied to Bioelectric Data

John J. Benedetto

Department of Mathematics, University of Maryland, College Park, MD
and The MITRE Corporation, McLean, VA

Abstract   Signal processing methods are developed which utilize frame, wavelet, and Fourier methods. Applications are made to noise reduction, and seizure localization and prediction problems. MRI and ECoG data are used in the experiments.

18.1 Introduction

We shall give two signal processing methods, which are independent of each other, but which are related to the theory of frames. The methods are frame multiresolution analysis (Section 18.4) and a variation of the classical Laplacian method related to Gaussian frames (Section 18.6). Background on the theory of frames is the subject of Section 18.3. We shall also use these ideas and related Fourier and wavelet methods to examine bioelectric data. MRI data is considered in Section 18.5; and we illustrate how to achieve signal reconstruction of such data, when it is contaminated with the broadband noise that arises in coding or quantization. ECoG data is analyzed in Section 18.7, with a view to comparing time-frequency and time-scale information as a method for dealing with seizure localization and prediction problems.

The Appendix provides mathematical details related to Section 18.6.

18.2   Notation

Besides the standard notation from mathematical analysis, we use the following conventions. $\int f(t)\,dt$ designates $\int_{\mathbb{R}^d} f(t)\,dt$, where $\mathbb{R}^d$ is d-dimensional Euclidean space. The *Fourier transform* of $f \in L^1(\mathbb{R}^d)$ is $\hat{f}$ defined by $\hat{f}(\gamma) \equiv \int f(t)e^{-2\pi it\gamma}\,dt$, where $t \in \mathbb{R}^d$, $\gamma \in \hat{\mathbb{R}}^d$ $(\equiv \mathbb{R}^d)$, and "$\equiv$" is the symbol we use in defining notation. The L^1-norm of $f \in L^1(\mathbb{R}^d)$ is $\|f\|_{L^1(\mathbb{R}^d)} \equiv \int |f(t)|\,dt$. *Translation* is denoted by τ, and so $\tau_n f(t)$ indicates $f(t-n)$, where $t \in \mathbb{R}$, $n \in \mathbb{Z}$ (the integers). The *circle group* is $\mathbb{T} = \mathbb{R}/\mathbb{Z}$. The set of finite linear combinations of a sequence $\{f_k\}$ of functions is denoted by $sp\{f_k\}$, and its closure in a given space is $\overline{sp}\{f_k\}$.

18.3   The Theory of Frames

18.3.1   Gabor and Wavelet Systems

Let $g \in L^2(\mathbb{R})$ and let a, $b > 0$. The *Gabor system* is the sequence $\{g_{m,n} : (m,n) \in \mathbb{Z} \times \mathbb{Z}\}$, where

$$g_{m,n}(t) \equiv e^{2\pi itmb}g(t-na) = e_{mb}(t)\tau_{na}g(t),$$

$$e_\gamma(t) \equiv e^{2\pi it\gamma}, \quad \text{and} \quad \tau_x g(t) \equiv g(t-x).$$

Clearly,

$$\hat{g}_{m,n}(\gamma) = e^{2\pi inamb}e^{-2\pi ina\gamma}\hat{g}(\gamma - mb) = \tau_{mb}(e_{-na}\hat{g})(\gamma).$$

Let $\psi \in L^2(\mathbb{R})$, the *affine system* or *wavelet system* is the sequence $\{\psi_{m,n} : (m,n) \in \mathbb{Z} \times \mathbb{Z}\}$, where $\psi_{m,n}(t) \equiv 2^{m/2}\psi(2^m t - n)$. Clearly,

$$\hat{\psi}_{m,n}(\gamma) = 2^{-m/2}e^{-2\pi in(\gamma/2^m)}\hat{\psi}(\gamma/2^m) = 2^{-m/2}(e_{-n}\hat{\psi})(\gamma/2^m).$$

18.3.2   Frames

A sequence $\{\phi_n : n \in \mathbb{Z}^d\}$ in a separable Hilbert space H is a *frame* for H if there exist $A, B > 0$ such that

$$\forall v \in H, \quad A\|v\|^2 \leq \sum |\langle v, \phi_n\rangle|^2 \leq B\|v\|^2,$$

where the norm of $v \in H$ is $\|v\| \equiv \langle v, v\rangle^{1/2}$. A and B are the *frame bounds*, and a frame is *tight* if $A = B$. A frame is *exact* if it is no longer a frame whenever any one of its elements is removed. The theory of frames is due to Duffin and Schaeffer [13], cf., [10–12, 14, 22].

The *frame operator* of the frame $\{\phi_n\}$ is the function $S : H \to H$ defined as $Sv \equiv \sum \langle v, \phi_n\rangle \phi_n$.

Let $\{\phi_n\} \subseteq H$ be a frame with frame bounds A and B. The *frame decomposition theorem* asserts that S is a topological isomorphism with inverse $S^{-1} : H \to H$, $\{S^{-1}\phi_n\}$ is a frame with frame bounds B^{-1} and A^{-1}, and

$$\forall v \in H, \quad v = \sum \langle v, S^{-1}\phi_n\rangle \phi_n = \sum \langle v, \phi_n\rangle S^{-1}\phi_n.$$

Let $H \equiv L^2(\mathbb{R})$, $g \in L^2(\mathbb{R})$, and $a, b > 0$. If the Gabor system $\{g_{m,n}\}$ defined above is a frame, then it is a *Gabor frame*. Let $H \equiv L^2(\mathbb{R})$ and $\psi \in L^2(\mathbb{R})$. If the wavelet system $\{\psi_{m,n}\}$ defined above is a frame, then it is a *wavelet frame*.

Let $H \equiv L^2[-\Omega, \Omega]$ and let $\{t_n\} \subseteq \mathbb{R}$ be a sequence of distinct points. The sequence $\{e^{2\pi i t_n \gamma}\} \subseteq L^2[-\Omega, \Omega]$ is a *Fourier system*, and results of Duffin and Schaeffer, H. Landau, and S. Jaffard allow a characterization of *Fourier frames* in terms of a density condition, e.g., [1, Theorem 7.44]. Fourier frames are useful in the design of auditory models for the purpose of speech compression [9], and in irregular sampling theory, e.g., [1, Section 7.7] which includes results proved with William Heller.

THEOREM 1

A sequence $\{\phi_n : n \in \mathbb{Z}^d\}$ in a separable Hilbert space H is a frame for H with frame bounds A and B if and only if the mapping

$$L : H \longrightarrow \ell^2(\mathbb{Z}^d), \quad y \longmapsto \{\langle v, \phi_n\rangle\},$$

is a well-defined topological isomorphism onto a closed subspace of $\ell^2(\mathbb{Z}^d)$. In this case,

$$\|L\| \leq B^{1/2} \quad and \quad \|L^{-1}\| \leq A^{-1/2},$$

where L^{-1} is defined on the range $L(H)$.

See [1, Theorem 7.15]

THEOREM 2

A sequence $\{\phi_n : n \in \mathbb{Z}^d\}$ in a separable Hilbert space H is a frame for H if and only if there is $C > 0$ such that for all $v \in H$,

(1) $\sum |\langle v, \phi_n \rangle| < \infty$;

(2) $\exists c_v \equiv \{c_n\} \in \ell^2(\mathbb{Z}^d)$ such that $v = \sum c_n \phi_n$;

(3) $\|c_v\|_{\ell^2(\mathbb{Z}^d)} \leq C\|v\|$.

See [10, Remark 3.9]. We observed Theorem 2 with David Walnut.

18.4   Frame Multiresolution Analysis (FMRA)

DEFINITION 1   A frame multiresolution analysis (FMRA) of $L^2(\mathbb{R})$ is an increasing sequence of closed linear subspaces $V_j \subseteq L^2(\mathbb{R})$ and an element $\phi \in V_0$ for which the following hold:

(i) $\overline{\cup_j V_j} = L^2(\mathbb{R})$ and $\cap_j V_j = \{0\}$,

(ii) $f(t) \in V_j$ if and only if $f(2t) \in V_{j+1}$,

(iii) $f \in V_0$ implies $\tau_k f \in V_0$, for all $k \in \mathbb{Z}$, where $\tau_k f(t) \equiv f(t-k)$,

(iv) $\{\tau_k \phi : k \in \mathbb{Z}\}$ is a frame for the subspace V_0.

We shall say that an FMRA is of *inexact/exact type* if $\{\tau_k \phi \in \mathbb{Z}\}$ is an inexact/exact frame for the subspace V_0. For a detailed analysis and construction of FMRAs, see [6, 7]. The *frame multiresolution subspaces* are the subspaces $V_j \equiv \overline{sp}\{\phi_{jk}\}_k$ defined in an FMRA, where

$$\phi_{jk} \equiv \sqrt{2^j}\phi(2^j t - k).$$

The redundancy inherent in frame decompositions can be used for noise reduction. In fact, the following results from an elementary calculation.

PROPOSITION 1

Let $\{\phi_n\}$ be a tight frame for H with frame bounds $A = B > 1$, and suppose each $\|\phi_n\| = 1$. Let $\{e_n\}$ be an orthonormal basis (ONB) of H, and let $\{w_n\}$ be a sequence of uncorrelated random variables with 0 mean and such that $\sum Var(w_n) = 1$. Consider the respresentation of a signal in H in terms of the ONB and the frame, i.e.,

$$\forall f \in H, \quad f = \sum \langle f, e_n \rangle e_n,$$

and

$$\forall f \in H, \quad f = \frac{1}{A} \sum \langle f, \phi_n \rangle \phi_n,$$

respectively. If the coefficients $\{\langle f, e_n \rangle\}$ and $\{\langle f, \phi_n \rangle\}$ are both perturbed componentwise by the "random noise" $\{\epsilon w_n\}$, then the expected reconstruction error due to the noise is less in the frame expansion than in the ONB expansion. In fact, there is a gain of $(1 - \frac{1}{A^2})$ in the frame case over the ONB case.

For $\phi \in L^2(\mathbb{R})$, we consider the 1-periodic function,

$$\Phi(\gamma) \equiv \sum_k |\hat{\phi}(\gamma + k)|^2.$$

Li and I proved the following result which is fundamental to our theory of FMRAs and the applications to noise reduction. A proof appears in [10].

THEOREM 3

Let $\phi \in L^2(\mathbb{R})$ and let V be the closed span of $\{\tau_k \phi : k \in \mathbb{Z}\}$ in $L^2(\mathbb{R})$, i.e., $V \equiv \overline{sp}\{\tau_k \phi\}$. The sequence $\{\tau_k \phi\}$ is a frame for V if and only if there are positive constants A and B such that

$$A \leq \Phi \leq B \quad a.e. \text{ on } \mathbb{T} \backslash N,$$

where $N = \{\gamma \in \mathbb{T} : \Phi(\gamma) = 0\}$. (Note that N is defined only up to sets of measure zero.)

The analogues of Theorem 3 for orthonormal bases ($\Phi = 1$ a.e.) and exact frames ($A \leq \Phi \leq B$ a.e. on $\mathbb{T}$) are elementary to prove.

Just as a multiresolution analysis leads to a subband coding system, e.g., [11], so too does an FMRA lead to a subband coding system, e.g., Figure 18.1.

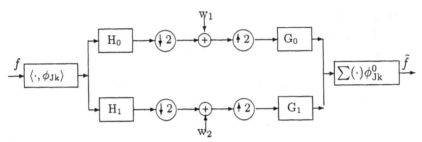

Figure 18.1
A subband processing system associated with an FMRA for ana-
log signals f; w_1 and w_2 model the quantization noise in subbands.

In order to explain Figure 18.1, we note that properties *(ii)* and *(iv)* of Definition 1 give rise to a filter H_0 defined on $\mathbb{T}$. For the case of FMRAs this filter is not necessarily unique. H_1 is then chosen so that the supports of H_0 and H_1 essentially cover the support of Φ on $\mathbb{T}$. By Theorem 3, the support of Φ does not necessarily cover $\mathbb{T}$. This feature allows for signal reconstruction in the presence of broadband noise added to the output from the analysis filters of the coefficient data $\{\langle f, \varphi_{Jk}\rangle\}$ for a given signal $f \in L^2(\mathbb{R})$.

H_0 and H_1 are analysis filters, and the general theory of FMRAs provides a means of constructing synthesis filters G_0, G_1 so that $\tilde{f}$ is f in the case $f \in V_J$, $\varphi^0 = S^{-1}\varphi$, and $w_1 = w_2 = 0$. Verification of this claim is found in [6, 7].

18.5   Noise reduction

Let
$$\hat{\varphi} = \mathbf{1}_{[-1/4,1/4)}$$

be the characteristic function of the interval $[-1/4, 1/4)$. By Theorem 3, $\{\tau_k\varphi\}$ is a frame for the subspace $V_0 \equiv \overline{sp}\{\tau_k\varphi\} \subseteq L^2(\mathbb{R})$. We define V_j by part *(ii)* of Definition 1, and can conclude that $\{V_j\}$ and φ give rise to an FMRA [6, Theorem 6]. We can then calculate that

$$\hat{\varphi}(\gamma) = \frac{1}{\sqrt{2}} H_0\left(\frac{\gamma}{2}\right) \hat{\varphi}\left(\frac{\gamma}{2}\right),$$

for some 1-periodic trigonometric polynomial H_0. In fact, because of our definition of $\hat{\varphi}$, we see that we can choose

$$H_0 = \sqrt{2}\,\mathbf{1}_{[-1/8,1/8)}. \tag{18.1}$$

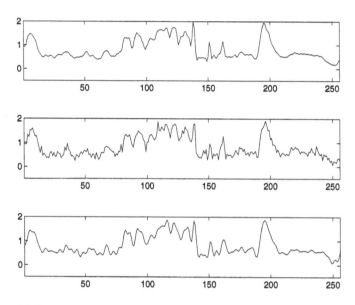

Figure 18.2

Because of our remarks about H_0 and H_1 at the end of Section 18.4, we let

$$H_1 = \sqrt{2}\,\mathbf{1}_{[-1/4,-1/8)} + \sqrt{2}\,\mathbf{1}_{[1/8,1/4)} \tag{18.2}$$

for this example.

The first graph f of Figure 18.2 is a line of 256 MRI data points taken from a square array. We have then added broadband noise n to the output of the analysis filters. The particular noise has mean 0 and variance 0.01. The second graph of Figure 18.2 is a quadrature mirror filter (QMF) subband coding reconstruction of f, contaminated by n at the coding level. The particular QMF is defined by Daubechies' wavelet with four vanishing moments [11]. The third graph of Figure 18.2 is the FMRA reconstruction of f, contaminated by n at the coding level. The particular FMRA is defined by (18.1) and (18.2).

REMARK 1 The FMRA reconstruction in Figure 18.2 is better than the QMF-wavelet reconstruction. This fact is predicted by Proposition 1, since the QMF gives rise to an ONB.

Intuitively, we also know that our FMRA reconstruction method will be better than the QMF-wavelet method since the QMF pair covers the whole frequency band. This means that the QMF-wavelet method will reconstruct all of the frequency content of the available signal, which in this case includes the noise n. On the other hand, since the noise is a

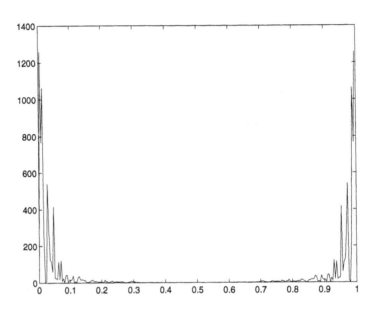

Figure 18.3
This is $|FFTf|$, f **of Figure 18.2, without** dc **component.**

broadband signal and the data f is narrowband (Figure 18.3), our FMRA
method will only reconstruct from the frequency content of a narrowband,
thereby excluding most of the broadband noise. In fact, since $H_0 + H_1$ is
relatively narrowband, our theory assures that the synthesis filters G_0, G_1
will have a similar property [6, 7].   ■

REMARK 2   The filters H_0 and H_1 are ideal filters, and in particular
have infinitely many taps. Even in implementation, for example in dealing
with a $2^9 - FFT$, the impulse responses have 2^9 points. If H_0 and H_1 are
modified into trapezoids, then we still have infinite tap filters, but faster
implementation. The greater speed arises since trapezoids are differences
of triangles, and the impulse responses, even for the DFT, have quadratic
decay. There is a new theory of pseudo-frames, proposed by Shidong Li,
which accomplishes a similar increase in efficiency [18].   ■

Example 1
Many important signals are narrowband, and therefore can be reconstructed
from a noisy (broadband) environment by our FMRA method. For example, spread spectrum calculations are frequently based on narrowband
jamming interference [16, 17]; and the α and θ (along with δ) rhythms of
Section 18.7 have narrow bands.   ▯

18.6   The Laplacian Method and Gaussian Frames

The L^1-*dilation* of a function $f : \mathbb{R}^d \to \mathbb{C}$, with dilation $\lambda > 0$, is the function f_λ defined as $f_\lambda(x) = \lambda^d f(\lambda x)$. If $f \in L^1(\mathbb{R}^d)$ then $\|f_\lambda\|_{L^1(\mathbb{R}^d)} = \|f\|_{L^1(\mathbb{R}^d)}$.

DEFINITION 2   Continuous wavelet transform
Let $\psi : \mathbb{R}^d \to \mathbb{C}$ be the impulse response of the filter $\hat{\psi}$, and let $f : \mathbb{R}^d \to \mathbb{C}$ be a given signal. The wavelet transform $W_\psi f$ of f is the function

$$W_\psi f : \mathbb{R}^d \times (0, \infty) \longrightarrow \mathbb{C}, \quad where \ (x, s) \longmapsto f * \psi_s(x).$$

Example 2
Laplacian of the Gaussian. Let $x \equiv (x_1, \dots, x_d) \in \mathbb{R}^d$, and let

$$g(x) \equiv \frac{1}{\pi^{d/2}} e^{-|x|^2}, \quad |x|^2 = x_1^2 + \cdots + x_d^2,$$

be the *Gaussian* defined on $\mathbb{R}^d$. Generally, by properties of convolution, differentiation, and approximate identities, we have

$$\Delta(h * k) = \Delta h * k = h * \Delta k,$$

and

$$\lim_{s \to \infty} \left(\Delta g_{\sqrt{1/(4s)}} \right) * f = \Delta f, \tag{18.3}$$

where $\Delta = \sum \partial_j^2$ is the Laplacian on R^d.   ▯

Example 3
In computer vision a standard method of feature extraction is to "pass a Laplacian Δ" over a planar image f in $\mathbb{R}^2$ to detect edges, homogeneous areas, and orientation. Digitally, we compute $\Delta_d f \equiv \Delta_d * f$, where Δ_d is the matrix

0	1	0
1	−4	1
0	1	0

Because of (18.3), the image f is often filtered by the Laplacian of the Gaussian, e.g., [15, 19]. Consistent with the above 3×3 matrix "mask", we note that $\int \Delta g(x) \, dx = 0$, cf., [11] for Gaussian wavelet frames. It is easy to see that $\{\tau_n g^{(2)}\}$ is not orthonormal on $\mathbb{R}$; thus, Δg will not lead to orthonormal wavelet bases, but will in fact yield wavelet frames.   ☐

Example 4
The *heat equation* initial value problem is

$$\Delta u(x,t) = \partial_t u(x,t), \quad (x,t) \in \mathbb{R}^d \times (0,\infty),$$

$$u(x,0) = f(x),$$

where $f(x)$ is given initial data. We know that

$$\Delta g_\sigma(x) = \partial_s g_\sigma(x), \tag{18.4}$$

where $\sigma \equiv \sqrt{1/(4s)}$, e.g., (18.12).   ☐

Example 5
Because of (18.4), it is natural to approximate Δg_σ in (18.3) by an approximation of $\partial_s g_\sigma$.   ☐

Using the heat equation and assuming natural hypotheses on the signal f, we obtain the following theorem, whose proof is found in the Appendix.

THEOREM 4
(Passing the Laplacian—a wavelet generalization)
  If $f : \mathbb{R}^d \longrightarrow \mathbb{C}$ is a signal, then

$$\lim_{s \to 0} \partial_s W_{\Delta g} f \left(x, \sqrt{\frac{1}{4s}} \right) = 4\Delta f. \tag{18.5}$$

DEFINITION 3   Spatio-temporal Laplacian
  Let $f(x_1, x_2, t)$ be a time-varying planar image. The spatio-temporal Laplacian *(STL) of f is*

$$STL(f)(x_1, x_2, t) = \Delta f(x_1, x_2, t) \partial_t^2 f(x_1, x_2, t),$$

where Δ is the 2-dimensional Laplacian on the (x_1, x_2)-plane, e.g., [8].

Because of Theorem 4 we define the *generalized spatio-temporal Laplacian* (GSTL) of f as

$$GSTL(f)(x_1, x_2, t, s) = \frac{1}{4}\partial_s W_{\Delta g} f(x_1, x_2, t, \sigma)\partial_t^2 f(x_1, x_2, t), \qquad (18.6)$$

where g and Δ are defined on the (x_1, x_2)-plane, and $W_{\Delta g} f$ is defined on $\mathbb{R}^2 \times \mathbb{R} \times (0, \infty)$. $\mathbb{R}^2$ is the (x_1, x_2)-plane, $\mathbb{R}$ is the time axis, and the computation of $W_{\Delta g} f$ is made for each fixed t, i.e., for a fixed t we write $f(x_1, x_2, t)$ as $f(x_1, x_2)$ so that $W_{\Delta g} f(x_1, x_2, t, \sigma)$ is really $W_{\Delta g} f(x_1, x_2, \sigma)$.

Note that (18.6) is s-dependent, and, because of (18.5), GSTL is STL in the limiting case $s = 0$. Thus, with notation as in part b, and for large m where $\lim_{m \to \infty} s_m = 0$, we have

$$\Delta f(x_1, x_2, t) \approx \frac{1}{4}\left\{ \frac{W_{\Delta g} f(x_1, x_2, t, \sigma_m) - W_{\Delta g} f(x_1, x_2, t, \sigma_{m+1})}{s_m - s_{m+1}} \right\}$$

for each fixed t, where $\sigma_m \equiv \sqrt{1/(4s_m)}$.

For implementation, GSTL(f) has the form

$$GSTL(f)(x_1, x_2, n, m)$$

$$= \frac{1}{4}\left\{ \frac{W_{\Delta g} f\left(x_1, x_2, t_n, \sqrt{\frac{1}{4s_m}}\right) - W_{\Delta g} f\left(x_1, x_2, t_n, \sqrt{\frac{1}{4s_{m+1}}}\right)}{s_m - s_{m+1}} \right\}$$

$$\times \frac{1}{(t_{n+1} - t_n)^2}\left\{ f\left(x_1, x_2, t_{n+1}, \sqrt{1/4s_m}\right) \right.$$

$$\left. -2f\left(x_1, x_2, t_n, \sqrt{1/4s_m}\right) + f\left(x_1, x_2, t_{n-1}, \sqrt{1/4s_m}\right) \right\}$$

18.7 An Interpretation of Spectral ECoG Data

The bioelectric trace at the top of Figure 18.4 is electrocorticogram (ECoG) data which is typical of the type we have been analyzing at The MITRE Corporation, e.g., [3–5]. This analysis is part of the program at The MITRE Corporation devoted to digital signal processing of ECoG and EEG data, and is inspired by the work of Schiff, e.g., [21].

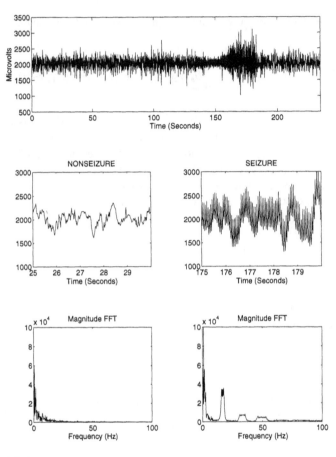

Figure 18.4

The length of the trace is 240 seconds, and it includes (epileptic) seizure activity as well as significant nonseizure activity. Typical of the latter type is activity f_{ns} in the time interval from 25 to 30 seconds, extracted from the original trace; it is reproduced in the left graph on the second line of Figure 18.4. The ordinate is a microvolt measurement of the potential of the electric field at the surface of the brain relative to a referential electrode. The right graph on the second line of Figure 18.4 is activity f_s extracted from seizure data in the original trace. (We admit to begging the question of what precisely is seizure data.) The third line of Figure 18.4 contains absolute values of the fast Fourier transforms (FFTs) of f_{ns} and f_s, respectively. The dc components $\int f_{ns}(t)\,dt$ and $\int f_s(t)\,dt$ have been removed from the FFTs since, as can be seen from line 2, these values are so large as to affect the readability of nonzero-frequency information. The left graph on the third line is indicative of $1/f$ noise, whereas the right graph exhibits some periodic behavior. We shall now look at this latter issue a little more closely.

The right graph on the second line of Figure 18.4 exhibits a high frequency almost periodic signal f "riding-on" a low frequency wave. This latter wave is usually in the θ-band (4–8 Hz) or the α-band (8–13 Hz) of brain activity. The θ-band is the spectral range of drowsiness or light sleep, and the α-band is the spectral range of rhythmic activity in an awake person. The amplitude of the bioelectric trace for the α-band is typically between 5 and 100 microvolts, e.g., [20].

A close look at f, including counting peaks of the trace over the duration of the seizure activity, justifies our labeling of f as an almost periodic signal. In fact, if we write $f = f_1$ at the beginning of the seizure and if we write $f = f_2$ near the end, then the period p_1 of f_1 is less than the period p_2 of f_2.

Assuming each f_j is periodic on $\mathbb{R}$, even though it is only periodic on a portion of the seizure interval, we have the Fourier series representation,

$$Sf_j(t) \equiv \sum_n a_{j,n} e^{2\pi i n t / p_j}; \tag{18.7}$$

and we further assume that $f_j = Sf_j$. Because of (18.7), the Fourier transform of each f_j is

$$\hat{f}_j = \sum_n a_{j,n} \delta_{n/p_j}. \tag{18.8}$$

As such, if we consider the (t, γ)-phase plane, and if we fix a value t_1 at the beginning of the seizure, then because of (18.8) we expect spectral ordinate data (corresponding to t_1) at the points $\{n/p_1 : n \in \mathbb{Z}\}$. A similar remark holds at other parts of the seizure. In particular, at the end of the seizure we expect spectral ordinate data at the points $\{n/p_2 : n \in \mathbb{Z}\}$.

Finally, for a fixed $n > 0$, we expect the graph of this spectral data in the seizure interval to be a decreasing function of t since $1/p_1 > 1/p_2$, cf., (7.2). This time varying spectral activity can be described in terms of elementary chirps, e.g., [2, Section 2.10].

If the previous discussion is too discursive, then experimental data reflected by Figure 18.5 tell the same story pictorially. In fact, the region of the (t, γ)-phase plane determined by the seizure time interval [170, 180] bears out the previous analysis (and handwaving).

The *prediction problem* is an important aspect of ECoG data analysis. This problem is to predict the onset of seizure sufficiently far in advance in order to take beneficial action. Such action may also require the solution of the *localization problem*, e.g., chemical response to *specific local* regions of the brain can temper seizure intensity. Of course, sufficient time prior

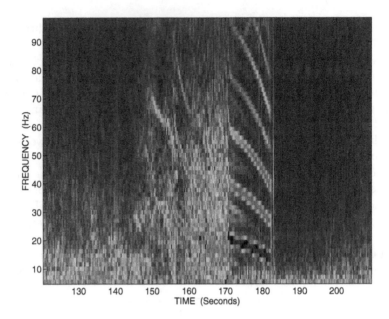

Figure 18.5

to seizure is required to make such a response, whence the interest in prediction. Our interpretation of Figure 18.4 and spectograms such as Figure
18.5 lead to cautious observations about the prediction problem. For example, the definitive chirps in the seizure time interval [170,180] of Figure
18.5 have as precursors the periodic chirp-like activity in the time interval [155,162]. One can even detect some such activity in the time interval
[150,155]. A close look at the trace on the top line of Figure 18.4 shows
that these precursors are imbedded in low amplitude data.

Another tool to deal with issues such as prediction and localization is the
scaleogram, e.g., [4]. This, along with a variety of other signal processing
tools, has been implemented by The MITRE Corporation as an EEG Analysis Workstation. The scaleogram in Figure 18.6 provides information on a
time-scale (t, s)-plane, and comes from the wavelet transform $W_h f$ for the
Haar function h. The wavelet transform was defined in Definition 18.6.1.

Figure 18.6 reflects a discretized version of $W_h f$. For a given scale s,
$W_h f(n, s)$ is the inner product of f with $\tau_n h_s$, where n is the nth sample of
the signal f; h is the Haar function, and, in the discrete case, $h(-1) = 1$,
$h(0) = -1$, and $h = 0$ otherwise. Information near the top of Figure 18.6
comes from inner products of f with translates of h, h_1, ...; information at
the bottom of Figure 18.6 comes from inner products of f with translates
of h_s for s large, e.g., [4].

We close this section by commenting on information garnered from Figure
18.6 that corroborates the evidence for chirps in Figure 18.5.

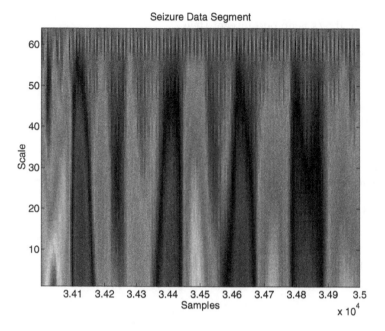

Figure 18.6

From our discussion of (18.7) and (18.8), we see that much of the seizure activity f can be written as a trigonometric polynomial, at least in an interval N of any point $t \in [170, 180]$. The lowermost chirp of Figure 18.5 for the time interval N corresponds to the low frequency component of f on the domain N. This behavior is reflected by the behavior of the bottom part of Figure 18.6, where there are "long" stretches of the same color. In fact, for large s, h_s has a long stretch of s values, followed by an equally long stretch of $-s$ values. Consequently, the inner product of $\tau_n h_s$ with the low frequency component of f will change slowly as n changes whereas, such inner products (for large s) with high frequency components will change values more rapidly. In this latter case, the ideal situation is 2-valued for the Haar dilation h_s since $\langle f, \tau_n h_s \rangle$ is near 0 on the long $\pm s$ stretches and contributes a sign change in going from n to $n + 1$. [4] quantifies this explanation of Figure 18.6.

A relationship, relating time-frequency and timescale analyses, can be observed in the following way. Consider the continuous wavelet transform $W_h f$ of Definition 6.1 for $f(t) = \sin 2\pi(t\gamma + \theta)$ and the ± 1 Haar function centered at 0 and supported by $[-1, 1]$. Then

$$W_h f(x, s) = \frac{2s}{\pi\gamma} \sin^2 \frac{\pi\gamma}{2s} \cos 2\pi(x\gamma + \theta).$$

As such, if γ/s is an odd integer then

$$W_h f(x, s) = \frac{2}{\pi(2k+1)} \cos 2\pi(x\gamma + \theta).$$

This is the simplest example of our ongoing work relating time-frequency and timescale methods.

18.8   Appendix

The following results are elementary, but they do establish the relationships between Laplacian masking techniques and the wavelet transform that was the main assertion of Section 18.6.

Let $x = (x_1, \ldots, x_d) \in \mathbb{R}^d$ and let

$$g(x) = \frac{1}{\pi^{d/2}} e^{-|x|^2}, \quad |x|^2 = x_1^2 + \cdots + x_d^2,$$

be the Gaussian defined on $\mathbb{R}^d$. Thus, $\int g(x)\, dx = 1$, e.g., [2, Chapter 1].

THEOREM 5
Let $h, k : (0, \infty) \to (0, \infty)$ be differentiable functions, and define

$$G(x, s) = h(s)g(k(s)x_1, \ldots, k(s)x_d)$$

for all $x \in \mathbb{R}^d$ and $s > 0$. If

$$\forall s > 0, \quad k'(s) = -2k(s)^3 \quad and \quad h'(s) = -2h(s)k(s)^2 \qquad (18.9)$$

then

$$\forall x \in \mathbb{R}^d \quad and \quad \forall s > 0, \quad \Delta G(x, s) = \partial_s G(x, s). \qquad (18.10)$$

PROOF   We calculate

$$\Delta G(x, s) = h(s) \sum_j \partial_j^2 g(k(s)x_1, \ldots, k(s)x_d)$$

$$= -\frac{2h(s)k(s)^2}{\pi^{d/2}} \sum_j \partial_j \left(x_j e^{-|k(s)x|^2} \right)$$

$$= -\frac{2h(s)k(s)^2}{\pi^{d/2}} e^{-|k(s)x|^2} \left[d - 2k(s)^2|x|^2 \right].$$

Also,

$$\partial_s G(x,s) = \frac{1}{\pi^{d/2}} e^{-|k(s)x|^2} \left[h'(s) - 2h(s)k(s)k'(s)|x|^2 \right]. \qquad (18.11)$$

Substituting (18.9) into (18.11) gives (18.10). ∎

THEOREM 6
If $C > 0$ and

$$G(x,s) = Cs^{-d/2} g \left(\frac{x_1}{2s^{1/2}}, \cdots, \frac{x_d}{2s^{1/2}} \right),$$

for all $x \in \mathbb{R}^d$ and $s > 0$ then

$$\forall x \in \mathbb{R}^d \quad and \quad \forall s > 0, \quad \Delta G(x,s) = \partial_s G(x,s).$$

PROOF   Let $h(s) = s^{-d/2}$ and let $k(s) = \frac{1}{2}s^{-1/2}$. Then (18.9) is satisfied and the result is obtained. ∎

As a corollary we have

$$\Delta g_\sigma(x) = \partial_s g_\sigma(x), \quad (x,s) \in \mathbb{R}^d \times (0,\infty). \qquad (18.12)$$

THEOREM 7
Let $f : \mathbb{R}^d \to \mathbb{C}$ have the property that $\Delta^2 f$ exists on $\mathbb{R}^d$ and $\Delta f, \Delta^2 f \in L^1(\mathbb{R}^d)$. Then

$$\lim_{s \to 0} \partial_s W_{\Delta g} f(x,\sigma) = 4\Delta f(x). \qquad (18.13)$$

PROOF   We calculate

$$W_{\Delta g} f(x,\sigma) = \sigma^d \int f(x-t)\Delta g(\sigma t)dt$$

$$= \int \Delta g(u)f(x - \sqrt{4s}u)du$$

$$= 4s(g_\sigma * \Delta f)(x).$$

Thus,

$$\partial_s W_{\Delta g} f(x, \sigma) = 4(g_\sigma * \Delta f)(x) + 4s\partial_s(g_\sigma * \Delta f)(x). \qquad (18.14)$$

By the heat equation (18.12), the second term on the right side of (18.14) is

$$4s(g_\sigma * \Delta^2 f)(x). \qquad (18.15)$$

Since $\{g_\sigma\}$ is an L^1-approximate identity (as $s \to 0$), e.g., [2, Chapter 1], (18.14) and (18.15) combine to give (18.13). The convergence in (18.13) is in L^1-norm as well as in other convergence criteria depending on the behavior of f. ∎

Clearly, the "proof" of Theorem 7 requires that f and its partial derivatives are not allowed to increase too rapidly at infinity.

References

[1] J. Benedetto, Frame decomposition, sampling, and uncertainty principle inequalities, Chapter 7 of *Wavelets: Mathematics and Applications*, J. Benedetto and M. Frazier, editors, CRC Press, Boca Raton, FL, 1994.

[2] J. Benedetto, *Harmonic Analysis and Applications*, CRC Press, Boca Raton, FL, 1996.

[3] G. Benke, M. Bozek-Kuzmicki, D. Colella, G. Jacyna, and J. Benedetto, Wavelet-based analysis of EEG signals for detection and localization of epileptic seizures, *SPIE 1995*, Orlando.

[4] J. Benedetto and D. Colella, Wavelet analysis of spectrogram seizure chirps, *SPIE 1995*, San Diego.

[5] M. Bozek-Kuzmicki, D. Colella, and G. Jacyna, Feature-based epileptic seizure detection and prediction from ECoG recordings, *IEEE-SP Int. Symp. Time-Frequency and Time-Scale Analysis*, Philadelphia, 1994.

[6] J. Benedetto and S. Li, Multiresolution analysis frames with applications, *IEEE-ICASSP*, Minneapolis, III(1993), 304–307.

[7] J. Benedetto and S. Li, Narrow band frame multiresolution analysis with perfect reconstruction, *IEEE-SP Int. Symp. Time-Frequency and Time-Scale Analysis*, Philadelphia, 1994.

[8] A. Barreto, J. Principe, and S. Reid, STL: A spatio-temporal characterization of focal interictal events, *Brain Topography*, **5** (1993), 215–228.

[9] J. Benedetto and A. Teolis, A wavelet auditory model and data compression, *Appl. Comp. Harmonic Analysis*, **1** (1993), 3–28.

[10] J. Benedetto and D. Walnut, Gabor frames for L^2 and related spaces, Chapter 3 of *Wavelets: Mathematics and Applications*, J. Benedetto and M. Frazier, editors, CRC Press, Boca Raton, FL, 1994.

[11] I. Daubechies, *Ten Lectures on Wavelets*, CBMS-NSF Reg. Conf. Ser. Appl. Math SIAM, **61**, 1992.

[12] I. Daubechies, A. Grossmann, and Y. Meyer, Painless nonorthogonal expansions, *J. Math. Physics*, **27** (1986), 1271–1283.

[13] R. J. Duffin and A. C. Schaeffer, A class of nonharmonic Fourier series, *Trans. Amer. Math. Soc.*, **72**:341–366, 1952.

[14] C. Heil and D. Walnut, Continuous and discrete wavelet transforms, *SIAM Rev.*, **31** (1989), 628–666.

[15] R. Hummel and R. Moniot, Reconstructions from zero crossings in scale space, *IEEE Trans. ASSP*, **37** (1989), 2111–2130.

[16] R. Iltis and L. Milstein, Performance analysis of narrow-band interference rejection techniques in DS spread spectrum systems, *IEEE Trans. Commun.*, **32** (1984), 1169–1177.

[17] J. Ketchum and J. Proakis, Adaptive algorithms for estimating and suppressing narrowband interference in PN spread spectrum systems, *IEEE Trans. Commun.*, **30** (1982), 913–923.

[18] S. Li, General frame decompositions, pseudo-duals and its application to Weyl-Heisenberg frames, *Numerical Functional Analysis and Optimization*, to appear.

[19] D. Marr, *Vision*, W. H. Freeman, San Francisco, 1982.

[20] P. Nunez, *Electric Fields of the Brain: The Neurophysics of EEG*, Oxford University Press, 1981.

[21] S. J. Schiff and J. Milton, Wavelet transforms for electroencephalographic spike and seizure detection, *SPIE*, 1993.

[22] R. M. Young, *An Introduction to Nonharmonic Fourier Series*, Academic Press, New York, 1980.

19

Diagnosis of Coronary Artery Disease Using Wavelet-Based Neural Networks

Metin Akay

Biomedical Engineering Department, Rutgers University, Piscataway, New Jersey

Abstract   This chapter examines the utility of wavelet-based neural networks for detecting coronary artery disease noninvasively by using the clinical examination variables and extracting useful information from the diastolic heart sounds associated with coronary occlusions.

It has been widely reported that coronary stenoses produce sounds due to the turbulent blood flow in these vessels. These complex and highly attenuated signals taken from recordings made in both soundproof and noisy rooms were detected and analyzed to provide feature set based on extrema representation of the fast wavelet transform coefficients. In addition, some physical exam variables such as sex, age, body weight, smoking condition, diastolic pressure, systolic pressure, and derivation from them were included in the feature vector. This feature vector was used as the input pattern to the neural network.

19.1   Introduction

Coronary artery disease (CAD) is one of the leading causes of death in the world, with one third of all deaths attributed to this disease [1, 15, 16].

For this reason, early detection of coronary artery disease is a most important medical research area. Several methods exist for the diagnosis of coronary artery disease. Noninvasive methods include the physical exam and history, ECG techniques (electrocardiograms, exercise testing, vector-cardiograms, apex cardiogram), ultrasounds (echocardiography), imaging (roentgenograms, tomography, nuclear magnetic resonance). These methods appear to be moderately useful noninvasive methods to detect CAD [1, 15, 16, 18, 19]. Another approach is the thalium test. In the thalium test, thalium-201, which is a radio-pharmaceutical substance with biological properties similar to potassium, is used to detect myocardial ischemia in patients with CAD. When given invasively, its myocardial distribution is proportional to myocardial blood flow. Therefore, low blood flow regions accumulate less thalium and appear as cold spots on the image obtained from a camera set over the precordium [18]. Although the sensitivity of the thailum test is 83%, and its specificity is 90%, it is costly and time-consuming [18].

As far as invasive techniques are concerned, the most reliable way to diagnose CAD is with cardiac catherization (cath) [1–3]. In this method, a catheter is inserted into an artery (usually brachial or femoral) and advanced to the heart. Once in the heart, dye can be released to observe the coronary arteries. Although direct assessment of a coronary occlusion is conclusive using cardiac catheterization, this method is expensive, painful, time-consuming, and has an element of risk (the mortality rates range from 0.2%–7%) [1]. For these reasons, a reliable noninvasive method is required for **early detection of coronary artery disease**.

In 1967 it was first reported that coronary stenosis can cause a diastolic murmur [21]. Later two patients were reported with diastolic murmurs associated with a severe, localized narrowing of the left anterior descending (LAD) coronary artery due to coronary stenosis [21]. Three cases with diastolic murmurs associated with coronary artery disease (CAD) were later reported. For these cases, stenosis at the site of the murmur was proven by catheterization, and the diastolic murmur was modified after surgery [22].

Studies involving turbulent blood flow have been carried out in many components of the cardiovascular system and it has been widely reported that turbulence produced by stenoses produce sounds due to the vibration of the surrounding structures [1–3]. These sounds have been detected and analyzed, and results generally showed that the high frequency energy increased when the degree of stenosis was increased [3]. However, for severe obstructions, (above 95% occlusion), sounds may not be produced due to very low blood flow. At the lower end, occlusions as small as 25% narrowing have been detected [3] and used as a noninvasive measure to assess arterial narrowing in vessels of the neck, thorax, and abdomen [3]. The auditory component associated with coronary stenosis is similar to that found in partially occluded carotid arteries, but is much attenuated by the intervening tissue. It is also masked by the comparatively loud valve sounds. It is during diastole that coronary blood flow is maximum and the sounds associated with turbulent blood flow through partially occluded coronary arteries would be loudest. These can be eliminated by isolating diastolic portions of the acoustic signal using a time window synchronized with the cardiac cycle [2].

The principal objective of this study is to use the combination of the additional signal components found in heart sounds of patients with coronary artery disease and the physical exam variables to improve the diagnostic accuracy of noninvasive detection of coronary artery disease.

These added components in hearts sounds of patients with CAD form the basis of our approach to noninvasive detection of coronary artery disease. Since the application of parametric modeling methods to signal identification problems results in a better estimation of spectral features, particularly for low signal-to-noise ratios (SNR), such model-based methods were employed to analyze the recordings of diastolic heart sounds and to detect features associated with coronary stenosis [3–7]. From the many model-based methods, the adaptive AR method was chosen to represent the diastolic signal source, since it does not require prior knowledge of the signal characteristics and it can track changes in signal characteristics. Initial analyses were carried out on 15 patients (10 abnormal, 5 normal patients) using two fast adaptive AR methods, the recursive least square lattice (RLSL) and the gradient adaptive lattice (GAL) method [3]. Spectra obtained from individual diastolic cycles showed some variation. To obtain representative frequency information, averages were calculated from an ensemble of 20–30 individual diastolic spectra. Results showed that the percentage of spectral power above 300 Hz differed between normal and diseased patients with the energy over 400 Hz being greater in diseased patients [3]. The poles of the AR model were also calculated and used as a discriminant criterion. In all subjects, the second and usually the third poles were farther from the unit circle in normal patients than in diseased patients [3].

Since the diastolic sound components associated with occlusive coronary stenosis contain narrow frequency bands, Eigenvector methods were also applied to six angioplasty patients [4]. In that application diastolic heart sounds were represented as a number of sinusoids along with background noise. Frequency peaks were first identified; then the power level of each peak was calculated. The relative power of the second (or in some patients, the third) peak was found to change in a consistent manner when the coronary stenosis was modified by angioplastic surgery [4].

Both applications of advanced signal processing techniques mentioned above demonstrated good performance in identifying diastolic heart sounds associated with coronary occlusion.

After the preliminary normal/abnormal and angioplasty studies, modified Yule-Walker (MYW) AR and ARMA methods were employed, using data obtained from angioplasty patients before and after angioplasty, and from the normal and diseased patients. These studies were carried out using **a blind protocol**. Both the AR and ARMA methods showed similar performance in differentiating abnormal from normal patients, and pre-angioplasty from post-angioplasty patients [3, 4].

The principal objective of the **angioplasty study** was to investigate the fundamental assumptions of the acoustical approach in the detection of **coronary artery disease**. The changes in decision parameters obtained from the angioplasty patients before and after angioplasty proved the basic acoustic concept, that coronary stenoses have an auditory correlate.

Details of the other evaluations using recordings taken in **a soundproof and patient's bedside (noisy room)** room have been described elsewhere [5–7]. Results from these studies showed that the percentage of spectral power above 300 Hz is associated with coronary artery disease. Again, in almost all subjects, it was found that the second and usually the third poles of normal patients and many post-angioplasty patients were farther from the unit circle than those of CAD patients [5–7].

In this study, the neural network was applied to noninvasive detection of coronary artery disease, using the extrema points of the detail signals obtained with the fast wavelet transform method applied to isolated diastolic heart sounds associated with coronary artery disease, as well as the physical exam variables of the patients in order to fully capture all relevant information related to the disease state of the patients, relying on their nonlinear and multilayered architecture.

19.2   Method

19.2.1   Fast Wavelet Transform

Wavelet transforms provide an important new tool in signal analysis [8–10]. Most information of a biomedical signal is carried by irregular structures and transient phenomena. The Fourier transform is global and provides a description of the overall regularity of signals. However, it may not be appropriate for finding the location and the spatial distribution of singularities [10]. The local maxima of the wavelet transform modulus represent the locations of irregular structures [10]. In this study, the fast wavelet transform proposed by Mallat and Zhong [10] was used in the analysis of diastolic heart sounds.

As described elsewhere [10], the integral of a smoothing function, $\phi(t)$, is equal to 1 and converges to 0 at infinity. The smoothing function can be assumed to be a Gaussian. It can be differentiable, where $\psi(t)$ is the first-order derivative of $\phi(t)$, to obtain the mother wavelet $\phi(t)$:

$$\psi(t) = \frac{d\phi(t)}{dt} \tag{19.1}$$

In this study, we used the redundant discrete wavelet transform in which the scales $a_j = 2^j$, $j \geq 0$ and the translations $b_k = k$, $k \in Z$ have been used (see Chapter 1.2 and [10], and Chapter 2).

Note that the constants λ_i compensate for the discretization errors. The complexity of this discrete wavelet transform is $O(N \log(N))$ [10].

19.2.2 Fuzzy Min-Max Neural Networks

Recent developments in the field of artificial neural networks have made them a powerful tool to analyze signals [11–13]. The application of artificial neural networks (ANNs) has opened a new area for solving problems that are ill-posed by other signal-processing techniques. A number of ANN algorithms and their applications have been widely reported [11, 12]. A multilayer perceptron can be trained by adjusting the connection weights and changing the unit threshold values. These networks have been widely trained using a **backpropagation** algorithm which has proven to be useful in training these networks.

Recently there has been a great interest in the combination of neural networks and fuzzy systems, by using neural network nodes as fuzzy sets and using fuzzy set operations during learning to replace the crisp decision boundaries of the perceptron neural network by the fuzzy hyperplane decision boundaries of the fuzzy neural networks [13]. Among the many fuzzy neural network models, **fuzzy min-max neural networks** proposed by Simpson will be summarized and used in this chapter [13]. Fuzzy min-max neural networks are constructed using hyperbox fuzzy sets. A hyperbox determines a region of n-dimensional pattern space that has patterns with full class membership. Each hyperbox is defined by its min and max points. A hyperbox membership function is determined by these min-max points. The combination of these hyperbox membership functions constitutes a fuzzy set. Learning in the fuzzy min-max classification neural network can be done by placing and adjusting hyperboxes in the pattern space [13].

Figure 19.1 shows the three-layer neural network that implements the fuzzy min-max neural network used here. Note that the input layer has n processing elements. The input nodes are connected to the second layer consisting of the m hyperbox fuzzy set nodes by two sets of connections— the min and max point vectors. The connections between the hyperbox and the output layers are binary. Finally, each node in the output layer represents a pattern class.

Fuzzy min-max learning is a series of an extension and contraction process. It works by finding a hyperbox for the same class that can expand (if necessary) to include the input. If a hyperbox that meets the expansion criteria is not included, a new hyperbox is included and added to the neural network. As described elsewhere, the fuzzy min-max classification learning algorithm can be summarized as follows [13]:

1. Expansion: Find the hyperbox that can be expanded and expand it. Otherwise, add a new hyperbox for that class.

2. Contraction: Find if any overlap exists between hyperboxes from different classes. If any overlap exists between hyperboxes that represent different classes, eliminate the overlap by minimally adjusting the hyperboxes.

Details of the fuzzy min-max neural networks have been described elsewhere [13].

19.2.3   Patient Analysis

The object of this study was to evaluate an improved method for the acoustical detection of diastolic heart sounds associated with the diagnosis of coronary artery disease. The heart sound study was carried out in a blind fashion without knowledge of whether a given recording was made before or after angioplastic surgery. Diastolic heart sounds were recorded in a soundproof room at the patient's bedside. Patients were selected from those undergoing catherization and/or angioplasty at the Cardiodynamics Laboratory of Robert Wood Johnson University Hospital. Diastolic heart sounds were recorded from the 4th intercostal space on the chest of patients using a specially designed high sensitivity accelerometer [23] in conjunction with a portable digital pulse code modulation (PCM) data recorder (TEAC, RD-11OT). The output of a finger plethysmograph was also recorded as a timing reference to aid in locating the diastolic period. Next, the data were loaded from the digital tape to a computer (HP 9000) using standard data acquisition system (3852A, HP). These sounds were recorded while the patients held their breath and were supine [2, 3].

Before analysis, the data quality was checked. Those records which contain artifacts such as stomach sounds, respiratory noise, unusual background noise, or tape dropouts were eliminated using an automated system. The data were normalized by dividing the overall system gain. For each patient, 10 cardiac cycles were digitized (sampling frequency, $f_s = 4$ kHz). As detailed elsewhere [2, 3] the diastolic heart sounds were passed through an anti-aliasing analog filter set for a cutoff frequency of 1200 Hz and a highpass digital filter set for a cutoff frequency of 200 Hz.

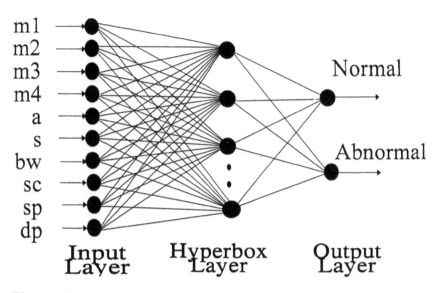

Figure 19.1
The fuzzy min-max neural network classifier: m1, m2, m3, and
m4 represent the first four moments of the extrema of the wavelet
transform coefficients a, s, bw, sc, sp and dp represent the age,
sex, body weight, smoking condition, systolic, and diastolic blood
pressure, respectively.

19.3   Results

As a first step, the extrema of the fast wavelet transform coefficients of
diastolic heart sounds were calculated for a period. Then, the first four
moments were averaged over 10 cardiac cycles for each patient.

19.3.1   Feature Extraction

For each patient, the feature pattern consists of 10 parameters. Of these
parameters, four were obtained from the analysis of the diastolic heart
sounds associated with CAD. The parameters obtained from the diastolic
heart sounds were the first four moments of the extrema of the detail signal at the third scale. The detail signal at the third scale was chosen since
this band was the most discriminative in separating normals from abnormal
subjects in our previous studies. Then, the first four moments were averaged over ten cardiac cycles for each patient. Figures 19.2a and b show the
diastolic heart sounds for a typical disease subject and the corresponding
extrema of four wavelet bands. Figures 19.3a and b show similar features
for a normal subject. Note that for diagnosis we only used the second and

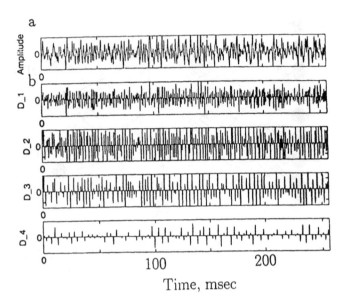

Figure 19.2
**The diastolic heart sounds for a typical disease subject (a) and
the corresponding extrema of four wavelet bands (b).**

third wavelet bands. These four parameters with the six parameters taken
from clinical examination records were used, providing a 10-point (for each
recording) feature vector as the input to the neural networks. Note that
each of the parameters was normalized with respect to the highest value of
this parameter in the data base.

The remaining six parameters were taken from physical exam records.
The physical exam parameters of the feature pattern were sex (s), age
(a), systolic blood pressure (sp), diastolic blood pressure (dp), smoking
habit (sc), and body weight (bw). These parameters are significant to the
diagnosis of coronary artery disease [1, 14–17].

The parameters a, dp, bw, and sp were coded as analog values between
0 and 1. The remaining physical exam parameters s, and smoking habit sc
were coded in binary manner where 1 represents a male as well as smoker
since the risk factor for a man and a smoker is much higher than that of a
woman and a nonsmoker.

The feature pattern, all parameters inclusive, was utilized as the input
to the neural network. There were 30 patients randomly selected for use
as training cases for the neural network. Of these 15 were normal, and 15
were abnormal patients. A three-layer **fuzzy min-max** network was used.
The network was run on a Sun system. Several configurations were tested.

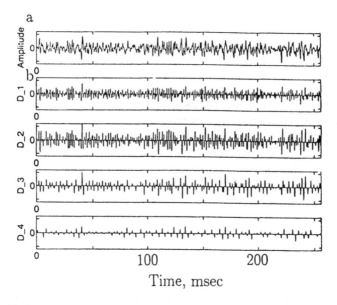

Figure 19.3
The diastolic heart sounds for a typical normal subject (a) and
the corresponding extrema of four wavelet bands (b).

19.3.2 Network Output Representation

The testing of the network was achieved by using the hyperbox derived
in the training test and applying the new patterns to the network to which
it has not been exposed. The network was tested on the 112 patients. Of
the 112 patient test cases, 30 were selected for use as training cases for the
neural networks. Of these, 15 were normal and 15 were abnormal subjects.
Another 55 abnormal and 27 normal subjects were used as testing cases
for the neural network. All of these patients, except for 5 pseudo-normals
(which were not cath-proven) were either cath-proven normal or abnormal
patients. All training was done in a supervised fashion, which means that
the inputs and desired outputs were known during the training process.

Results showed that sensitivity and specificity of the NNs using only
moments were 78% and 89%, respectively. Therefore, 43 of 55 abnormal and
24 of 27 normal cases were correctly diagnosed. Sensitivity and specificity of
the NNs using only physical examination parameters were 73% and 79%,
respectively. Therefore, 40 out of 55 abnormal and 21 out of 27 normal
subjects were correctly identified. Finally, sensitivity and specificity of the
NNs using the combination of the physical examination parameters and
the moments of the third wavelet bands of diastolic heart sounds were 85%
and 89%, respectively. Therefore, 47 out of 55 abnormal and 24 out of 27
normal subjects were correctly identified.

19.4   Conclusion

In this study, neural networks were applied to the combination of the physical exam variables and the moments of the extrema of the detail signals obtained with the redundant discrete wavelet transform method applied to the diastolic heart sounds associated with coronary artery disease. The network had a detection rate 85.5% and a false alarm rate of 11.2% (1-*specificity*), whereas the previous study, using only the PSD characteristics of the AR method, showed a detection rate 76% and a false alarm of 16% [3].

These results compare quite favorably with other noninvasive methods for detecting CAD, since our approach is very quick and inexpensive. For example, the sensitivity of the Cardiointegram (CIG) technique developed by Teichholtz [19] was found to be 73%, with a specificity of 78%. This approach was considered to be a moderately useful noninvasive method to detect CAD. However, the diagnostic capability of this approach should be compared with other noninvasive methods for detecting CAD using the same data base.

This new approach described above is based on the diastolic heart sound measurements associated with turbulence due to stenoses and the physical exam variables such as age, sex, diastolic and systolic blood pressures, and weight.

Results showed that neural networks were potentially capable of differentiating normal patients from abnormal patients.

In order to further explore the extraction of the useful information regarding the complex diastolic heart sounds produced by single and multi-lesions, the analysis of the diastolic heart sounds will be approached using **fuzzy min-max neural networks**.

19.5   Acknowledgment

The author wishes to thank Drs. W. Welkowitz, J. L. Semmlow, and J. Kostis for providing data and technical assistance, and J. Redling, D. Shen, A. Smith, and V. Padmanabhan for collecting and preprocessing the data used in this study. This work was supported by a grant from Colin Medical Instrument Corporation. The author can be reached at the Biomedical Engineering Department, Rutgers University, Piscataway, NJ 08855, e-mail: akay@gandalf.rutgers.edu.

References

[1] M. A. Krupp. *Current Medical Diagnosis and Treatment*, Lange Medical Publications, Los Altos, CA, 1982, 193–210.

[2] J. L. Semmlow, W. Welkowitz, J. Kostis, and J. M. Mackenzie. Coronary artery disease-correlates between diastolic auditory characteristic and coronary artery stenoses, *IEEE Trans. Biomed. Eng.*, 30:136–139, 1983.

[3] M. Akay, J. L. Semmlow, W. Welkowitz, M. Bauer, and J. Kostis. Detection of coronary occlusions using AR modelling of diastolic heart sounds, *IEEE Trans. Biomed. Eng.*, 37:366–373, 1990.

[4] M. Akay, J. L. Semmlow, W. Welkowitz, M. Bauer, and J. Kostis. Noninvasive detection of coronary occlusions using Eigenvector methods before and after angioplasty, *IEEE Trans. Biomed. Eng.*, 37: 1095–1104,1990.

[5] M. Akay. Noninvasive diagnosis of coronary artery disease using a neural network algorithm, *Biol. Cybernetics*, 67:361–367, 1992.

[6] M. Akay, W. Welkowitz. Acoustical detection of coronary artery disease using neural networks, *J. Biomed. Eng.*, 15:469–473, 1993.

[7] Y. M. Akay, M. Akay, W. Welkowitz , J. L. Semmlow, and J. Kostis. A comparative study of advanced signal processing techniques for detection of coronary artery disease, *IEEE Trans. BME*, 40:571–578, 1993.

[8] A. Grossman and J. Morlet. Decomposition of Haar functions into square integrable wavelets of constant shape, *SIAM. J. Math.*, 15, 723–736.

[9] I. Daubechies. Orthonormal bases of compactly supported wavelets, *Commun. Pure Appl. Math.*, 909–996, 1988.

[10] S. G. Mallat and S. Zhong, Characterization of signals from multiscale edges. *IEEE Trans. PAMI*, 10:710–732, 1992.

[11] R. Lipmann. Introduction to computing with Neural Nets, *IEEE ASSP Mag.*, 4:2,4–22, 1988.

[12] D. Rumelhart, G. E. Hunton, and R. J. Williams. Learning inter-
      nal representations by error propagation. In *Parallel Distributed Pro-
      cessing; Explorations in the Microstructure of Cognition*, Vol. I, MIT
      Press, Cambridge, MA, 1986, 318–362.

[13] P. K. Simpson. Fuzzy Min-Max Neural Networks—Part 1: Classifica-
      tion, 3:776–786, 1992.

[14] A. Blinowska, G. Chatellier, J. Bernier, and M. Larvil. Bayesian statis-
      tics as applied to hypertension diagnosis, *IEEE Trans. BME*, 38, 699–
      706, 1991.

[15] W. F. Ganong. *Review of Medical Physiology*, Lange Medical Publi-
      cations, Los Altos, CA, 485–488, 1991.

[16] A. C. Guyton. *Textbook of Medical Physiology*, W. B. Saunders Com-
      pany, Philadelphia, 1987.

[17] H. C. Sox, M. A. Blatt, M. C. Higgins, and K. I. Marton. *Medical
      Decision Making*, Butterworth, London, 1988.

[18] J. Stolzenberg. Stress-thalium-201 scanning in CAD, *Med. Clin. North
      Am.*, 64(2):149–162, 1980.

[19] L. E. Teichholtz. Cardiointegram detection CAD using in normal rest-
      ing electrocardiograms, *J. Am. Coll. Cardio.*, 3, 598, 1984.

[20] J. Chen, J. Vandewalle, W. Sansen, G. Vantrappen, and J. Janssens.
      Adaptive method for cancellation of respiratory artifact in electrogas-
      tic measurements, *Med. Biol. Eng. Comp.*, 27, 57–63, 1989.

[21] W. Dock and S. Zoneraich. A diastolic murmur arising in a stenosed
      coronary artery, *Am. J. Med.*, 42, 617, 1967.

[22] J. F. Sangster et al. Diastolic murmur of coronary artery stenosis, *Br.
      Heart J.*, 35, 840–844, 1973.

[23] V. Padmanabhan, R. Fisher, J. L. Semmlow, W. Welkowitz, and J.
      Kostis. High sensitivity PCG transducer for extended frequency ap-
      plications, *Proc. IEEE Frontiers in Med.*, Seattle, 57–59, 1989.

Part IV

Wavelets and Mathematical Models in Biology

20

A Nonlinear Squeezing of the
Continuous Wavelet
Transform Based on Auditory
Nerve Models

Ingrid Daubechies[1] and Stéphane Maes[2]

[1] *Program in Applied and Computational Mathematics and Department of Mathematics, Princeton University, Princeton, NJ*
[2] *IBM T. J. Watson Research Center, Human Language Technologies, Acoustic Processing Department, Yorktown Heights, NY*

20.1 Introduction

The approach presented in this chapter resulted from a concrete problem in speaker identification. Our goal was to incorporate the wavelet transform and auditory nerve-based models into a tool that could be used for speaker identification (among other applications), in the hope that the results would be more robust to noise than the standard methods.

This chapter is organized as follows. Sections 20.2 to 20.4 present background material, explaining, respectively, (1) how the (continuous) wavelet transform comes up "naturally" in our auditory system; (2) a heuristic approach (the ensemble interval histogram of O. Ghitza [1]) based on auditory nerve models, which eliminates much of the redundancy in the first-stage transform; and (3) the modulation model, valid for large portions of (voiced) speech, and which is used for speaker identification.[1] In Section 20.5 we put all this background material to use in our own synthesis, an approach that we call "squeezing" the wavelet transform; with an extra refinement this becomes "synchrosqueezing." The main idea is that the wavelet transform itself has "smeared" out different harmonic components, and that we need to "refocus" the resulting time-frequency or timescale picture. How this is done is explained in Section 20.5. Section 20.6 deals with various implementation issues, which are touched upon rather than explained in detail; for details, we refer to the various articles [2–6]. Finally, Section 20.7 shows some results: the "untreated" wavelet transform of a speech segment, its squeezed and synchrosqueezed versions, and the extraction of the parameters used for speaker identification. We conclude with some pointers to and comparisons with similar work in the literature, and with sketching possible future directions.

20.2   The Wavelet Transform as an Approach to Cochlear Filtering

When a sound wave hits our eardrum, the oscillations are transmitted to the basilar membrane in the cochlea. The cochlea is rolled up like a spiral; imagine unrolling it (and with it the basilar membrane), and putting an axis y onto it, so that points on the basilar membrane are labeled by their distance to one end. (For simplicity, we use a one-dimensional model, neglecting any influence of the transverse direction on the membrane, or its thickness.) If a pure tone, i.e., an excitation of the form $e^{i\omega t}$ (or its real part) hits the eardrum, then the response at the level of the basilar membrane, as observed experimentally or computed via detailed models, is in first approximation given by $e^{i\omega t} F_\omega(y)$ — a temporal oscillation with the same frequency as the input, but with an amplitude localized within a specific region in y by the function $F_\omega(y)$. In a first approximation, the dependence of F_ω on ω can be modeled by a logarithmic shift: $F_\omega(y) = F(y - \log \omega)$. (Strictly speaking, this model is only good for frequencies above say, 500 Hz; for low frequencies, the dependence of F_ω on ω is approximately linear.)

---

[1]Some of our descriptions of the auditory system may well look naïve and distorted to the more informed reader. They are in no way meant as an accurate description of what we realize is a very complex system. Rather, they are snapshots that motivated our mathematical construction further on, and they should be taken only as such.

The response to a more complicated $f(t)$ can then be computed as follows:

$$f(t) = \frac{1}{2\pi} \int_{-\infty}^{\infty} \hat{f}(\omega) e^{i\omega t} \, d\omega$$

$$\implies \quad \text{response } B(t, y) = \frac{1}{2\pi} \int_{-\infty}^{\infty} \hat{f}(\omega) e^{i\omega t} F(y - \log \omega) \, d\omega.$$

(Note that we are assuming linearity here — a superposition of inputs leading to the same superposition of the respective responses. This is again only a first approximation; richer and more realistic auditory models contain significant nonlinearities [7].) If we relabel the axis along the basilar membrane by defining $y := -\log a$ with $a > 0$ and $B'(t, a) = B(t, -\log a)$, and if we moreover define a function G by putting $F(x) =: \hat{G}(e^{-x})$, then the response can be rewritten as

$$B'(t, a) = \frac{1}{2\pi} \int_{-\infty}^{\infty} \int_{-\infty}^{\infty} f(t') e^{i\omega(t-t')} \hat{G}(a\omega) \, dt' \, d\omega \qquad (20.1)$$

$$= \int_{-\infty}^{\infty} f(t') \frac{1}{a} G\left(\frac{t - t'}{a}\right) \, dt'.$$

By taking $\psi(t) := G(-t)$, we find that $B'(t, a) = |a|^{-\frac{1}{2}} (W_\psi f)(a, t)$, where W_ψ is the continuous wavelet transform as defined by formula (1.23) in Chapter 1. In this sense, the cochlea can be seen as a "natural" wavelet transformer; all this is of course a direct consequence (and nothing but a reformulation) of the logarithmic dependence on ω of F_ω.

20.3   A Model for the Information Compression after the Cochlear Filters

The cochlear filtering, or the continuous wavelet transform that approximates it, transforms the one-dimensional signal $f(t)$ into a two-dimensional quantity. If we were to sample this two-dimensional transform like an image, then we would end up with an enormous number of data, far more than can in fact be handled by the auditory nerve. Some compression therefore has to take place immediately. The ensemble interval histogram (EIH) method of Oded Ghitza [1] gives such a compression, inspired by auditory nerve models. We describe it here in a nutshell, with its motivation.

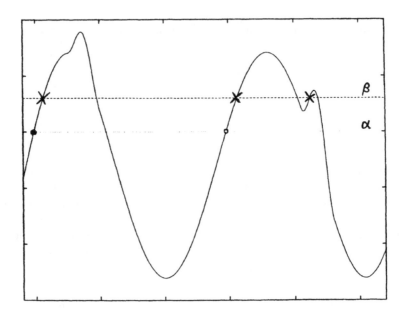

Figure 20.1
Displacement of the basilar membrane, at one fixed point y**, as**
a function of time. The horizontal lines α **and** β **represent the**
thresholds for bristles of different stiffness.

Near the basilar membrane, and over its whole length, one finds series
of bristles of different stiffness. As the membrane moves near a particular
bristle, it can, if the displacement is sufficiently large, "bend" the bristle.
For different degrees of stiffness, this happens for different thresholds of
displacement. Every time a bristle is bent, we think of this as an "event";
we also imagine that events only count when the bristle is bent away from its
equilibrium position, not when it moves back. Figure 20.1 gives a schematic
representation of what this means. The curve represents the movement of
the membrane, as a function of time, at one particular location y.

The two horizontal lines, labeled by α and β, represent two different bristle thresholds, and the dots and crosses mark the corresponding "events"
in the timespan represented in the figure. Replacing the information contained in all the curves (for different y) by only the coordinates (level, time,
location) of these events would already be a formidable compression. Yet
the EIH model reduces the information even more, by another transformation. Start by setting a certain resolution level ΔT, and a "window width"
t_0. Then, for a given t, look back in time and count within the interval
$[t - t_0, t]$, the number $N_{\alpha,y}(T)$ of successive events (for the bristle at position y and with stiffness α) that were spaced apart by an interval between
T and $T + \Delta T$. Next, compute $S(t, T)$, the sum over all α and y of these
$N_{\alpha,y}(T)$. This new representation $S(t, T)$ of the original signal is still two-

dimensional, like the original cochlear or wavelet filtering output; it is, however, often sampled more coarsely than the continuous wavelet transform.
More important, from our point of view, than the compression that this
represents, is the very nonlinear and adaptive transformation represented
by $S(t, T)$, which can again be viewed as a time-frequency representation
(a second look at the construction of $S(t, T)$ shows that T^{-1} plays the role
of an instantaneous frequency). O. Ghitza [1] compared the performance
of EIH-based tools for several types of discrimination tests (such as word
spotting) with the results obtained from LPC (linear predictive coding, a
hidden Markov model for speech); for clean speech, LPC performed better,
but the EIH-based schemes were, like the human auditory system itself,
much more robust when the noise level was raised, and provided still useful
results at noise levels where LPC could no longer be trusted. The nonlinear
squeezing of the continuous wavelet transform that we describe in Section
20.5 is inspired by the EIH-construction.

20.4 The Modulation Model for Speech

The modulation model represents speech signals as a linear combination
of amplitude and phase modulated components,

$$f(t) = \sum_{k=1}^{K} A_k(t) \cos[\theta_k(t)] + \eta(t),$$

where $A_k(t)$ is the instantaneous amplitude and

$$\omega_k(t) = \frac{d}{dt} \theta_k(t)$$

the instantaneous frequency of component (or formant) k; $\eta(t)$ takes into
account the errors of modeling [8, 9]. In a slightly more sophisticated model,
the components are viewed as "ribbons" in the time-frequency plane rather
than "curves," and one also associates instantaneous bandwidths $\Delta\omega_k(t)$
to each component. The parameters $A_k(t)$, $\omega_k(t)$, and $\Delta\omega_k(t)$ are all assumed to vary in time (as the notation indicates), but we assume that this
variation is slow when compared with the oscillation time of each component, measured by $[\omega_k(t)]^{-1}$. For large parts of speech, the modulation
model is very satisfactory, and one can take $\eta(t) \simeq 0$; for other parts (e.g.,
fricative sounds) it is completely inadequate. The parameters $A_k(t)$, $\omega_k(t)$,
and $\Delta\omega_k(t)$ (for those portions of speech where they are meaningful) can

be used for speaker recognition. The basic idea is as follows. Imagine that the speech signal can be well represented by, say, $K = 8$ components. For each component, we have 3 parameters that vary in time. The signal can thus be viewed as a path in an $8 \times 3 = 24$-dimensional space. This path depends of course on both the speaker and the utterance. During certain portions (such as within one vowel), the 24 parameters remain in the same neighborhood, after which they make a rapid transition to another neighborhood, where they then dwell for a while, and so on. The order in which these "islands" appear depends on the utterance, but their location in our 24-dimensional space is believed to be independent of the utterance, and can be used to characterize the speaker. To use this for a speaker identification project, one must thus do two things: (1) extract the $A_k(t)$, $\omega_k(t)$, $\Delta\omega_k(t)$ (or a subset of these parameters) from the speech signal; and (2) process this information in a classification scheme in order to identify the speaker. When LPC methods are used for this purpose [10–12], one determines in fact only the $\omega_k(t)$ and $\Delta\omega_k(t)$, not the amplitudes $A_k(t)$. They are incorporated into one complex number,

$$z_k(t) = e^{i[\omega_k(t) + i\Delta\omega_k(t)]};$$

the $z_k(t)$ are the poles of the vocal tract transfer function

$$\mathcal{H}(z, t) = \sum_{k=1}^{K} \frac{1}{1 - z/z_k(t)}.$$

It is not always straightforward to label the $z_k(t)$ correctly with the LPC method, i.e., to decide which of the poles, determined separately, belongs to which component. To circumvent this, one works not with the $z_k(t)$ themselves, but with the so-called LPC-derived cepstrum,

$$c_n(t) = \frac{1}{n} \sum_{k=1}^{K} [z_k(t)]^n,$$

for which the exact attribution of the $z_k(t)$ does not matter; this formula is due to Schroeder [16]. This speaker identification program was developed at CAIP (Center for Aids to Industrial Productivity) at Rutgers University, by K. Assaleh, R. Mammone, and J. Flanagan [10–12]. Once the cepstrum is extracted, they use a neural network to do the classification and identification part. They fine-tuned it until it performed so well that it could perfectly distinguish identical twins, when starting from clean speech signals, thus outperforming most humans!

20.5 Squeezing the Continuous Wavelet Transform

Our goal is to use the continuous wavelet transform to extract reliably the different components of the modulation model (when it is applicable) and the parameters characterizing them. Our first problem is that the wavelet transform gives a somewhat "blurred" time-frequency picture. Let us take, for instance, a purely harmonic signal,

$$f(t) = A \cos \Omega t.$$

We compute its continuous wavelet transform $(W_\psi f)(a, b)$, using a wavelet ψ that is concentrated on the positive frequency axis (i.e., support $(\hat\psi) \subset [0, \infty)$, or $\hat\psi(\xi) = 0$ for $\xi < 0$; note that this means that ψ is complex):

$$(W_\psi f)(a, b) = \int f(t) \frac{1}{\sqrt{a}} \overline{\psi\left(\frac{t-b}{a}\right)} \, dt \tag{20.2}$$

$$= \frac{1}{2\pi} \int \hat f(\xi) \sqrt{a} \, \overline{\hat\psi(a\xi)} \, e^{ib\xi} \, d\xi$$

$$= \frac{1}{2\pi} \int \frac{A}{2} [\delta(\xi - \Omega) + \delta(\xi + \Omega)] \sqrt{a} \, \overline{\hat\psi(a\xi)} \, e^{ib\xi} \, d\xi$$

$$= \frac{A}{4\pi} \sqrt{a} \, \overline{\hat\psi(a\Omega)} \, e^{ib\Omega}.$$

If $\hat\psi(\xi)$ is concentrated around $\xi = 1$, then $(W_\psi f)(a, b)$ will be concentrated around $a = \Omega^{-1}$, as expected. But it will be spread out over a region around this value (see Figure 20.2), and not give a sharp picture of what was a signal very sharply localized in frequency.

In order to remedy this blurring, the "Marseilles group" developed the so-called "ridge and skeleton" method [13]. In this method, special curves (the ridges) are singled out in the (a, b)-plane, depending on the wavelet transform $(W_\psi f)(a, b)$ itself (for each b, one finds the values of a where the oscillatory integrand in $(W_\psi f)(a, b)$ has "stationary phase"; for the signals considered here, this amounts to $\partial_b[\text{phase of } (W_\psi f)(a, b)] = \omega_0/a$, where ω_0 is the center frequency for ψ). From the restriction of $W_\psi f$ to these ridges (the "skeleton" of the wavelet transform), one can then read off the important parameters, such as the instantaneous frequency. This method has been used with great success for various applications, such as reliably

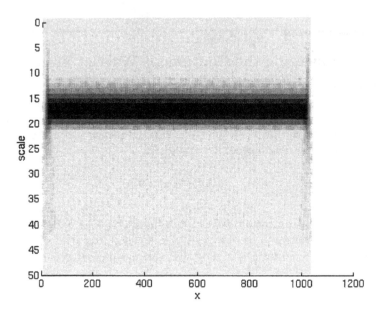

Figure 20.2
Absolute value $|W_\psi f(a,b)|$ of the wavelet transform of a pure tone
f.

identifying and extracting spectral lines of widely different strengths [13].
In our speech signals, we have many components, some of which can remain
very close for a while, to separate later again; components can also die or
new components can suddenly appear out of nowhere. For these signals,
the ridge and skeleton method does not perform as well. For this reason, we
developed a different approach, where we try to squeeze back the defocused
information in order to gain a sharper picture; in so doing, we try to use
the whole wavelet transform instead of concentrating on special curves.

Let us look back at the wavelet transform (20.2) of a pure tone. Although
it is spread out over a region in the a-variable around $a = \Omega^{-1}$, the b-
dependence still shows the original harmonic oscillations with the correct
frequency, regardless of the value of a. This suggests that we compute, for
any (a,b), the instantaneous frequency $\omega(a,b)$ by

$$\omega(a,b) = -i[W_\psi f(a,b)]^{-1}\frac{\partial}{\partial b}W_\psi f(a,b),$$

and that we transfer the information from the (a,b)-plane to a (b,ω)-plane,
by taking for instance,

$$S_\psi f(b,\omega_\ell) = \sum_{a_k \text{ such that } |\omega(a_k,b) - \omega_\ell| \le \Delta\omega/2} |W_\psi f(a_k,b)|. \qquad (20.3)$$

We have assumed here that both the old a-variable and the new ω-variable have been discretized. (A continuous formulation would be to introduce, for every b, a measure $d\mu_b$ in the ω-variable, which assigns to Borel sets A the measure

$$\mu_b(A) = \int |W_\psi f(a,b)| \chi_A(\omega(a,b)) \, da,$$

where χ_A is the indicator function of A, $\chi_A(u) = 1$ if $u \in A$, $\chi_A(u) = 0$ if $u \notin A$.) This has *exactly* the same flavor as the EIH transform described in Section 20.3: we transform to a different time-frequency plane by reassigning contributions with the same instantaneous frequency to the same bin, and we give a larger weight to components with large amplitude $|W_\psi f|$ (just as components with large amplitude in the EIH would give rise to several level crossings and would therefore contribute more). Our S_ψ is also close to the SBS (in-synchrony bands spectrum, a precursor of the EIH) [14] or to the IFD (instantaneous frequency distribution) [15]. For good measure, one can also sum the $|a_k|^{-\alpha} |W_\psi f(a_k, b)|$ rather than the $|W_\psi f(a_k, b)|$, thus renormalizing the fine-scale regions where often $|W_\psi f(a, b)|$ is much smaller.

When this squeezing operation is performed on the wavelet transform of a pure tone, we find a single horizontal line in the (b, ω)-plane, at $\omega = \Omega$, as expected.

We can, however, refine the operation even further, and define a particular type of squeezing, which we call *synchrosqueezing*, that still allows for reconstruction, even after the (highly nonlinear!) transformation. To see this, we first have to observe that the reconstruction formula of f from $W_\psi f$, given by formula (1.25) in Chapter 1, is not the only one. We also have, again assuming support $\hat{\psi} \subset [0, \infty)$,

$$\int_0^\infty W_\psi f(a,b) \, a^{-3/2} \, da = \int \int \hat{f}(\xi) \, e^{ib\xi} \, \overline{\hat{\psi}(a\xi)} \, a^{-1} \, da \, d\xi \qquad (20.4)$$

$$= \left[\int_0^\infty \hat{\psi}(\xi) \frac{d\xi}{\xi} \right] \cdot \int \hat{f}(\xi) e^{ib\xi} \, d\xi$$

$$= \left[2\pi \int_0^\infty \hat{\psi}(\xi) \frac{d\xi}{\xi} \right] f(b).$$

This suggests that we define

$$(S_\psi f)(b, \omega_\ell) = \sum_{a_k \text{ such that } |\omega(a_k, b) - \omega_\ell| \leq \Delta\omega/2} W_\psi f(a_k, b) a_k^{-3/2} \qquad (20.5)$$

(without absolute values!); with ω_ℓ spaced apart by $\Delta\omega$, we then still have

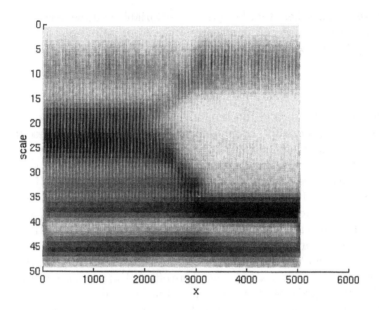

Figure 20.3
Absolute value $|W_\psi f(a,b)|$ of the sound /a–a–i–i/. A colored noise
is present with SNR = 15 dB. The horizontal axis is sampled
at 8 kHz. The vertical axis represents different subbands (five
octaves, split into eight equally spaced suboctaves); low indices
are associated to high frequencies.

(in the assumption that the discretizations are sufficiently fine to be good
approximations to integrals)

$$\sum_\ell (\mathcal{S}_\psi f)(\omega_\ell, b) = C_\psi^\# f(b). \tag{20.6}$$

Having the exact reconstruction (20.6) will be useful to us later on (see
the end of this section); note that such an exact reconstruction is not available for the EIH, SBS, or IFD. There is an added bonus to *synchro*squeezing.
The process of reassigning components from the (a,b)-plane to the (b,ω)-
plane is not perfect, especially when noise is present, and occasionally parts
of components that are truly different get assigned to the same ω_ℓ-bin.
When this happens, the two pieces from different components are often
out of phase with each other, and cancellation takes place in the computation of $\mathcal{S}_\psi$ (but not in S_ψ!). Figures 20.3 and 20.4 show the unprocessed
wavelet transform and the synchrosqueezed wavelet transform, respectively,
of the speech signal consisting of the two vowels /a-a–i-i/; clearly, the different components can be distinguished much more clearly after the (syn-

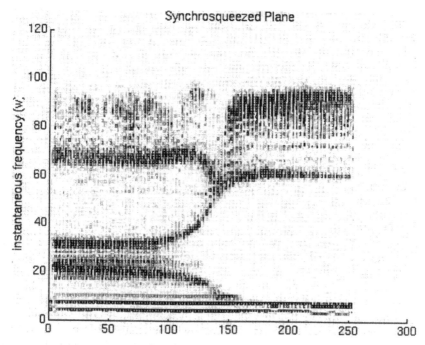

Figure 20.4
Synchrosqueezed representation of /a-a–i-i/ (same signal, same noise level as in Figure 20.3). The components can be distinguished much more clearly than in Figure 20.3. (Note that because the scale a corresponds to ω^{-1}, there is also a distortion of the vertical axis when compared to Figure 20.3.)

chro)squeezing. The extra focusing of the synchrosqueezing over squeezing can be seen in an example in Section 20.7.

One remark is in order here. Both the squeezing and synchrosqueezing operations can be defined with any arbitrary reassigning rule — it does not have to be governed by the instantaneous frequency. In particular, the reconstruction property from $S_\psi f$ does not depend on the physical interpretation of the reassignment rule. This means that we should not worry about the parts of f where the modulation model does not apply — true, the reassignment will not be as meaningful, because instantaneous frequency does not make much sense there, but we still haven't "hurt" the information that was there. In fact, as the synchrosqueezed representation of "august" in Figure 20.5 shows, the "s" part is still nicely localized in the upper frequencies, where it belongs, so in practice we don't seem to displace such nonmodulated parts in the time-frequency plane. Of course, the refocusing that we see in the squeezed and synchrosqueezed transform *does* depend on the physical interpretation — an arbitrary reassignment rule would give a messy picture.

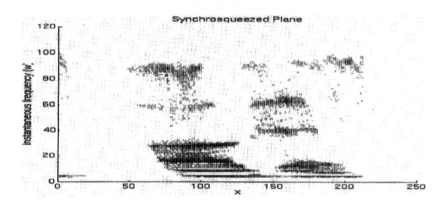

Figure 20.5
Synchrosqueezed representation of /ow-g-λ-s-t/. A colored noise
is present with SNR of 15 dB. The "s" part is the cloud in the
upper right corner.

After synchrosqueezing, the components are well-separated and can be
identified. From the synchrosqueezed representation, we can determine the
central frequencies $\omega_k(t)$ and the bandwidths $\Delta\omega_k(t)$. How can we find
the $A_k(t)$? Remember our exact reconstruction formula (20.6)! If a postprocessing step separates the different components in the synchrosqueezed
plane, then we can carve out the component under consideration in the
synchrosqueezed plane, delete all the rest, and reconstruct from only this
component; this is called the selective fusion algorithm [2, 4]. The direct
summation method (20.6) provides fast and relatively accurate results; a
slightly slower but even more accurate method uses double integrals (see
[2, 4]). This is carried out for speech signals, within the modulation model
framework, in [2, 5]. From every reconstructed single component, we can
then determine $A_k(t)$, $\theta_k(0)$ so that $A_k(t)\cos(\theta_k(t))$ fits this reconstructed
component, within the constraint $\frac{d}{dt}\theta_k(t) = \omega_k(t)$.

This finishes our program of extracting the modulation model parameters
from an EIH-analog based on the wavelet transform. After a (very summary) discussion of some implementation issues, we shall return to results
in Section 20.7.

20.6   Short Discussion of Some Implementation Issues

First of all, the whole construction is based on a continuous wavelet
transform. In practice, this is of course a discrete but very redundant
transform, heavily oversampled both in time and in scale. In order to be

practical, we need a fast implementation scheme. This was achieved by borrowing a leaf from (nonredundant) wavelet bases, i.e., by using subband filtering schemes. For a given profile $\hat{\psi}(\xi)$ (close to that of a Morlet wavelet), we identified a function $\hat{\phi}$ and trigonometric polynomials $\hat{h}, \hat{g}_\ell$; $\ell = 1, \ldots, L$, so that

$$\hat{\psi}(2^{(\ell-1)/L}\omega) \simeq \hat{g}_\ell(\omega)\hat{\phi}(\omega)$$

$$\hat{\phi}(2\omega) \simeq \hat{h}(\omega)\hat{\phi}(\omega).$$

This means that the Fourier coefficients of $\hat{h}, \hat{g}_\ell$ can be used for an iterated FIR filtering scheme that gives the redundant wavelet transform in linear time. For details on the algorithm and on the construction of the filters, see [2, 6], or Chapter 2, Section 2.5 in this book.

Next we note that the squeezing and synchrosqueezing operations entailed first the determination of the instantaneous frequency $\omega(a, b)$. This was done by a logarithmic differentiation of $W_\psi f(a, b)$. This is of course very unstable when $|W_\psi f(a, b)|$ is small; note however that these regions will contribute very little to either $S_\psi f$ or $\mathcal{S}_\psi f$ (defined by (20.3) and (20.5), respectively), so that we can safely avoid this problem by putting a lower threshold on $|W_\psi f(a, b)|$. On the other hand, differentiation itself is also a tricky business when the data are noisy; in practice, a standard numerical difference operator was used, involving a weighted differencing operator, spread out over a neighborhood of samples. Again, details can be found in [2, 4].

In the previous section, we also glossed over the extraction of the $\omega_k(t)$, $\Delta\omega_k(t)$ from the synchrosqueezed picture. In fact, although we can often clearly see the different components with our eyes, extracting them and their parameters automatically is a different matter. For instance, in "How are you?", an example shown in Section 20.7, the components are much weaker in some spots than in others, yet we want our "extractor" to bridge those weak gaps. The approach we use, developed with Trevor Hastie [18], views $|\mathcal{S}_\psi f(b, \omega)|$ as a probability distribution in ω, for every value of b, which can be modeled as a mixture of Gaussians, and which evolves as b changes; moreover, we impose that the centers of the Gaussians follow paths given by splines (cubic or linear). We also allow components to die or to be born. In order to find an evolution law that fits the given $|\mathcal{S}_\psi f(b, \omega)|$, a few steps of an iterative scheme suffice; for details, see [2, 18]. The resulting centers of the Gaussians in the mixture give us the frequencies $\omega_k(t)$, their widths give us the $\Delta\omega_k(t)$.

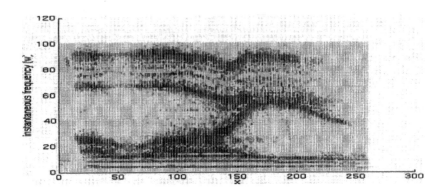

Figure 20.6
Squeezed plane representation for /h-δ-w-a-r-j-u?/. A colored
noise is present with SNR = 15 dB.

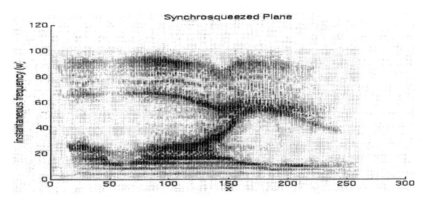

Figure 20.7
Synchrosqueezed plane representation for /h-δ-w-a-r-j-u?/. A colored noise is present with SNR = 15 dB.

20.7   Results on Speech Signals

We start by illustrating the enhanced focusing of the synchrosqueezed
representation when compared to the squeezed representation of a different
example, namely, the utterance, "How are you?" or /h-δ-w-a-r-j-u?/; see
Figures 20.6 and 20.7.

Figure 20.8 shows the curves for the corresponding extracted central frequencies $\omega_k(t)$. In this case, the original signal was somewhat noisy; the
(pink) noise had an SNR of about 15 dB.

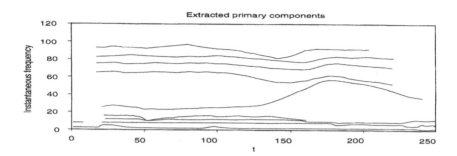

Figure 20.8
Curves for the central frequencies $\omega_k(t)$ for /h-δ-w-a-r-j-u?/. A colored noise is present with SNR = 15 dB.

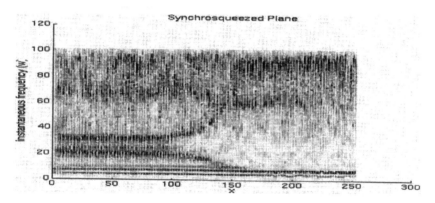

Figure 20.9
Synchrosqueezed plane representation for /···-a-a–i-i-···/. A colored noise is present with SNR = 15 dB. An additional white noise is added with SNR = 11 dB.

Next, we illustrate the robustness of our analysis under higher noise levels. We return to the signal /a-a–i-i/, this time with an additional white noise with SNR of 11 dB. Figure 20.9 shows the synchrosqueezed representation of this noisier signal; although the representation is noisier as well, the different components can still be identified clearly, and they haven't moved. This is borne out by a comparison of the extracted central frequency curves. Figure 20.10 shows the extracted frequency curves for the slightly noisy original of Figure 20.4. Figure 20.11 shows the extracted frequency curves for the much noisier version given in Figure 20.9.

Finally, we also show results of a first test of the use of the synchrosqueezed representation for speaker identification. For this first test, we did not use the full strength of the representation, and we did not develop our own classification either. Instead, we took our $\omega_k(t)$, $\Delta\omega_k(t)$ values,

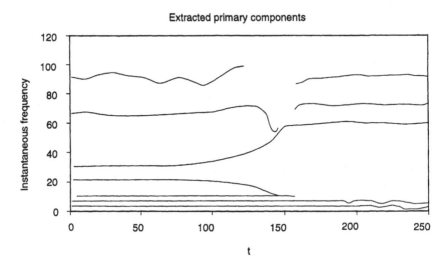

Figure 20.10
Curves for the central frequencies $\omega_k(t)$ for /a-a–i-i/, extracted
from Figure 20.4.

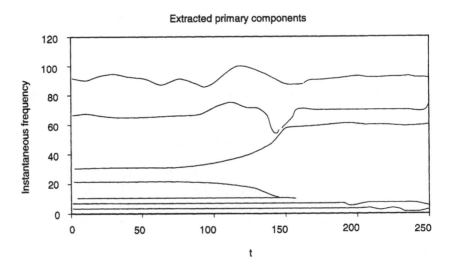

Figure 20.11
Curves for the central frequencies $\omega_k(t)$ for /a-a–i-i/ with additional white noise; see Figure 20.9.

and constructed an analog to the LPC-derived cepstrum by defining

$$z_k^w(t) = \exp[i\omega_k(t) - \Delta\omega_k(t)]$$

$$c_n^w(t) = \frac{1}{n} \sum_{k=1}^{K} [z_k^w(t)]^n \, ;$$

we called this the "wastrum." We then used the wastrum as input for the classification scheme that had been developed at CAIP. For the experiment we performed, the input data come from the narrowband part of the *KING* database, released by ITT Aerospace/Communications Division, in April 1992. It is a telephone network database built with 52 American speakers, among whom the first 26 speakers are from the San Diego region. For each speaker, ten sessions have been recorded. The first five sessions were recorded at intervals of 1 week. Each session is narrowband, with the bandwidth of a telephone channel. Each session consists of roughly 50 to 75 seconds of conversational speech which contains roughly 40% of silences. The sessions are recorded from the interlocutor's side. The first five sessions are within the Great Divide, which means on the West Coast. The SNR is about 15 dB to 20 dB. This noise is introduced by the phone network. The five remaining sessions are recorded across the Great Divide at intervals of 1 month and they are much noisier. These last sessions were not used in this experiment. The signal is sampled at 8 kHz and quantized over 12 bits.

For the experiment, the first session of the first 26 speakers is used for training and the following four within divide sessions are used for testing.

The classifier is a vector quantizer. Decisions are made on the basis of the cumulated distances obtained in each frame relative to the codebooks associated to the different speakers.

Table 20.1 summarizes the results in closed-set speaker identification obtained with the LPC-derived cepstrum and the wastrum. The long-term mean is removed from the features, in agreement with [10]. The silence frames are removed on the basis of energy thresholds for the primary components. The same frames are removed for the LPC approach, in order to compare exactly the same utterances.

The performances of the wastrum are comparable to the LPC-derived cepstrum for the relatively clean speech, which is reassuring: we aim to extract the same cepstral-like information, albeit with very different methods, and so we expect similar performance! The wastrum method is, however, more robust to noise when the noise can not be considered as negligible, since we get a lower error rate even though the noise level is significantly higher (12 dB versus 15 dB).

Table 20.1
Summary of the results obtained on *KING* database, within the Great Divide, 26 speakers, first section used for training, four other sessions used for testing. Long-term mean removal is used.

Method	additional SNR	error rate
LPC-derived cepstrum	none	~ 0.22
wastrum	none	0.23
LPC-derived cepstrum	15 dB	0.33
wastrum	12 dB	0.3

Note that we are comparing here a suboptimal version of our approach (the $A_k(t)$ are not taken into account, and the $\omega_k(t)$, $\Delta\omega_k(t)$ are transformed into the wastrum, that is then put through a classification scheme not specially tailored to our different approach) with a very much optimized version of the LPC-based method. Yet even so, the wastrum method leads to fewer errors for noisy speech than the LPC-derived cepstrum. This indicates that we have indeed inherited (some of) the robustness that characterizes true auditory systems.

The following is a short list of promising future directions to be explored: include the amplitude information $A_k(t)$ (obtained by selective fusion [5]) as well; develop a more direct classification scheme, without the detour of the wastrum, and maybe even directly from the synchrosqueezed plane, without extraction of the parameters first; and finally, use of this approach for other tasks in speech analysis.

There is some similarity between our squeezing and synchrosqueezing methods and a technique of "reassignment" developed by Auger and Flandrin [17], with the same goal of "refocusing" in the time-frequency plane; we first heard of their method after the work described here was completed. Auger and Flandrin typically work with Wigner-Ville or similar time-frequency distributions, and their reassignment method is not limited to one direction only (we don't change the b variable in our scheme); on the other hand, their scheme is not linked to an exact reconstruction formula such as our (20.6).

20.8   Acknowledgments

Both authors would like to thank CAIP (Rutgers University) and especially Prof. R. Mammone and his group for their hospitality and advice. Ingrid Daubechies also wants to thank NSF (grant DMS-9401785) and AFOSR (grant F49620-95-1-0290) for partial support.

References

[1] O. Ghitza. Auditory models and human performances in tasks related to speech coding and speech recognition. *IEEE Trans. Speech Audio Proc.*, 2(1):115–132, 1994; see also O. Ghitza. Advances in speech signal processing, in *Advances in speech signal processing*, S. Furui and M. Sondhi, editors. Marcel Dekker, New York, NY 1991.

[2] S. Maes. The wavelet transform in signal processing, with application to the extraction of the speech modulation model features. Ph.D. thesis, Université Catholique de Louvain, Louvain-la-Neuve, Belgium, 1994.

[3] S. Maes. The synchrosqueezed representation yields a new reading of the wavelet transform. In *Proc. SPIE 1995 on OE/Aerospace Sensing and Dual Use Photonics – Wavelet Applications for Dual Use – Session on Acoustic and Signal Processing, Wavelet Applications II*, Vol. 2491, H. H. Szu, editor, Orlando, FL, April 1995. Part I, 532–559

[4] S. Maes. The wavelet-derived synchrosqueezed plane representation yields a new time-frequency analysis of 1-D signals, with application to speech. *Preprint submitted to IEEE Trans. Speech and Audio Processing.*

[5] S. Maes. The wavelet-derived synchrosqueezed plane representation yields new front-ends for automated speech recognition. *Preprint submitted to IEEE Trans. Speech and Audio Processing.*

[6] S. Maes. Fast quasi-continuous wavelet algorithms for analysis and synthesis of 1-D signals. *Preprint submitted to SIAM J. Appl. Math.*

[7] J. B. Allen. Cochlear modeling. *IEEE ASSP Magazine*, 2(1):3–29, 1985.

[8] C. D'Alessandro. Time-frequency speech transformation based on an elementary waveform representation. *Speech Commun.*, 9:419–431, 1990.

[9] J. S. Liénard. Speech analysis and reconstruction using short-time, elementary, waveforms. In *IEEE Proc. ICASSP*, Dallas, TX, 1987, 948–951

[10] K. Assaleh. *Robust features for speaker identification.* Ph.D. thesis, CAIP Center – Rutgers University, The State University of New Jersey, New Brunswick, NJ, 1993.

[11] K. Assaleh, R. J. Mammone, and J. L. Flanagan. Speech recognition using the modulation model. In *IEEE Proc. ICASSP*, Vol. 2, 1993, 664–667

[12] K. T. Assaleh and R. J. Mammone. New LP-derived features for speaker identification. *IEEE Trans. Speech Audio Proc.*, 2(4):630–638, 1994.

[13] N. Delprat, B. Escudié, P. Guillemain, R. Kronland-Martinet, Ph. Tchamitchian, and B. Torrésani. Asymptotic wavelet and Gabor analysis: extraction of instantaneous frequencies. *IEEE Trans. Inf. Theory*, 38(2 Part II):644–664, 1992.

[14] O. Ghitza. Auditory nerve representation criteria for speech analysis/synthesis. *IEEE Trans. ASSP*, 6(35):736–740, 1987.

[15] D. H. Friedman. Instantaneous-frequency distribution vs. time: an interpretation of the phase structure of speech. In *IEEE Proc. ICASSP*, 1985, 1121–1124.

[16] M. Schroeder. Direct (non-recursive) relations between cepstrum and predictor coefficients. *IEEE Trans. ASSP*, 29:297–301, 1981.

[17] F. Auger and P. Flandrin. Improving the readablilty of time-scale representations by the reassignment method. *IEEE Trans. Signal Process.*, 43(5):1068–1089, 1995.

[18] T. Hastie and S. Maes. The maximum-likelihood-estimation-based living cubic spline extractor and its application to saliency grouping in the time-frequency plane. Preprint.

21

The Application of Wavelet Transforms to Blood Flow Velocimetry

Lora G. Weiss

The Pennsylvania State University, Applied Research Laboratory, State College, PA

Abstract   This chapter presents a technique for blood flow velocimetry using wavelet transforms and wideband signals. Ultrasonic signals with high fractional bandwidths and large time-bandwidth products are processed with wideband/wavelet transform methods. This approach removes many of the narrowband assumptions typically invoked when measuring blood flow. The received signals are assumed to be reflected from particles moving in the blood stream. Instead of measuring the Doppler shift associated with the reflection, the time-scaling of the signal is obtained along with the round trip travel time of the signal. This time-scaling more accurately reflects the effects of motion on the signals than does a Doppler shift since a Doppler shift is an approximation to time-scaling. The continuous wavelet transform is then used to obtain the axial velocity of scatterers.

21.1   Introduction

The goal of blood flow velocimetry is to obtain an accurate measurement of the velocity of the blood as it flows through a blood vessel. Accuracy is

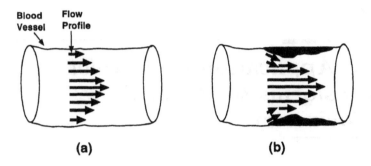

Figure 21.1
Vector lengths indicate speed. (a) Laminar flow through blood
vessel, (b) Flow through a partially blocked vessel. An obstructed
vessel will have a higher flow rate (b) than an unobstructed vessel
(a). Underestimating the velocity in (b) may yield the same velocity measurement as an accurate measurement of the velocity
in (a).

a crucial element of this measurement. For example, if a blood vessel has a
partial occlusion, then the velocity in the vessel will increase. If the measurement technique underestimates the blood flow velocity (as is often the
case), then the measurement may appear normal and the occlusion may go
undetected. See Figure 21.1. To prevent an incorrect diagnosis, researchers
continually seek new devices and improved processing techniques to obtain
accurate measurements of the hemodynamic state of the vessel.

It has been shown [27] that scattering of ultrasound by blood is at-
tributable almost entirely to red blood cells which are uniformly distributed
within most vessels. A typical red blood cell is approximately 7 μ in diameter and 1–2 μ thick. Red blood cells occupy approximately 40–50% of
the total blood volume in an individual and are therefore a major source
of ultrasonic scattering from the blood. Blood velocities average from approximately 20 cm/s in the aorta to approximately 0.2 cm/s in capillary
beds.

In this work, we focus on one-dimensional (1-D) ultrasonic blood flow
measurement techniques, and we remove some of the assumptions generally applied with the current signal processing methods. In particular, if
the particles in the blood stream are moving rapidly or if the transmitted
ultrasound signal has a large time-bandwidth product, then the narrowband processing methods currently in use may not be valid and wideband
methods may be required. We describe wavelet transform processing of
wideband signals reflected from particles moving in the blood stream. The
wavelet transform is applied since it is a natural tool for processing wideband signals, and by doing so, it allows for the removal of several assumptions currently invoked.

The situation considered is shown in Figure 21.2, where particles in the

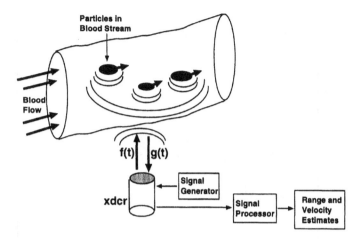

Figure 21.2
Widebandsignal, $f(t)$, insonifying particles in the blood stream.
Arrows on particles indicate motion.

blood stream are insonified by the wideband signal $f(t)$ and where $g(t)$ is the received signal. The goal is to appropriately process the transmitted and received signals to accurately measure the range and the velocity of the particles in the blood stream.

This chapter is organized as follows: Section 21.2 presents ultrasound devices that are currently used for 1-D blood flow velocimetry; Section 21.3 briefly describes 1-D velocimetry methods and their limitations, and Section 21.4 describes new wideband/wavelet transform techniques that remove some of the current assumptions; Section 21.4 also presents an example and compares wavelet processing of wideband signals to the current narrowband Doppler approach.

21.2   1-D Measurement Devices

Ultrasound involves transmitting a sound wave whose frequency is greater than 20 kHz. Blood flow velocimetry devices generally operate at a frequency of approximately 5 MHz with a 2.5 MHz bandwidth. This corresponds to a 50% fractional bandwidth for the transmitted signal. A signal whose fractional bandwidth is greater than 10% is generally considered to be wideband. Figure 21.3 shows a typical transmitted signal for a commercial 2.3 MHz single element transducer with a 45% fractional bandwidth; Figure 21.4 shows the frequency response of this transducer.

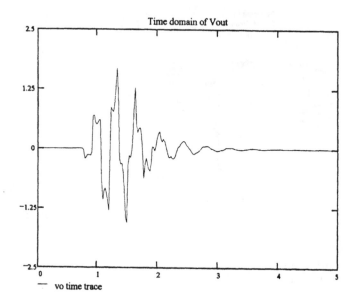

Figure 21.3
Transmit signal of a 2.3-MHz transducer.

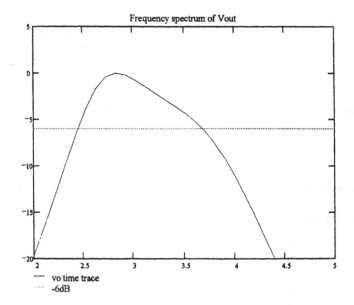

Figure 21.4
Frequency response of 2.3-MHz transducer with ~45% fractional bandwidth.

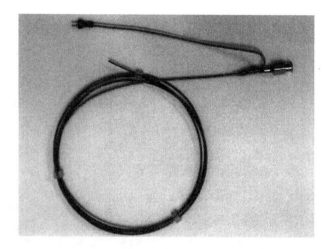

Figure 21.5
Newer devices with higher center frequencies. Courtesy of Millar Instruments, Inc.

There is a trade-off when determining which center frequency, f_c, to use. The trade-off is between the backscattering energy, which is proportional to f_c^4, and attenuation losses, which are proportional to f_c. Increasing the operational frequency obviously yields a stronger reflected signal. Recently, devices have been developed to operate at 20 MHz and even 60 MHz and 80 MHz with correspondingly larger fractional bandwidths. The higher frequency and larger time-bandwidth products result in improved resolution, as well as an increase in gain. It is therefore desirable to use devices with higher center frequencies and larger time-bandwidth products. Figure 21.5 shows a commercial 20-MHz Doppler catheter, and Figure 21.6 shows a close-up view of its 0.014″ guidewire.

As newer devices continue to be developed with higher center frequencies and larger fractional bandwidths, newer processing methods are needed to accommodate and exploit the features of these devices. One approach is the wideband/wavelet transform method presented in Section 21.4.

21.3   1-D Velocimetry Methods

One-dimensional methods for estimating blood flow velocity are usually accomplished by transmitting an ultrasound wave and receiving a signal that has scattered off the moving red blood cells. The transmitted and received signals are processed to extract various properties of the scatterers,

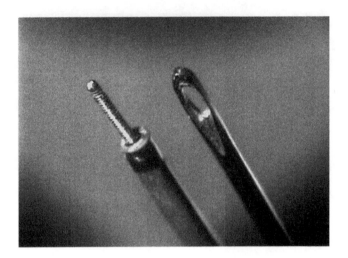

Figure 21.6
Close-up of guide wire for catheter in Figure 21.5. Courtesy of Millar Instruments, Inc.

namely, range and velocity. One of two approaches to do this is usually taken: Doppler processing or time domain correlation processing. Section 21.4 presents a third approach: wavelet transform processing, which is somewhat of a hybrid of these two techniques and removes some of their assumptions and limitations.

21.3.1 Doppler Methods

By transmitting an ultrasound wave and processing the received signal that has scattered off the moving red blood cells, one can extract the distance to the particles as well as the Doppler shift of the signal [2, 26, 28, 32]. The transmitted and received signals are processed with a narrowband correlation receiver:

$$N_f g(f_d', \tau') = \int_{-\infty}^{\infty} g(t) \, \overline{f(t - \tau')} \, e^{-2\pi i f_d' t} \, dt, \qquad (21.1)$$

where $f(t)$ is the transmit signal, $g(t)$ is the receive signal, and f_d' and τ' are the hypothesized values of Doppler and delay; $\overline{(\cdot)}$ denotes complex conjugation. The measured delay, τ, and Doppler, f_d, associated with the scatterers are values of $N_f g$ that maximize the magnitude of this correlator:

$$\max_{f_d', \tau'} |N_f g(f_d', \tau')|^2. \qquad (21.2)$$

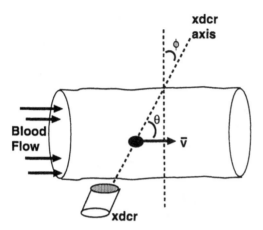

Figure 21.7
Transducer and vessel geometry for measuring Doppler.

The distance, R, to the particles is then computed from the round trip travel time, τ, of the signal: $R = c\tau/2$, where c is the speed of sound ($c \simeq 1500$ m/s in blood). The Doppler shift, f_d, is proportional to the velocity of the moving red blood cells. If the transmitted center frequency is f_c and the particles are moving with velocity $\bar{v}$, then the Doppler shift, f_d, is given by

$$f_d = \frac{2|\bar{v}|}{c} f_c \cos \theta. \tag{21.3}$$

Here $|\bar{v}|$ is the speed of the particle. The quantity $v_a = |\bar{v}| \cos \theta$ is called the axial velocity of the particle, which is the velocity of the particle along the transducer axis, θ is the angle the particle's velocity vector, $\bar{v}$, makes with the transducer axis. It is often assumed that the particles are moving parallel to the walls of the blood vessel so that $\theta = 90° - \phi$, where ϕ is the transducer angle, which is the angle between the transducer axis and the line orthogonal to the vessel wall. It is also often assumed that ϕ (and therefore θ) is known. See Figure 21.7. Assumed knowledge of θ is one shortfall of this approach. Solving (21.3) for v_a yields

$$v_a = \frac{cf_d}{2f_c}, \tag{21.4}$$

which is the axial velocity of the particular red blood cell from which the signal scattered. A number of Doppler systems employing this technique have been built and used for measuring blood flow.

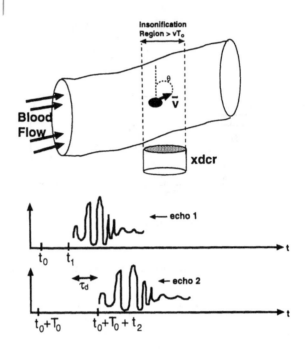

Figure 21.8
Transducer and vessel geometry for time domain correlation methods.

21.3.2 Time Domain Correlation Methods

A second approach to estimating the axial velocity of the particles in the blood stream is to use time domain correlation methods to track a group of scatterers [3, 11–14]. This method uses either two ultrasonic echoes or two ultrasonic transducers. At time t_0, the first pulse is transmitted. Let t_1 be its roundtrip travel time. At time $t_0 + T_0$, transmit the next pulse, and let t_2 be its round-trip travel time. Letting $\tau_d = t_2 - t_1$, then the axial distance, d_a, the scatterers move is given by $d_a = \tau_d c/2$, and the axial velocity is given by

$$v_a = \frac{\tau_d c}{2T_0}. \tag{21.5}$$

The actual distance and speed are:

$$d = \frac{d_a}{\cos\theta}, \quad |\bar{v}| = \frac{\tau_d c}{2T_0 \cos\theta}. \tag{21.6}$$

(See Figure 21.8.) For the case of two transducers, τ_d is the difference in time between the received echos.

This processing assumes that the scattering volume does not move out of the region of insonification, thus requiring the pulse period, T_0, to be chosen so that the dominant scattering remains common to both pulses. This ensures a similar echo in both returns. When the red blood cells move out of the ultrasonic beam during the processing interval so that the same reflection is not seen in both echos, the resulting effect is called the *transit time effect*, and it poses one limitation to this approach. In [15] a simulation describing transit time effects is presented.

21.3.3 Limitations

Both the Doppler shift and the time domain correlation approaches to measuring blood flow assume minimal motion of the scatterers. Doppler methods assume that the particles do not move out of the range resolution cell corresponding to the transmitted signal. Time domain correlation methods assume the particles do not move out of the scattering region of insonification. In both cases, the duration of insonification (pulse length), T, is limited by the velocity of the scatterers.

For Doppler processing, this limitation can be summarized by the condition called the *narrowband condition* [6]:

$$\frac{2v}{c} \ll \frac{1}{TB}, \tag{21.7}$$

where $v = |\bar{v}|$ is the maximum speed of any particular scatterer, c is the speed of sound, B is the bandwidth of the transmit signal, and TB is the time-bandwidth product of the signal.

This is a condition not only on the bandwidth of the signal, but more so on the time-bandwidth product of the signal relative to the motion of the scatterers. Rewriting this equation as

$$vT \ll \frac{c}{2B}, \tag{21.8}$$

the restriction becomes clear: in time T, the particles move a distance vT and the processing assumes that the movement of the scatterers is less than the positional resolution of the signal, $c/2B$ (slowly fluctuating scatterers).

For time domain correlation, the condition becomes

$$vT_o < I, \tag{21.9}$$

where I is the insonification region or 3-dB beam width of the transducer's focal region.

Table 21.1
Some Limitations

Method	Limitations
Doppler	• sensitive to phase measurements of f_d • dependent on f_c and f_d • multiple Doppler shifts for broadband signal are not measured • requires knowledge of transducer angle • limited by velocity • measures axial velocity, not vector velocity
Time Domain	• suffers from transit time effects • duration of pulse is limited • requires multiple pulses to make measurmenet • limited by velocity • measures axial velocity, not vector velocity

Another limitation for the Doppler approach is the reliance on the center frequency, f_c, and the Doppler shift, f_d, when computing axial velocity from (21.4). With a wideband transmit signal, the definition of center frequency becomes vague [24]. The center frequency is also affected by various aspects of pulse propagation in tissue. Frequency-dependent attenuation lowers the center frequency while Rayleigh scattering raises the center frequency. Acoustic speckle can either increase or decrease the center frequency. These frequency changes introduce errors into the measurement of axial velocity when using

$$f_d = \frac{2v}{c} f_c.$$

In addition, for a wideband signal, a single scatterer may give rise to a spectrum of Doppler shifts of the transmit signal (frequency-dependent frequency shifts) so that a single Doppler shift is an inaccurate measurement of the compression or dilation a signal undergoes. Therefore, it is desirable to apply a technique whose measurement is independent of f_c and f_d.

These issues with Doppler measurements lead to the use of time domain correlation techniques. As noted above, they too have their limitations. The main shortfall is the transit time effect. The assumption that the scattering volume does not change from pulse to pulse is a major assumption. To meet it, pulse durations must remain short, thereby limiting potential benefits from new signal designs.

Table 21.1 summarizes some of the limitations of these two approaches.

As new devices become available with higher center frequencies and larger time-bandwidth products, along with a desire to increase the processing interval, T, for improved frequency resolution, the narrowband condition and the processing assumptions become easier and easier to violate. Since velocity resolution is proportional to $1/T$ and since transit time effects are dependent on T, a long time duration is desired. Similarly, since range resolution is proportional to $1/B$, a large bandwidth is desired. But increasing TB makes it easier to violate the narrowband condition and processing assumptions. Thus, new approaches to signal processing of ultrasound signals for blood flow measurements are needed that do not have limitations on the velocity of the scatterers.

In the next section, we describe a wideband/wavelet transform approach where the processing interval is no longer limited by the velocity of the particles. Instead, in the wideband/wavelet case, the processing is limited by the acceleration of the particles, with the *wideband condition* being [30, 33]:

$$T < \sqrt{\frac{c}{2Ba}}. \tag{21.10}$$

Here $a = |\bar{a}|$ is the maximum acceleration of the particles. This condition allows for signals with higher time-bandwidth products to be used.

21.3.4 Summary of Desirable Signal Characteristics

(i) *Large bandwidth, B*: range resolution is inversely proportional to B.

(ii) *Long pulse duration, T*: Doppler resolution is inversely proportional to T, and transit time effects decrease with larger T.

(iii) *High time-bandwidth product, TB*: energy, gain, and SNR increase with TB.

21.4 Wideband/Wavelet Transform Processing

21.4.1 Wavelet Transform Processing

As new devices evolve whose transmit signals have larger fractional bandwidths, along with the benefits from increasing the processing duration T (and therefore TB) for improved resolution and increased gain, the conventional narrowband approaches may need to be replaced by wideband techniques [3]. Such techniques have been investigated recently by [9, 23], but in [9] only the envelope of the signal is scaled, as opposed to the entire time-series as presented below. In [23], these ideas were not pursued.

The wideband/wavelet transform approach does not use f_c nor f_d in the calculation of axial velocity as the Doppler technique does, and it does not require two pulses as time domain correlation does. It still applies a cross-correlation to obtain robustness as in time domain correlation; however, it does not limit the pulse length, T. Therefore, wavelet processing attains some immunity to transit time effects as desired. Finally, since ultrasound signals for blood flow measurements are wideband by design, the wideband/wavelet transform approach applies the necessary wideband processing.

A wideband signal is a signal whose fractional bandwidth (B/f_c) is greater than approximately 10%. Wideband processing is also required when the narrowband condition $(vT \ll c/(2B))$ is violated. If $f(t)$ is a wideband signal that is transmitted and reflected off a point scatterer with uniform radial velocity, v, then the received signal, $g(t)$, is approximated by [16]

$$g(t) \simeq \sqrt{s}\, f(s(t - \tau)), \tag{21.11}$$

where $s = (c-v)/(c+v)$ is the time-scaling (compression or dilation) of the signal and τ is the round-trip travel time. The factor $\sqrt{s}$ is used to maintain energy normalization between the transmitted and received signals. This approximation is derived in the Appendix.

When the transmitted signal is scattered from a continuous distribution of scatterers, the acoustic velocity potential at the receiver is simply a superposition of contributions from each scale, s, and delay, τ. Writing this superposition as an integral yields the received acoustic velocity potential:

$$g(t) \simeq \int\int S(s,\tau)\sqrt{s}f(s(t-\tau))\,ds\,d\tau, \tag{21.12}$$

where the weight $S(s,\tau)$ describes the distribution of scatterers in s and τ. The integration is over the delay and scale values corresponding to the range and velocity of the scattering volume of interest. It can be shown [29] that this expression for $g(t)$ is in the form of an inverse wavelet transform.

This equation shows that the received acoustic velocity potential is a weighted integration of replicas of the source signal. In deriving this equation, the incident wave was *not* assumed to be planar, the scattering volume was *not* assumed to be in the far field, and the medium was *not* assumed to be at rest, and thus provides a more general relationship between the transmitted and received signals.

For narrowband signals, the Doppler shift, f_d, is an approximation to the time-scaling, s, a signal undergoes when reflected from a moving object:

$$f_d \simeq (s-1)f_c \tag{21.13}$$

where f_c is the center frequency of the transmitted signal. For truly wideband signals, different frequencies in the band will have different Doppler

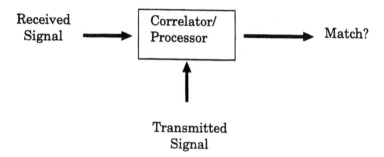

Figure 21.9
Input/Output correlation approach to measuring delay and scale.

shifts, and a single Doppler shift will not accurately reflect the collection
of Doppler shifts the signal undergoes. This Doppler measurement is then
inaccurate, and instead, the compression or dilation, s, of the signal should
be used.

The approach to measuring values of scale, s, and delay, τ, for the wideband case is similar to that of the Doppler shift methods. In both cases,
the transmitted and received signals are fed through a correlator processor
and the peak correlation value is sought. See Figure 21.9.

In narrowband Doppler processing, the received signal is correlated with
time-delayed and Doppler-shifted replicas of the transmitted signal:

$$N_f g(f_d, \tau) = \int_{-\infty}^{\infty} g(t) \overline{f(t-\tau)} e^{-i2\pi f_d t} \, dt. \qquad (21.14)$$

For wideband processing, the received signal is correlated with time-delayed
and time-scaled replicas of the transmitted signal:

$$W_f g(s, \tau) = \frac{1}{\sqrt{s}} \int_{-\infty}^{\infty} g(t) \overline{f\left(\frac{t-\tau}{s}\right)} \, dt, \qquad (21.15)$$

Here, the change of variables $s \to 1/s$ is applied to (21.11).

This last equation is the definition of the *continuous wavelet transform*
of $g(t)$ with respect to $f(t)$, denoted $W_f g$. It assumes that $f, g \in L_2(\mathbb{R})$,
where $L_2(\mathbb{R})$ is the space of finite energy signals and that the signal $f(t)$ is
admissible [10] as described in Chapter 1.

In much of the wavelet transform literature, orthogonal dyadic wavelet
transforms are chosen [7]. These transforms have proven very effective in
speech and image processing, data compression, subband coding, and many
other areas [1, 4, 5, 17–20, 25]. They are not only effective but also efficient:
wavelet transform computations are on the order of $O(N)$ (cf. Chapter 2);

recall that the fast Fourier transform is $O(N \log(N))$. However, for certain applications such as wideband processing, the mother wavelet must not only be a specific function, namely, the transmitted signal, but it must also assume a continuous range of delay and scale values. Although orthogonal mother wavelets could, theoretically, be applied to wideband processing, the efficiencies they offer are usually lost [31]. Instead, continuous wavelet transforms are required.

By using this wideband/wavelet transform approach to blood flow velocimetry, three advantages result:

(i)   The narrowband assumption is removed:

$$\frac{2v}{c} \ll \frac{1}{TB}.$$

Acceleration, not velocity is now the limiting factor of the processing.

(ii) The actual scale value, s, is used, not f_d: $f_d \simeq (s-1)f_c$, so that a more accurate measurement of the compression/dilation effects that the moving particles have on the signal results. For wideband signals, this is important, since different frequencies will have different Doppler shifts.

(iii) The wideband/wavelet transform processing accounts for first order time variations; the argument of $f(s(t - \tau))$ is of the form $\alpha t + \beta$ with αt accounting for the first order time variations.

The goal now is to obtain estimates of the values of delay, τ, and scale, s, corresponding to scatterers in the environment.

21.4.2   Parameter Estimation

To determine values of s and τ for each scatterer, one must correlate the received signal $g(t)$ with hypothesized replicas of the transmitted signal $f(t)$. The hypothesized delay and scale values are denoted by τ' and s', respectively. The correlation is a wideband correlation, which under a change of variables, is a continuous wavelet transform of $g(t)$ with respect to the mother wavelet $f(t)$:

$$W_f g(s', \tau') = \frac{1}{\sqrt{s'}} \int_{-\infty}^{\infty} g(t) \overline{f\left(\frac{t - \tau'}{s'}\right)} \, dt. \qquad (21.16)$$

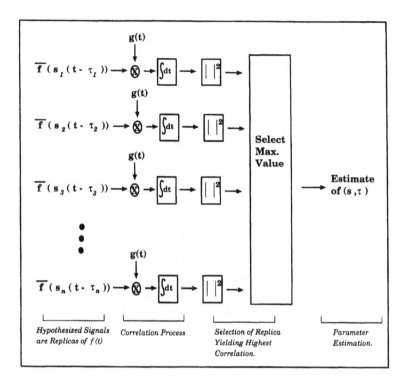

Figure 21.10
Parameter estimation process.

The magnitude of this correlation peaks at values of $s = s'$ and $\tau = \tau'$ associated with scatterers in the blood vessel. Figure 21.10 shows a block diagram of the correlation process. Shown are n hypothesized delay and scale values. The output with the greatest magnitude determines the values of delay, τ, and scale, s, corresponding to scatterers. For a point scatterer, this is the maximum likelihood estimate of delay and scale in the presence of white Gaussian noise. From these values, the associated range, R, and axial velocity, v_a, of each scatterer can be determined. For a distributed scatterer, an estimate of $S(s, \tau)$ results. Dixon and Sibul [8] describe estimating S when the distributed object is a sphere.

By computing the wavelet transform of the received signal with respect to the transmitted signal, one obtains a value of delay, τ, and scale, s, for each scatterer (point scattering) in the blood vessel. These delay and scale values map to range and axial velocity as follows:

$$R = \frac{c\tau}{2}, \quad v_a = \frac{c(1-s)}{1+s}. \tag{21.17}$$

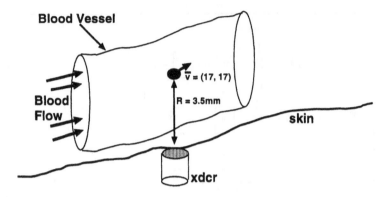

Figure 21.11
Transducer and vessel geometry for example.

The axial velocity is no longer computed using the center frequency and Doppler shift as in Doppler processing. This measurement uses the scale value, s, which accounts for all of the frequency shifts in the wideband signal. In addition, this processing occurs over one observation interval, thereby not requiring multiple transmits as in time domain correlation.

21.4.3 Example

Point Scattering: We provide an example of scattering from a particle in the blood stream. A red blood cell is traveling through the blood vessel at 3.5 mm from the transmitter and with an axial velocity of $v_a = 17$ cm/s as shown in Figure 20.11. Here, $c \simeq 1500$ m/s. The transmitted signal has a center frequency of 5 MHz with a 2.5 MHz bandwidth. This transmitted signal is a linear FM ramping up over the 2.5 MHz bandwidth. The received signal is sampled at 50 MHz and is a time-delayed and time-scaled replica of the transmitted signal. The first 8 μs (400 samples) of the transmitted and received signals are shown in Figure 20.12 and Figure 20.13. Effects of transducer losses, propagation losses, and attenuation have been ignored for now.

The time-bandwidth product of the signal is $TB = 1000$ so that the narrowband condition is violated. The wavelet transform of the received signal with respect to the transmitted signal is then computed using (21.15). Theoretically, the correlation of these two signals should be a delta function located at the position corresponding to the particle in the blood stream. Unfortunately, signal effects broaden the correlation surface so that ambiguities result.

Figure 21.14 shows the resulting wavelet transform plotted on a 25 dB vertical axis. The scale axis is plotted logarithmically. The peak of the wavelet transform is at $(\tau, s) = (4.7\mu s, 0.99977)$. Inserting these values into

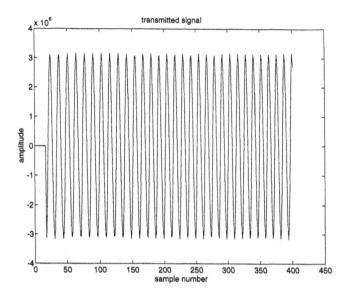

Figure 21.12
First 8 μs of transmit signal.

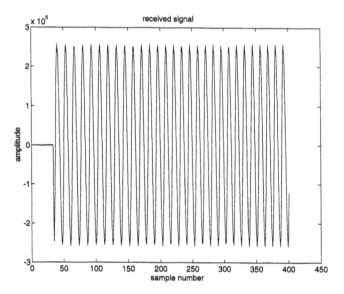

Figure 21.13
First 8 μs of received signal.

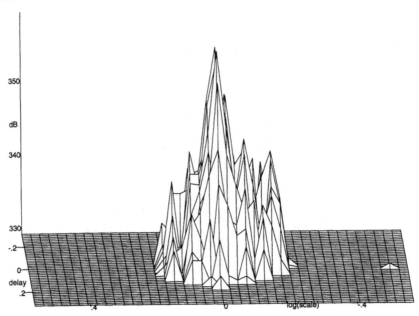

Figure 21.14
Wavelet transform of signal reflected from particle on a 25 dB vertical axis.

(21.17) yields the estimate R' of range and the estimate v_a' of axial velocity:

$$R' = 3.525 \text{ mm} \quad v_a' = 17.25 \text{ cm/s}. \tag{21.18}$$

The errors associated with these estimates are:

$$\text{range error} = 0.7\% \quad \text{axial velocity error} = 1.5\%. \tag{21.19}$$

We now compare this with narrowband processing of these wideband signals. If the same wideband transmit and receive signals are processed using the narrowband Doppler correlator in (21.1), the delay-Doppler surface that results is shown in Figure 21.15. As with the wavelet transform, this figure is plotted on a 25 dB vertical axis and theoretically should be a delta function. Resolution in delay is seen to be acceptable; however, an unacceptable amount of spectral broadening can be seen, which makes it difficult to determine the correct Doppler shift to insert in (21.4). The reason for this broadening is the narrowband condition (21.7) is violated, yet narrowband processing was applied. In cases such as this, the wideband/wavelet transform approach is required.

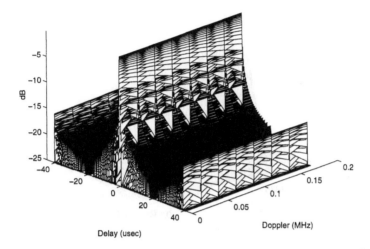

Figure 21.15
Narrowband Doppler processing of same wideband signals.

Distributed Scattering: When the transmitted signal is reflected from a distribution of scatterers, the wavelet transform describes the distribution of scatterers in delay and scale. Figure 21.16 shows the wavelet transform that results when the distributed scatterer is a rotating sphere [29]. This example is not from a distribution of red blood cells, but rather a simulation of a wideband signal reflected from a sphere rotating under water and then processed as above. In the case of a distribution of red blood cells, the wavelet transform assumes a shape that corresponds to the velocity profile of the distribution of cells. The principles are generally the same as for a distribution of particles in the blood stream; the figure is included for illustrative purposes and is plotted on a 25 dB vertical axis.

The large peak indicates the return from the front of the sphere closest to the transducer, while the decrease in amplitude on both sides of the peak indicates weaker acoustic returns from the sides of the sphere. The spread across the scale axis measures the different axial velocities of the rotating sphere relative to the transducer axis. Again, many important acoustic affects such as creeping waves were ignored for this example.

21.5   Conclusions

It was shown that range and axial velocity measurements of particles in the blood stream can be obtained by using wideband/wavelet transform techniques. This processing allows for several assumptions to be removed.

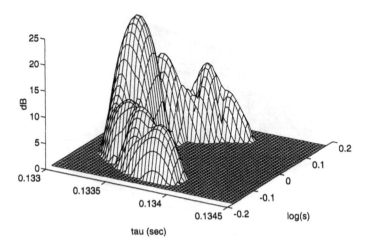

Figure 21.16
Wavelet transform of wideband signal reflected from rotating sphere.

Instead of measuring the Doppler shift associated with the reflection, the time-scaling of the signal is obtained. This time-scaling more accurately reflects the effects of motion on a signal than does a Doppler shift since a Doppler shift is an approximation to time-scaling.

By computing a continuous wavelet transform of the received echo with respect to the transmitted signal, the processing is no longer limited by transit time effects or spectral broadening as are the conventional techniques of time domain correlation or Doppler processing. An example was provided comparing the conventional Doppler approach to the wavelet transform approach. This example shows that when the narrowband assumption is violated, the standard blood flow measurement methods are lacking, while the wavelet transform approach is not, since wavelet transform processing of high time-bandwidth signals more accurately accounts for the effects of compression and dilation in a signal when reflected from moving red blood cells.

21.6   Acknowledgment

The author thanks Ken L. Hillsley for many helpful comments on this manuscript.

21.7 Appendix

Here, we derive (21.11), showing that the received signal is a time-scaled replica of the transmitted signal.

If the transmitter is moving along the x axis towards the scatterer with uniform speed, v, relative to the surrounding fluid, then the wave equation for the acoustic velocity potential, g, at the scatterer is [21]:

$$\nabla^2 g - \frac{1}{c^2} \frac{\partial^2 g}{\partial t^2} = -f(t)\delta(x - vt)\delta(y). \qquad (21.20)$$

Using a sequence of coordinate transformations as presented in Morse and Ingard [21], this wave equation for a moving transmitter can be reduced to that of the equivalent problem of radiation from a stationary source.

The new wave equation is then:

$$\nabla''^2 g - \frac{1}{c^2} \frac{\partial^2 g}{\partial t''^2} = -\gamma^2 f(t'')\delta(x'')\delta(y''), \qquad (21.21)$$

where $''$ denotes the new coordinates,

$$\gamma = \frac{1}{\sqrt{1 - \beta^2}}, \quad \beta = \frac{v}{c},$$

and c is the speed of sound. The solution to this wave equation is

$$g(r'', t'') = \frac{\gamma^2}{4\pi r''} f\left(t'' - \frac{r''}{c}\right), \qquad (21.22)$$

where, $r'' = \sqrt{x''^2 + y''^2}$, and subsonic motion of the transmitter is assumed. Transforming back to the initial variables, x, t, the argument of f in (21.22), which describes the scattering effects on the transmitted signal, becomes:

$$t'' - \frac{r''}{c} = t - \frac{\beta(x - vt) + \sqrt{(x - vt)^2 + (1 - \beta^2)y^2}}{c(1 - \beta^2)}. \qquad (21.23)$$

When the source and the scatterer are colocated on the x axis (transducer axis) so that $y = 0$, then the argument (21.22) becomes:

$$t'' - \frac{r''}{c} = \frac{t - \frac{x}{c}}{1 - \beta} = s't - s'\tau, \qquad (21.24)$$

where

$$s' = \frac{1}{1 - \beta} \quad \text{and} \quad \tau = \frac{x}{c}$$

is the propagation delay corresponding to the scatterer's range at the time the signal is transmitted. For two-way propagation where the (moving) transmitter and receiver are colocated, the argument (21.24) becomes:

$$t'' - \frac{r''}{c} = \frac{1 - \frac{v}{c}}{1 + \frac{v}{c}}\left(t - \frac{x}{c}\right) = st - s\tau, \quad \text{with } s = \frac{1 - \frac{v}{c}}{1 + \frac{v}{c}} \tag{21.25}$$

This yields

$$g(r'', t) = \tilde{\gamma}(x'')\sqrt{s}f(st - s\tau). \tag{21.26}$$

Here, $\tilde{\gamma}(x'')$ accounts for γ and the range-dependent propagation effects. By reciprocity, when the scatterer is moving and the transmitter is stationary, the received velocity potential remains unchanged. Suppressing the range-dependent propagation effects on g in (21.26) then yields (21.11). This says the received acoustic velocity potential, $g(t)$, is an attenuated, delayed, and scaled replica of the transmitted signal, $f(t)$.

References

[1] M. Antonini, M. Barlaud, D. Mathieu, and I. Daubechies. Image Coding Using Wavelet Transform. *IEEE Trans. on Image Proc.*, 1(2):205–220, 1992.

[2] D. W. Baker. Pulsed Ultrasonic Doppler Blood-Flow Sensing. *IEEE Trans. on Sonics and Ultrasonics*, SU-17(3):170-185, 1970.

[3] O. Bonnefous and P. Pesque. Time-domain formulation of pulse-doppler ultrasound and blood velocity estimation by cross correlation. *Ultrasonic Imaging*, 8:73-85, 1986.

[4] R. R. Coifman. Multiresolution Analysis in Nonhomogeneous Media. In *Wavelets: Time-Frequency Methods and Phase Space*, J. M. Combes, et al., eds., 2nd Edition, Springer-Verlag, New York, 1989.

[5] R. R. Coifman. Wavelet Analysis and Signal Processing. In *Signal Processing, Part I: Signal Processing Theory*, L. Auslander et al. eds., IMA, Vol. 22, Springer-Verlag, New York, 1990.

[6] C. E. Cook and M. Bernfeld. *Radar Signals, An Introduction to Theory and Applications*, Academic Press, 1967.

[7] I. Daubechies. *Ten Lectures on Wavelets*, SIAM, Philadelphia, 1992.

[8] T. L. Dixon and L. H. Sibul. Wideband imaging of the rotating sphere: A wavelet transform approach, *Proc. 27th Ann. Asilomar Conf. Signals, Systems, and Computers*, Pacific Grove, CA, Nov. 1–3, 1993.

[9] K. W. Ferrara and V. R. Algazi. A new wideband spread target maximum likelihood estimator for blood velocity estimation — Part I: Theory, and Part II: Evaluation of Estimators with Experimental Data, *IEEE Trans. Ult., Ferr, and Freq. Cont.*, 38(1):1–16, 17–26, 1991.

[10] A. Grossmann and J. Morlet. Decomposition of Hardy functions into square integrable wavelets of constant shape. *SIAM J. Math. Anal.*, 15(4):723–736, 1984.

[11] I. Hein and W. O'Brien, Jr. Volumetric measurement of pulsatile flow via ultrasound time-domain correlation. *J. Cardiovascular Tech.*, 8(4):339–348, 1989.

[12] I. Hein, V. Suorsa, J. Zachary, R. Fish, J. Chen, W. Jenkins, and W. O'Brien, Jr. Accurate and precise measurement of blood flow using ultrasound time-domain correlation. *Ultrasonics Symp.*, 881–886, 1989.

[13] I. Hein, J. Zachary, R. Fish, and W. O'Brien, Jr. In vivo measurement of blood flow using ultrasound time-domain correlation. *Acoustical Imaging*, 19:311–315, 1992.

[14] I. Hein and W. O'Brien, Jr. Current time-domain methods for assessing tissue motion by analysis from reflected ultrasound echoes — a review. *IEEE Trans. Ultrasonics, Ferr., Freq. Control*, 40(2):84–102, 1993.

[15] S. Jones and D. Giddens. A simulation of transit time effects in doppler ultrasound signals. *Ultrasound in Med. and Biol.*, 16(6):607–619, 1990.

[16] E. J. Kelly and R. P. Wishner. Matched-filter theory for high-velocity targets. *IEEE Trans. Military Elect.*, 9:56–69, 1965.

[17] S. G. Mallat. A theory for multiresolution signal decomposition: The wavelet representation. *IEEE Trans. Pattern Anal. Mach. Intel.*, 11(7):674–693, 1989.

[18] S. G. Mallat. Multifrequency channel decompositions of images and wavelet models. *IEEE Trans. Acoust. Speech Signal Proc.*, 37(12): 2091–2110, 1989.

[19] S. G. Mallat. Multiresolution approach to wavelets in computer vision. In *Wavelets: Time-Frequency Methods and Phase Space*, J. M. Combes et al., eds., 2nd ed., Springer-Verlag, New York, 313–327, 1989.

[20] S. G. Mallat. Multiresolution approximations and wavelet orthonormal bases of $L_2(\mathbb{R})$. *Trans. Amer. Math. Soc.*, 315(1):69–87, 1989.

[21] P. M. Morse and K. U. Ingard. *Theoretical Acoustics*, Princeton University Press, New Jersey, 1968, Chapter 11.

[22] H. Naparst. Dense target signal processing. *IEEE Trans. Inf. Theory*, 37(2):317–327, 1991.

[23] M. de Olinger. Ultrasonic blood flow imaging using correlation processing. Ph.D. thesis, Michigan State University, 1981.

[24] A. W. Rihaczek. *Principles of High Resolution Radar*, McGraw Hill, 1969.

[25] O. Rioul and M. Vetterli. Wavelets and signal processing. In *Signal Process. Mag.*, 8(4):14–38, 1991.

[26] S. Satomura. Ultrasonic doppler method for the inspection of cardiac function. *JASA*, 29:1181–1185, 1957.

[27] K. K. Shung. Physics of blood echogenicity. *J. Cardiocasc. Ultrasonography*, (2):401–406,1983,

[28] K. K. Shung, M.B. Smith, and B. Tsui. *Principles of Medical Imaging*, Academic Press, Inc., 1992.

[29] L. H. Sibul, L. G. Weiss, and T. L. Dixon. Characterization of stochastic propagation and scattering via Gabor and wavelet transforms. *J. Computational Acoustics*, 345–369, 1994.

[30] J. L. Stewart and E. C. Westerfield. A theory of active sonar detection. *Proc. IRE*, 872–881, 1959.

[31] L. G. Weiss. Wavelets and wideband correlation processing. *IEEE Signal Process. Mag.*, 1994.

[32] P. Wells. A range-gated ultrasonic doppler system. *Med. Biol. Eng.*, 7:641–652, 1969.

[33] R. K. Young. *Wavelet Theory and Its Applications*, Kluwer Academic Publishers, Boston, 1993.

22

Wavelet Models of Event-Related Potentials

Jonathan Raz[1] and Bruce Turetsky[2]

[1] *Department of Biostatistics, School of Public Health, University of Michigan, Ann Arbor, MI*
[2] *Department of Psychiatry, University of Pennsylvania, Philadelphia, PA*

22.1 Introduction

Event-related potentials (ERPs) are the brain electrical potentials associated with sensory and cognitive processing. In an ERP experiment, a sensory stimulus is presented to a human subject or experimental animal, and the brain electrical activity is recorded by electrodes on the scalp or implanted in the skull or brain. We refer to the brain electrical response to the stimulus as the "evoked potential." Following Vaughan [13], we use the general term "ERP" to include potentials associated with cognitive, rather than strictly sensory, processing.

Analysis of ERP data requires separation of the recorded potentials into component waveforms and estimation of the effects of experimental conditions and disease states on the components. There are two conventional approaches to decomposition and statistical analysis of ERPs: (i) frequency domain filtering followed by identification of peaks and statistical analysis of peak amplitudes, and (ii) principal component analysis (PCA) with varimax rotation followed by statistical analysis of the factor scores [5, 9, 14]. The first approach assumes complete separation of components in time or frequency, while the second assumes factor scores that are uncorrelated and "components" (factor loadings) that are constrained by the varimax criterion. This chapter describes a wavelet approach that allows components to overlap in time and frequency while avoiding the unrealistic mathematical constraints of PCA. We estimate changes in the amplitudes of entire component waveforms, rather than the individual time points used in peak analysis.

Wavelets are useful in analysis of ERPs, because wavelets, like ERP components, are localized in both time and frequency. Another advantage is that by construction fine-scale wavelets have narrow support, while coarse-scale wavelets have wide support. This is generally true of ERP components, which suggests that wavelets provide a parsimonious representation of ERPs. Our approach uses orthogonal wavelets, but the models still allow for overlap of components in both time and frequency and for nonorthogonal ERP components.

In this chapter we describe a preliminary version of the "single channel wavelet model," and its application to cat auditory evoked potentials. The single channel wavelet model represents ERPs as linear combinations of component waveforms. The decomposition is uniquely determined by prior information about times and frequencies of the components and differential effects of the experimental conditions. Thus, the single channel wavelet gives a decomposition based on scientific knowledge about ERPs, rather than on the mathematically convenient but sometimes unrealistic constraints imposed by PCA. The traditional approach of measuring peak amplitudes in filtered ERPs also requires prior knowledge of times and frequencies for identification of peaks and choice of filter settings. However, the prior knowledge required by peak analysis must be very specific and the components must not overlap in both time and frequency. In contrast, the prior knowledge required by the single channel wavelet model can be quite vague, because uncertainty about component boundaries can be expressed as overlap among the components.

We also describe a preliminary version of the "topographic wavelet model," which generalizes the single channel wavelet model to multichannel data. We give an application to human cognitive ERPs recorded from nine scalp electrodes. In the topographic wavelet model, both time/frequency and topographic information can be used for decomposition of the recorded waveforms and estimation of condition effects. Under the assumptions of a multilinear model [6, 8], the decomposition is unique even if no prior time/frequency information is available; however, using prior time/frequency information yields substantial data reduction and provides numerical stability.

22.2 The Single Channel Wavelet Model

This section presents a preliminary version of the single channel wavelet model that is restricted to two components. We assume that the ERP components are partly separated in time and/or frequency, and that the amplitudes of the two components respond differently to the experimental conditions.

Define $\{y_i(k), k = 0, \ldots, N_0-1\}$ to be the recorded ERP for experimental condition i ($i = 1, \ldots, I$). Also define $\{\gamma_q(k), k = 0, \ldots, N_0 - 1\}$ to be component q ($q = 1, 2$) at the sampled time points, $\boldsymbol{\beta}_q$ to be a vector of amplitude parameters for component q, $\mathbf{x}_i$ to be a design vector defining experimental condition i, and $\{\epsilon_i(k), k = 0, \ldots, N_0 - 1\}$ to be a discrete time random process with mean zero. The parameters $\boldsymbol{\beta}_1$, $\boldsymbol{\beta}_2$, $\{\gamma_1(k), k = 0, \ldots, N_0 - 1\}$, and $\{\gamma_2(k), k = 0, \ldots, N_0 - 1\}$ are unknown quantities to be estimated from the data. In the time domain, the model has the form:

$$y_i(k) = \sum_{q=1}^{2} \exp \langle \boldsymbol{\beta}_q, \mathbf{x}_i \rangle \gamma_q(k) + \epsilon_i(k), \qquad (22.1)$$

$$i = 1, \ldots, I, \quad k = 0, \ldots, N_0 - 1,$$

The exponential $\exp \langle \boldsymbol{\beta}_q, \mathbf{x}_i \rangle$ constrains the condition effects to be positive; we thus incorporate into the model an assumption that experimental conditions do not change the sign of a component waveform. This assumption is based on a premise that each ERP component arises from the activity of a fixed anatomical generator.

We derive the wavelet representation of the model by applying an orthogonal wavelet transformation to each of the I recorded ERPs. Assume $N_0 = 2^J$ for a positive integer J, and define

$$\left\{ d_{ij}(k), j = 1, \ldots, J, k = 1, \ldots, N_0/2^j \right\}$$

to be the detail wavelet coefficients of the recorded ERP $\{y_i(k), k = 0, \ldots, N_0 - 1\}$. Further define

$$\left\{ \delta_{qj}(k), j = 1, \ldots, J, k = 1, \ldots, N_0/2^j \right\}$$

to be the wavelet coefficients of the component $\{\gamma_q(k), k = 0, \ldots, N_0 - 1\}$, and

$$\left\{ \eta_{ij}(k), j = 1, \ldots, J, k = 1, \ldots, N_0/2^j \right\}$$

to be the (random) wavelet coefficients of the noise $\{\epsilon_i(k), k = 0, \ldots, N_0 - 1\}$. Taking the wavelet transform of both sides of model (22.1) gives the representation

$$d_{ij}(k) = \sum_{q=1}^{2} \exp \langle \boldsymbol{\beta}_q, \mathbf{x}_i \rangle \, \delta_{qj}(k) + \eta_{ij}(k), \qquad (22.2)$$

$$i = 1, \ldots, I, \quad j = 1, \ldots, J, \quad k = 1, \ldots, N_0/2^j.$$

For notational simplicity, we omit the lowpass coefficient c_J, but it can be included in the model in the same manner as the detail coefficients.

Note that the unknown model parameters are not necessarily uniquely defined. If $I = 2$, the number of parameters exceeds the number of data points. Even if $I \geq 2$, a unique solution may not exist, because the model may admit an infinite number of equally valid parameter estimates through rotation.

An essential feature of the single channel wavelet model is the assumption that prior information about the components can be used to specify times and frequencies (as represented by the wavelets) that are unique to each component, as well as times and frequencies that may be shared by both components. Assume that there are nonempty sets W_1 and W_2 of scale/translate pairs (j, k) that represent the times/frequencies unique to components 1 and 2, and a possibly empty set $W_{1,2}$ of scale/translate pairs that are shared by both components. Then the single channel model can be written

$$d_{ij}(k) = \begin{cases} \exp \langle \boldsymbol{\beta}_1, \mathbf{x}_i \rangle \, \delta_{1j}(k) + \eta_{ij}(k), & (j,k) \in W_1, i = 1, \ldots, I, \\ \exp \langle \boldsymbol{\beta}_2, \mathbf{x}_i \rangle \, \delta_{2j}(k) + \eta_{ij}(k), & (j,k) \in W_2, i = 1, \ldots, I, \\ \sum_{q=1}^{2} \exp \langle \boldsymbol{\beta}_q, \mathbf{x}_i \rangle \, \delta_{qj}(k) + \eta_{ij}(k), & (j,k) \in W_{1,2}, i = 1, \ldots, I. \end{cases}$$

In this representation, the unknown model parameters to be estimated are $\boldsymbol{\beta}_1, \boldsymbol{\beta}_2, \{\delta_{1j}(k), (j,k) \in W_1 \cup W_{1,2}\}$, and $\{\delta_{2j}(k), (j,k) \in W_2 \cup W_{1,2}\}$. The parameters still are not uniquely defined since we can multiply the factor $\exp \langle \boldsymbol{\beta}_q, \mathbf{x}_i \rangle$ by a positive constant and divide $\delta_{qj}(k)$ by the same constant. Setting the absolute value of one of the $\delta_{qj}(k)$ equal to an arbitrary constant makes all model parameters uniquely defined, even if $I = 2$, assuming that $\boldsymbol{\beta}_1 \neq \boldsymbol{\beta}_2$ (that is, the conditions have different effects on the two components). We can achieve substantial data reduction, because the union of the sets W_1, W_2, and $W_{1,2}$ need not contain all N_0 scale/translate pairs. Although the wavelets are orthogonal, the single channel wavelet model does not assume orthogonal ERP components, since the two components share wavelets with indices in $W_{1,2}$.

We implemented an algorithm for computing ordinary least squares estimates of the model parameters using the Gauss-Newton method.

22.3 Application of the Single Channel Wavelet Model to Cat Auditory Evoked Potentials

We applied the single channel wavelet model to data from a study of the auditory system of cats [4]. Figure 22.1 shows auditory evoked potentials acquired from cats with identification codes JN and NK; each waveform is the average of responses to 2000 stimulus presentations. These plots contrast the responses to low and high stimulus rates (0.2/s and 2/s for JN, and 0.1/s and 5/s for NK). Cat auditory evoked potentials typically exhibit characteristic peaks and troughs called the auditory brainstem response (ABR), wave 7, wave A, wave N_A, and wave C; these features are labeled in Figure 22.1.

In auditory evoked potentials collected from most cats, including cat JN, the wave A peak precedes the wave N_A trough [3, 4], but these two components are completely superimposed in the data recorded from cat NK. To illustrate the ability of the single channel wavelet model to decompose overlapping ERP components, we analyzed the responses of cat NK at six different stimulus rates: 0.1, 0.2, 0.5, 1, 2, and 5 stimuli per second. We defined x_i to be a 6×1 vector with element i equal to 1 and the other elements equal to 0, so that each of the six conditions had a separate amplitude parameter. Before analysis, we took a subset of 256 points between 15.50 and 53.25 milliseconds and extracted every fourth time point to create a data set containing 64 time points for each of six conditions.

We defined sets of scale/translate pairs that assigned the lowest frequencies to wave N_A and higher frequencies to wave A, but constrained wave A to times less than 44 ms, and allowed for a great deal of overlap in frequency. The wavelet coefficients were computed using Daubechies' extremal phase wavelet transform with 6 filter coefficients [2, pp. 194–197], and the single channel wavelet model was fit to the data based on the prior definitions of the sets of scale/translate pairs. We also applied PCA with varimax rotation to the same six waveforms. We rotated the first four principal components, which explained most of the variance, and then extracted the two rotated eigenvectors (factor loadings) that mostly closely resembled the component waveforms generated by the wavelet model.

Figure 22.2 shows the fitted wavelet model (after transformation to the time domain) overlaid on the data, while Figures 22.3(a) and 22.3(b) show the estimated wavelet components and the factor loadings. The wave A

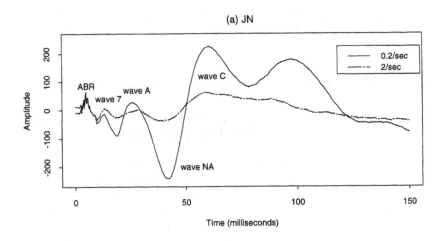

(a) JN

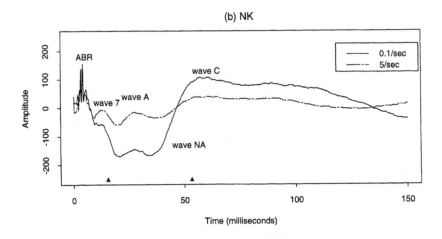

(b) NK

Figure 22.1

Auditory evoked potentials elicited by a click stimulus. (a) Cat JN: stimulus rates of 0.2/s and 2/s. (b) Cat NK: stimulus rates of 0.1/s and 5/s. Positive amplitudes are up. Each waveform is the average of 2000 responses recorded from the vertex. In response to a click stimulus, the cat auditory evoked potential exhibits characteristic peaks and troughs that are called the auditory brainstem response (ABR), wave 7, wave A, wave N_A, and wave C. The amplitudes of wave N_A and C are greatly diminished by the faster stimulus rate. In NK's data, wave A appears to completely overlap the wide trough of wave N_A. We applied the single channel wavelet model to the data in the interval between 15.50 and 53.25 ms poststimulus; the endpoints of the interval are indicated by triangles in plot (b).

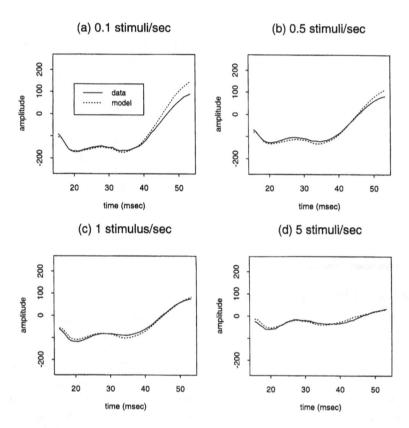

Figure 22.2
Auditory evoked potentials for cat **NK** at four stimulus rates with fitted wavelet model. Wave N_A (the low frequency negative wave) and wave **A** (the higher frequency positive deflection near **30 ms**) are completely superimposed. We separated these components by fitting the single channel wavelet model to data recorded at six stimulus rates. The data and fitted model for four of these experimental conditions are displayed; a similar excellent fit was obtained for the other two conditions. The amplitude of wave N_A clearly decreases with increasing stimulus rate, but inspection of these figures suggests little change in wave **A** amplitude. Analysis with the wavelet model, however, showed a decrease in the amplitude of both components, which is consistent with the results from previous studies.

component shown in Figure 22.3(a) is very similar to that seen in typical recordings [3, Figure 1], while the corresponding factor loadings (the dotted line in Figure 22.3(b)) show a peak that is much broader than the typical cat wave A.

Figure 22.3(c) shows the estimated condition-specific weights $\exp\langle\boldsymbol{\beta}_q, \mathbf{x}_i\rangle$ of each component as a function of stimulus rate, while Figure 22.3(d) shows the factor scores as a function of stimulus rate. The wavelet model clearly indicates that the amplitude of both wave A and wave N_A is a monotonically decreasing function of stimulus rate, which is consistent with previous research [3, 4]. The factor scores indicate a nonmonotonic decrease in wave N_A amplitude with increasing stimulus rate, as well as a very confusing relationship between wave A amplitude and stimulus rate. These results are not surprising, since PCA requires that the condition effects on wave A be uncorrelated with the effects on wave N_A, which contradicts a monotonic decrease in amplitude for both components.

22.4 The Topographic Wavelet Model

We extended the single channel wavelet model to multichannel data by assuming that each component is associated with a topography (pattern of potentials among the scalp locations of the recording electrodes) that does not vary with time or the experimental condition. Like the assumption of positive condition effects, the assumption of invariant topography is motivated by the idea that ERP components represent the activity of fixed anatomical generators. Let α_{lq} be a weight specific to component q and channel l ($l = 1, \ldots, L$), so that the set $\{\alpha_{lq}, l = 1, \ldots, L\}$ defines the topography of component q. In the time domain, our preliminary version of the topographic wavelet model has the form:

$$y_{il}(k) = \sum_{q=1}^{2} \alpha_{lq} \exp\langle\boldsymbol{\beta}_q, \mathbf{x}_i\rangle \gamma_q(k) + \epsilon_{il}(k), \tag{22.3}$$

$$i = 1, \ldots, I, \quad k = 1, \ldots, N_0, \quad l = 1, \ldots, L.$$

where $\{y_{il}(k), k = 0, \ldots, N_0-1\}$ is the set of potentials recorded in channel l under condition i, $\{\epsilon_{il}(k), k = 0, \ldots, N_0-1\}$ is a mean zero random process, and $\boldsymbol{\beta}_q$ and $\mathbf{x}_i$ are defined as in equation (22.1). If we were to replace $\exp\langle\boldsymbol{\beta}_q, \mathbf{x}_i\rangle$ by a single real-valued parameter, say β_{iq}^*, then model (22.3) would have the same trilinear form as the topographic components model (TCM) of Möcks [7, 8] with condition effects replacing subject effects. Since

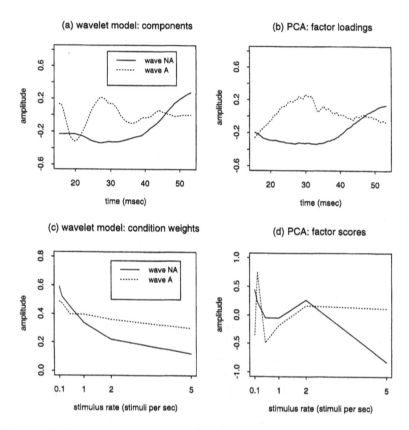

Figure 22.3
Results of wavelet and principal components analyses of the auditory evoked potentials for cat NK. (a) Estimated component waveforms generated by the single channel wavelet model. (b) Varimax-rotated factor loadings for the two principal components that most closely resemble the wavelet components. (c) Estimated condition-specific weights $\exp \langle \beta, x \rangle$ as a function of stimulus rate for each wavelet component. (d) Factor scores corresponding to factor loadings given in (b). The wavelet model shows a monotonic decrease in the amplitude of both components with increasing stimulus rate, which is consistent with previous studies. The factor scores suggest a more confusing relationship between amplitude and stimulus rate. All estimates were rescaled to facilitate comparison between the wavelet model and PCA.

under mild conditions [8], the parameters of TCM are uniquely defined up
to a constant factor, and the topographic wavelet model imposes additional
positivity constraints, the parameters of (22.3) are uniquely defined up to a
constant factor. By setting one of the parameters α_{lq} and the absolute value
of one of the parameters $\gamma_q(k)$ equal to arbitrary constants, we uniquely
define all model parameters.

After wavelet transformation of (22.3), as described for the single channel
wavelet model, we can easily incorporate prior time/frequency information
into the model, thus achieving considerable data reduction and ease of
model-fitting. We successfully implemented the Gauss-Newton method for
fitting the topographic wavelet model to real ERP data. In comparison,
Möcks [7, 8] reported serious algorithmic difficulties when fitting TCM.

22.5   Application of the Topographic Wavelet Model to Human Cognitive ERPs

We applied the topographic wavelet model to analysis of cognitive potentials from a study conducted by Turetsky and Fein [12]. ERPs were
acquired from 10 subjects before and after administration of clonidine in
a three-tone auditory discrimination experiment. Recordings were made
from $L = 9$ mid-saggital electrodes referenced to the left ear and sampled
at 250 Hertz. For each channel and condition, we computed the grand average of all subjects' waveforms. We included $I = 6$ experimental conditions
representing three stimulus types (standard, target, and rare nontarget) for
each of two drug conditions (predrug vs. postdrug), and extracted the 64
time points between 268 and 520 ms post-stimulus. The positive wave in
this interval is called the P300 and has been shown to be related to cognitive processing [1, 10, 11]. Figure 22.4 shows the data recorded at the Fz
(frontal) and Oz (occipital) electrodes for the target and nontarget, predrug
and postdrug conditions.

We defined time/frequency restrictions on the two components based on
previous research that identified a slightly earlier higher frequency component denoted P3a and a slightly lower frequency component denoted P3b
[1, 11, 12]. We allowed a great deal of overlap in both time and frequency.
A total of 12 wavelet coefficients represented the 64×2 time points in
the P3a and P3b components. These two components are known to have
different topographies, with P3b having greater amplitude at more posterior locations. The model included no constraints on the channel weights
α_{lq}, which allowed us to compare the estimated topographies to the known
topographic structure of these components.

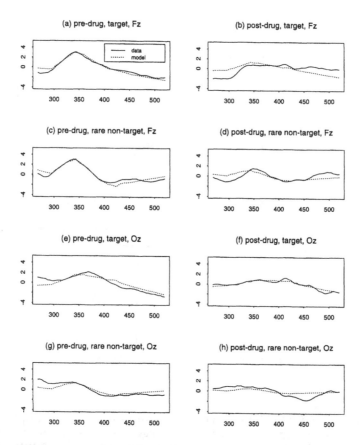

Figure 22.4

Grand average P300 waveforms recorded under four experimental conditions from the Fz (Frontal) and Oz (Occipital) electrodes, with fitted wavelet model. The horizontal axis in each plot gives time in milliseconds, and the vertical axis gives amplitude in microvolts. We applied the topographic wavelet model to recordings from nine mid-saggital electrodes under six experimental conditions. The fit of the model at the other seven electrodes and under the predrug and postdrug standard conditions is similar to that shown here. Even though P3a and P3b are completely superimposed, the wavelet model successfully separated these components. Each of the waveforms generated by the model (dashed lines) is the weighted sum of the two waveforms shown in Figure 22.5(a), with weights that depend on the channel and the condition. The lack of model fit at the beginning and end of the time window suggests the presence of earlier and later components that were not included in the model.

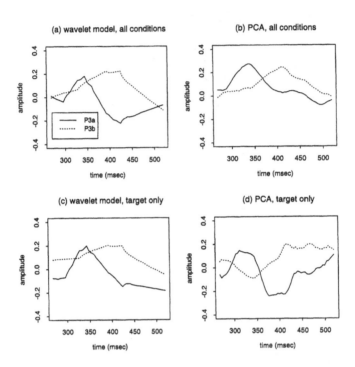

Figure 22.5
Analysis of P300 data: estimated components from applications
to all six conditions and to the target conditions only. (a) Estimated P3a and P3b components generated by applying the
topographic wavelet model to all six conditions. (b) Varimax-
rotated factor loadings that most closely resemble the wavelet
components, generated by applying PCA to all six conditions.
(c) Estimated components generated by applying the topographic
wavelet model to the target conditions only. (d) Varimax-rotated
factor loadings that most closely resemble the wavelet components, generated by applying PCA to the target conditions only.
Separation of P3a and P3b using all conditions is easy, because
P3b appears to be nearly absent in responses to the standard
and rare nontarget stimuli. The wavelet model gave very similar results when applied to the much more difficult problem of
separating the components based only on the target conditions.
All estimates were rescaled to facilitate comparison between the
wavelet model and PCA.

We applied Daubechies' extremal phase wavelet transform with four filter coefficients [2, pp. 194–197], and then fit the topographic wavelet model both with and without an interaction effect between stimulus type and drug condition. Since we obtained quite similar results in the two analyses, we chose the simpler model that excludes the interaction effect.

Figure 22.4 shows the fitted topographic wavelet model (after transformation to the time domain) overlaid on the data, while Figure 22.5(a) shows the estimated P3a and P3b components. Each model waveform given as a dashed line in Figure 22.4 is the weighted sum of the two components in Figure 22.5(a), which are completely superimposed to create only one major peak. The lack of fit near the beginning and the end of the time window suggests the presence of the earlier N250 and later slow wave components.

Compared to the response to the target stimulus, P3a amplitude was reduced by 59% in response to the standard stimulus, and slightly increased in response to the rare non-target stimulus. P3b had essentially zero weight at the standard and rare non-target conditions. This pattern of response is typical of these components [1, 11, 12].

Clonidine reduced P3a amplitude by 62%, while having little effect on P3b amplitude. This result is qualitatively similar to the result reported by Turetsky and Fein [12] using very different statistical methods.

Figure 22.6(a) shows the estimated topography of each component, that is, the estimated α_{lq} plotted against l for $q = 1, 2$. P3a clearly shows a frontocentral topographic peak, while P3b is widely spread over the central to occipital regions. These results are consistent with previous reports of differing P3a and P3b topography [1, 11, 12].

Separation of P3a and P3b in this data set is easy, because P3b appears to be nearly absent in responses to the standard and rare nontarget conditions. To further demonstrate the ability of the topographic wavelet model to separate overlapping components, we analyzed a subset of these data that included only the responses to the target stimulus, both predrug and postdrug. The P3a and P3b components are both present in these responses, and they overlap in time and frequency, so that separation of the components is much more difficult. Nevertheless, the results of this analysis were very similar to the results of the analysis of the full data set. Figure 22.5(c) shows the estimated component waveforms, while figure 22.6(c) show the estimated topographies.

We also applied PCA with varimax rotation to all six conditions (54 waveforms) and to the subset that included only the responses to the target stimulus (18 waveforms). The rotation was applied to the first four PCs, which explained most of the variance. Two of the rotated eigenvectors (factor loadings) were similar to the wavelet components; these loadings are illustrated in Figures 22.5(b) and 22.5(d).

PCA does not define a unique topography for each component, since a separate set of factor scores are generated for each condition. The predrug

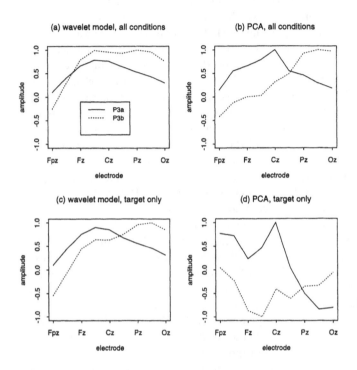

Figure 22.6
Analysis of P300 data: estimated topographies from applications
to all six conditions and to the target conditions only. (a) Estimated channel-specific weights α plotted as a function of scalp location for each of the wavelet components given in Figure 22.5(a).
(b) Factor scores corresponding to the factor loadings given in
Figure 22.5(b). (c) Estimated channel-specific weights for each of
the wavelet components given in Figure 22.5(c). (d) Factor scores
corresponding to the factor loadings given in Figure 22.5(d). The
electrode placements range from the most anterior (Fpz) to the
most posterior (Oz) locations along the midline. The wavelet estimates of P3a and P3b topography are consistent with previous
reports of these components. PCA gave nearly zero weight to
the P3b component at the vertex (Cz) in the application to all
conditions, and gave greatly distorted topography for the target
only data set. All estimates were rescaled to facilitate comparison
between the wavelet model and PCA.

target condition had the ERP with the greatest amplitude, and the factor scores for this condition defined a topography most like that generated by the wavelet model. These factor scores are plotted in Figures 22.6(b) and 22.6(d). As shown in Figure 22.6(b), the factor scores based on the full data set are somewhat similar to the topographies defined by the wavelet model in Figure 22.6(a), although PCA gives little weight to the P3b component at the central electrodes. We conjecture that this result is a distortion arising from the constraints on the factor scores.

Figure 22.6(d) shows that the topographies are greatly distorted in the application to the target only data set. This result was not due to our selection of these particular factor scores: no other sets of factor scores looked more like the topographies we would expect for these components.

22.6 Discussion

This chapter presented preliminary versions of the single channel and topographic wavelet models of event-related potentials. In applications to cat auditory evoked potentials and human cognitive potentials, we contrasted the results of the wavelet analyses to the results of PCA. The wavelet analysis yielded results more consistent with previous studies of these ERPs, and more internally consistent (as in the comparison of the analyses of the full human data set and the subset). We presented models with two ERP components, but the single channel and topographic wavelet models can be generalized easily to more than two components by defining additional sets of scale/translate pairs.

The methods presented here are restricted to analyses of data from one individual (such as cat NK) or data sets constructed by averaging ERPs from many individuals (such as the human cognitive ERPs). We are extending the preliminary versions of the wavelet models to account for variability among individuals.

The ordinary least squares estimators presented here are the maximum likelihood estimators when the noise process is Gaussian white noise. The noise in ERP data is mainly due to background EEG, which is highly correlated, so ordinary least squares estimators may be inefficient, and estimators of their statistical variability will be biased. We also are generalizing the wavelet models and the model-fitting algorithm to account for the noise correlation.

22.7   Acknowledgments

This work was supported by NIH award # 1 R29 MH51310 01A2. We are grateful to Drs. Linda Dickerson and Jennifer Buchwald for providing the cat evoked potentials and for many helpful suggestions.

References

[1] E. Courchesne. Changes in P3 waves with event repetition: long-term effects in scalp distribution and amplitude. *Electroencephalogr. Clin. Neurophysiol.*, 45:754–766, 1978.

[2] I. Daubechies. *Ten Lectures on Wavelets*. SIAM, Philadelphia, 1992.

[3] L. W. Dickerson and J. S. Buchwald. Midlatency auditory-evoked responses: effect of scopolamine in the cat and implications for brain stem cholinergic mechanisms, *Exp. Neurol.*, 112:229–239, 1991.

[4] L. W. Dickerson, and J. S. Buchwald. Long-latency auditory evoked potentials: role of polysensory association cortex in the cat. *Exp. Neurol.*, 202:313–324, 1992.

[5] E. Donchin. A multivariate approach to the analysis of average evoked potentials. *IEEE Trans. Biomed. Eng.*, 13:131–139, 1966.

[6] S. Leurgans and R. T. Ross. Multilinear models: applications to spectroscopy. *Stat. Sci.*, 7:289–319, 1992.

[7] J. Möcks. Decomposing event-related potentials: a new topographic components model. *Biol. Psych.*, 26:199–215, 1988.

[8] J. Möcks. Topographic components model for event-related potentials and some biophysical considerations. *IEEE Trans. Biomed. Eng.*, 35:482–484, 1988.

[9] J. Möcks and R. Verleger. Principal component analysis of event-related potentials: A note on misallocation of variance. *Electroencephalogr. Clin. Neurophysiol.*, 65:393–398, 1986.

[10] D. Regan. *Human Brain Electrophysiology*. Elsevier, New York, 1989.

[11] N. K. Squires, K. C. Squires, and S. A. Hillyard. Two varieties of long-latency positive waves evoked by unpredictable auditory stimuli in man. *Electroencephalogr. Clin. Neurophysiol.*, 38:387–401, 1975.

[12] B. Turetsky, and G. Fein. α_2-noradrenergic effects on ERP and behavioral indices of auditory information processing. Submitted.

[13] H. Vaughan. Relationship of brain activity to scalp recording of event-related potentials. In *Average Evoked Potentials*, E. Donchin and D. B. Lindsley, editors, NASA, Washington, D.C., 1969, 45–94

[14] C. C. Wood, and G. McCarthy. Principal component analysis of event-related potentials: Simulation studies demonstrate misallocation of variance across components. *Electroencephalogr. Clin. Neurophysiol.*, 59:249–260, 1982.

23

Macromolecular Structure Computation Based on Energy Function Approximation by Wavelets

Eberhard Schmitt

IMB-Institute for Molecular Biotechnology, Beutenbergstraße, Jena, Germany

Abstract   We outline an approach using domain decomposition and wavelet techniques to analyze the geometry of macromolecules and to investigate important physical properties by means of simulations. The classical method of force field calculations requires minimizing of the energy as a function of the Cartesian coordinates of all atoms. Presently this method is limited to relatively small molecules due to the large number of degrees of freedom, which leads to severe problems in the minimization procedure. In our approach, we reduce the number of free variables by assembling certain groups of atoms into configurational structures with considerably less degrees of freedom. In this way, a whole hierarchy of coordinate spaces with decreasing dimensions is defined. Furthermore, approximations to the energy function with respect to these variables are constructed using methods from the theory of splines and wavelets. The problem of global approximation on the parameter manifolds leads to a unified approach to constructing wavelets on $SO(3)$, S^3, and S^2. Therefore we also address another subject related to biological and medical applications, namely, the representation of surfaces, for example in tomography.

23.1   Introduction

The analysis of the 3-D structure of macromolecules, especially of biologically interesting proteins, nucleic acids, and DNA-protein complexes, has become more and more important within the last few years due to questions arising in the fields of protein engineering, drug design, and gene transcription. Rapid progress in the areas of biochemistry, molecular biology, and biophysics calls for new methods in the theoretical computation of macromolecular structures to reduce efforts and costs in the design of experiments for understanding enzymes and biocatalysis or the structural basis of genetic expression.

Presently, the methods to compute the 3-D structure of macromolecules concentrate mainly on two approaches based on the knowledge of the energy function of the molecule: force field minimization and molecular dynamics simulations. In the first method, one tries to find a minimum of the total internal energy of the molecule. In the second approach, a trajectory of the equations of motion near an equilibrium structure is computed and statistically evaluated. The motivation comes from the laws of classical and quantum mechanics.

The structure of a molecule in space is determined by the interaction of its n atoms having the Cartesian coordinates $\mathbf{x}_i \in \mathcal{R}^3$, $1 \leq i \leq n$. Interaction energies are described by analytical functions derived theoretically from quantum mechanics and empirically from experiments. The energy functions depend on distances between bonded and nonbonded atoms as well as on bond and torsion angles which are computed from the coordinates $\mathbf{x}_i$. The total internal energy E of the molecule consists of four contributions (see, e.g., [10, 19, 21])

$$E = E_{bond} + E_{angle} + E_{torsion} + E_{NB}, \qquad (23.1)$$

namely, the bonding energy, the angle energy, the torsion angle energy, and the nonbonding energy contributions. There exist slightly different approximations for these four energy functions ([11, 21]), especially for E_{NB}. In specific examples, we always refer to the implementation of the consistent force field as done in the AMBER program package [21]. Here, for example,

$$E_{bond} = \sum_{(i,j) \in I_{bond}} K_{Bij} (\|\mathbf{x}_i - \mathbf{x}_j\| - R_{0ij})^2$$

denotes the energy contribution of all pairs of bonded atoms. Energies E_{angle} of bonding angles between three atoms connected by two bonds are described by quadratic potentials as well. Truncated Fourier series

$$E_{torsion} = \sum_{I_{torsion}} \left(E_{1-4} + \sum_{\nu=1}^{6} K_{\theta ijkl\nu} \left(1 + \cos(\nu\theta_{ijkl} + \delta_{\nu ijkl}) \right) \right)$$

denote the energy contributions arising from torsion angles. In this expression, $I_{torsion}$ denotes the index set of all torsion angles θ_{ijkl} formed by all sequences of four consecutively bonded atoms i, j, k, and l. Here θ_{ijkl} depends on the position of the four atoms i, j, k, and l. The phase factor $\delta_{\nu ijkl}$ and the force constant $K_{\theta ijkl\nu}$ are defined by the force field. All the constants depend on the atoms involved as well as on their structural neighbors. The nonbonding energy $E_{NB} = E_C + E_{HB} + E_{vdW}$ is a sum over all pairs of nonbonded atoms and includes the long-range Coulomb forces E_C, the hydrogen bond potentials E_{HB}, and the van der Waals forces E_{vdW}. The potentials are inverse powers of the respective atomic distances (r^{-1} for E_C, combinations of r^{-6}, r^{-10}, r^{-12} for E_{HB} and E_{vdW}).

A stable three-dimensional structure of the molecule corresponds to a minimum of the total internal energy E_{total}. In consistent force field calculations, the minimum of the total internal energy is usually computed iteratively by means of gradient methods. The location of atoms is described by their Cartesian coordinates. Thus a function of $3n$ variables

$$E : \mathcal{R}^{3n} \longrightarrow \mathcal{R}$$

has to be minimized. It is clear that this configuration space is far too large, as only a small part of the configurations is feasible. Within the minimization step, the function and its partial derivatives have to be evaluated and a new improved estimate for the actual configuration with a lower total internal energy is calculated. The high dimension (approximately $100 - 10,000$) of the space of free variables leads to severe problems in the minimization process, as observed, e.g., in [19]. It is therefore a major goal to reduce the large number of parameters significantly.

We will describe the application of domain decomposition (cf. [2]) and approximation by wavelets in the case of force field minimization. But the method can also be applied to molecular dynamics simulations. Here, one should keep in mind, that the motion of atoms in biological macromolecules cover a wide range of time scales. The fastest vibrations consist in the motion of pairs of chemically bonded atoms oscillating around their average distance with periods in the order of 10^{-15} seconds. This type of motion is highly localized and largely independent of the global conformation of the molecule. The other extreme is found in the folding of proteins, which range in the time scale of 10^{-3} to 10^2 seconds or even longer. The biological function is mostly related to the slower type of motions covering the time scales from 10^{-9} seconds and above. Here, many atoms are always involved. For any structure $\mathbf{R} \in \mathcal{R}^{3n}$, one can identify directions related to fast and slow motions, respectively. The space of motion, the tangent space $\mathcal{T}$ to $\mathbf{R}$, can therefore be decomposed into subspaces $\mathcal{T}_F$ (fast) and $\mathcal{T}_S$ (slow)

$$\mathcal{T} = \mathcal{T}_F \oplus \mathcal{T}_S.$$

The method described here takes advantage of the fact that for large molecules the dimension of $\mathcal{T}_S$, which we are interested in, is considerably smaller compared to the dimension of $\mathcal{T}_F$. This fact has also been used by Amadei et al. [1] in their approach to reduce the number of degrees of freedoms dynamically in molecular simulations.

One can furthermore expect that the hierarchical features of wavelet decompositions are the appropriate counterpart on the function level to deal with the principal difficulty of interrelating rather different physical scales. Though we are interested mainly in the macroscopic effects, local effects on the atomic level should not be neglected. It should therefore be important to choose mathematical representations that reflect such hierarchies of scales in an appropriate fashion. If the energy function is approximated by wavelets, the costs of evaluating the energy function at a point remain independent of the discretization level. Efficient and stable subdivision techniques facilitate local refinements. Data compression techniques can be used to evaluate the function with variable accuracy in the optimization procedure. This provides a most natural framework for employing adaptive methods which are ultimately indispensable for handling problems of interesting size.

In the following sections, we will describe the reduction of the number of degrees of freedom by domain decomposition and the approximation of the energy functions by wavelets. As we have in mind the computation of minima, we are mainly interested in differentiable wavelets.

23.2 Hierarchical Domain and Function Decomposition

23.2.1 Reduction of the Degrees of Freedom

To reduce the number of free variables, we assemble certain groups of atoms into one configurational structure which can be described by fewer variables than the number of all atom coordinates involved. This process

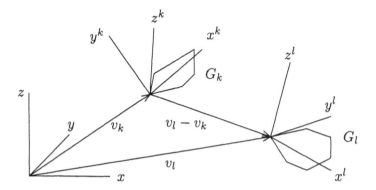

Figure 23.1
Two molecular subunits G_l and G_k in the global coordinate system (x, y, z). The positions of the atoms are defined by their local coordinates in the systems (x_l, y_l, z_l) and (x_k, y_k, z_k), respectively. The global atom coordinates are therefore given by the transformation $(x, y, z)^T = A_i \cdot (x_i, y_i, z_i)^T + v_i$ for $i \in \{l, k\}$.

will be iterated to yield a whole hierarchy of coordinate spaces of decreasing dimensions.

The position of the atoms of a single subunit is defined in a local Cartesian coordinate system (compare Figure 23.1). In the easiest case, the substructure is rigid. Then all its atoms have a fixed position, and the respective substructure is completely described by giving the atomic coordinates in the local coordinate system. As examples for this case, we mention the bases and the phosphate group in DNA molecules, or some of the small amino acids in proteins. All these configurational substructures can be regarded as rigid, at least for a first approximation.

But there are also subunits of macromolecules which demand a certain flexibility in their description. Examples are the ribose group in DNA or those amino acids which have side chains of significant length or special affinity properties. Here we have to introduce a parameter space which allows the subunit to take different conformations. So it is known that the configuration of the ribose group in DNA can be described as a function of a periodic variable, the so called pseudorotation angle $p \in S^1$ (cf., e.g., [6, 9, 12, 13, 15]). So the state of the structure is parameterized by

$$S^1 = \{x \in \mathcal{R}^2 : \|x\| = 1\}.$$

Thus, in our local coordinate system for the ribose subunit, the atom coordinates are functions of the angle $p \in S^1$. Here, we identify points in S^1 with the corresponding angle. For larger amino acids and bigger subunits, such as complete nucleotides, one will have to introduce more complicated parameter manifolds P to describe the flexibility of the substructure in local coordinates.

The 3-D structure of the whole molecule is given by specifying the coordinates of all its atoms in a global Cartesian coordinate system. As we have defined the atom coordinates of a specific subunit in a local coordinate system, we have to describe its location within the global system (compare Figure 23.1). This is done by specifying the vector coordinates $v \in \mathcal{R}^3$ of a specific point (the origin of the local system) and the rotation of the local system with respect to the global one. The set of rotations is given by $SO(3) = \{A \in \mathcal{R}^{3 \times 3} : A^T A = I, \det A = 1\}$. The set of all possible positions of a local coordinate system within the global system is parameterized by $\mathcal{R}^3 \times SO(3)$, the set of Euclidean motions, which has six degrees of freedom. Thus, a rigid substructure of several atoms can be characterized by the Cartesian coordinates of one atom and three additional variables defining the relative position of the whole rigid structure in space within the global coordinate frame. The parameter space for a rigid subunit is $\mathcal{R}^3 \times SO(3)$, whereas the parameter space for flexible subunits is $P \times \mathcal{R}^3 \times SO(3)$, where P denotes the space of parameters defining the possible deformations of the substructure in the local coordinates. Thus, position and state of ribose is parameterized by $\mathcal{R}^3 \times SO(3) \times S^1$, a manifold of dimension 7. In the case of guanine, for example, which is described as a rigid subunit, the number of free parameters is reduced from 33 to 6.

Let us assume that we have a molecule that is partitioned into N subunits. Then the space of all parameters of all subunits is given by

$$U = V_1 \times \cdots \times V_N, \tag{23.2}$$

where $V_i = P_i \times \mathcal{R}^3 \times SO(3)$ denotes the parameter space of substructure G_i. The parameters of a subunit determine the coordinates of all its atoms. Therefore, we have a map

$$\rho : U \longrightarrow \mathcal{R}^{3n},$$

which assigns to every point of the parameter space U the sequence of the coordinates of all n atoms of the configuration. For instance, for DNA molecules with M nucleotides, we can use the four bases A, T, G, C, the ribose, and the phosphate group as subunits. Therefore $N = 3M$, and $V_{3k-2} = V_{3k-1} = \mathcal{R}^3 \times SO(3)$ and $V_{3k} = S^1 \times \mathcal{R}^3 \times SO(3)$ describe phosphate, base, and ribose of nucleotide k, respectively.

Thus ρ itself is a Cartesian product of mappings $\rho^{(i)}$ acting on the respective components V_i. As the above example of guanine indicates, the image $\rho(U)$ is a subset of $\mathcal{R}^{3n}$ of significantly lower dimension, which, in effect, is a proper reduction of degrees of freedom.

The process of introducing spaces of coordinates can be iterated to establish a whole hierarchy of coordinate sets U_i satisfying

$$\rho_m(U_m) \subset \rho_{m-1}(U_{m-1}) \subset \cdots \subset \rho_0(U_0) = U_0 = \mathcal{R}^{3n}$$

and

$$\dim(U_i) < \dim(U_{i-1}) \quad \text{for } 1 \leq i \leq m,$$

describing the molecule on different levels of accuracy. Again each manifold

$$U_i = V_1^{(i)} \times \cdots \times V_{N_i}^{(i)}$$

is a product of parameter manifolds

$$V_k^{(i)} = \mathcal{R}^3 \times \mathrm{SO}(3) \times P_k^{(i)}$$

describing groups of atoms $G_k^{(i)}$, respectively, on the hierarchical coordinate level i. $P_k^{(i)}$ denotes the flexibility parameter space of group $G_k^{(i)}$.

For DNA, the next step in this hierarchy are complete nucleotides or base pairs. A slightly different hierarchical approach was already successfully applied to the calculation of curved DNA [20] and Holliday junctions [7].

The actual definition of groups $G_k^{(i)}$ and corresponding parameter manifolds U_i is motivated by experimental results. In general, the parameters in U_i should consist of the most relevant degrees of freedom. The existence of a decomposition of the parameter space of macromolecules into an "essential" subspace of only a few degrees of freedom and a "physically constrained" remaining space has been shown recently by extended molecular dynamics simulations [1].

23.2.2 Representation of the Energy Function

We now consider one particular coordinate space U representing N groups of atoms and hence having the form (23.2). In (23.1), the total internal energy E was defined as a sum of functions depending on the Cartesian coordinates of two, three, or four atoms [10]. If the subunits are defined in such a way that those sequences of atoms which contribute to bond or torsion angle energies belong to at most two subunits, then the terms in the expression (23.1) for E can be rearranged so that E has the form

$$E = \sum_{i=1}^{N} f_i(w_i) + \sum_{1 \leq i < j \leq N} f_{ij}(w_i, w_j). \tag{23.3}$$

Here, f_i is the internal energy of group G_i and can be neglected for rigid subunits. For nonrigid groups, it is dependent on the flexibility parameters $p \in P_i$ only.

The interaction energy f_{lk} between two groups G_l and G_k depends only on the relative position of these groups (compare Figure 23.1), described by a point in $\mathcal{R}^3 \times \mathrm{SO}(3)$, and possible flexibility parameters. In particular, if the coordinates of subunit G_i, $i \in \{l, k\}$, are denoted by

$$w_i = (p_i, v_i, A_i) \in P \times \mathcal{R}^3 \times \mathrm{SO}(3),$$

then the position y_i within the global coordinate system of an atom with coordinates x_i in the local coordinate system is given by

$$y_i = A_i x_i + v_i.$$

From elementary linear algebra, we find that the relative position of subunit G_k with respect to subunit G_l is defined by the equation

$$x_k = A_k^T A_l \cdot x_l + A_k^T (v_l - v_k),$$

where x_k are the coordinates with respect to the local system k of a point with coordinates x_l in system l. Therefore, f_{lk} can be written as a function $f_{lk}(p_l, p_k, v, A)$ of $v = A_k^T(v_l - v_k) \in \mathcal{R}^3$ and $A = A_k^T A_l \in \mathrm{SO}(3)$, which is more convenient than using the original form $f_{ij}(w_i, w_j)$. Making use of this invariance, we reduce the parameter space by six more dimensions.

Expression (23.3) for E can be evaluated at any point of the coordinate space U, using formula (23.1) and the map ρ. We now turn to discussing efficient evaluation strategies for the energy function E, regarding the individual terms f_{ij} of the sum as functions on $\mathcal{R}^3 \times \mathrm{SO}(3)$. It is then clear how the method can be extended, if additional flexibility parameters have to be considered.

The energy between two groups has to be expressed in these new variables. This can be done on a relatively fine grid in the corresponding parameter space $\mathcal{R}^3 \times \mathrm{SO}(3)$ by computing the usual Cartesian coordinates of all atoms using ρ and then evaluating the analytical expression (23.1) for the total energy of the two groups under consideration. As a result, the exact value of the total internal energy is known at the grid points. To evaluate the energy at arbitrary points of the parameter space, an approximating or interpolating function to these data has to be computed. This can be done on the whole grid or on parts of it. Due to the structure of the energy function, several choices of function types are possible. Here we will concentrate on the use of wavelets.

23.3   Approximation by Wavelets

The energy function in the form (23.3) is a sum of functions defined on product manifolds, consisting of $\mathcal{R}^3$, SO(3), and in some cases additional special manifolds. It is the main goal to derive efficient evaluation strategies for the energy function. It is sufficient to explain the method for the function f_{lk}. As already mentioned, the function f_{lk} will be evaluated on a fine grid of the parameter manifold $\mathcal{R}^3 \times$ SO(3) and a suitable approximation will be calculated. This has to be done only once, and the coefficients of the approximation can be stored. On the other hand, the reconstruction of function values has to be done fast and efficiently.

We will mention two different ways how to deal with $\mathcal{R}^3$ and SO(3). The manifold SO(3), the group of rotations in $\mathcal{R}^3$, is a three-dimensional space. Therefore one can use any type of interpolation or approximation procedure on $\mathcal{R}^3$ to approximate a function on SO(3) locally. Global approximation is much more complicated due to the topological structure of SO(3).

In our local and global approximation procedures, we will use tensor products of functions on the individual parts $\mathcal{R}^3$ and SO(3).

23.3.1   Local Approximation by Cubic B-Spline Wavelets

A natural and convenient parameterization of SO(3) are Euler angles. There are different versions in the literature. We prefer to use the following map τ on the 3-dimensional cube $C := [0, 2\pi] \times [0, 2\pi] \times [-\pi/2, \pi/2]$

$$\tau : C \ni (\alpha, \beta, \theta) \mapsto M(\alpha, \beta, \theta) \in \text{SO}(3)$$

where $M(\alpha, \beta, \theta)$ is defined by

$$\begin{pmatrix} \cos\beta\cos\theta - \cos\alpha\sin\beta - \sin\alpha\cos\beta\sin\theta & \sin\alpha\sin\beta - \cos\alpha\cos\beta\sin\theta \\ \sin\beta\cos\theta & \cos\alpha\cos\beta - \sin\alpha\sin\beta\sin\theta & -\sin\alpha\cos\beta - \cos\alpha\sin\beta\sin\theta \\ \sin\theta & \sin\alpha\cos\theta & \cos\alpha\cos\theta \end{pmatrix}$$

This map is a diffeomorphism on the interior of C. The angles α and β can be extended periodically. But this is not true for θ. In fact, it is easily seen that

$$\tau(\alpha, \beta, \pm\pi/2) = \begin{pmatrix} 0 & \mp\sin(\alpha\pm\beta) & \mp\cos(\alpha\pm\beta) \\ 0 & \cos(\alpha\pm\beta) & -\sin(\alpha\pm\beta) \\ \pm 1 & 0 & 0 \end{pmatrix},$$

so that for $\theta = \pi/2$ lines $\{\alpha+\beta =\text{const}\}$ are mapped to one point in SO(3). The same holds for $\theta = -\pi/2$ and lines $\{\alpha - \beta =\text{const}\}$. Nevertheless, because of this definition of Euler angles, the identity in SO(3) has a regular neighborhood and those rotations describing the usual relative positions in the DNA double helix, which is our present test example, have well-defined pre-images. Furthermore, in this way one can cover the whole manifold by one coordinate chart. Therefore, if the function values near the singular points $\theta = \pm\pi/2$ are not needed, one can use any approximation method on C for functions $f_{lk}(\alpha, \beta, \theta)$ which correspond to functions $f_{lk}(A)$ via the map τ.

On $\mathcal{R}^3$ we are also interested in local approximations only. Therefore a function $f_{lk}(v, A)$ can be approximated locally by a six-dimensional tensor product function and the corresponding wavelets. As we are interested in piecewise differentiable wavelets, which can be used in minimization procedures using gradient methods, we have implemented a tensor product of one-dimensional cardinal spline-wavelets, based on the cubic B-spline N_4. A full characterization of semi-orthogonal spline wavelets with all implementation details can be found in [18]. The extension to the tensor product case is straightforward. But as there are 63 types of tensor product wavelets, the handling of the coefficients and the design of data compression algorithms is a considerable problem.

23.3.2   Global Approximation by Tensor Products

In some cases the relative position of two molecular subunits is described by a matrix which is the image of a point near the singular set of the map τ. Then the local approximation can lead to errors in the function value. Furthermore, this can happen on the minimization path or during a molecular dynamics simulation. Then one would like to have a global approximation, at least on SO(3), or one would have to change the chart describing the manifold, which again is not easy to handle.

It also turns out, that the Euler angle parameterization leads to another problem. If we want to construct a differentiable function F on SO(3), then its coordinate representation $f(\alpha, \beta, \theta)$ has to respect the topological properties of the manifold and the map τ. The following theorem, which can be proved in the same way as the corresponding theorems [3] on S^2 and S^3, characterizes the functions $f : C \longrightarrow \mathcal{R}$ that lead to differentiable functions F on SO(3) if we define $f = F \circ \tau$.

THEOREM 1

F is C^1 if and only if f and its derivatives are periodic in α and β and there are real-valued 2π-periodic C^1 functions $F_\pm$ as well as 2π-periodic continuous functions $A_\pm$, $B_\pm$ such that for $0 \leq \alpha \leq 2\pi$ and $0 \leq \beta \leq 2\pi$:

1. $f(\alpha, \beta, \pm\pi/2) = F_\pm(\alpha \pm \beta)$

2. $f_\theta(\alpha, \beta, \pm\pi/2) = A_\pm(\alpha \pm \beta)\cos\alpha + B_\pm(\alpha \pm \beta)\sin\alpha$

3. $(f_\alpha \mp f_\beta)_\theta(\alpha, \beta, \pm\pi/2) = -A_\pm(\alpha \pm \beta)\sin\alpha + B_\pm(\alpha \pm \beta)\cos\alpha.$

Condition 1 just means that f defines a function on SO(3), because then f has to be constant on those points in C which are mapped to the same point on SO(3). Condition 3 is a condition on the mixed second derivatives in the singular points, where $\theta = \pm\pi/2$. Fortunately, this condition is automatically satisfied for a tensor product function, if condition 2 is satisfied. So, to construct differentiable scaling functions and wavelets on SO(3), we must only meet conditions 1 and 2. Another problem is that the functions depend on mixed variables $\alpha \pm \beta$. Introducing the variables $x = \alpha + \beta$ and $y = \alpha - \beta$, one can in principle separate the two angles using the formulae for cos- and sin-function and define tensor products of polynomial splines B_i and trigonometric splines T_j

$$f(\alpha, \beta, \theta) := \sum_{i=1}^{l_1}\sum_{j=1}^{l_2}\sum_{k=1}^{l_3} c_{ijk} B_i(\theta)\, T_j\left(\frac{1}{2}(\alpha + \beta)\right) T_k\left(\frac{1}{2}(\alpha - \beta)\right)$$

on C. Yet, it is not clear how one can derive a multiresolution analysis in this case.

We therefore use a different parameterization of SO(3), namely by quaternions of modulus 1. Essentially, this is a parameterization by $S^3 = \{x \in \mathcal{R}^4 : \|x\| = 1\}$, the three-dimensional sphere. The whole construction of this parameterization uses largely the fact, that S^3 can be seen as the set of units of the multiplication of the skew symmetric quaternion field. Explicitly, the parameter correspondence is given by the following map. If $x = (\chi, \xi, \eta, \zeta)$ is a point in S^3 then

$$M(x) := \begin{pmatrix} \xi^2 - \eta^2 - \zeta^2 + \chi^2 & 2(\xi\eta - \zeta\chi) & 2(\xi\zeta + \eta\chi) \\ 2(\xi\eta + \zeta\chi) & -\xi^2 + \eta^2 - \zeta^2 + \chi^2 & 2(\eta\zeta - \xi\chi) \\ 2(\xi\zeta - \eta\chi) & 2(\eta\zeta + \xi\chi) & -\xi^2 - \eta^2 + \zeta^2 + \chi^2 \end{pmatrix}$$

is an element of SO(3). Furthermore, $M(p) = M(q)$ if and only if $p = \pm q$. So under this map $M : S^3 \to$ SO(3) the sphere S^3 is a twofold cover of SO(3). Each matrix in SO(3) has two pre-images, which are antipodal points in S^3. M is a local diffeomorphism. This means that SO(3) looks locally like S^3. In fact, in a certain sense one can even say that the metric properties are locally the same.

Thus, if we want to construct a multiresolution analysis on SO(3), we can use a multiresolution analysis on S^3 and apply it to functions which have the same value in antipodal points. These are exactly the functions on S^3 which define functions on SO(3). Furthermore, the function on SO(3) is differentiable if and only if the corresponding function on S^3 is differentiable.

Technically, the procedure is as follows. Each function $F : SO(3) \to \mathcal{R}$ can be lifted to a function G on S^3 defining $G : S^3 \to \mathcal{R}$ by $G(x) = y$ if $F(M(x)) = y$ for $x \in S^3$ and $M(x) \in SO(3)$. If we want to approximate or analyze a function F on $SO(3)$ with some wavelet type technique, we can first define its extension G to S^3 in the way indicated and apply a multiresolution analysis on S^3 to G. Of course, one has to take care that the antipodal point condition is satisfied.

The disadvantage of this parameterization lies in the fact, that we deal with four parameters (χ, ξ, η, ζ) and one side condition, namely, $\chi^2 + \xi^2 + \eta^2 + \zeta^2 = 1$.

We will now shortly review how one can get a multiresolution analysis on S^3. The detailed construction is given in [3]. The construction is based on a special parameterization which differs form the usual polar coordinates on S^3. In particular, S^3 is covered by the chart $\rho : U := [0,1]^3 \to S^3$ defined by

$$\alpha = (\alpha_1, \alpha_2, \theta) \mapsto \begin{pmatrix} \cos(2\pi\alpha_1)\cos(\frac{\pi}{2}\theta) \\ \sin(2\pi\alpha_1)\cos(\frac{\pi}{2}\theta) \\ \cos(2\pi\alpha_2)\sin(\frac{\pi}{2}\theta) \\ \sin(2\pi\alpha_2)\sin(\frac{\pi}{2}\theta) \end{pmatrix}.$$

Again, a function $f(\alpha_1, \alpha_2, \theta)$ in these coordinates has to satisfy differentiability conditions according to the following theorem.

THEOREM 2

Let F be a real-valued function on S^3 and $f = F \circ \sigma$ its coordinate representation. Then F is C^1 if and only if f is C^1, if $f_{\alpha_1}(0, \alpha_2, \theta) = f_{\alpha_1}(1, \alpha_2, \theta)$ and $f_{\alpha_2}(\alpha_1, 1, \theta) = f_{\alpha_2}(\alpha_1, 1, \theta)$ and

(i)   there are real-valued 1-periodic C^1-functions F_i as well as 1-periodic continuous functions a_i, b_i for $i = 1, 2$ such that for $0 \le \alpha_1 \le 1$ and $0 \le \alpha_2 \le 1$:

$$f(\alpha_1, \alpha_2, i - 1) = F_i(\alpha_i) \tag{23.4}$$

$$f_\theta(\alpha_1, \alpha_2, 0) = a_1(\alpha_1)\cos 2\pi\alpha_2 + b_1(\alpha_1)\sin 2\pi\alpha_2 \tag{23.5}$$

$$f_\theta(\alpha_1, \alpha_2, 1) = a_2(\alpha_2)\cos 2\pi\alpha_1 + b_2(\alpha_2)\sin 2\pi\alpha_1 \tag{23.6}$$

(ii) and $f_{\alpha_2,\theta}(\alpha_1,\alpha_2,0)$ and $f_{\alpha_1,\theta}(\alpha_1,\alpha_2,1)$ exist for all (α_1,α_2) and are given by

$$f_{\alpha_2,\theta}(\alpha_1,\alpha_2,0) = 2\pi[-a_1(\alpha_1)\sin 2\pi\alpha_2 + b_1(\alpha_1)\cos 2\pi\alpha_2]$$

$$f_{\alpha_1,\theta}(\alpha_1,\alpha_2,1) = 2\pi[-a_2(\alpha_2)\sin 2\pi\alpha_1 + b_2(\alpha_2)\cos 2\pi\alpha_1].$$

We use a tensor product construction and need not care about satisfying conditions ii. But we see from condition i, that we have to be able to generate the cos- and sin-function. This is done by using periodized E-splines [5] as scaling functions and the corresponding wavelets. Furthermore, as there is no direct periodicity in the variable θ, we use scaling functions and wavelets on the interval $[0,1]$ for this variable, in particular the B-spline wavelets [14]. A detailed description of these constructions is given in [3]; see also the references therein.

A tensor product function $\varphi \in V_j$ has the form

$$\varphi(\underline{\alpha},\theta) = \sum_{\beta_1=0}^{2^j-1}\sum_{\beta_2=0}^{2^j-1}\sum_{\gamma=-m+1}^{2^j-1} \lambda_{\underline{\beta},\gamma} C_{\mu/2^j}(2^j\alpha_1 - \beta_1)\cdot \qquad (23.7)$$

$$C_{\mu/2^j}(2^j\alpha_2 - \beta_2)B_{\gamma,m,j}(\theta)$$

Here $C_{\mu/2^j}$ denotes an E-spline with parameter μ and $B_{\gamma,m,j}$ a spline function on the interval. It should be remarked that E-splines give rise to a nonstationary multiresolution analysis.

The differentiability conditions in the theorem now translate into a system of linear equations for the coefficients $\lambda_{\underline{\beta},\gamma}$, which is explicitly given in [3]. So, if we want to compute an approximating function $\varphi \in V_j$, we have to solve a system of equations arising from the approximation problem and from the differentiability conditions.

The wavelet spaces W_j are direct sums of seven tensor products of three one dimensional spaces each (where at least one of the spaces is a wavelet space). We set $E := \{0,1\}^2$, $E^* = E \setminus \{0,0\}$. For $e \in E$, let ψ^e be defined by

$$\psi^e(\underline{\alpha}) := \psi^{e_1}(\alpha_1)\psi^{e_2}(\alpha_2)$$

where

$$\psi^{e_i} = \begin{cases} C_{\mu/2^j}, & e_i = 0 \\ \psi_{\mu/2^j}, & e_i = 1 \end{cases} \qquad (23.8)$$

and $\psi_{\mu/2^j}$ denotes the wavelet corresponding to the E-spline $C_{\mu/2^j}$. Then

$\psi \in W_j$ is given by

$$\psi(\underline{\alpha}, \theta) = \sum_{e \in E^*} \sum_{\underline{\beta}} \sum_{\tilde{\beta}} \lambda^{e,0}_{\underline{\beta}, \tilde{\beta}} \psi^e (2^j \underline{\alpha} - \underline{\beta}) B_{\tilde{\beta}, m, j}(\theta) \tag{23.9}$$

$$+ \sum_{e \in E} \sum_{\underline{\beta}} \sum_{\tilde{\beta}} \lambda^{e,1}_{\underline{\beta}, \tilde{\beta}} \psi^e (2^j \underline{\alpha} - \underline{\beta}) \psi_{j, \tilde{\beta}}(\theta).$$

Again, the coefficients $\lambda^{e,m}_{\underline{\beta}, \tilde{\beta}}$ have to satisfy a system of linear equations, if ψ is to define a function on S^3. So the multiresolution analysis on S^3 is the restriction of the tensor product multiresolution analysis of two copies of periodized E-splines and E-wavelets and one factor of B-spline wavelets on an interval, to a subspace defined by a system of linear equations. One has to study carefully the effects of this projection map.

23.4   Further Applications: Surface Representation

As a further example that fits into this framework, we mention the problem of surface representation in medicine, e.g., in tomography. Suppose the surface S is the surface of an organ like the heart or the head. If S is sphere-like, it can be represented by specifying a radius function $r(\alpha, \theta)$ on S^2, where $R := \{(\alpha, \theta) : 0 \leq \alpha \leq 1, 0 \leq \theta \leq 1\}$ defines a parameterization of S^2, e.g., by polar coordinates. Of course, the properties of the surface define the properties of the function r and vice versa. If, for example, r is continuously differentiable, then S has a continuously varying tangent plane. Furthermore, one might have measurements on the surface of the organ considered, for example values of electric potentials. Again, they are represented by a function $f(\alpha, \theta)$. In general, one wants to find a function f which is globally defined on S and which can be easily computed from the measured data points $\{g(\alpha_i, \theta_i) : i = 1, \ldots, N\}$. Thus, one has to consider the problem of fitting a smooth function f to regularly distributed or scattered data $\{g(\alpha_i, \theta_i) : i = 1, \ldots, N\}$ on a sphere-like surface, such that $f(\alpha_i, \theta_i) = g(\alpha_i, \theta_i)$ or $f(\alpha_i, \theta_i) \approx g(\alpha_i, \theta_i)$. This problem has been considered quite frequently, see [17] for a nice solution using trigonometric splines and for further references. The methods described in the previous section can also be used to construct an MRA ([3], [16]) for the analysis of the geometry or structure of data on sphere-like surfaces.

Similar to the case of S^3, one has differentiability conditions for functions depending on the usual polar coordinates for S^2

$$(\alpha, \theta) \mapsto (\cos(2\pi\alpha)\sin(\pi\theta), \sin(2\pi\alpha)\sin(\pi\theta), \cos(\pi\theta)) . \quad (23.10)$$

By analogy to the case of S^3, we define

$$V_j = V_j^1 \otimes V_j^2 = \overline{\mathrm{span}\{C_{\mu/2^j}(2^j \cdot -\alpha_1)B_{\alpha_2,m,j}(\cdot)\}},$$

where $0 \le \alpha_1 \le 2^j - 1$ and $-m + 1 \le \alpha_2 \le 2^j - 1$. For the wavelet spaces we have

$$W_j = V_j^1 \otimes W_j^2 \oplus W_j^1 \otimes V_j^2 \oplus W_j^1 \otimes W_j^2, \quad (23.11)$$

where the spaces W_j^i are the wavelet spaces associated to the MRA generated by the corresponding V_j^i. The characterization of those functions in V_j and W_j that satisfy the differentiability conditions and therefore define smooth functions on S^2, again leads to linear conditions on the coefficients of the functions. So the situation is completely analogous to the case of S^3.

23.5 Discussion

The methods of local and global approximation of energy functions by wavelets should facilitate the computation of molecular structure. The possibility of combining the hierarchical organization of molecular substructures described above with the hierarchical features of wavelet decompositions is particularly promising. The design of an optimization procedure can make use of both hierarchies to evaluate the energy function with a specially adapted accuracy determined by the minimization path. Finally, one expects (e.g., from [4]) that such wavelet expansions are particularly well suited for preconditioning gradient methods for optimization purposes.

To make efficient use of the wavelet decomposition, one has to design appropriate data compression algorithms. This is a challenging problem, as we are dealing with wavelets on at least six-dimensional spaces. One should also be aware of the fact that it takes quite some time to compute the coefficients of approximation functions and their wavelet decomposition up to a prescribed level. This is presently done for the 27 possible pairs of DNA subunits (ribose, phosphate, bases ATGC; binding and nonbinding substructures) in the local cubic B-spline and wavelet approximation. We hope that this approach will reduce drastically the computation time for the interesting biological macromolecules, which presently for a 40-base pair DNA molecule is several months of CPU-time.

For further computations, one will also need the global approximation. Global approximation can also be interesting for applications in robotics or biomedical engineering. Here the manifold SO(3) plays an important role in mechanical problems.

In a further step one could try to combine the advantages of wavelet expansions with the features of radial basis functions, which particularly well describe the long range Coulomb potentials. This can be done by a homotopy of the form

$$f_t(x, \alpha) = \sigma(|x|) \cdot R(x) + (1 - \sigma(|x|)) \cdot w(x, \alpha), \quad (x, \alpha) \in \mathcal{R}^3 \times \text{SO}(3).$$

Here $\sigma : \mathcal{R}_{\geq 0} \to [0, 1]$ is some suitable sigmoidal function satisfying $\sigma(r) \to 1$ for $r \to \infty$ and $\sigma(r) \to 0$ for $r \to 0$. R should be a linear combination of just a few radial basis functions, while $w(x, \alpha)$ should be an expansion of wavelet type basis functions which, in view of the form of σ, have to be determined only on essentially bounded domains. Calculations with radial basis functions and positive definite functions have proved to be successful in model calculations of small molecules [8].

References

[1] A. Amadei, A. B. M. Linssen, and H. J. C. Berendsen. Essential dynamics of proteins. *Proteins*, 17:412–425, 1993.

[2] M. Butzlaff, W. Dahmen, S. Diekmann, A. Dress, E. Schmitt, and E. V. Kitzing. A hierarchical approach to force field calculations through spline approximations. *J. Math. Chem.*, 15:77–92, 1994.

[3] S. Dahlke, W. Dahmen, I. Weinreich, and E. Schmitt. Multiresolution analysis and wavelets on S^2 and S^3. *Numer. Funct. Anal. Optimiz.*, 16(1&2):19–41, 1995.

[4] W. Dahmen and A. Kunoth. Multilevel preconditioning. *Numer. Math.*, 63:315–327, 1992.

[5] W. Dahmen and C. A. Micchelli. On multivariate E-splines. *Adv. Math.*, 76:33–93, 1989.

[6] H. P. M. de Leeuw, C. A. G. Haasnoot, and C. Altona, Empirical correlations between conformational parameters in β-D-Furanoside fragments derived from a statistical survey of crystal structures of nucleic acid constituents. Full description of nucleoside molecular geometries in terms of four parameters. *Isr. J. Chem.*, 20:108–126, 1980.

[7] D. R. Duckett, A. I. H. Murchie, R. M. Clegg, E. von Kitzing, S. Diekmann, and D. M. J. Lilley. The structure of the Holliday junction. In *Structure and Methods*, R. H. Sarma and M. H. Sarma, editors, Vol. 1, Adenine Press, Schenectady, NY, 1990, 157–181.

[8] T. Gutzmer and E. Schmitt. Domain decomposition and approximation by positive definite functions in biomolecular structure calculations. In *High Performance Computing*, A. Tentner, editor, The Society for Computer Simulation, San Diego, 1995, 82–87.

[9] M. Levitt and A. Warshel. Extreme conformational flexibility of the furanose ring in DNA and RNA. *J. Am. Chem. Soc.*, 100:2607–2613, 1978.

[10] S. R. Niketic and K. Rasmussen, *The Consistent Force Field* (Lecture Notes in Chemistry 3, Springer, Berlin, 1977).

[11] L. Nilsson and M. Karplus. Empirical energy functions for energy minimization and dynamics of nucleic acids. *J. Comput. Chem.*, 7:591–616, 1986.

[12] D. Pearlman and S.-H. Kim. Conformational studies of nucleic acids. I. A rapid and direct method for generating furanose coordinates from the pseudorotation angle. *J. Bio. Struc. Dyn.*, 3:85–98, 1985.

[13] D. Pearlman and S.-H. Kim. Conformational studies of nucleic acids. II. The conformational energetics of commonly occurring nucleosides. *J. Bio. Struc. Dyn.*, 3:99–125, 1985.

[14] E. Quak and N. Weyrich. Wavelets on the interval. In *Approximation Theory, Wavelets and Applications*, S. P. Singh, editor, Kluwer Academic Publishers, Dordrecht, 1995, 247–283.

[15] T. Schlick, C. Peskin, S. Broyde, and M. Overton. An analysis of the structural and energetic properties of desoxyribose by potential energy methods. *J. Comput. Chem.*, 8:1199–1224, 1987.

[16] E. Schmitt. Wavelets and multiresolution analysis on sphere-like surfaces. In: *Mathematical Imaging: Wavelet Applications in Signal and Image Processing* III, SPIE Proc. Vol. 2569, A. F. Laine, A. Aldroubi, and M. Unser, editors, SPIE — The International Society for Optical Engineering, Bellingham, WA, 1995.

[17] L. L. Schumaker and C. Traas. Fitting scattered data on sphere-like surfaces using tensor products of trigonometric and polynomial splines. *Numer. Math.*, 60:133–144, 1991.

[18] M. Unser, A. Aldroubi, and M. Eden. A family of polynomial spline wavelet transforms. *Signal Process.*, 30:141–162, 1993.

[19] E. von Kitzing, Molekülsimulation mit Hilfe von Kraftfeldrechnungen am Beispiel der Aggregation von Nukleinsäuren verschiedener Konformation zu einem Komplex mit Übersetzungsfunktion. Dissertation, Rader Verlag, Aachen, Germany, 1986.

[20] E. von Kitzing and S. Diekmann. Molecular Calculations of $d(A)_{12}*d(A)_{12}$ and of the Curved Molecule $d(GCTCGAAAAA)_4*$ $d(TTTTTCGAGC)_4$. *Eur. Biophys. J.*, 15:13–26, 1987.

[21] S. J. Weiner, P. A. Kollman, D. A. Case, U. C. Singh, C. Ghio, G. Alagona, S. Profeta, Jr., and P. Weiner, A new force field for molecular mechanical simulation of nucleic acids and proteins. *J. Am. Chem. Soc.*, 106:765–784, 1984.

Index